PROGRESS IN BRAIN RESEARCH

VOLUME 86

MOLECULAR AND CELLULAR MECHANISMS OF NEURONAL PLASTICITY IN
NORMAL AGING AND ALZHEIMER'S DISEASE

Other volumes in PROGRESS IN BRAIN RESEARCH

PROGRESS IN BRAIN RESEARCH

VOLUME 86

MOLECULAR AND CELLULAR MECHANISMS OF NEURONAL PLASTICITY IN NORMAL AGING AND ALZHEIMER'S DISEASE

EDITED BY

PAUL D. COLEMAN

Department of Neurobiology and Anatomy, University of Rochester Medical Center, 601 Elmwood Avenue, Rochester, NY 14642, U.S.A.

GERALD A. HIGGINS

Molecular Neurobiology, National Institute on Aging, 4940 Eastern Avenue, Baltimore, MD 21224, U.S.A.

and

CREIGHTON H. PHELPS

Division of Medical and Scientific Affairs, Alzheimer's Association, 70 East Lake Street, Suite 600, Chicago, IL 60601, U.S.A.

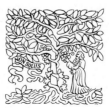

ELSEVIER
AMSTERDAM – NEW YORK – OXFORD
1990

© 1990, Elsevier Science Publishers B.V. (Biomedical Division)

All rights reserved. No part of this publication may be reproduced, stored in a retrieval system or transmitted in any form or by any means, electronic, mechanical, photocopying, recording or otherwise without the prior written permission of the publisher, Elsevier Science Publishers B.V. (Biomedical Division), P.O. Box 1527, 1000 BM Amsterdam, The Netherlands.

No responsibility is assumed by the Publisher for any injury and/or damage to persons or property as a matter of products liability, negligence or otherwise, or from any use of operation or any methods, products, instructions or ideas contained in the material herein. Because of the rapid advances in the medical sciences, the Publisher recommends that independent verification of diagnoses and drug dosages should be made.

Special regulations for readers in the USA:
This publication has been registered with the Copyright Clearance Center Inc. (CCC), Salem, Massachusetts. Information can be obtained from the CCC about conditions under which the photocopying of parts of this publication may be made in the USA. All other copyright questions, including photocopying outside of the USA, should be referred to the copyright owner, Elsevier Science Publishers B.V. (Biomedical Division) unless otherwise specified.

ISBN 0-444-81121-4 (volume)
ISBN 0-444-80104-9 (series)

This book is printed on acid-free paper

Published by:
Elsevier Science Publishers B.V. (Biomedical Division)
P.O. Box 211
1000 AE Amsterdam
The Netherlands

Sole distributors for the USA and Canada:
Elsevier Science Publishing Company, Inc.
655 Avenue of the Americas
New York, NY 10010
USA

Library of Congress Cataloging-in-Publication Data

Molecular and cellular mechanisms of neuronal plasticity and
  Alzheimer's disease / edited by Paul D. Coleman, Gerald A. Higgins,
  Creighton H. Phelps.
     p. cm. -- (Progress in brain research ; v. 86)
    Includes bibliographical references and index.
    ISBN 0-444-81121-4 (alk. paper)
    1. Alzheimer's disease--Molecular aspects. 2. Alzheimer's
disease--Pathophysiology. 3. Neuroplasticity. I. Coleman, Paul D.
II. Higgins, Gerald A. III. Phelps, Creighton A. IV. Series.
    [DNLM: 1. Aging--physiology--congresses. 2. Alzheimer's Disease-
-physiopathology--congresses. 3. Gene Expression Regulation-
-physiology--congresses. 4. Growth Substances--physiology-
-congresses. 5. Neuronal Plasticity--physiology--congresses.   W1
PR667J v. 86 / WE 102 M718]
RC523.M65 1990
616.8'3107--dc20
DNLM/DLC
for Library of Congress   90-14087
                                 CIP

Printed in The Netherlands

List of Contributors

J.G. Altin, Department of Biological Chemistry, College of Medicine, University of California, Irvine, CA 92717, U.S.A.

D.M. Armstrong, Department of Neurosciences, University of California at San Diego, La Jolla, CA 92093, U.S.A.

M.A. Armstrong-Jones, Neuroscience Group, The London Hospital Medical College, University of London, Turner Street, London E1 2AD, U.K.

J.M. Baraban, Departments of Neuroscience, Neurology, Psychiatry and Behavioral Sciences, Johns Hopkins University School of Medicine, 725 North Wolfe Street, Baltimore, MD 21205, U.S.A.

C.A. Barnes, Department of Psychology, Campus Box 345, University of Colorado, Boulder, CO 80309, U.S.A.

L.I. Benowitz, McLean Hospital, MRC 315, 115 Mill Street, Belmont, MA 02178, U.S.A.; and Department of Psychiatry, Program in Neuroscience, Harvard Medical School, Boston, MA, U.S.A.

M. Blaber, Department of Biological Chemistry, College of Medicine, University of California, Irvine, CA 92717, U.S.A.

J. Boulter, Molecular Neurobiology Laboratory, The Salk Institute, P.O. Box 85800, San Diego, CA 92138, U.S.A.

R.A. Bradshaw, Department of Biological Chemistry, College of Medicine, University of California, Irvine, CA 92717, U.S.A.

V.F. Castellucci, Laboratory of Neurobiology and Behavior, Clinical Research Institute of Montreal, Montreal, Quebec, Canada.

K.P. Cavanaugh, Department of Biological Chemistry, College of Medicine, University of California, Irvine, CA 92717, U.S.A.

B. Chamak, CNRS URA 1414, Département de Biologie, ENS, 46 rue d'Ulm, 75005 Paris, France.

L.J. Chandler, Department of Pharmacology and Therapeutics, College of Medicine, Box J-267, J.H.M. Health Center, Gainesville, FL 32610, U.S.A.

K.S. Chen, Department of Neurosciences, University of California at San Diego, La Jolla, CA 92093, U.S.A.

A.J. Cole, Departments of Neuroscience, Neurology, Psychiatry and Behavioral Sciences, Johns Hopkins University School of Medicine, 725 North Wolfe Street, Baltimore, MD 21205, U.S.A.

P.D. Coleman, Department of Neurobiology and Anatomy, University of Rochester Medical Center, 601 Elmwood Avenue, Rochester, NY 14642, U.S.A.

J. Connolly, Molecular Neurobiology Laboratory, The Salk Institute, P.O. Box 85800, San Diego, CA 92138, U.S.A.

L.C. Cork, Departments of Pathology, Division of Comparative Medicine, Neuropathology Laboratory, 509 Pathology Building, Johns Hopkins University School of Medicine, 600 North Wolfe Street, Baltimore, MD 21205-2181, U.S.A.

C.W. Cotman, Department of Psychobiology, University of California, Irvine, CA 92717, U.S.A.

F.T. Crews, Department of Pharmacology and Therapeutics, College of Medicine, Box J-267, J.H.M. Health Center, Gainesville, FL 32610, U.S.A.

T. Curran, Departments of Neuroscience and Molecular Oncology, Roche Institute of Molecular Biology, Roche Research Center, Nutley, NJ 07110, U.S.A.

L.R. Dawes, The Children's Hospital, 300 Longwood Avenue, Boston, MA 02115, U.S.A.; and Department of Pediatrics, Harvard Medical School, Boston, MA, U.S.A.

P. Delrée, Service de Physiologie Humaine et de Physiopathologie, Institut Léon Frédéricq, Place Delcour 17, B-4020 Liège, Belgium.

E. Deneris, Molecular Neurobiology Laboratory, The Salk Institute, P.O. Box 85800, San Diego, CA 92138, U.S.A.

R. Duvoisin, Molecular Neurobiology Laboratory, The Salk Institute, P.O. Box 85800, San Diego, CA 92138, U.S.A.

F.F. Ebner, Neurobiology Section and Center for Neural Science, Brown University, Providence, RI 02912, U.S.A.

D.D. Eveleth, Department of Biological Chemistry, College of Medicine, University of California, Irvine, CA 92717, U.S.A.

S.E. Fahrbach, Department of Entomology, University of Illinois, Urbana, IL 61801, U.S.A.

D.G. Flood, Department of Neurology, University of Rochester Medical Center, 601 Elmwood Avenue, Rochester, NY 14642, U.S.A.

T. Friedmann, Department of Pediatrics, University of California at San Diego, La Jolla, CA 92093, U.S.A.

F.H. Gage, Department of Neurosciences, University of California at San Diego, La Jolla, CA 92093, U.S.A.

J.W. Geddes, Division of Neurosurgery, University of California, Irvine, CA 92717, U.S.A.

P.B. Guthrie, Program in Neuronal Growth and Development, and Department of Anatomy and Neurobiology, Colorado State University, Ft. Collins, CO 80523, U.S.A.

R.C. Hayes, Department of Neurosciences, University of California at San Diego, La Jolla, CA 92093, U.S.A.

F. Hefti, Andrus Gerontology Center, University of Southern California, University Park, MC 0191, Los Angeles, CA 90089-0191, U.S.A.

S. Heinemann, Molecular Neurobiology Laboratory, The Salk Institute, P.O. Box 85800, San Diego, CA 92138, U.S.A.

G.A. Higgins, Molecular Neurobiology, National Institute on Aging, 4940 Eastern Avenue, Baltimore, MD 21224, U.S.A.

G. Jackson, Department of Human Biological Chemistry and Genetics, University of Texas Medical Branch, 436 Gail Borden, F52, Galveston, TX 77550-2777, U.S.A.

S.B. Kater, Program in Neuronal Growth and Development, and Department of Anatomy and Neurobiology, Colorado State University, Ft. Collins, CO 80523, U.S.A.

K. Kimura, Department of Zoology, NJ-15, University of Washington, Seattle, WA 98195, U.S.A.

M. Klein, Department of Psychobiology, University of California, Irvine, CA 92717, U.S.A.

B. Knusel, Andrus Gerontology Center, University of Southern California, University Park, MC 0191, Los Angeles, CA 90089-0191, U.S.A.

S. Koh, Department of Neurobiology and Anatomy, University of Rochester Medical Center, 601 Elmwood Avenue, Rochester, NY 14642, U.S.A.

V.E. Koliatsos, Departments of Pathology and Neurology, Neuropathology Laboratory, 509 Pathology Building, Johns Hopkins University School of Medicine, 600 North Wolfe Street, Baltimore, MD 21205-2181, U.S.A.

E.H. Koo, Departments of Pathology and Neurology, Neuropathology Laboratory, 509 Pathology Building, Johns Hopkins University School of Medicine, 600 North Wolfe Street, Baltimore, MD 21205-2181, U.S.A.

H.I. Kornblum, Department of Pharmacology, College of Medicine, University of California, Irvine, CA 92717, U.S.A.

P.P. Lefebvre, Service de Physiologie Humaine et de Physiopathologie, Institut Léon Frédéricq, Place Delcour 17, B-4020 Liège, Belgium.

P. Leprince, Service de Physiologie Humaine et de Physiopathologie, Institut Léon Frédéricq, Place Delcour 17, B-4020 Liège, Belgium.

F.M. Leslie, Department of Pharmacology, College of Medicine, University of California, Irvine, CA 92717, U.S.A.

F.M. Longo, Departments of Neurology and the Neuroscience Program, University of California, School of Medicine, San Francisco, CA 94143-0114, U.S.A.

D. Marchetti, Department of Human Biological Chemistry and Genetics, University of Texas Medical Branch, 436 Gail Borden, F52, Galveston, TX 77550-2777, U.S.A.

D.R. Marshak, Cold Spring Harbor Laboratory, Cold Spring Harbor, NY 11724, U.S.A.

L.J. Martin, Department of Pathology, Neuropathology Laboratory, 509 Pathology Building, Johns Hopkins University School of Medicine, 600 North Wolfe Street, Baltimore, MD 21205-2181, U.S.A.

M.P. McKinley, Department of Neurology, University of California School of Medicine, San Francisco, CA 94143-0114, U.S.A.

P.P. Michel, Andrus Gerontology Center, University of Southern California, University Park, MC 0191, Los Angeles, CA 90089-0191, U.S.A.

F.D. Miller, Department of Anatomy and Cell Biology, University of Alberta, Edmonton T6G 2H7, Canada.

L.R. Mills, Program in Neuronal Growth and Development, and Department of Anatomy and Neurobiology, Colorado State University, Ft. Collins, CO 80523, U.S.A.

W.C. Mobley, Departments of Neurology, Pediatrics and the Neuroscience Program, University of California, School of Medicine, San Francisco, CA 94143-0114, U.S.A.

G. Moonen, Service de Physiologie Humaine et de Physiopathologie, Institut Léon Frédéricq, Place Delcour 17, B-4020 Liège, Belgium.

B. Morgan, Department of Human Biological Chemistry and Genetics, University of Texas Medical Branch, 436 Gail Borden, F52, Galveston, TX 77550-2777, U.S.A.

J.I. Morgan, Departments of Neuroscience and Molecular Oncology, Roche Institute of Molecular Biology, Roche Research Center, Nutley, NJ 07110, U.S.A.

E.J. Mufson, Christopher Center for Parkinson's Research, Institute for Biogerontology Research, Sun City, AZ 85351, U.S.A.

N.A. Muma, Department of Pathology, Neuropathology Laboratory, 509 Pathology Building, Johns Hopkins University School of Medicine, 600 North Wolfe Street, Baltimore, MD 21205-2181, U.S.A.

R.L. Neve, Division of Genetics, The Children's Hospital, 300 Longwood Avenue, Boston, MA 02115, U.S.A.; Department of Psychobiology, University of California at Irvine, Irvine, CA 92127, U.S.A.; and Department of Pediatrics, Program in Neuroscience, Harvard Medical School, Boston, MA, U.S.A.

J.W. Olney, Departments of Psychiatry and Neuropathology, Washington University Medical School, St. Louis, MO 63110, U.S.A.

R. Papke, Molecular Neurobiology Laboratory, The Salk Institute, P.O. Box 85800, San Diego, CA 92138, U.S.A.

J. Patrick, Baylor College of Medicine, Houston, TX, U.S.A.

J. R. Perez-Polo, Department of Human Biological Chemistry and Genetics, University of Texas Medical Branch, 436 Gail Borden, F52, Galveston, TX 77550-2777, U.S.A.

N.I. Perrone-Bizzozero, Department of Psychiatry, Mailman Research Center, McLean Hospital, 115 Mill Street, Belmont, MA 02178, U.S.A.; and Department of Psychiatry, Harvard Medical School, Boston, MA, U.S.A.

C.H. Phelps, Division of Medical and Scientific Affairs, Alzheimer's Association, 70 East Lake Street, Suite 600, Chicago, IL 60601, U.S.A.

N.J. Pontzer, Department of Pharmacology and Therapeutics, College of Medicine, Box J-267, J.H.M. Health Center, Gainesville, FL 32610, U.S.A.

D.L. Price, Departments of Pathology, Neurology and Neuroscience, Neuropathology Laboratory, 509 Pathology Building, Johns Hopkins University School of Medicine, 600 North Wolfe Street, Baltimore, MD 21205-2181, U.S.A.

A. Prochiantz, CNRS URA 1414, Département de Biologie, ENS, 46 rue d'Ulm, 75005 Paris, France.

S.B. Prusiner, Departments of Neurology, Biochemistry and Biophysics, University of California, School of Medicine, San Francisco, CA 94143-0114, U.S.A.

S. Raffioni, Department of Biological Chemistry, College of Medicine, University of California, Irvine, CA 92717, U.S.A.

F. Rahbar, Department of Neurology, University of California, San Francisco, CA 94143-0114, U.S.A.

J.M. Rigo, Service de Physiologie Humaine et de Physiopathologie, Institut Léon Frédéricq, Place Delcour 17, B-4020 Liège, Belgium.

E. Roberts, Department of Neurobiochemistry, Beckman Research Institute of the City of Hope, Duarte, CA 91010, U.S.A.

W. Rodriguez, Mailman Research Center, McLean Hospital, 115 Mill Street, Belmont, MA 02178, U.S.A.

K.E. Rogers, Department of Neurobiology and Anatomy, University of Rochester Medical Center, 601 Elmwood Avenue, Rochester, NY 14642, U.S.A.

B. Rogister, Service de Physiologie Humaine et de Physiopathologie, Institut Léon Frédéricq, Place Delcour 17, B-4020 Liège, Belgium.

M.B. Rosenberg, Department of Pediatrics, University of California at San Diego, La Jolla, CA 92093, U.S.A.

A. Rousselet, CNRS URA 1414, Département de Biologie, ENS, 46 rue d'Ulm, 75005 Paris, France.

D.W. Saffen, Departments of Neuroscience, Neurology, Psychiatry and Behavioral Sciences, Johns Hopkins University School of Medicine, 725 North Wolfe Street, Baltimore, MD 21205, U.S.A.

R.M. Sapolsky, Department of Biological Sciences, Stanford University, Stanford, CA 94305, U.S.A.

S. Schacher, Center for Neurobiology and Behavior, Columbia University, New York, NY, U.S.A.

J. Schoenen, Service de Physiologie Humaine et de Physiopathologie, Institut Léon Frédéricq, Place Delcour 17, B-4020 Liège, Belgium.

S.S. Sisodia, Department of Pathology, Neuropathology Laboratory, 509 Pathology Building, Johns Hopkins University School of Medicine, 600 North Wolfe Street, Baltimore, MD 21205-2181, U.S.A.

A.M. Spiegel, Molecular Pathophysiology Branch, National Institutes of Diabetes, Digestive, and Kidney Diseases, National Institutes of Health, Bethesda, MD 20892, U.S.A.

B.R. Stevens, Department of Pharmacology and Therapeutics, College of Medicine, Box J-267, J.H.M. Health Center, Gainesville, FL 32610, U.S.A.

L. Thorpe, Department of Human Biological Chemistry and Genetics, University of Texas Medical Branch, 436 Gail Borden, F52, Galveston, TX 77550-2777, U.S.A.

J.W. Truman, Department of Zoology, NJ-15, University of Washington, Seattle, WA 98195, U.S.A.

M.H. Tuszynski, Department of Neurosciences, University of California at San Diego, La Jolla, CA 92093, U.S.A.

J. Ulas, Department of Psychobiology, University of California, Irvine, CA 92717, U.S.A.

J.S. Valletta, Department of Neurology, University of California, San Francisco, CA 94143-0114, U.S.A.

L.C. Walker, Department of Pathology, Neuropathology Laboratory, 509 Pathology Building, Johns Hopkins University School of Medicine, 600 North Wolfe Street, Baltimore, MD 21205-2181, U.S.A.

K. Werrbach-Perez, Department of Human Biological Chemistry and Genetics, University of Texas Medical Branch, 436 Gail Borden, F52, Galveston, TX 77550-2777, U.S.A.

P.F. Worley, Departments of Neuroscience, Neurology, Psychiatry and Behavioral Sciences, Johns Hopkins University School of Medicine, 725 North Wolfe Street, Baltimore, MD 21205, U.S.A.

B.A. Yankner, The Children's Hospital, 300 Longwood Avenue, Boston, MA 02115, U.S.A.; and Department of Neuropathology, Harvard Medical School, Boston, MA, U.S.A.

K. Yoshida, Department of Neurosciences, University of California at San Diego, La Jolla, CA 92093, U.S.A.

Preface

The chapters included in this volume are derived from presentations made at the National Institute on Aging Symposium on Molecular and Cellular Mechanisms of Neuronal Plasticity in Aging and Alzheimer's Disease, which was held May 1 through May 3, 1989 in Bethesda, Maryland. The symposium was organized to bring together specialists from many disciplines to discuss issues important for the understanding of the molecular mechanisms underlying plasticity in the nervous system during normal aging and in dementia. Talented neuroscientists, who do not work directly on aging or dementia, were included to provide valuable expertise in research areas not usually considered central to aging or Alzheimer's research. The program was designed to critically analyze mechanisms of neuronal cell death, synaptic plasticity, the role of glia in plasticity, inter- and intracellular molecular signalling, and changes in gene expression and protein processing during aging and dementia. The program was arranged to allow many opportunities for both formal and informal discussion. As a result, many new collaborative research efforts have germinated and we hope future scientific meetings on neuroplasticity will include the fruits of these collaborations.

The symposium was supported by a major gift from the Sigma-Tau Foundation of Rome, Italy, a philanthropic organization dedicated to the advancement and interaction of culture and science. Additional support was received from G.D. Searle and Company, Cortex Pharmaceuticals, Abbott Laboratories, Bristol Myers, and Sterling Drug. The organizers would like to express their gratitude to these sponsors and to T. Franklin Williams, Director, and Zaven Khachaturian, Associate Director, of the National Institute on Aging for their advice and support.

Paul D. Coleman
Gerald A. Higgins
Creighton H. Phelps

Contents

SECTION I

Introductory Overview

P. Coleman, G. Higgins and C. Phelps (Eds.)
Progress in Brain Research, Vol. 86
© 1990 Elsevier Science Publishers B.V. (Biomedical Division)

CHAPTER 1

Neural plasticity in aging and Alzheimer's disease: some selected comments

Creighton H. Phelps

Division of Medical and Scientific Affairs, Alzheimer's Association, Chicago, IL 60601, U.S.A.

Increasing birth rate and decreasing mortality have led to dramatic increases in the number of older people. It is estimated that the world's elderly population is currently growing at a rate of 2.4%/year from an estimated 290 million over age 65 in 1987 to an anticipated 410 million in the year 2000 (Torrey et al., 1987). The number of "oldest old" (aged 80 and over) is growing even more rapidly. With longer lifespans, diseases associated with old age will become more prevalent. While tremendous advances in the treatment of cancer, heart disease, and stroke have allowed people to live longer, progress has been slower in the treatment of other diseases of later life, particularly brain diseases associated with aging. Among these diseases, the dementias present a particularly difficult research problem, one which many neuroscientists are actively investigating.

Neural plasticity can be defined as adaptive changes in structure and function of the nervous system occurring during all stages of development, as a result of experience, or following injury. Many levels of complexity have been attached to the concept of plasticity with time spans ranging from seconds to years; from very precise modifications in behavior related to learning and memory to global responses such as attempts to recover function following environmental insult. The immature central nervous system (CNS) is considered to be extremely plastic but, until recently, the mature and aging CNS were thought to have very little plastic capability. We now know axonal sprouting, dendritic growth, and glial changes occur in older animal and human brains.

The most consistent changes described in normally aging brain are decreased brain weight accompanied by cortical atrophy, loss of cortical neurons, accumulation of lipofuscin storage granules in neurons and glia, and hypertrophic changes in neuroglia (Landfield, 1982). Neuron loss in non-cortical areas is less consistent with some brain stem nuclei showing significant reductions in cell numbers while others appear normal (reviewed in Coleman and Flood, 1987). Earlier work described decreased neuronal density with age in several cortical areas (Brody, 1970), but more recent studies indicate that the losses may not be as great as the earlier work indicated. While the number of large neurons decreases, smaller neurons are more numerous. This suggests that the changes previously reported may be due partially to shrinkage of the large cells (Terry et al., 1987). With glial cell density also increasing, the overall decrease in cortical volume probably results from both cell loss and reduction in volume of cells and neurites. It is important to discover the molecular mechanisms underlying the processes of cell shrinkage and cell death in normal aging.

Reports on changes in dendritic extent with advancing age depend on the area of brain examined, and the method of tissue preparation. Using the rapid Golgi technique, Scheibel et al. (1975)

4

reported losses of dendrites and dendritic spines in pyramidal cells of the frontal and temporal lobe neocortex and hippocampus while Coleman's group (Buell and Coleman, 1979) using the Golgi – Cox method, described increased dendritic branching and growth in pyramidal cells of the parahippocampal gyrus and suggested that dendritic growth may be an attempt to compensate for loss of neighboring neurons. A larger dendritic surface area would provide new synaptic sites for afferent axons formerly connected to the now missing cells. However, in the very old, Flood et al. (1985) found that there was regression of dendritic extent in pyramidal cells of the dentate gyrus while in still other areas of the hippocampus, dendritic extent in pyramidal cells was unchanged. Thus even in the so-called plastic areas of the brain, dendritic changes with aging are variable.

Cotman and his group (reviewed in Cotman and Anderson, 1988) have investigated reactive synaptogenesis in the aging brain and determined that hippocampal afferent axons in the brains of aged rodents demonstrate a remarkable capacity for sprouting and synaptogenesis although the response may not be as rapid as in younger animals (Scheff et al., 1980). Synaptic regrowth is slower and less complete in older animals. Whether the reconnection is adaptive remains to be demonstrated.

Neuroglia, astrocytes in particular, play a dynamic role in brain function by modulating the extraneuronal microenvironment. Astrocytes have specific receptors for neurotransmitters and a complement of enzyme systems which aid in the processing of neurotransmitters and metabolites released during neuronal activity. These cells are exquisitely sensitive to changes in the brain environment and, after injury to the central nervous system, demonstrate dramatic reactive properties. Very few studies of physiological properties of aging astrocytes have been conducted. However, beginning in middle age and increasing into old age, marked astrocyte hypertrophy occurs in the vicinity of terminal synaptic fields in the hippocampus (Lindsey et al., 1979). This results in increased glial volume but not number. Other studies have noted increases in the glial – neuronal ratio and glial reactivity with advancing age in a number of species including man (Hansen et al., 1987).

Because memory loss is a hallmark of Alzheimer's disease, much attention has been focused on the physiological basis of memory and the changes that occur during aging. Basic understanding of memory decline (reduced plasticity) in normal aging may provide insight into memory losses in dementia. There is convincing evidence that aging leads to impairment of tasks requiring behavioral plasticity (reviewed in Landfield et al., 1986). This impairment relates primarily to recall of recent events and includes faster rates of forgetting. Studies of the granule cells in the hippocampus of younger animals show an activity-dependent long-term enhancement (LTE) or potentiation (LTP) of synaptic strength that may represent a mechanism for information storage. This stimulation-induced effect shows some evidence of decline in older animals (Sharp et al., 1987; Barnes, this volume).

Dementia is a clinical state characterized by the development of memory and learning impairments, loss of intellectual and cognitive functions, and disorientation (Katzman, 1986). This complex of symptoms can be caused by a number of disorders, but the most common cause of dementia is Alzheimer's disease accounting for 60 – 70% of all cases.

It was in 1907 that Alois Alzheimer published the first case report, "about a peculiar disease of the cerebral cortex" (Alzheimer, 1907). He described a 51-year-old patient whose ability to encode information was severely disturbed and had compromised language functions. At autopsy the brain was atrophic and demonstrated "abnormal accumulations of neurofibrillary bundles", "miliary foci" (neuritic plaques) and "deposits of a peculiar substance" (amyloid) in the cerebral cortex. There was also cell loss in the upper layers of the cerebral cortex accompanied by changes in glia. These findings have been confirmed and studied more intensely in many cases of dementia of the Alzheimer type.

Estimates vary for the prevalence of Alzheimer's disease in the U.S. but recent studies indicate that as many as 4 million Americans are afflicted. Since the primary risk factor is age, by the year 2040 the prevalence of dementia is expected to be as much as 5 times greater if significant progress is not made in treatment or prevention.

In order to understand the changes that occur in the brains of demented patients, it is first necessary to distinguish them from changes occurring in the brain during normal aging in disease-free individuals and from changes seen in other brain diseases not related to dementia. The pathological changes in Alzheimer's disease appear to be particularly severe in those areas of the brain that are considered to be plastic including areas closely associated with cognitive processing such as the hippocampus, amygdala, and other limbic structures as well as the neocortical association areas. Basal forebrain and brain stem neurons are also affected. The cognitive deficits associated with the dementias stem from dysfunction of these brain areas and, therefore, much of the research on dementias focuses on structure and function of these plastic areas, particularly the hippocampus and the neocortex. Study of these areas in non-demented individuals and in experimental animals has contributed valuable information about synaptic plasticity and its relation to learning and memory during normal aging (See Barnes, this volume).

When the disease process is superimposed on the aging process, cortical atrophy, cell loss and proliferation of neuroglia are even more pronounced than with aging alone. Similar histological changes exist in normal and Alzheimer's brains but differ in degree. In very old patients and in late onset disease differences are particularly difficult to identify; this may explain why neurochemical differences between age-matched controls and Alzheimer's subjects are not always obvious (Hauw et al., 1988). An important finding in AD brains is specific loss of cells in association areas of the neocortex, limbic structures, nucleus basalis, and

locus coeruleus accompanied by reductions in levels of neurotransmitters including acetylcholine, serotonin, norepinephrine, GABA (gamma-aminobutyric acid), aspartate, and corticotrophin releasing factor. Transmitter reductions stem from dysfunction or death of specific cell types. For example the reduction of acetylcholine is closely correlated with the shrinkage and loss of cholinergic cells in nucleus basalis and reduction of norepinephrine reflects loss of cells in the nucleus of the locus coeruleus. It is not yet clear which transmitter(s) are associated with the specific cells lost in the neocortex although glutamate is a prime candidate.

The molecular mechanisms underlying selective cell death are under study in a number of different laboratories. Some forms of neuronal cell death result from a cascade of events set in motion by stimulation of receptors on the cell membrane leading to abnormal phosphorylation of proteins. The details of these events are still not known but it is thought that changes in calcium homeostasis, gene expression and protein processing lead to dysfunction and eventual cell death. One class of receptor implicated in cell death is the NMDA receptor which is normally stimulated by excitatory amino acids such as glutamate. However, under certain circumstances excitatory amino acids or other endogenous factors can be excitotoxic, causing overstimulation of the receptors and activation of the events leading to cell death (see Olney, this volume). Receptor and channel blockers or other compounds that might interrupt the subsequent cascade of events leading to cell death may serve to protect vulnerable cells. These compounds would need to be delivered to the appropriate cells while not interfering with normal cell function. Among the compounds being considered are the calcium channel blocker, nimodipine, and NMDA receptor blockers. If vulnerable cells can be protected, the progress of Alzheimer's disease might be slowed.

The role of neurotrophic factors in the normal aging brain and in Alzheimer's disease is a topic of great interest. Nerve growth factor (NGF) is the only neurotrophic factor demonstrated to protect a specific class of neurons in the brain affected by AD, the basal forebrain cholinergic neurons. Other trophic factors are less specific in their actions and influence neuroglia and cells associated with brain vessels as well as neurons (Hefti, this volume). NGF exerts its influence by binding to specific receptors on the surface of the axon terminal and after internalization is retrogradely transported to the perikaryon where it influences gene expression and stimulates both cell maintenance and neurite outgrowth. In the mature nervous system, cell maintenance requires a balance of synthesis and degradation of molecular constituents in the cell. Normal turnover allows the cell to remodel and repair axons and dendrites and to modify synaptic structure in response to changes in activity. Withdrawal or absence of NGF inhibits neurite outgrowth and can lead to neuronal cell death by an active death program (Martin et al., 1988).

Studies of reactive synaptogenesis and dendritic remodeling in Alzheimer's disease show that the entorhinal projection neurons and the perforant pathway are destroyed by neurofibrillary tangles and neuritic plaques in AD (Hyman et al., 1984). To investigate whether this degeneration led to any plastic response such as reactive sprouting, Geddes et al. (1985) and Hyman et al. (1987) examined the hippocampus and described changes in Alzheimer brains that looked very similar to the reorganization seen in animals following experimental lesions. This surprising result indicates that patients with AD do demonstrate neuroplasticity. On the other hand Coleman and his colleagues noted that dendritic remodeling in AD does not occur as it does in the normal aging brain leading to the suggestion that there is some failure of plasticity in AD. The results from these two sets of studies are not necessarily inconsistent (see Coleman, this volume).

Astrocytic proliferation and hypertrophy (gliosis) have been noted in the course of normal aging and in Alzheimer's disease. Gliosis is widely assumed to occur as a reaction to toxic or traumatic injury to the brain. Current hypotheses suggest that the astrocytic reaction is triggered by lymphokines such as interleukin-1 (IL-1) which are released either from resident microglia or macrophages derived from the blood (Giulian and Lachman, 1985; Giulian et al., 1986). Activation of phagocytes is one of the earliest events described during insults to the nervous system seen before or accompanying proliferation and hypertrophy of the astrocytes. Reactive astrocytes have the capacity to synthesize many factors which could have positive or negative influences on other cells in the vicinity of the wound. Reactive astrocytes express the message for beta nerve growth factor, and after injury to the brain the wound cavity is bordered by astrocytes expressing NGF as demonstrated by in situ hybridization (see Gage et al., this volume). Presumably NGF or other factors could stabilize the cells around the lesion and prevent further dysfunction or death of those neurons capable of responding. It has not yet been demonstrated whether NGF message is elevated in the cerebral cortex where gliosis has been described during aging.

In Alzheimer's disease, basal forebrain cholinergic neurons are one of the populations of neurons specifically vulnerable; these neurons along with their axons degenerate resulting in a loss of neocortical and hippocampal choline acetyl transferase (ChAT), a marker of cholinergic activity (Whitehouse et al., 1982). This loss, in turn, correlates with decreased cognitive function (Francis et al., 1985; Katzman et al., 1986). Attempts to treat AD with drugs which increase cholinergic function have had very limited success. As mentioned above NGF specifically acts on basal forebrain cholinergic neurons and intracerebral administration of NGF selectively induces an increase in the activity of choline acetyltransferase (Gnahn et al., 1983; Will and Hefti, 1985; Mobley et al., 1986). A report from a recent workshop held at the National Institute on Aging concluded that there is sufficient evidence to pursue studies on NGF as a potential treatment for Alzheimer's disease (Phelps et al., 1989). The evidence included the following: (1) memory loss associated with AD is correlated with cholinergic dysfunction in the basal forebrain (Perry et al., 1978; Francis et al., 1985; Katzman et al., 1986); (2) markers of cholinergic activity co-localize with NGF receptors on basal forebrain neurons in all species examined (Korsching et al., 1985; Richardson et al., 1986; Taniuchi et al., 1986; Goedert et al., 1989); and (3) rodent studies demonstrate that NGF rescues basal forebrain cholinergic neurons from death in normal aging (Fischer et al., 1987) and following experimental lesions of the fimbria-fornix (Hefti, 1986; Williams et al., 1986; Kromer, 1989). Despite the compelling rationale for the use of NGF in the treatment of AD there are investigators who caution against its use (Butcher and Woolf, 1989). They argue that exogenous administration of trophic factors may lead to aberrant neuronal growth and exacerbate rather than retard the disease process. For these reasons much more animal research especially in non-human primates is needed before moving on to human trials (Phelps et al., 1989).

While it is highly likely that astrocytes are a source of NGF in the central nervous system, they may also be the source of endogenous excitotoxins such as quinolinic acid. The excitotoxins are the subject of much interesting research on mechanisms of neuronal cell death (see Olney, this volume). The excitotoxins are glutamate analogs but, except for glutamate itself, aspartate and quinolinic acid, they do not normally exist in the brain. There has been much speculation that excessive release of glutamate or aspartate may lead to death of neurons. However, in several studies the amount of glutamate necessary to trigger cell death in vivo was far beyond physiological levels (Stone et al., 1987). This can be explained by the very efficient buffering mechanisms for glutamate. On the other hand, quinolinic acid is not as efficiently removed by the uptake mechanisms that rapidly remove glutamate and aspartate. As a result, quinolinic acid causes neuron death after application in much smaller concentrations (Schwarz et al., 1983). The enzymes responsible for synthesis of quinolinic acid are localized in astrocytes (Kohler et al., 1987). Therefore, it is possible that neuronal cell death may be caused by release of quinolinic acid from astrocytes triggered by some as yet unknown stimulus. Interestingly, it has been reported that the concentration of brain quinolinic acid increases markedly in old animals (Moroni et al., 1984). Whether this reflects the increased number of glial cells present in older animals or upregulation of synthesis is not yet known.

The neuroglia play a more complex role in central nervous function than was previously recognized. They are exquisitely sensitive to changes in their environment and help maintain a relatively constant environment for neurons by participation in the inactivation of neurotransmitters and toxic metabolites resulting from neuronal activity (reviewed in Vernadakis, 1988). Changes in glial structure and function are evident following insults to the brain usually before any demonstrable changes are apparent in the neurons. With the more recent findings of both toxic and trophic factors localized to astrocytes in the adult nervous system (see Moonen, this volume), it now appears that glia may, under the appropriate circumstances, participate in the stimulation of normal or aberrant growth as well as degenerative changes in the adult and aging brain. Astrocytes are highly plastic themselves and have the metabolic capabilities to influence the plasticity of neurons.

Plasticity in the adult and aging brain is now an established fact. However, the molecular mechanisms underlying both neuronal and glial plasticity require much further study. By exploiting the tools of molecular and cellular biology, communication within and between cells of the brain will gradually be better understood. This will enhance our ability to investigate the dynamic regulation of plasticity during normal aging and in brain diseases such as dementia. The remaining chapters in this volume direct our attention to the wealth of new information and technology now available to pursue this quest.

References

Alzheimer, A. (1907) Über ein eigenartige Erkrankung der Hirnrinde. *Allg. Z. Psychiat.,* 64: 146 – 148.

Brody, H. (1970) Structural changes in the aging nervous system. In: H.T. Blumenthal (Ed.), *The Regulatory Role of the Nervous System in Aging,* Karger, Basel, pp. 9 – 21.

Buell, S.J. and Coleman, P.D. (1979) Dendritic growth in the aged human brain and failure of growth in senile dementia. *Science,* 206: 854 – 856.

Buell, S.J. and Coleman, P.D. (1981) Quantitative evidence for selective dendritic growth in normal human aging but not in senile dementia. *Brain Res.,* 214: 23 – 41.

Butcher, L.L. and Woolf, N.J. (1989) Neurotrophic agents exacerbate the pathological cascade of Alzheimer's disease. *Neurobiol. Aging,* 10: 557 – 570.

Coleman, P.D. and Flood, D.G. (1987) Neuron number and dendritic extent in normal aging and Alzheimer's disease. *Neurobiol. Aging,* 8: 521 – 545.

Cotman, C.W. and Anderson, K.J. (1988) Synaptic plasticity and functional stabilization in the hippocampal formation: possible role in Alzheimer disease. *Adv. Neurol.,* 47: 313 – 335.

Fischer, W., Wictorin, K., Björklund, A., Williams, L.R., Varon, S. and Gage, F.H. (1987) Amelioration of cholinergic neuron atrophy and spatial memory impairment in aged rats by nerve growth factor. *Nature,* 329: 65 – 68.

Flood, D.G., Buell, S.J., DeFiore, C.H., Horwitz, G.J. and Coleman, P.D. (1985) Age-related dendritic growth in dentate gyrus of human brain is followed by regression in the "oldest old". *Brain Res.,* 345: 366 – 368.

Flood, D.G., Buell, S.J., Horwitz, G.J. and Coleman, P.D. (1987) Dendritic extent in human dentate gyrus cells in normal aging and senile dementia. *Brain Res.,* 402: 205 – 216.

Francis, P.T., Palmer, A.M., Sims, N.R., Bowen, D.M., Davison, A.N., Esiri, M.M., Neary, D., Snowden, J.S. and Wilcock, G.C. (1985) Neurochemical studies of early-onset Alzheimer's disease: possible influence on treatment. *New Engl. J. Med.,* 313: 7 – 11.

Geddes, J.W., Monaghan, D.T., Cotman, C.W., Lott, I.T., Kim, R.C. and Chui, H.C. (1985) Plasticity of hippocampal circuitry in Alzheimer's disease. *Science,* 230: 1179 – 1181.

Giulian, D. and Lachman, L.B. (1985) Interleukin-1 stimulation of astroglial proliferation after brain injury. *Science,* 228: 497 – 499.

Giulian, D., Baker, T.J., Shih, L.C. and Lachman, L.B. (1986) Interleukin 1 of the central nervous system is produced by ameboid microglia. *J. Exp. Med.,* 164: 594 – 604.

Gnahn, H., Hefti, F., Heumann, R., Schwab, M.E. and Thoenen, H. (1983) NGF-mediated increase of choline acetyltransferase (ChAT) in the neonatal rat forebrain: evidence for a physiological role of NGF in the brain. *Dev. Brain Res.,* 9: 45 – 52.

Goedert, M., Fine, A., Dawbarn, D., Wilcock, G.K. and Chao, M.V. (1989) Nerve growth factor receptor mRNA distribution in human brain: normal levels in basal forebrain in Alzheimer's disease. *Mol. Brain Res.,* 5: 1 – 7.

Hansen, L.A., Armstrong, D.M. and Terry, R.D. (1987) An immunohistochemical quantification of fibrous astrocytes in the aging human cerebral cortex. *Neurobiol. Aging,* 8: 1 – 6.

Hauw, J.J., Duyckaerts, C. and Delaere, P. (1988) Neuropathology of aging and DAT. In: A.S. Henderson and J.H. Henderson (Eds.), *Etiology of Dementia of Alzheimer's Type,* Wiley, New York, pp. 195 – 211.

Hefti, F. (1986) Nerve growth factor promotes survival of septal cholinergic neurons after fimbria transection. *J. Neurosci.,* 6: 2155 – 2162.

Hefti, F. and Weiner, W.J. (1986) Nerve growth factor and Alzheimer's disease. *Ann. Neurol.,* 20: 275 – 281.

Hyman, B.T., Van Hoesen, G.W., Damasio, A.R. and Barnes, L.L. (1984) Alzheimer's disease: cell specific pathology isolates the hippocampal formation. *Science,* 225: 1168 – 1170.

Hyman, B.T., Kromer, L.J. and Van Hoesen, G.W. (1987) Reinnervation of the hippocampal perforant pathway zone in Alzheimer's disease. *Ann. Neurol.,* 24: 259 – 267.

Katzman, R. (1986) Alzheimer's disease. *New Engl. J. Med.,* 314: 964 – 973.

Katzman, R., Brown, T., Field, P., Thal, L., Davies, P. and Terry, R. (1986) Significance of neurotransmitter abnormalities in Alzheimer disease? In: J.B. Martin and J.D. Barchas (Eds.), *Neuropeptides in Neurologic and Psychiatric Disease,* Raven Press, New York, pp. 279 – 280.

Kohler, C., Okuno, E., Flood, P.R. and Schwarcz, R. (1987) Quinolinic acid phosphoribosyltransferase: preferential glial localization in the rat brain visualized by immunocytochemistry. *Proc. Natl. Acad. Sci. U.S.A.,* 84: 3491 – 3495.

Korsching, S., Auburger, G., Heumann, R., Scott, J. and Thoenen, H. (1985) Levels of nerve growth factor receptor and its mRNA in the central nervous system of the rat correlate with cholinergic innervation. *EMBO J.,* 4: 1389 – 1393.

Kromer, L.F. (1989) Nerve growth factor treatment after brain injury prevents neuronal death. *Science,* 235: 214 – 217.

Landfield, P.W. (1982) Measurement of brain aging: conceptual issues and neurobiological indices. In: R. Adelman and G. Roth (Eds.), *Endocrine and Neuroendocrine Mechanisms of Aging,* CRC Press, Boca Raton, FL, pp. 183 – 207.

Landfield, P.W., Pitler, T.A. and Applegate, M.D. (1986) The aged hippocampus. In: R.L. Isaacson and K.H. Pribram (Eds.), *The Hippocampus,* Plenum, New York, pp. 323 – 367.

Lindsey, J.D., Landfield, P.W. and Lynch, G. (1979) Early onset and topographical distribution of hypertrophied astrocytes in hippocampus of aging rats: a quantitative study. *J. Gerontol.,* 34: 661 – 671.

Martin, D.P., Schmidt, R.E., DiStefano, P.S., Lowry, O.H.,

Carter, J.G. and Johnson, E.M., Jr. (1988) Inhibitors of protein synthesis and RNA synthesis prevent neuronal death caused by nerve growth factor deprivation. *J. Cell Biol.,* 106: 829 – 844.

Mobley, W.C., Rutkowski, J.L., Tennekoon, G.I., Gemski, J., Buchanan, K. and Johnston, M.V. (1986) Nerve growth factor increases choline acetyltransferase activity in developing basal forebrain neurons. *Mol. Brain Res.,* 1: 53 – 62.

Moroni, F., Lombardi, G., Moneti, G. and Aldino, C. (1984) The excitotoxin quinolinic acid is present in the brain of several mammals and its cortical content increases during the aging process. *Neurosci. Lett.,* 47: 51 – 55.

Perry, E.K., Tomlinson, B.E., Blessed, G., Bergman, K., Gibson, P.H. and Perry, R.H. (1978) Correlation of cholinergic abnormalities with senile plaques and mental test scores in senile dementia. *Br. Med. J.,* 2: 1457 – 1459.

Phelps, C.H., Gage, F.H., Growden, J.H., Hefti, F., Harbaugh, R., Johnston, M.V., Khachaturian, Z.S., Mobley, W.C., Price, D.L., Raskind, M., Simpkins, J., Thal, L.J. and Woodcock, J. (1989) Potential use of nerve growth factor to treat Alzheimer's disease. *Neurobiol. Aging,* 10: 205 – 207.

Richardson, P.M., Verga Issa, V.M.K. and Riopelle, R.J. (1986) Distribution of neuronal receptors for nerve growth factor in the rat. *J. Neurosci.,* 6: 2312 – 2321.

Scheff, S.W., Benardo, L.S. and Cotman, C.W. (1980) Decline in reactive fiber growth in the dentate gyrus of aged rats as compared to young adult rats following entorhinal cortex removal. *Brain Res.,* 199: 21 – 38.

Scheibel, M.E., Lindsay, R.D., Tomiyasu, U. and Scheibel, A.B. (1975) Progressive dendritic changes in aging human cortex. *Exp. Neurol.,* 47: 392 – 403.

Schwarz, R., Whetsell, W.O. and Mangano, R.M. (1983) Quinolinic acid: an endogenous metabolite that produces axon-sparing lesions. *Science,* 21: 316 – 318.

Sharp, P.E., Barnes, C.A. and McNaughton, B.L. (1987) Effects of aging on environmental modulation of hippocampal evoked responses. *Behav. Neurosci.,* 101: 170 – 178.

Stone, T.W., Connick, J.H., Winn, P., Hastings, M.H. and English, M. (1987) Endogenous excitotoxic agents. *Ciba Found. Symp.,* 126: 204 – 220.

Taniuchi, M., Schweitzer, J.B. and Johnson, E.M., Jr. (1986) Nerve growth factor receptor molecules in rat brain. *Proc. Natl. Acad. Sci. U.S.A.,* 83: 1950 – 1954.

Terry, R.D., DeTeresa, R. and Hansen, L.A. (1987) Neocortical cell counts. *Ann. Neurol.,* 21: 530 – 539.

Torrey, B.B., Kinsella, K. and Taeuber, C.M. (1987) An aging world. *Int. Populat. Rep.,* 78: 1 – 85.

Vernadakis, A. (1988) Neuron-glia interrelations. *Int. Rev. Neurobiol.,* 30: 149 – 224.

Whitehouse, P.J., Price, D.L., Struble, R.G., Clark, A.W., Coyle, J.T. and DeLong, M.R. (1982) Alzheimer's disease and senile dementia: loss of neurons in the basal forebrain. *Science,* 215: 1237 – 1239.

Will, B. and Hefti, F. (1985) Behavioral and neurochemical effects of chronic intraventricular injections of nerve growth factor in adult rats with fimbria lesions. *Behav. Brain Res.,* 17: 17 – 24.

Williams, L.R., Varon, S., Peterson, G.M., Wictorin, K., Fischer, W., Björklund, A. and Gage, F.H. (1986) Continuous infusion of nerve growth factor prevents basal forebrain neuronal death after fimbria fornix transection. *Proc. Natl. Acad. Sci. U.S.A.,* 83: 9231 – 9235.

SECTION II

Cell Death

P. Coleman, G. Higgins and C. Phelps (Eds.)
Progress in Brain Research, Vol. 86
© 1990 Elsevier Science Publishers B.V. (Biomedical Division)

CHAPTER 2

Glucocorticoids, hippocampal damage and the glutamatergic synapse

Robert M. Sapolsky

Department of Biological Sciences, Stanford University, Stanford, CA 94305, U.S.A.

Introduction

Organisms are often subject to stressors which disrupt homeostasis; such perturbations produce a set of endocrine and neural adaptations that form the stress-response. Central to this is the secretion of glucocorticoids (GCs) by the adrenal cortex. These steroid hormones are secreted as the final step in an endocrine cascade beginning with the perception of stress in the brain. The hypothalamus, within seconds, secretes corticotropin releasing factor (CRF) along with a number of other minor secretagogues which augment CRF action. These collectively stimulate the pituitary release of ACTH, within approximately 15 sec. ACTH, in turn, stimulates the adrenal secretion of GCs within minutes. The GCs divert energy to muscles by blocking glucose utilization in other tissues and promoting the breakdown of stored energy; they increase blood pressure in synergy with catecholamines. Finally, they suppress costly anabolic processes such as growth, reproduction, and the immune and inflammatory responses until more auspicious times. These GC actions are highly catabolic, underscoring the dramatic responses needed in adapting to stress. Thus when exposure to GCs is prolonged (due to stress, pathologic hypersecretion, or exogenous administration), the deleterious consequences can include myopathy, steroid diabetes, hypertension, impotency, amenorrhea and immunosuppression

(Krieger, 1982; Munck et al., 1984).

It has become clear that the deleterious consequences of GC overexposure can also include damage to neurons of the hippocampus. The structure is a principal neural target site for GCs. It (and the septum) are the only regions with appreciable concentrations of the type I corticosteroid receptor, and it has concentrations of the type II receptor equal to any other brain region (Reul and De Kloet, 1985). Moreover, hippocampal neurochemistry and electrophysiology, and hippocampal-dependent behavior are very sensitive to GCs (Meyer, 1985; McEwen et al., 1986). This paper will review the current knowledge concerning the cell biology of how GCs damage hippocampal neurons.

The first evidence of this neurotoxicity was that pharmacologic concentrations of GCs preferentially damage the guinea pig hippocampus (Aus der Muhlen and Ockenfels, 1979). This observation was difficult to interpret at the time, as it predated the first demonstration of corticosteroid receptors in the brain, at which time GCs and the hippocampus were linked together. A decade later, GCs were implicated in playing a physiological role in hippocampal aging in the rat. The first evidence was correlative. Aged male rats typically have elevated basal GC concentrations (reviewed in Sapolsky et al., 1987), and it was shown that the more severe the GC hypersecretion in aged rats, the more pronounced the hippocampal degeneration (Landfield et al., 1978). Subsequently, the same authors showed that removal of GCs (via adrenalectomy) at mid-age (12 months) prevented the hippocampal neuron loss and cognitive impairments typical of old age in the rat (Landfield et al., 1981). Thus, some adrenal-derived hormone caused hippocampal neuronal aging. We strengthened the case for the hormone being GCs, showing that prolonged exposure to GC concentrations in the upper physiologic range (equivalent to those of major stressors) accelerates hippocampal neuron loss (Sapolsky et al., 1985). The pattern of degeneration resembled that seen in the aged hippocampus: pyramidal neurons of Ammon's horn with high concentrations of corticosteroid receptors were preferentially lost. Moreover, this was accompanied by glial proliferation and infiltration, classic neuropathologic markers of neuronal degeneration. It was then demonstrated that prolonged stress itself could also damage the hippocampus (Kerr et al., 1986).

Research then focused on the mechanisms of GC hippocampal neurotoxicity. It was reasoned that GCs need not be directly toxic but need only be as catabolic as in many peripheral tissues. GCs may, in effect, leave the neurons on the "edge" of a metabolic cliff. With no further challenge, the period of GC exposure passes uneventfully. However, a co-incident challenge might be less readily survived. This idea predicted that varied neurological insults that damage the hippocampus should become more toxic in the presence of more GCs (Sapolsky, 1985a). Work by ourselves and others supports this idea. Insults as varied as excitotoxic seizures due to kainic acid (Sapolsky, 1985a, 1986a; Theoret et al., 1985), the antimetabolite 3-acetylpyridine (Sapolsky, 1985a, b), hypoxia – ischemia (Sapolsky and Pulsinelli, 1985; Koide et al., 1986; James Davis, personal communication) and the oxygen radical generator paraquat (Sapolsky et al., 1988) are worsened by GCs. In vivo, reduction of GCs (by adrenalectomy) reduces hippocampal damage, while elevating GC concentrations to the stress range (via GC administration) increases damage. The extremes vary as much as 10-fold, emphasizing the potency of this effect.

These studies on the GC exacerbation of the toxicity of varied insults make it uncertain what the precise role is of the steroids in hippocampal degeneration during aging. Do the GCs *kill* hippocampal neurons outright, or do they *endanger* them and compromise their ability to survive insults? The latter would appear to be unlikely, given that GCs contribute to hippocampal senescence even in the absence of overt neurological crises such as hypoxia – ischemia or seizure. However, the GCs may induce a sufficient vulnerability in the neurons such that the insults that now become damaging are so subtle as to be difficult to detect – perhaps a brief period of vasospasm, or the mild hypoglycemia induced when an animal technician feeds the rats late may be sufficient to damage an aged hippocampal neuron, with its lifetime of cumulative GC exposure. As is obvious, the latter model – one of an extremely lowered threshold for damage – would be extremely difficult to test, especially in the prolonged circumstances of an aging study. The question is not yet settled.

Features of glucocorticoid endangerment of hippocampal neurons

In attempting to uncover the mechanisms by which GCs endanger the hippocampal neurons, it became important to determine whether it was the GC molecule itself which acted upon the neuron to endanger it, or whether the GCs' effects arose secondarily, from one of their many peripheral actions. One study implicating GCs in damaging the hippocampus suggested that it was via secondary GC actions. Specifically, the authors suggested that it was not the chronic hippocampal exposure to GCs themselves which was destructive, but rather the chronic diminution of ACTH secretion (which is typically inhibited by elevated GC concentrations, via the negative feedback effects of the steroid (Keller-Wood and Dallman, 1984). Conversely, given this view, the protective effects of long-term adrenalectomy were not so much from the elimination of the GCs, but rather from the resultant elevation of ACTH concentrations. In support of that idea, it was shown that sustained exposure of aging rats to an ACTH analogue protected the hippocampus in much the same manner as did adrenalectomy (Landfield et al., 1981). In contrast to the predictions of that scenario, however, is the fact that in the aging rat, ACTH concentrations are elevated and, in fact, are the driving force for the elevated basal GC concentrations (Tang and Phillips, 1978). As an alternative model that we have favored, GCs could be endangering the neurons directly, independent of any secondary physiological effects. The first support for this view was somewhat indirect — the GC exacerbation of damage by the various insults was exclusive to, or occurred preferentially in the hippocampus. The atypically high concentration of corticosteroid receptors in that structure suggested a direct, receptor-mediated GC effect. Stronger support for the view of direct GC endangerment comes with the observation that GCs can exacerbate the damaging effects of these various insults when studied in vitro with primary hippocampal cultures (Sapolsky et al., 1988). Much as with the in vivo model, damage was exacerbated by concentrations of GCs that were, themselves, not toxic. Hypothalamic or cerebellar cultures were not sensitive to the GC insult synergy. The endangerment was not triggered by other steroids such as testosterone, estradiol or progesterone. This suggests that it is not a generalized steroid effect, but rather is specific to GCs, and mediated by their receptors. This was further supported by the finding that the GC endangerment could be prevented with GC receptor antagonists in the culture system (in preparation).

In then exploring the mechanisms by which the GCs might endanger the hippocampus, it became important to test whether a very attractive model of cell death was relevant. One of the hallmarks of the stress-response is the suppression of immune function, and GCs are central to this process. Among the numerous catabolic actions of GCs in the immune system, the steroids can trigger lysis of lymphocytes and thymocytes (reviewed in Munck et al., 1984; Bateman et al., 1989). Recent work has uncovered the mechanism by which GCs trigger this instance of "apoptosis", or programmed cell death. The steroids induce the synthesis of protein(s); it is either an endonuclease itself, or activates an endonuclease. The result is that DNA is cleaved at internucleosomal sites, producing a characteristic "ladder" of DNA fragments which are multiples of 180 base pairs (Wyllie, 1980; Umansky et al., 1981; Cohen and Duke, 1984; Compton and Cidlowski, 1986, 1987; Compton et al., 1988). The DNA fragmentation precedes the loss of cell viability. Apparently, during this process, the cell even attempts to repair its DNA in a futile attempt to stop the degradation; as evidence, poly(ADP-ribosyl)ation is activated, NAD concentrations fall, and the GC-induced lymphocytolysis is exacerbated by inhibition of poly(ADP-ribose)synthetase (Wielckens and Delfs, 1986). Moreover, it appears that this mechanism can potentially be provoked in a broad range of cell types, since cytotoxic T cells also promote DNA cleavage in target cells (Ucker, 1987). These observations suggested that GCs might provoke a similar process in the hippocampus. However, we have recently obtained evidence suggesting that this is not the case. Under conditions in which GCs exacerbate the damaging effects of the excitotoxin kainic acid, we observed no evidence of DNA cleavage. Moreover, the viability of the hippocampal neurons was not exacerbated by inhibition of poly(ADP-ribose)synthetase (Masters et al., 1989). In hindsight, this finding seems reasonable and comforting. Instances of apoptosis — during development, immunosuppression, cytotoxic attack — tend to be rapid, all-or-none in nature, and highly stereotyped in the patterns of damage. It seems logical that the underlying mechanisms should be fairly discrete, linear cascades of damage. In contrast, the GC toxicity during aging, and the insults whose toxicities are exacerbated by GCs, emerge slowly, are more selective, and are relatively ideosyncratic. Teleologically, it would seem surprising if the underlying mechanism would turn out to be a fairly discrete "suicide switch". The present evidence suggests that the mechanisms of GC endangerment are anything but discrete.

Energy availability and the glutamatergic synapse

How then do GCs compromise neuronal viability? The insults made worse by GCs are extremely varied in their mechanisms of action — cutting off of oxygen and glucose availability to the brain (hypoxia – ischemia), greatly accelerating the rate of action potentials (seizures), disrupting energy production by uncoupling electron transport (3-acetylpyridine). This suggests that whatever the GCs are doing, it is a broad and generalized vulnerability that they are inducing. Yet, as will be reviewed here, these differing neurological insults appear to have two common threads. All appear to damage hippocampal neurons via a cascade that involves excessive synaptic concentrations of excitatory amino acid neurotransmitters which, through the NMDA receptor, leads to mobilization of damaging concentrations of free cytosolic calcium. Second, this excitatory/calcium cascade seems to be highly sensitive to energy depletion. Very recent work suggests that the GC endangerment is involved with both of these themes.

Currently, there is tremendous excitement concerning the role of glutamate and other excitatory amino acid neurotransmitters (EAAs) as a common pathway by which hypoxia – ischemia, seizure and hypoglycemia are neurotoxic. The hippocampus is rich in EAAs and their receptors, which include the kainic acid, quisqualate, and N-methyl-D-aspartate (NMDA) receptor. The NMDA receptor is immensely complex; there is an allosteric binding site for glycine, and a receptor-gated channel that allows the flow of sodium and calcium only under conditions of depolarization, since at resting potential, the channel is typically blocked by magnesium in a voltage-dependent manner (MacDermott and Dale, 1987). It is the NMDA receptor which has been most implicated in

neuronal damage. The EAAs can be neurotoxic, and their synaptic concentrations rise to excessive levels following hypoxia – ischemia, hypoglycemia or seizures. These excessive levels appear both as enhanced release of the EAAs from the presynaptic neuron, as well as failure of reuptake back into the neuron, or of uptake into glia. Commensurate with the excitatory effects of these EAAs, all of these insults lead to a period of neuronal excitation. As the most direct evidence available that the EAAs mediate the neurotoxicity of these insults via the NMDA receptor, damage induced by hypoxia – ischemia, incomplete ischemia, anoxia (in cultured neurons), excitotoxic seizures, brain trauma, hypoglycemia and electron transport uncouplers can all be prevented by silencing the NMDA synapse. This can be done with antagonists that directly block the NMDA receptor, such as aminophosphonovaleric acid (APV). This can also be brought about with non-competitive antagonists that block the receptor-gated channel (such as magnesium, MK-801, dextromethorphan, or dissociative anesthetics such as phencyclidine or ketamine). Finally, it can be brought about by destruction of glutamatergic projections to the vulnerable neurons. With these varied paradigms, there is usually protection, as measured by the numbers of volume of neurons lost, by biochemical or electrophysiological markers of injury, or by functional indices of damage. Collectively, these numerous studies represent a near consensus that EAAs, via the NMDA receptor, can mediate much of the damaging effects in the hippocampus of these neurological insults (reviewed in Rothman and Olney, 1987; Choi, 1988).

The most accepted mechanism by which EAA-activation of the NMDA receptor damages neurons is via increased free cytosolic concentrations of calcium. Both EAAs and the varied insults discussed increase calcium conductance, decrease extracellular calcium concentrations, and cause intracellular calcium accumulation, and these effects can be blocked with NMDA receptor antagonists. Moreover, the toxicity of EAAs and these various insults in vitro is diminished by removing calcium from the medium (cf. Choi, 1988). There are a number of possible routes by which the calcium is mobilized. Of primary interest is the calcium channel gated to the NMDA receptor. In addition, the depolarization by the EAAs will lead to opening of voltage-gated calcium channels. As an additional mechanism, the excessive sodium influx during sustained depolarization will increase free cytosolic calcium via a cell surface membrane sodium/calcium exchanger, as well as via similar exchangers that liberate calcium from organelles. Finally, the sequestering and efflux of the calcium is apparently impaired during these insults. Thus, the excessive cytosolic calcium concentrations are derived from both increased entry of the ion into that cellular compartment, as well as impaired removal from it (McBurney and Neering, 1987; Choi, 1988). Excessive levels of such calcium are among the broadest of routes by which cells can be damaged, potentially via generation of oxygen radicals, and activation of proteases, lipases and nucleases (Cheung et al., 1986). At present, it is not clear which routes of damage are relevant in these cases of neurological crisis.

Thus, considerable evidence suggests that hypoxia – ischemia, hypoglycemia and seizure damage the hippocampus via this EAA/NMDA/calcium cascade. Critically, the cascade seems extremely sensitive to energy depletion. All three of the insults deplete hippocampal neurons of energy, as measured by declining ATP and phosphocreatine concentrations. In general, the order of severity of depletion is hypoxia – ischemia > hypoglycemia > seizure (Auer and Siesjo, 1988). Moreover, the damaging effects of all of the insults can be attenuated by supplementing neurons with energy. That is obviously the case with hypoglycemia, where the insult is, by definition, attenuated with additional glycose. It is also the case with seizure where limited energy availability compromises neuronal viability (Meldrum, 1983; Johansen and Diemer, 1986; Sapolsky and Stein, 1989). Hypoxic – ischemic damage also seems sensitive to energy, although the issue there is com-

plicated by the issue of lactate-induced acidosis. A long-standing observation is that hypoxic – ischemic damage to the hippocampus is exacerbated in vivo by glucose pre-loading (Myers and Yamaguchi, 1977; Siemkowicz and Hansen, 1978; Ginsberg et al., 1980; Kalimo et al., 1981; Pulsinelli et al., 1982). The most convincing explanation for this is that this allows the neuron to enter the crisis with more glycogen stores and thus carry on more anerobic metabolism during that time. A major consequence of this is elevated lactate production, leading to damaging acidosis. As evidence for this scenario, exposure of normoxic neurons to the concentrations of lactate or hydrogen ions generated during such hypoxia – ischemia is damaging (Kraig et al., 1987). In this view then, hypoxia – ischemia is damaging not so much for its disruption of energy production, but for the kind of energy produced during the crisis. This is turning out to be somewhat of a simplification, however, and there is also a route of damage during hypoxia – ischemia which is energy-dependent; this has most readily been demonstrated with in vitro systems of primary dispersed neurons or hippocampal slices, and where the insult is anoxia, rather than hypoxia. With these experimental paradigms, under circumstances where the acidosis is, itself, not sufficient to be damaging, glucose can protect against both neuron death and dysfunction (Schurr et al., 1987; Tombaugh and Sapolsky, 1988).

Thus, all of these insults seem to damage, in at least in part, because of their disruptive effects upon neuronal energetics. It is clear that such disruptions exacerbate the damaging effects of the glutamate/NMDA/calcium cascade just outlined. There are numerous mechanisms potentially underlying this. To begin with, glutamate release will be enhanced and uptake blocked. The latter can fail in at least two ways. Pre-synaptic reuptake is mediated by a glutamate/sodium cotransporter, which is driven by a steep extracellular/intracellular sodium gradient. With energy failure, Na-K-ATPase fails, the gradient is lost, and reuptake fails; for example, this occurs after hypoxia–ischemia (Drejer et al., 1985). As evidence of the importance of this component, EAA toxicity is enhanced when neuronal reuptake is blocked (either by poisoning the pump, or destruction of pre-synaptic neurons (Kohler and Schwarcz, 1981; Choi, 1987b)). In addition, glial uptake is also dependent on energy (as manifested by maintaining gradients of both sodium and potassium in order to transport glutamate (Barbour et al., 1988)). Thus, various NMDA-mediated insults to neuronal cultures are more toxic in the absence of glia (Vibulsreth et al., 1987). *Enhanced release* occurs in at least two ways. With energy scarcity neurons depolarize, increasing calcium-dependent release of EAAs. Second, the sodium/glutamate cotransporter used for neuronal reuptake is bidirectional; with failing energy and increased intracellular sodium concentrations, the transport reverses, causing calcium-independent EAA leakage (Drejer et al., 1985; Dagani and Erecsinka, 1987). Evidence suggests that the calcium-independent component is the major route by which energy failure leads to excessive release of glutamate. Thus, a paucity of energy will enhance glutamatergic tone in a variety of ways. The implications of this are shown most explicitly with the recent demonstration in cerebellar cultures that glutamate toxicity via the NMDA receptor is energy-dependent (Novelli et al., 1988).

Energy failure is likely to lead to more post-synaptic calcium mobilization, simply because of more EAA interaction with the NMDA receptor. There are many reasons to believe that the calcium signal will be further enhanced because of energetic constraints in the post-synaptic neuron itself: (1) The calcium channel gated to the NMDA receptor is blocked by magnesium in a voltage-dependent manner. With depolarization in states of energy depletion, the blockade is released, allowing enhanced calcium influx. (2) With loss of the membrane potential, intracellular sodium concentrations rise, releasing calcium from intracellular storage sites, via a sodium/calcium exchanger. (3) Sequestering of calcium into mitochondria or SER will be compromised, as the process is energy-dependent (relying either on ATP directly, or on a steep sodium gradient). (4) The efficiency of efflux should also be compromised, as it is similarly energy-dependent. Moreover, one route of efflux is through a sodium/calcium exchanger; as intracellular sodium concentrations rise, not only should calcium efflux be blocked, but the exchanger can reverse, providing an additional route of calcium influx (reviewed in McBurney and Neering, 1987; Blaustein, 1988; Choi, 1988).

Glucocorticoids and the glutamatergic synapse

This preceding section has outlined, at some length, the considerable evidence that hypoxia–ischemia, seizure and hypoglycemia damage the hippocampus via the interacting components of energy depletion and the glutamate/NMDA/calcium cascade. We are beginning to obtain evidence that GCs exacerbate these three insults by exacerbating this cascade.

The first potential route by which this might occur is rather specific to glutamate trafficking in the synapse. A large percentage of neurotransmitter glutamate cycles through a shuttle involving astrocytes. Synaptic glutamate, after dissociating from the post-synaptic receptor, can be taken up by glia and converted to glutamine (by the enzyme glutamine synthetase), which is then shuttled back to the pre-synaptic neuron for conversion to glutamate. This shuttle has been viewed as a protective mechanism to remove highly excitatory glutamate from the synapse and return it to the neuron as "deactivated" glutamine (Hertz et al., 1983). The potential for the glutamine to be converted back to glutamate is shown with the recent demonstration that glutamine increases anoxic damage to cortical cultures, and this augmentation is NMDA receptor-dependent (Monyer et al., 1988). It has been estimated that as much as 80% of neurotransmitter glutamate cycles this way (Hertz et al., 1983). This suggests that the total availability of glutamine to neurons via this cycle is an important determinant of the amount of glutamate that the neurons can release. This is supported by several recent studies. In one, glutamate release from striatal slices increased when the glucose concentrations in the media were dropped. This fits nicely with the previous discussion about EAA release being exacerbated by energy failure. Importantly, this hypersecretion could only be sustained when the neurons were supplied with glutamine (Szerb, 1988). In another study, when glutamine cycling was blocked with the glutamine synthetase inhibitor methionine sulfoximine, glutamate release declined (Rothstein and Tabakoff, 1985).

Thus, given that EAA release will be exacerbated by energy failure and neurological insults, the extent of hypersecretion can be sensitive to the extent that glutamine can be generated and supplied to the neurons. In that context, it is of importance to note that GCs stimulate the synthesis of glutamine synthetase, the rate-limiting state in glutamine production. This is a well-characterized genomic effect in the developing brain, and in both developing and adult muscle (Martinez-Hernandez et al., 1977; Pishak and Phillips, 1980; Holbrook et al., 1981; Juurlink et al., 1981; Kumar et al., 1984; Smith et al., 1984; Patel and Hunt, 1985; Max et al., 1987); less attention has been focused on whether this also occurs in the adult brain. However, it has recently been shown that GCs increase amounts of mRNA for activity of glutamine synthetase in the adult hippocampus (Nichols et al., 1989; Tombaugh and Sapolsky, in preparation). This suggested that GCs could potentially endanger the hippocampus by indirectly fueling the generation of more glutamate. However, we are not sanguine about the importance of this regulatory link in the adult hippocampus. In the two studies just cited, animals were exposed to GC concentrations in the upper (stressed) physiological range constantly for days. Under such conditions, hippocampal glutamine synthetase activity was increased by approximately 25%, a not particularly robust amount. We then examined whether more physiological circumstances of GC hypersecretion could increase the enzyme's activity. We observed that one day of status epilepticus seizures (which provokes approximately 12 h of GC hypersecretion; Stein and Sapolsky, 1988), and three days of intermittent and shifting stressors both failed to significantly elevate glutamine synthetase activity (while being sufficient to cause moderate rises in muscle activity of the enzyme). Thus, our present sense is that while this could theoretically be a route for GC's exacerbating the glutamate/NMDA/calcium cascade, it can only apply to stressors more severe or prolonged than these rather major ones.

The most plausible route by which GCs endanger the hippocampus is by disrupting energy storage. Previous work implied this (Sapolsky, 1986b). In it, I reasoned that the common thread among the insults worsened by GCs was a problem of energy — either pathologic disruption of energy production (hypoxia – ischemia, antimetabolites), or pathologically-elevated demands for energy (excitotoxic seizures). I reasoned that the broad vulnerability induced by GCs might be an energetic one; supporting this, I found that supplementing neurons with energy substrates such as glucose, mannose or ketone bodies reduce the endangering effects of GCs (Sapolsky, 1986b). We subsequently found that this also worked in vitro (Sapolsky et al., 1988). What remained was to demonstrate how GCs disrupt hippocampal energetics. The hormones appear to inhibit glucose transport; this is not a particularly radical observation, given that GCs have long been known to inhibit glucose transport in peripheral tissues (Munck, 1971), and the molecular biology of the effect is well-characterized (Horner et al., 1987). The first evidence that this was occurring in the brain was the finding that GCs inhibit local cerebral glucose utilization in many brain regions, with the hippocampus being among the most sensitive (Bryan and King, 1988; Kadekaro et al., 1988). A number of mechanisms could account for this, and it could be occurring at a number of possible cell types. Clarifying these issues, we have found that nanomolar concentrations of corticosterone (the rat GC) inhibit approximately 20 – 35% of glucose transport in both cultured hippocampal neurons and glia (Horner and Sapolsky, 1988). This inhibition is time- and protein synthesis-dependent. It is not triggered by non-GC steroids, but is triggered by other GCs, such as cortisol and dexamethasone. The inhibition is mediated by the type II GC receptor; as evidence, the type II ligand dexamethasone inhibits glucose transport, 50% inhibition occurs around the Kd of the receptor, and the inhibition is blocked with a type II receptor antagonist. Finally, the effect does not occur in cultures from other brain regions. The steroid and receptor specificity, and protein synthesis dependence agree with what is known about GC inhibition of glucose transport in peripheral tissues (Munck, 1971).

Neurons are notorious for their metabolic vulnerability — they consume enormous amounts of energy, it must come almost exclusively in the form of glucose, and it is not stored as glycogen in particularly large amounts (Siesjö, 1981). Nevertheless, it seems unlikely that a 20 – 35% inhibition of glucose transport is sufficient to, in effect, get the hippocampus into trouble under resting conditions. However, a similar inhibition during a period of major energetic crisis for the neuron — i.e., one of the neurological insults discussed — could well exacerbate the insult. Critically, the consequences of the small inhibition of glucose transport need not be dramatic; it must merely be multifaceted. At the pre-synaptic end of the picture, a bit more EAAs may be released and a bit less taken up again. Neighboring glia may be somewhat impaired in their ability to take up EAAs, to act as a proton sink, or to detoxify ammonia. Finally, at the post-synaptic end, there might be a small bias towards more calcium entering the free cytosolic compartment, less being cleared from it and less export of protons. Collectively, these steps may bias a neuron in energetic trouble towards death, rather than survival. If so, this would be a metabolic explanation for the capacity of GCs to synergize with these insults under conditions where the GCs are, themselves, not damaging. Only a few of these steps have been tested yet, but they support this scenario. In one

study, GCs appeared to inhibit glutamate reuptake in the hippocampus (Halpain and McEwen, 1988). In addition, GCs increase calcium-dependent afterhyperpolarizations in hippocampal pyramidal neurons, accounting for the phenomenon in the aged hippocampus (Kerr and Landfield, 1988). Neither of these studies examined whether the GC effects arise from their effects on glucose transport or from any of their many other actions. Clearly, a great deal of work needs to be done to test the ideas just outlined.

The most specific prediction from these ideas is that if GCs endanger hippocampal neurons by exacerbating the glutamate/EAA/calcium cascade, GC endangerment of the hippocampus should be reversed by blocking the NMDA receptor. We have recently observed just that (Armanini et al., 1989). In order to test this, we had to find an insult which was exacerbated by GCs, but was not, itself, working via the NMDA receptor; we would then see if receptor blockade would subtract out the GC component of the synergy. We tested 3AP, the electron transport uncoupler. At a high concentration, the hippocampal damage that it induced was indeed NMDA receptor-dependent and was reversed by APV. We interpreted this as showing that the profound energy failure caused by the high 3AP concentrations triggered the glutamate/EAA/ calcium cascade. At lower concentrations of 3AP, however, lesser but still consistent hippocampal damage occurred, which was insensitive to APV. This implies an additional mechanism by which 3AP damages, which is the predominant route at these lower concentrations. Working with this lesser 3AP insult, we replicated our prior observation that GCs synergized with the toxin. Specifically, the volume of hippocampal damage in animals exposed to high physiological GC concentrations for a week before and after the insult was about 75% greater than in rats adrenalectomized and GC-free during that period. We then found that microinfusion of APV completely eliminated the GC exacerbation of damage; again, this was without changing the toxicity of 3AP in the adrenalectomized rats. Although preliminary, this represents strong support for the model of GCs exacerbating the glutamate/ NMDA/calcium cascade. We are currently pursuing the mechanisms underlying this exacerbation, along the lines outlined above.

Conclusions

These studies suggest that GCs, at least in part through their disruptive effects on glucose transport, leave hippocampal neurons in a state of metabolic vulnerability. In the absence of a co-incident metabolic challenge, this vulnerability is survived readily. However, when co-incident insults occur, neuronal viability is compromised, at least in part via exacerbation of the EAA cascade of damage. These observations are of some potential relevance, in that they suggest that exogenous GCs, in the aftermath of some insults, can potentially exacerbate hippocampal damage, and should be avoided if possible. Moreover, they suggest that strategies to decrease endogenous GC secretion after such insults, or over the course of the lifespan, can protect the hippocampus from damage. It has recently been shown that inhibiting the GC stress response in the aftermath of status epilepticus seizures, by administering the adrenal steroidogenesis inhibitor metyrapone, diminishes hippocampal damage (Stein and Sapolsky, 1988). In an approach meant to decrease the total lifetime exposure to GCs, we demonstrated that a neonatal behavioral intervention which reduces adult basal GC concentrations in the rat prevents some the neuron loss and spatial learning deficits that characterize aging in the rat (Meaney et al., 1988). In considering whether these interventions may be of any clinical relevance, the question remains whether any of the findings described here apply to the human hippocampus. This remains an open question at this point, and should be a focus of research in coming years.

Acknowledgements

The studies were made possible by the technical support of Mark Armanini, Heidi Horner, Chris Hutchins, Elicia Morrow, Desta Packan, Becky Stein, Geoffrey Tombaugh and Charles Virgin.

Financial support was provided by NIH RO1 AG06633, The Klingenstein Fund, the Alzheimer's Disease and Related Disorders Association, a Presidential Young Investigator's Award, and a MacArthur Fellowship.

References

Armanini, M., Hutchins, C., Stein, B. and Sapolsky, R. (1989) Corticosterone endangers hippocampal neurons via the NMDA-receptor. *Soc. Neurosci. Abstr.,* in press.

Auer, R. and Siesjö, B. (1988) Biological differences between ischemia, hypoglycemia, and epilepsy. *Ann. Neurol.,* 24: 699 – 714.

Aus der Muhlen, K. and Ockenfels, H. (1979) Morphologische Veranderungen in Diencephalon und Telencephalon nach Störungen des regelkreises Adrenohypophyse-Nebennierenrinde. III. Ergebnisse beim Meerschweinchen nach Verabrechung von Cortison und Hydrocortison. *Z. Zellforsch.,* 93: 126 – 135.

Barbour, B., Brew, H. and Attwell, D. (1988) Electrogenic glutamate uptake in glial cells is activated by intracellular potassium. *Nature,* 335: 433 – 435.

Bateman, A., Singh, A., Kral, T. and Solomon, S. (1989) The immune-hypothalamic-pituitary-adrenal axis. *Endocr. Rev.,* 10: 92 – 106.

Blaustein, M. (1988) Calcium transport and buffering in neurons. *Trends Neurosci.,* 11: 438 – 442.

Bryan, R. and King, J. (1988) Glucocorticoids modulate the effect of plasma epinephrine on regional cerebral glucose utilization (rCMRgl). *Soc. Neurosci. Abstr.,* 399.11.

Cheung, J., Bonventre, J., Malis, C. and Leaf, A. (1986) Calcium and ischemic injury. *New Engl. J. Med.,* 26: 1670 – 1676.

Choi, D. (1987a) Glutamate neurotoxicity in cortical cell culture. *J. Neurosci.,* 7: 357 – 368.

Choi, D. (1987b) Ionic dependence of glutamate neurotoxicity. *J. Neurosci.,* 7: 369 – 375.

Choi, D. (1988) Calcium-mediated neurotoxicity: relationship to specific channel types and role in ischemic damage. *Trends Neurosci.,* 11: 465 – 472.

Cohen, J. and Duke, J. (1984) Glucocorticoid activation of a calcium dependent endonuclease in thymocyte nuclei leads to cell death. *J. Immunol.,* 132: 38 – 44.

Compton, M. and Cidlowski, J. (1986) Rapid in vivo effects of glucocorticoids on the integrity of rat lymphocyte genomic DNA. *Endocrinology,* 118: 38 – 42.

Compton, M. and Cidlowski, J. (1987) Identification of a glucocorticoid-induced nuclease in thymocytes: a potential "lysis gene" product. *J. Biol. Chem.,* 262: 8288 – 8293.

22

Compton, M., Haskill, J. and Cidlowski, J. (1988) Analysis of glucocorticoid actions on rat thymocyte deoxyribonucleic acid by fluorescence-activated flow cytometry. *Endocrinology,* 122: 2158 – 2263.

Dagani, F. and Erecsinka, M. (1987) Relationship among ATP synthesis, potassium gradients, and neurotransmitter amino acid levels in isolated rat brain synaptosomes. *J. Neurochem.,* 49: 1229 – 1235.

Drejer, J., Benveniste, H., Diemer, N. and Schousboe, A. (1985) Cellular origin of ischemia-induced glutamate release from brain tissue in vivo and in vitro. *J. Neurochem.,* 34: 145 – 153.

Ginsberg, M., Welsh, F. and Budd, W. (1980) Deleterious effect of glucose pretreatment on recovery from diffuse cerebral ischemia in the cat. I. Local cerebral blood flow and glucose utilization. *Stroke,* 11: 347 – 355.

Halpain, S. and McEwen (1988) *Neuroendo,* in press.

Hertz, L., Kvamme, E., McGreer, E. and Schousboe, A. (1983) *Glutamate and GABA in the Central Nervous System,* A.R. Liss, New York, NY.

Holbrook, N., Grasso, R. and Hackney, J. (1981) Glucocorticoid receptor properties and glucocorticoid regulation of glutamine synthetase activity in sensitive C6 and resistant C6H glial cells. *J. Neursci. Res.,* 6: 75 – 81.

Horner, H. and Sapolsky, R. (1988) Glucocorticoids decrease glucose transport in cultured hippocampal neurons. *Soc. Neurosci. Abstr.,* 372.11.

Horner, H., Munck, A. and Lienhard, G. (1987) Dexamethasone causes translocation of glucose transporters from the plasma membrane to an intracellular site in human fibroblasts. *J. Biol. Chem.,* 262: 17696 – 17700.

Johansen, F. and Diemer, N. (1986) Influences of the plasma glucose level on brain damage after systemic kainic acid injection in the rat. *Acta Neuropathol.,* 71: 46 – 54.

Juurlink, B., Schousboe, A., Jørgensen, O. and Hertz, L. (1981) Induction by hydrocortisone of glutamine synthetase in mouse primary astrocyte cultures. *J. Neurochem.,* 36: 136 – 142.

Kadekaro, M., Ito, M. and Gross, P. (1988) Local cerebral glucose utilization is increased in acutely adrenalectomized rats. *Neuroendocrinology,* 47: 329 – 336.

Kalimo, H., Rehncrona, S., Söderfeldt, B., Olsson, Y. and Siesjö, B. (1981) Brain lactic acidosis and ischemic cell damage. II. Histopathology. *J. Cereb. Blood Flow Metab.,* 1: 313 – 319.

Keller-Wood, M. and Dallman, M. (1984) Corticosteroid inhibition of ACTH secretion. *Endocr. Rev.,* 5: 1 – 24.

Kerr, D. and Landfield, P. (1988) A corticosteroid-sensitive component of the hippocampal calcium-dependent afterhyperpolarization increases with aging. *Soc. Neurosci. Abstr.,* 509.17.

Kerr, D., Applegate, M., Campbell, L., Goliszek, A., Brodish, A. and Landfield, P. (1986) Chronic stress-induced acceleration of age-related hippocampal neurophysiological changes.

Soc. Neurosci. Abstr., 12: 274.

Kohler, C. and Schwarcz, R. (1981) Monosodium glutamate: increased neurotoxicity after removal of neuronal re-uptake sites. *Brain Res.,* 211: 485 – 491.

Koide, T., Wieloch, T. and Siesjö, B. (1986) Chronic dexamethasone pretreatment aggravates ischemic neuronal necrosis. *J. Cereb. Blood Flow Metab.,* 6: 395 – 406.

Kraig, R., Petito, C., Plum, F. and Pulsinelli, W. (1987) Hydrogen ions kill brain at concentrations reached in ischemia. *J. Cereb. Blood Flow Metab.,* 7: 379 – 386.

Kreiger, D. (1982) Cushing's syndrome. In: *Monographs in Endocrinology,* Springer-Verlag, Berlin.

Kumar, S., Weingarten, D., Callagan, J., Schar, K. and De Vellis J. (1984) Regulation of mRNA's for three enzymes in the glial cell model C6 cell line. *J. Neurochem.,* 43: 1455 – 1460.

Landfield, P., Waymire, J. and Lynch, G. (1978) Hippocampal aging and adrenocorticoids: a quantitative correlation. *Science,* 202: 1098 – 1101.

Landfield, P., Baskin, R. and Pitler, T. (1981) Brain-aging correlates: retardation by hormonal – pharmacological treatments. *Science,* 214: 581 – 585.

MacDermott, A. and Dale, N. (1987) Receptors, ion channels and synaptic potentials underlying the integrative actions of excitatory amino acids. *Trends Neurosci.,* 10: 280 – 283.

Martinez-Hernandez, A., Bell, K. and Norenberg, M. (1977) Glutamine synthetase: glial localization in brain. *Science,* 195: 1356 – 1360.

Masters, J., Finch, C. and Sapolsky, R. (1989) Glucocorticoid endangerment of hippocampal neurons does not involve DNA cleavage. *Endocrinology,* in press.

Max, S., Thomas, J., Banner, C., Vitkovic, L., Konagaya, M. and Konagaya, Y. (1987) Glucocorticoid-receptor mediated induction of glutamine synthetase in skeletal muscle cells in vitro. *Endocrinology,* 120: 1179 – 1184.

McBurney, R. and Neering, I. (1987) Neuronal calcium homeostasis. *Trends Neurosci.,* 10: 164 – 168.

McEwen, B., De Kloet, E. and Rostene, W. (1986) Adrenal steroid receptors and actions in the nervous system. *Physiol. Rev.,* 66: 1121 – 1167.

Meaney, M., Aitken, D., Bhatnager, S., Van Berkel, C. and Sapolsky, R. (1988) Effect of neonatal handling on age-related impairments associated with the hippocampus. *Science,* 239: 766 – 769.

Meldrum, B. (1983) Metabolic factors during prolonged seizures and their relation to nerve cell death. In: A. Delgado-Escueta, C. Wasterlain, D. Treiman and R. Porter (Eds.), *Advances in Neurology, Vol 34,* Raven Press, New York, NY, pp. 261 – 275.

Meyer, J. (1985) Biochemical effects of corticosteroids on neural tissues. *Physiol. Rev.,* 65: 946 – 1020.

Monyer, H., Goldberg, M. and Choi, D. (1988) Glucose-deprivation cortical neuronal injury is strongly influenced by the availability of extracellular amino acids. *Soc. Neurosci.*

Abstr., 299.2.

Munck, A. (1971) Glucocorticoid inhibition of glucose uptake by peripheral tissues: old and new evidence, molecular mechanisms, and physiological significance. *Perspect. Biol. Med.*, 14: 265 – 281.

Munck, A., Guyre, P. and Holbrook, N. (1984) Physiological functions of glucocorticoids during stress and their relation to pharmacological actions. *Endocr. Rev.*, 5: 25 – 46.

Myers, R. and Yamaguchi, S. (1977) Nervous system effects of cardiac arrest in monkeys: preservation of vision. *Arch. Neurol.*, 34: 65 – 72.

Nichols, N., Masters, J., May, P., De Vellis, J. and Finch, C. (1989) Corticosterone-induced responses in rat brain mRNAs are also evoked in the hippocampus by acute vibratory stress. *Neuroendocrinology*, 49: 40 – 47.

Novelli, A., Reilly, J., Lysko, P. and Henneberry, R. (1988) Glutamate becomes neurotoxic via the NMDA receptor when intracellular energy levels are reduced. *Brain Res.*, 451: 205 – 210.

Patel, A. and Hunt, A. (1985) Observations on cell growth and regulation of glutamine synthetase by dexamethasone in primary cultures of forebrain and cerebellar astrocytes. *Dev. Brain Res.*, 18: 175 – 183.

Pishak, M. and Phillips, A. (1980) Glucocorticoid stimulation on glutamine synthetase production in cultured rat glioma cells. *J. Neurochem.*, 34: 866 – 872.

Pulsinelli, W., Waldman, S., Rawlinson, D. and Plum, F. (1982) Moderate hyperglycemia augments ischemic brain damage: a neuropathologic study in the rat. *Neurology*, 32: 1239 – 1246.

Reul, J. and De Kloet, E. (1985) Two receptor systems for corticosterone in rat brain: microdistribution and differential occupation. *Endocrinology*, 117: 2505 – 2511.

Rothman, S. and Olney, J. (1987) Excitotoxicity and the NMDA receptor. *Trends Neurosci.*, 10: 299 – 303.

Rothstein, J. and Tabakoff, B. (1985) Alteration of striatal glutamate release after glutamine synthetase inhibition. *J. Neurochem.*, 43: 1438 – 1444.

Sapolsky, R. (1985a) A mechanism for glucocorticoid toxicity in the hippocampus: increased neuronal vulnerability of metabolic insults. *J. Neurosci.*, 5: 1228 – 1332.

Sapolsky, R. (1985b) Glucocorticoid toxicity in the hippocampus: temporal aspects of neuronal vulnerability. *Brain Res.*, 359: 300 – 305.

Sapolsky, R. (1986a) Glucocorticoid toxicity in the hippocampus: synergy with kainic acid. *Neuroendocrinology*, 43: 386 – 392.

Sapolsky, R. (1986b) Glucocorticoid toxicity in the hippocampus: reversal by supplementation with brain fuels. *J. Neurosci.*, 6: 2240 – 2246.

Sapolsky, R. and Pulsinelli, W. (1985) Glucocorticoids potentiate ischemic injury to neurons: therapeutic implications. *Science*, 229: 1397 – 1399.

Sapolsky, R. and Stein, B. (1989) Status epilepticus-induced hippocampal damage is modulated by glucose availability. *Neurosci. Lett.*, 97: 157 – 163.

Sapolsky, R., Krey, L. and McEwen, B. (1985) Prolonged glucocorticoid exposure reduces hippocampal neuron number: implications for aging; *J. Neurosci.*, 5: 1221 – 1226.

Sapolsky, R., Armanini, M., Packan, D. and Tombaugh, G. (1987) Stress and glucocorticoids in aging. *Endocr. Metab. Clinics*, 16: 965 – 981.

Sapolsky, R., Packan, D. and Vale, W. (1988) Glucocorticoid toxicity in the hippocampus: in vitro demonstration. *Brain Res.*, 453: 367 – 372.

Schurr, A., West, C., Reid, K., Tseng, M., Reiss, S. and Rigor, B. (1987) Increased glucose improves recovery of neuronal function after cerebral hypoxia in vitro. *Brain Res.*, 421: 135 – 139.

Siemkowicz, E. and Hansen, A. (1978) Clinical restitution following cerebral ischemia hypo-, normo-, and hyperglycemic rats. *Acta Neurol. Scand.*, 58: 1 – 11.

Siesjö, B. (1981) Cell damage in the brain: a speculative synthesis. *J. Cereb. Blood Flow Metab.*, 1: 155 – 173.

Smith, R., Larson, S., Stred, S. and Durschlag, R. (1984) Regulation of glutamine synthetase and glutaminase activities in cultured skeletal muscle cells. *J. Cell Physiol.*, 120: 197 – 202.

Stein, B. and Sapolsky, R. (1988) Chemical adrenalectomy reduces hippocampal damage induced by kainic acid. *Brain Res.*, 473: 175 – 181.

Szerb, J. (1988) Changes in the relative amounts of asparate and glutamate released and retained in hippocampal slices during stimulation. *J. Neurochem.*, 50: 219 – 225.

Tang, G. and Phillips, R. (1978) Some age-related changes in pituitary-adrenal function in the male laboratory rat. *J. Gerontol.*, 33: 377 – 385.

Theoret, Y., Caldwell-Kenkel, J. and Krigman, M. (1985) The role of neuronal metabolic insult in organometal neurotoxicity. *Toxicologist*, 6: 491 (abstract).

Tombaugh, G. and Sapolsky, R. (1988) Anoxic hippocampal damage in primary cultures: protective effects of glucose are pH-dependent. *Soc. Neurosci. Abstr.*, 327.8.

Ucker, D. (1987) Cytotoxic T lymphocytes and glucocorticoids activate an endogenous suicide process in target cells. *Nature*, 327: 62 – 64.

Umansky, S., Korol, B. and Nelipovich, P. (1981) In vivo DNA degradation in thymocytes of gamma-irradiated or hydrocortisone-treated rats. *Biochim. Biophys. Acta*, 655: 9 – 16.

Vibulsreth, S., Hefti, F., Ginsberg, M., Dietrich, W. and Busto, R. (1987) Astrocytes protect cultured neurons from degeneration induced by anoxia. *Brain Res.*, 422: 303 – 308.

Wielckens, K. and Delfs, T. (1986) Glucocorticoid-induced cell death and poly[adenosine diphosphate (ADP)-ribosyl]ation: increased toxicity of dexamethasone on mouse S49.1 lymphoma cells with the poly (ADP-ribosyl)ation inhibitor benzamide. *Endocrinology*, 119: 2383 – 2388.

Wyllie, A. (1980) Glucocorticoid-induced thymocyte apoptosis is associated with endonuclease activation. *Nature*, 284: 555 – 558.

P. Coleman, G. Higgins and C. Phelps (Eds.)
Progress in Brain Research, Vol. 86
© 1990 Elsevier Science Publishers B.V. (Biomedical Division)

CHAPTER 3

Hormones and programmed cell death: insights from invertebrate studies

James W. Truman[1], Susan E. Fahrbach[2], and Ken-ichi Kimura[1]

Department of Zoology NJ-15, University of Washington, Seattle, WA 98195, U.S.A., and [2]Department of Entomology, University of Illinois, Urbana, IL 61801, U.S.A.

Introduction

Cell death occurs in the nervous system both during normal development and as a result of certain pathologies. At this time, though, it is unclear whether the neuronal death that accompanies certain diseases involves normal cell death mechanisms but expressed at inappropriate times or in the wrong neuronal populations, or whether the two types of death are completely unrelated. Our knowledge of the mechanisms that mediate naturally occurring cell death is too incomplete to resolve this issue at present. We have only fragmentary information on factors that predispose CNS neurons to die, the signals that actually trigger the death, and the molecular steps involved in the degeneration response.

This paper deals with the use of invertebrates to study cellular and molecular aspects of neuronal death. The identified neurons in these animals, which are well known for their stereotyped morphologies and patterns of connectivity, may likewise have stereotyped, predictable fates (e.g., Horvitz et al., 1982; Truman, 1983). Thus, one can examine not only the changes that occur after degeneration begins, but also the events that precede death. Much of this work has been done on insects, in which neuronal death plays a prominent role both during embryogenesis (Loer et al., 1983) and at metamorphosis. The neurons that die

during the latter period include both immature cells (Booker and Truman, 1987) and mature, functioning neurons which are used during larval life but then discarded (Truman, 1983; Weeks and Truman, 1985). The occurrence of cell death as part of metamorphosis means that these events have come under the control of the hormones that regulate metamorphosis. Besides being able to manipulate the timing of cell death by endocrine manipulations, hormones have also provided useful tools for probing cellular interactions in the degeneration response (Truman and Schwartz, 1984; Weeks, 1987). Large moths such as the giant silkmoth and the tobacco hornworm, *Manduca sexta*, have been used to gain insights into the physiology involved in degeneration. Recent extension of these studies to *Drosophila* will hopefully provide an avenue to discovering the underlying genetic and molecular mechanisms.

Patterns of neuronal and muscular degeneration during insect metamorphosis

Cell death plays a major role in transforming the neuromuscular system of the larva into that of the adult. In larval *Manduca*, for example, a typical abdominal segment has 50 paired muscle groups that are innervated by about 34 pairs of motoneurons (Taylor and Truman, 1974). After metamorphosis, the corresponding segment in the mature adult contains only 9 muscle groups supplied by about 10 pairs of motoneurons. The fates of motoneurons are closely matched to those of their muscles, but, as seen in Fig. 1, a number of fates are possible.

The internal muscles (the intersegmental muscles; ISMs) are large, segment-spanning muscles that are the major phasic muscles in the larval abdomen. Most ISMs persist through the larval–pupal transition, are used during adult development, and then rapidly die after adult emergence. The ISM motoneurons persist with little modification from the larval stage through metamorphosis but also abruptly degenerate during the first 2 days of adult life.

The larval external muscle groups are primarily postural muscles and their fates through metamorphosis are varied. They degenerate in two waves during the larval–pupal transition: some just prior to pupal ecdysis, while others die within the 2 days following adult ecdysis (Weeks and Truman, 1985). In some cases the muscles degenerate completely, but in others, a remnant of the muscle remains to provide a scaffold for the growth and differentiation of adult muscles (Nuesch, 1985). Most of these rebuilt muscles persist through adult life although a few, such as DE5, are used at adult ec-

dysis and then degenerate (Taylor and Truman, 1974). Motoneurons that supply muscles that degenerate completely during the larval–pupal transition also degenerate. They die 1–2 days after pupal ecdysis irrespective of the time of death of their target. Neurons that are associated with remodeled muscles are themselves remodeled, in terms both of central dendrites (Levine and Truman, 1985) and peripheral axon arbors (Nuesch, 1985). Most remodeled neurons persist through adult life but a few, such as MN-12 which supplies a short-lived adult muscle (DE5), degenerate following adult emergence.

The degeneration of motoneurons after adult emergence follows a stereotyped time course which has been best described for the D-IV motoneurons (Stocker et al., 1978). The first ultrastructural sign of degeneration in these cells is a disruption of the endoplasmic reticulum (ER) and the release of ribosomes from the rough ER and from polysome clusters. By about 20 h later, the nuclear membrane ruptures and membranous and granular organelles begin to segregate in different parts of the cell body. Shortly thereafter, fragments of degenerating neurons can be seen in vacuoles in the surrounding glial cells. The cell body is eventually reduced to a tightly wrapped collection of mem-

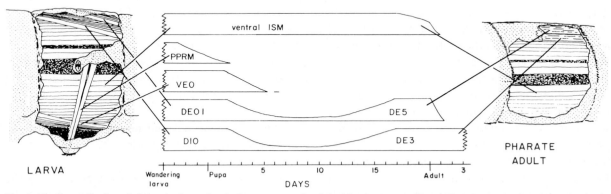

Fig. 1. The fates of selected abdominal muscles during metamorphosis in *Manduca sexta*, illustrating the types of changes that occur in the musculature. Diagrams are lateral views of segment A4 of a larva and a pre-emergence adult showing muscle positions. The central part of the figure shows relative changes in muscle size through this transition. The principal proleg retractor muscle (PPRM) and the ventral external oblique (VEO) die during the larval–pupal transition. The ventral intersegmental muscles (ISM) persist unchanged through most of metamorphosis to then die after adult emergence. The dorsal external oblique 1 (DEO1) and the dorsal internal oblique (DIO) regress early in metamorphosis but then regrow to become the adult dorsal external 5 (DE5) and DE3 respectively. DE5 dies after emergence of the adult.

branes that is apparently engulfed by glia.

All of the doomed motoneurons progress through a similar sequence of changes as they degenerate, but the time that they initiate this program differs from cell to cell. As seen in Fig. 2, the first motoneuron to die (MN-11) begins degeneration about 8 h post-ecdysis. The D-IV motoneurons start degeneration at 14 h, MN-2 at about 30 h, and the last cells to die, MN-12, at about 40 h. Thus, *Manduca* shows a reproducible, stereotyped sequence of cell death which is referenced to a discrete behavioral marker, the ecdysis of the adult.

Hormonal regulation of degeneration

Three hormones are involved in triggering neuronal or muscle death in holometabolous in-sects. These include a class of steroid hormones, the ecdysteroids, the sesquiterpenoid hormones, the juvenile hormones, and the neuropeptide, eclo-sion hormone. The ecdysteroids are responsible for driving the molting process during which a new exoskeleton is produced and the old one then shed (a process termed ecdysis). The ecdysteroid titers are typically high at the beginning of a molt but then decline as the molt nears completion (e.g., Bollen-bacher et al., 1981). Juvenile hormone (JH) acts in concert with the ecdysteroids to regulate the nature of the molt. When a molt occurs in the presence of JH, the insect makes the same type of exoskeleton it had before, e.g., a larva molts into another lar-val stage. In the absence of JH, a metamorphic molt ensues, such as a larva becoming a pupa or the pupa transforming into the adult. Ecdysis, which occurs at the end of each molt, is then trig-

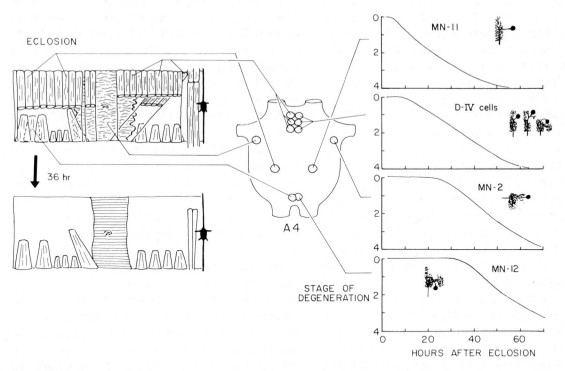

Fig. 2. Degeneration of selected muscles and their motoneurons after eclosion (emergence) of the adult moth. Middle: ganglion A4 showing the positions of the cell bodies of selected motoneurons. Left: drawing of an A4 hemisegment showing the position of the muscles innervated by the respective motoneurons. The muscles are dead within 36 h of eclosion. Right: time course of degeneration of 4 sets of motoneurons; stages progress from a normal cell (0), through the rupture of the nucleus (2), to the last remnants of the cell (4). Insets represent the dendritic morphology of the neurons.

gered by eclosion hormone (EH). This peptide acts on the CNS to evoke the motor patterns used during the shedding of the old cuticle (Reynolds and Truman, 1983). Although we will be concerned here with the regulation of post-metamorphic degeneration, considerable information is also available concerning the hormonal regulation of cell death during the larval – pupal transition (Runion and Pipa, 1973; Weeks and Truman, 1985; Weeks, 1987).

Muscle death

The abdominal ISMs of silkmoths such as *Antheraea polyphemus* and of *Manduca*, undergo a slow atrophy that begins about 3 days before emergence of the adult (Lockshin and Beaulaton, 1974), and then lysis after emergence (Finlayson, 1956). The atrophy is characterized by a gradual thinning of the muscle fibers and results from the waning ecdysteroid titers at the end of metamorphosis (Schwartz and Truman, 1983, 1984). Augmentation of ecdysteroid levels by either injection or infusion during the course of atrophy retards or arrests this process.

The rapid degeneration, by contrast, is an all-or-none event which is triggered in various ways depending on the species considered. In *Antheraea*, EH triggers muscle degeneration (Schwarz and Truman, 1982, 1984). When the abdominal muscles were denied exposure to EH by securing a blood-tight ligature between the thorax and abdomen, the rapid degeneration was blocked although the slow atrophy continued. Injection of EH into such isolated abdomens then caused the rapid dissolution of the muscles. In contrast to *Antheraea*, abdomen isolation in *Manduca* did not block rapid degeneration. Depending on the time of isolation, the degeneration process was either not affected in its time course or accelerated (Schwartz and Truman, 1983), implying that EH is not necessary. Degeneration was blocked or delayed by the infusion or injection of ecdysteroids. Thus, in *Manduca*, the withdrawal of ecdysteroids is sufficient to trigger the rapid

degeneration as well as the slow atrophy.

The regulation of muscle death in *Drosophila* resembles that seen in *Antheraea* (Kimura and Truman, 1990). In this fly abdomen isolation prevented the normal death of the intersegmental muscles but only if performed prior to 1 h before ecdysis. After this time the muscles degenerated despite the ligature. We believe that the timing of this switch-over coincides with the normal time of EH release.

Neuronal degeneration

Patterns of neuronal death vary widely amongst the species that have been studied. Adults of *Antheraea* show no death of motoneurons even though their target muscles degenerate (Lockshin and Beaulaton, 1974). In both *Manduca* (Truman, 1983) and *Drosophila* (Kimura and Truman, 1990), by contrast, a major bout of motoneuron death follows the muscle degeneration.

The withdrawal of ecdysteroids at the end of metamorphosis is required for the death of neurons as well as muscle in *Manduca* (Truman and Schwartz, 1984). Abdominal isolation had no effect on the time course of motoneuron death or accelerated it depending on the time of isolation. Injection or infusion of ecdysteroids into isolated abdomens or intact animals prevented degeneration as long as the steroid titer remained elevated, but once the titer was allowed to fall, the neurons then died. Thus, the ecdysteroid withdrawal is a necessary prerequisite for the degeneration of these cells.

An interesting feature of neuronal death is the stereotyped sequence of degeneration seen within the set of doomed motoneurons. Since specific cells commence degeneration at fixed times following adult ecdysis, it was possible to examine how steroid treatment at various times affects the subsequent fate of specific cells. For example, the D-IV motoneurons begin to die about 14 h after ecdysis (Fig. 2). A single injection of 20-HE delayed degeneration but this treatment became ineffective as the time of injection approached the normal onset of degeneration. The experimentally-determined switch point, when 50% of the cells show delays after the treatment, has been termed the "commitment point" (Truman and Schwartz, 1984). For the D-IV cells this commitment point occurs 3 h after ecdysis (10−12 h before the first ultrastructural signs of degeneration). Each motoneuron shows its own characteristic commitment point (Fig. 3): that for MN-11 is 5 h before ecdysis, whereas MN-12 is not committed until about 30 h after ecdysis (Fahrbach and Truman, 1987). A strikingly consistent pattern is seen: in each case the motoneurons become committed 10−12 h before they begin degeneration. What then is responsible for the commitment point and why does the time of commitment vary between cells? Also, what are the processes that occur during this 10−12 h span?

A simple hypothesis to explain the timing of the commitment points is that the doomed motoneurons differ in the levels of circulating steroid needed to maintain them. As the ecdysteroid titer declines, those having the highest thresholds would then be the first to commence degeneration. This hypothesis was tested by ex-

planting ganglia to organ culture where they were provided with an abrupt step-down in hormone concentration rather than a gradual, exponential decline (Bennett and Truman, 1983). The doomed neurons in the cultured ganglia survived in the presence of ecdysteroids but degenerated in their absence. Even after the abrupt removal of ecdysteroids, however, the cells showed their proper sequence of death. Thus, the sequencing of cell death is intrinsic to the ganglion and not a direct response to the shape of the ecdysteroid titer.

Role of neuronal interactions

Nerve − muscle interactions

In *Antheraea*, chronically denervated ISMs persist through adult development but then undergo prompt degeneration when challenged with EH at adult ecdysis (Schwartz and Truman, 1982). Thus, their death is a direct response to circulating cues and does not require CNS involvement. The CNS, however, can still influence the fate of the ISMs to some degree. Enhancement of motor activity to the ISMs either pharmacologically or through im-

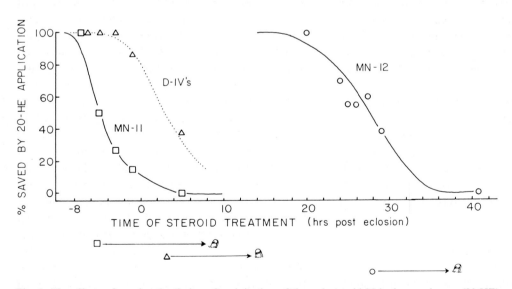

Fig. 3. The effects of varying the timing of an injection of the ecdysteroid 20-hydroxyecdysone (20-HE) on its ability to block the degeneration of specific motoneurons. The bottom portion compares the time of the commitment point (the time when 50% of the neurons are spared) with the subsequent onset of degeneration.

planted electrodes resulted in persistence of the muscles beyond their normal time of death (Lockshin and Williams, 1965a, b). A similar effect is also seen in *Drosophila*: when newly emerged flies are forced to display ecdysis behavior over an extended period of time (see below), their ecdysial muscles survive for a few hours longer than seen in controls (Kimura and Truman, 1990).

Various endocrine manipulations have been used in *Manduca* to explore the relationship between neurons and muscle during the period of cell death. Like for the neurons, a commitment point can be experimentally determined for the ventral ISMs, and it occurs at 12 h before ecdysis. Their motoneurons, the D-IV cells, by contrast, are not committed until about 3 h after ecdysis. When ecdysteroids were injected into animals within this 15 h period, the ISMs showed normal degeneration but death of the neurons was blocked (Truman and Schwartz, 1984). These results indicate that muscle death is not automatically followed by the degeneration of the respective motoneurons.

Whether muscle death is a necessary prerequisite for neuronal death was examined by topically applying a juvenile hormone (JH) mimic to a small patch of cuticle overlying a group of ISMs (Truman, unpublished manuscript). The local concentration of the JH mimic in the vicinity of these muscles was sufficient to prevent them from completing their metamorphosis; hence, they did not degenerate after the emergence of the adult. Their motoneurons, however, were not exposed to the JH mimic and typically died after emergence despite the survival of their target muscles. Thus, muscle and motoneuron deaths are coordinated in time because they are responding to the same endocrine cue (the decline in ecdysteroids) and not because the death of one causes the death of the other.

Neuron – neuron interactions

The possible role of neuron – neuron interactions in triggering neuronal death is harder to examine. Such interactions appear very important in causing neuronal death in *Drosophila* (Kimura and Truman, 1990). Neck ligation of newly emerged flies did not block muscle degeneration but it suppressed the motoneuron death. The results of ligations performed during the first 15 min after ecdysis depended on the subsequent behavior of the ligated (decapitated) fly. Those that showed wing inflation behavior also displayed the normal pattern of neuronal death, while those that did not perform the behavior showed reduced degeneration. When ligations were done after the behavior was completed, normal cell death always ensued.

In intact flies, inflation behavior can be prevented if ecdysing animals are positioned so that they enter an empty puparial case as they are leaving their own. These flies are trapped in the new case and show sustained ecdysis behavior. Those that were freed after 2 h subsequently performed the inflation behavior and showed a normal time course of neuronal death that was shifted by 2 h relative to controls. By contrast, animals permanently maintained in the puparial case showed little neuronal death. Besides these behavioral modifications of the death program, analysis of a mutant that fails to undergo inflation behavior after ecdysis reveals that it also shows reduced levels of neuronal death (Kimura and Truman, unpublished manuscript). These observations suggest that neural events associated with performing the inflation behavior are involved in triggering neuronal death in *Drosophila*. The nature of these interactions are unknown.

In *Manduca*, isolated abdomens show no ecdysis, expansion, or digging behaviors and yet their neuronal death is essentially normal with regard to its time course and extent (Truman and Schwartz, 1984). Consequently, the performance of a particular behavior is not a requirement for neuronal death in this moth. It should be noted, however, that forcing moths to show sustained ecdysis behavior delayed the death of certain motoneurons for a few hours although it did not prevent it (Truman, 1983). Thus, as described above for the muscles, sustained activity of particular cells may delay death that has been triggered by other means.

Although not linked to the performance of specific behaviors, neuronal death in *Manduca* may nevertheless involve local neuronal interactions. MN-12 is the last motoneuron to die. Transection of the intersegmental connectives in newly ecdysed animals spared the MN-12s that reside in the ganglion immediately posterior to the lesion. The neurons were not injured by the surgery (they project caudally) and the sparing was permanent. Transections performed up to about 30 h post-ecdysis were effective in saving the cells, whereas later treatments were ineffective. Interestingly, the time that connective transection lost its ability to save MN-12 coincided with the neuron's commitment point. These observations suggest that at 30 h there is a phasic signal from the next anterior ganglion that results in the death of MN-12.

Thus, there appears to be 2 events required for the death of MN-12: a blood-born signal, the withdrawal of ecdysteroids, is necessary but not sufficient for causing death. A cue arising in the next anterior ganglion and transmitted in the interganglionic connective then acts in concert with the ecdysteroid signal to determine the exact time of death. How are the two cues related? One possibility is that ecdysteroids block the transmission of the neural cue. Another possibility is that the ability of the neurons to respond to the neural cue requires the absence of steroids. We cannot discriminate between the two hypotheses at this time but we favor the latter. As detailed below, MN-12 possesses ecdysteroid receptors which is consistent with the steroid effects being directly on these cells. Also, the programmed death of muscles in *Antheraea* sets the precedent for a death-triggering signal (in this case the circulating peptide, EH) acting on target muscles that must be primed by steroid withdrawal (Schwartz and Truman, 1984).

Another question posed by MN-12 is whether this cell is unique in requiring both steroid withdrawal and a neuronal signal. The most parsimonious explanation is that MN-12 is unique only in the fact that the neuronal signal is supplied by an interganglionic neuron. Other neurons may receive similar inputs but from neurons that are intraganglionic. If other cells share this control with MN-12, then the temporal distribution of commitment points likely represents the times that the respective cells receive this neural input.

Steroid receptor distribution and cell fates

Whether working alone or in concert with neural factors, ecdysteroids play a key role in triggering neuronal death. A preliminary examination of the spatial distribution of ecdysteroid receptors in the CNS of *Manduca* has been carried out using [^{3}H]ponasterone, an ecdysone analogue (Fahrbach and Truman, 1989). Abdominal ganglia were removed about 2 h prior to adult ecdysis, exposed to radiolabeled ponasterone in vitro, and then quick frozen. Cryostat sections were mounted onto emulsion-coated slides and the distribution of label within the ganglion determined by autoradiography. Grains due to radiolabeled steroid were concentrated in neuronal nuclei and this accumulation was abolished by preincubation of the ganglia with excess unlabeled steroid. Importantly, only a subset of the neurons showed steroid accumulation. Identified neurons that were not fated to die (MN-1, 4, 5, the bursicon cells, the CAP cells), did not possess receptors as indicated by their failure to accumulate steroid. By contrast, the doomed neurons varied with some showing receptors while others did not.

We do not yet know the reason for the differences seen amongst the neurons in the doomed group. One possibility is that these cells are indeed heterogeneous in their ability to bind steroid. Alternatively, the doomed neurons might all have had receptors initially but as each cell approaches its appointed time to die, these receptors may be lost. Indeed, the nervous systems in this preliminary series were taken at 2 h before ecdysis, just prior to the commitment point of the D-IV cells but well before that of MN-2 and MN-12. The latter cells showed strong steroid accumulation whereas the D-IV cells showed no significant binding.

Priming of steroid sensitivity

An intriguing aspect of degeneration in *Manduca* is that the ISMs and their motoneurons die as a result of the withdrawal of ecdysteroids, but early in life these same cells show no steroid dependence. For example, under certain environmental conditions, the pupa enters a period of developmental arrest termed diapause which lasts for a number of months. This condition is maintained by the absence of ecdysteroids and both neurons and muscles persist through this period without ill effects (Truman, unpublished manuscript). During the subsequent transition from the pupa to the adult, however, the cells now become dependent on ecdysteroids for their continuing survival. The action of ecdysteroids to render neurons ecdysteroid-dependent appears due to the direct action of the steroids on the CNS. For example, when pupal ganglia were implanted into the body cavity of developing adults, the motoneurons of the implant developed the same steroid sensitivities as did those of the host despite the fact that the former were deprived of their normal targets during adult development (Truman and Schwartz, 1984).

The change in neurons and muscles that render them ecdysteroid-dependent requires that ecdysteroids act on these cells in the absence of JH. This was first shown for the muscles by applying a JH mimic early in the pupal – adult transition and producing muscles which did not then die (Lockshin and Williams, 1964). For the CNS of *Manduca*, application of JH mimics early in the pupal – adult transition likewise prevents the neurons from becoming ecdysteroid-dependent (Truman, unpublished manuscript). For example, JH treatment up to 5 days after pupal ecdysis routinely resulted in adults in which MN-12 did not die. Interestingly, the timing and dosage of JH treatment that are effective in preserving the cell do not interfere with the overall metamorphosis of the insect: they become morphologically normal adults that have superficially normal adult nervous systems. It is not yet known how such treatment alters the neurons in question, for instance by affecting their ecdysteroid receptor populations late in adult development.

Mechanism of degeneration

The signals that bring about death may vary (EH, ecdysteroid withdrawal, ecdysteroid withdrawal plus neuronal factors) but in all cases there is a substantial lag between the final signal and the onset of degeneration. A central question is what are the events that occur during this period? Two classes of mechanisms are possible. One is a trophic mechanism in which the presence of a factor, such as the ecdysteroids, promotes the production of something necessary for cell survival. Decline in steroid levels would then result in the loss of this necessary material and the cells would die. Alternatively, the appropriate cues could initiate synthesis of materials that would kill the cell. The earliest paper to direct attention to the latter mechanism of degeneration was that by Lockshin (1969) which focused on muscle death in silkmoths. He showed that the death of these cells could be prevented by treatment of animals with drugs that blocked RNA or protein synthesis. Similar experiments have been carried out in *Manduca* for both muscle (Schwartz and Kay, 1987) and neuronal degeneration (Fahrbach and Truman, 1988). In the case of the latter, the RNA synthesis inhibitor, actinomycin D, blocks degeneration but only if given prior to the commitment point. After the commitment point, the cells die irrespective of the presence or absence of the inhibitor. Protein synthesis inhibitors, such as cycloheximide, also block degeneration but their period of effectiveness extends 5 – 6 h beyond the commitment point. The timing of sensitivities to these drugs is consistent with the hypothesis that death is brought about through the activation of new genetic information. The respective hormonal and neural signals presumably result in transcription of this new information which commits the cell to its new pathway. The translation products would then mediate the death response.

The involvement of specific genes in mediating cell death is likely not limited to invertebrate systems. For example, the death of cultured embryonic sympathetic ganglion neurons that results from nerve growth factor deprivation can be prevented by inhibitors of protein synthesis (Martin et al., 1988). Likewise, inhibitors of RNA synthesis will depress the degeneration of motoneurons and dorsal root ganglion cells in the embryonic chick spinal cord (Oppenheim and Prevette, 1988).

The nature of these new products is presently unknown but they may be revealed by genetic and molecular approaches. In the nematode, *Caenorhabdites elegans*, a series of recessive mutations have been isolated which block programmed cell death in the CNS (Horvitz et al., 1982; Ellis and Horvitz, 1986). In two of the mutants, cell death-3 (*ced*-3) and *ced*-4, immature neurons that would normally die survive and mature into functional, supernumerary nerve cells. Thus, these two gene products seem to be essential for the normal death of cells. In *Drosophila*, no mutants have yet been isolated that prevent programmed cell death but there are two mutants that affect the dynamics of the degeneration process. Muscle cell death 1 (*mcd*-1) and *mcd*-2 retard the progression of degeneration of certain temporary head muscles after the emergence of the adult fly (Kimura and Tanimura, unpublished manuscript).

Conclusions

The signals that bring about death have been the focus of much investigation. They are varied and are a function of species, stage and tissue. Nevertheless, a common theme that is evident in the post-metamorphic death is the role of ecdysteroids. In all cases action by this hormone is required during the pupal – adult transition either to trigger the death itself or to prepare the tissue so that other factors (EH or neural-derived cues) can

act on the cells to bring about degeneration. A novel aspect of the system is that the death or preparation for death results from the removal of ecdysteroids rather than from the appearance of the hormone. A recent report suggests that a somewhat similar response may operate in the rodent hippocampus, as removal of corticosteroids by adrenalectomy results in selective loss of granule cells (Sloviter et al., 1989).

The factor that makes the moth neurons and muscles sensitive to the removal of ecdysteroids is the action of these steroids (in the absence of JH) during the pupal – adult transition. A possible model to explain how steroid exposure might then make cells sensitive to steroid withdrawal is provided by the studies by Ashburner et al. (1973) on the steroid-induced pattern of chromosomal puffing in the salivary gland of larval *Drosophila*. Ecdysteroids cause the activation of early genes whose products, in turn, are required for the activation of "late" genes. These late genes, however, are apparently inhibited by the ecdysteroid – receptor complex and hence can only be expressed after the steroid is removed.

Fig. 4 is a direct extension of the Ashburner et al. model in which the death-related genes are included as one of the late genes. Thus, the ecdysteroid – receptor complex would act as a positive regulator of the early genes but as a

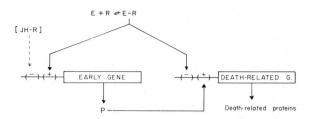

Fig. 4. A possible model by which death-related genes might be activated by the appearance and then withdrawal of ecdysteroids. E, ecdysteroids; JH-R, juvenile hormone in association with its receptor; P, product of the early activated gene which then interacts with later expressed genes; R, ecdysteroid receptor. The + and − refer to regulatory regions where factors might enhance or suppress, respectively, the transcription of the associated gene. See text for further explanation.

negative regulator of the genes related to cell death. The early gene product would act on enhancer elements of the latter but transcription of the genes would be blocked while the steroid – receptor concentrations remained elevated. Declining steroids, however, would then allow the genes to be activated. Under this type of model, juvenile hormone would most likely be involved in blocking the activation of the appropriate early genes since this hormone can only block death if given within the first few days of adult development.

The study of cell death is moving towards analysis on the genetic and molecular levels. But besides identifying the genes that may be involved in causing degeneration, one must also be concerned with issues of why some cells activate these genes in response to particular cues whereas others do not. Also, what predisposes a cell to respond to such cues at certain times in its life but not at others? Invertebrates, with their simplified nervous system, should continue to provide valuable insights into these problems.

Acknowledgements

The research in this paper was supported by grant NS 13079 from NIH.

References

Ashburner, M., Chihara, C., Meltzer, P. and Richards, G. (1973) Temporal control of puffing activity in polytene chromosomes. *Cold Spring Harbor Symp. Quant. Biol.,* 23: 655 – 662.

Bennett, K.L. and Truman, J.W. (1985) Steroid-dependent survival of identifiable neurons in cultured ganglia of the moth *Manduca sexta. Science,* 229: 58 – 60.

Bollenbacher, W.E., Smith, S.L., Goodman, W. and Gilbert, L.I. (1981) Ecdysteroid titer during larval – pupal – adult development of the tobacco hornworm, *Manduca sexta. Gen. Comp. Endocrinol.,* 44: 302 – 306.

Booker, R. and Truman, J.W. (1987) Postembryonic neurogenesis in the CNS of the tobacco hornworm, *Manduca sexta.* I. Neuroblast arrays and the fate of their progeny during metamorphosis. *J. Comp. Neurol.,* 255: 548 – 559.

Ellis, H.M. and Horvitz, H.R. (1986) Genetic control of programmed cell death in the nematode, *C. elegans. Cell,* 44: 817 – 829.

Fahrbach, S.E. and Truman, J.W. (1987) Possible interactions of a steroid hormone and neural inputs in controlling the death of an identified neuron in the moth *Manduca sexta. J. Neurobiol.,* 18: 497 – 508.

Fahrbach, S.E. and Truman, J.W. (1988) Cycloheximide inhibits ecdysteroid-regulated neuronal death in the moth *Manduca sexta. Soc. Neurosci. Abstr.,* 14: 368.

Fahrbach, S.E. and Truman, J.W. (1989) Autoradiographic identification of ecdysteroid-binding cells in the nervous system of the moth *Manduca sexta. J. Neurobiol.,* 20: 681 – 702.

Finlayson, L.H. (1956) Normal and induced degeneration of abdominal muscles during metamorphosis in the lepidoptera. *Q. J. Microsc. Sci.,* 97: 215 – 234.

Hamburger, V. and Oppenheim, R.W. (1982) Naturally occurring neuronal death in vertebrates. *Neurosci. Comment.,* 1: 39 – 55.

Horvitz, H.R., Ellis, H.M. and Sternberg, P.W. (1982) Programmed cell death in nematode development. *Neurosci. Comment.,* 1: 56 – 65.

Kimura, K.-I and Truman, J.W. (1990) Postmetamorphic cell death in the nervous and muscular systems of *Drosophila melanogaster. J. Neurosci.,* 10: 403 – 411.

Levine, R.B. and Truman, J.W. (1985) Dendritic reorganization of abdominal motoneurons during metamorphosis of the moth *Manduca sexta. J. Neurosci.,* 5: 2424 – 2431.

Lockshin, R.A. (1969) Programmed cell death. Activation of lysis by a mechanism involving the synthesis of protein. *J. Insect Physiol.,* 15: 1505 – 1516.

Lockshin, R.A. and J. Beaulaton, J. (1974) Programmed cell death. Cytochemical evidence for lysosomes during normal breakdown of the intersegmental muscles. *J. Ultrastruct. Res.,* 46: 43 – 62.

Lockshin, R.A. and Williams, C.M. (1964) Programmed cell death. II. Endocrine influences on the breakdown of the intersegmental muscles in saturniid moths. *J. Insect Physiol.,* 10: 643 – 649.

Lockshin, R.A. and Williams, C.M. (1965a) Programmed cell death. III. Neural control of the breakdown of the intersegmental muscles of silkmoths. *J. Insect Physiol.,* 11: 601 – 610.

Lockshin, R.A. and Williams, C.M. (1965b) Programmed cell death. IV. The influence of drugs on the breakdown of the intersegmental muscles of silkmoths. *J. Insect Physiol.,* 11: 803 – 809.

Loer, C.M., Steeves, J.D. and Goodman, C.S. (1983) Neuronal death in grasshopper embryos: variable patterns in different species, clutches, and clones. *J. Embryol. Exp. Morph.,* 78: 169 – 182.

Martin, D.P., Schmidt, R.E., DiStefano, P.S., Lowry, O.H., Carter, J.G. and Johnson, E.M. (1988) Inhibitors of protein synthesis and RNA synthesis prevent neuronal death caused by nerve growth factor deprivation. *J. Cell Biol.,* 106: 829 – 844.

Nuesch, H. (1985) Control of muscle development. In: G.A.

Kerkut and L.I. Gilbert (Eds.), *Comprehensive Insect Physiology, Biochemistry and Pharmacology, Vol 2,* Pergamon, Oxford, pp. 425–452.

Oppenheim, R.W. and Prevette, D.M. (1988) Reduction of naturally occurring neuronal death in vivo by the inhibition of protein and RNA synthesis. *Soc. Neurosci. Abstr.,* 14: 368.

Reynolds, S.E. and Truman, J.W. (1983) Eclosion hormone. In: R.G.H. Downer and H. Laufer (Eds.), *Endocrinology of Insects,* A.R. Liss, New York, pp. 217–233.

Runion, H.I. and Pipa, R. (1973) Electrophysiological and endocrinological correlates during the metamorphic degeneration of a muscle fibre in *Galleria mellonella* (L.). *J. Exp. Biol.,* 53: 9–24.

Schwartz, L.M. and Kay, B.K. (1987) De novo transcription and translation of new genes is required for the programmed death of the intersegmental muscles of the tobacco hawkmoth, *Manduca sexta. Soc. Neurosci. Abstr.,* 13: 8.

Schwartz, L.M. and Truman, J.W. (1982) Peptide and steroid regulation of muscle degeneration in an insect. *Science,* 215: 1420–1421.

Schwartz, L.M. and Truman, J.W. (1983) Hormonal control of rates of metamorphic development in the tobacco hornworm, *Manduca sexta. Dev. Biol.,* 99: 103–144.

Schwartz, L.M. and Truman, J.W. (1984) Hormonal control of muscle atrophy and degeneration in the moth *Antheraea polyphemus. J. Exp. Biol.,* 111: 13–30.

Sloviter, R.S., Valiquette, G., Abrams, G.A., Ronk, E.C., Sollas, A.L., Paul, L.A. and Neubort, S. (1989) Selective loss of hippocampal granule cells in the mature rat brain after adrenalectomy. *Science,* 243: 535–538.

Stocker, R.F., Edwards, J.S. and Truman, J.W. (1978) Fine structure of degenerating moth abdominal motoneurons after eclosion. *Cell Tissue Res.,* 191: 317–331.

Taylor, H.M. and Truman, J.W. (1974) Metamorphosis of the abdominal ganglia of the tobacco hornworm, *Manduca sexta:* changes in populations of identified motor neurons. *J. Comp. Physiol.,* 90: 367–388.

Truman, J.W. (1983) Programmed cell death in the nervous system of an adult insect. *J. Comp. Neurol.,* 216: 445–452.

Truman, J.W. (1984) Cell death in invertebrate nervous systems. *Ann. Rev. Neurosci.,* 7: 171–188.

Truman, J.W. and Schwartz, L.M. (1984) Steroid regulation of neuronal death in the moth nervous system. *J. Neurosci.,* 4: 274–280.

Weeks, J.C. (1987) Time course of hormonal independence for developmental events in neurons and other cell types during insect metamorphosis. *Dev. Biol.,* 124: 163–176.

Weeks, J.C. and Truman, J.W. (1985) Independent steroid control of the fates of motoneurons and their muscles during insect metamorphosis. *J. Neurosci.,* 5: 2290–2300.

P. Coleman, G. Higgins and C. Phelps (Eds.)
Progress in Brain Research, Vol. 86
© 1990 Elsevier Science Publishers B.V. (Biomedical Division)

CHAPTER 4

Excitotoxin-mediated neuron death in youth and old age

John W. Olney

Departments of Psychiatry and Neuropathology, Washington University Medical School, St. Louis, MO 63110, U.S.A.

Introduction

Glutamate (Glu), an amino acid found abundantly in the CNS, is a Jekyll/Hyde molecule, vitally important for its metabolic, neurotrophic and neurotransmitter roles, but ominously threatening in its neurotoxic potential. The neurotoxicity of Glu, although first described 30 years ago, was relatively ignored until studies in the early 1970's linked the phenomenon to an excitatory mechanism. Over the past decade, additional advances have been made in understanding the neurotoxic (excitotoxic) properties of Glu. Several receptor subtypes that mediate Glu excitotoxicity have been delineated, drugs with anti-excitotoxic actions have been identified and evidence for the potential complicity of excitotoxins in neurodegenerative disorders has begun to unfold. Here I will review evidence for such complicity and consider the possibility that neuronal vulnerability to excitotoxic injury may vary with age (for more detailed reviews pertaining to excitotoxicology, please see Robinson and Coyle, 1987; Choi, 1988; Olney, 1989).

The excitotoxic concept

Historical perspective

Three decades ago, Curtis and colleagues (1963) using newly developed microelectrophoretic techniques to examine the membrane-depolarizing properties of Glu and related compounds, characterized the structural requirements for interaction with an apparent excitatory amino acid (EAA) receptor. However, the myriad metabolic involvements of Glu, its ability to excite neurons throughout the CNS and the lack of any known mechanism for terminating its excitatory action led neuroscientists of the 1960's to reject Glu as a transmitter candidate. This view prevailed for 2 decades before yielding slowly to evidence suggesting that Glu satisfies the criteria for a transmitter. Finally, in the 1980's, Glu has gained widespread acceptance as the front-running transmitter candidate at the majority of excitatory synapses in the mammalian CNS.

Since Glu is found in very high concentrations in the CNS and serves a number of important metabolic functions, early reports that systemic administration of Glu to infant mice destroys neurons in the retina (Lucas and Newhouse, 1957; Olney, 1969a), or in certain regions of the brain (Olney, 1969b), were met with disbelief. However, CNS damage following either oral or subcutaneous administration was readily reproduced in a number of animal species, including primates (Olney et al., 1972). In addition, it was shown (Olney et al., 1971) that specific Glu analogs (Fig. 1) known to share the neuroexcitatory properties of Glu mimic its neurotoxic effects, that these analogs have a parallel order of potencies for their excitatory and toxic actions and that analogs lacking excitatory activity also lack neurotoxicity. Moreover, ultrastructural studies (Olney, 1969a, 1971) localized the apparent site of toxic action to post-synaptic

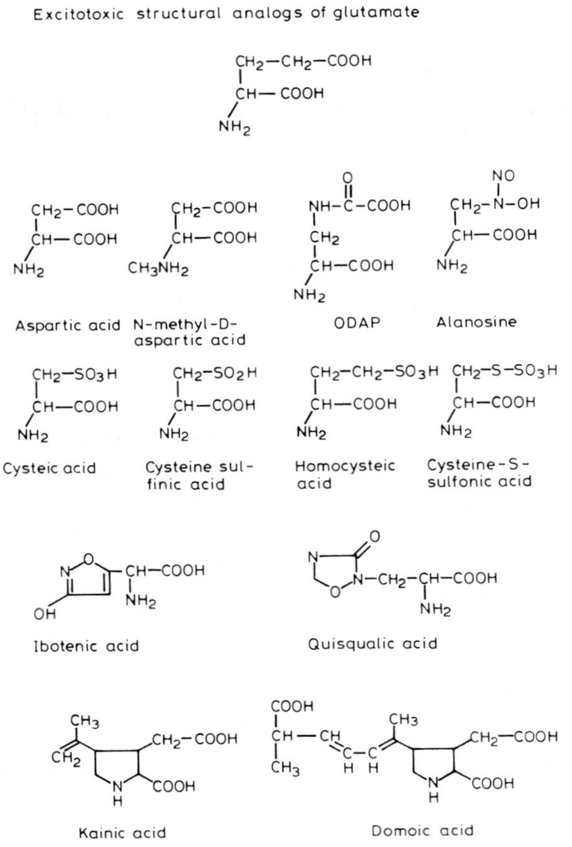

Excitotoxic structural analogs of glutamate

Fig. 1. Acidic amino acids which have been shown to mimic both the excitatory and neurotoxic properties of glutamate. ODAP = β-N-oxalylamino-L-alanine (also abbreviated BOAA).

dendrosomal membranes where Glu excitatory synaptic receptors are located. These and related observations gave rise to the excitotoxic concept that Glu destroys neurons by excessive activation of excitatory receptors on the dendrosomal surfaces of neurons.

Excitotoxin receptors and anti-excitotoxic drugs

Of major importance for developing better insight into the physiological and pathological properties of EAA transmitter systems was the identification of EAA receptor subtypes differentially sensitive to specific agonists (N-methyl-D-aspartate

(NMDA), quisqualic acid, kainic acid (KA)), and the discovery of antagonists that block the excitatory actions of EAA agonists at such receptors (Watkins, 1978; Watkins and Evans, 1981). Shortly after the first EAA antagonists were identified, it was shown that they protect neurons in the in vivo mouse hypothalamus against the neurotoxic actions of Glu or its more potent analog, NMDA (Olney et al., 1979, 1981). In further confirmation of the excitotoxic hypothesis, many EAA antagonist candidates have now been systematically screened in in vitro preparations and found to have anti-excitotoxic activities corresponding in potency and receptor specificity to their known anti-excitatory activities (Olney et al., 1986b, 1987a; Choi, 1988).

Evidence implicating excitotoxins in neurodegenerative disorders (see below), stimulated interest in the possibility that EAA antagonists might prove valuable as neuroprotective agents in clinical neurology. In Table I, the results of several EAA agonist/antagonist studies (Olney et al., 1986b, 1987a, b) are summarized. The first generation of EAA antagonists identified (Watkins and Evans, 1981) were competitive NMDA antagonists which compete with NMDA agonists for binding at NMDA receptors. Agents in this class, although possessing moderately potent antagonist properties, are of uncertain value for clinical applications as they do not readily penetrate blood brain barriers. The most powerful anti-excitotoxic drugs identified thus far are non-competitive NMDA antagonists which act at phencyclidine receptors to block both the excitatory (Lodge and Anis, 1982; Lodge et al., 1987) and toxic (Olney et al., 1986b, 1987a) actions of NMDA. MK-801, a drug developed by Merck, Sharp and Dohme, is the most potent known compound in this category. Since these compounds do penetrate blood brain barriers, they are of interest as potential therapeutic drugs. Certain currently marketed drugs, including dextromethorphan (Goldberg et al., 1987) and several anti-Parkinsonian agents (Olney et al., 1987b), are moderately potent non-competitive NMDA antagonists. Mixed an-

TABLE I

Potencies of antagonists in blocking NMDA or KA toxicity

Compounds were rated according to the minimal concentration (μM) required to provide total protection against NMDA (120 μM) or kainic acid (25 μM) toxicity. Antagonists were tested over a range of doses from 3000 μM downward. When no blocking was observed at 3000 μM, this is indicated by a dash ($-$).

Potential antagonist	vs. NMDA (120 μM)	vs. KA (25 μM)
Competitive NMDA antagonists	(μM)	(μM)
D-2-amino-5-phosphonopentanoate (AP5)	25	$-$
D-2-amino-5-phosphonoheptanoate (AP7)	75	$-$
D-alpha-aminoadipate	200	$-$
Non-competitive NMDA antagonists		
MK-801	0.1	$-$
Phencyclidine	0.5	$-$
Ketamine	5	$-$
($\pm$) Cyclazocine	5	$-$
($\pm$) SKF 10,047	10	$-$
Dextromethorphan	50	$-$
Anti-Parkinsonian agents		
Procyclidine (Kemadrin)	15	$-$
Ethopropazine (Parsidol)	25	$-$
Mixed EAA antagonists		
CNQX	100	15
Kynurenic acid	300	750
(+)-cis-2,3-piperidine dicarboxylate	1000	2000
Barbiturates		
Thiamylal	50	250
Thiopental	200	400

tagonists, such as kynurenic acid and cis-2,3-piperidine dicarboxylate, block the excitotoxic effects of both NMDA and non-NMDA agonists but are of limited interest because of their low potency and inability to penetrate blood brain barriers. CNQX, a recently described quinoxalinedione (Honore et al., 1988), has the important distinction of being the first agent found to block the excitatory (Honore et al., 1988) and excitotoxic (Price et al., 1988) actions of non-NMDA agonists more powerfully than it blocks those of NMDA. Certain thiobarbiturates penetrate blood brain barriers and are moderately potent against both NMDA and non-NMDA agonists.

Acute versus delayed excitotoxic cell death

In vitro ion substitution experiments have provided evidence for more than one mechanism by which excitotoxin-induced neuronal degeneration can occur. In hippocampal cell cultures (Rothman, 1985) or in the isolated chick retina (Olney et al., 1986c), neurons degenerate very rapidly when exposed continuously for 30 min to a toxic concentration of Glu or any of its excitotoxic analogs. In either of these preparations, this acute toxic reaction is abolished by the removal of Na$^+$ or Cl$^-$ from the incubation medium, but is not affected by the removal of Ca^{2+}. However, Choi (1985) has described a slow degenerative process triggered by brief (5 min) exposure of cultured neurons to Glu, a process which is facilitated by the presence of Ca^{2+} in the incubation medium. Thus, there is basis for believing that excitotoxins can destroy neurons by either an acute fulminating process which is Na^+ and Cl^- (but not Ca^{2+}) dependent, or by a slow process which is Ca^{2+} dependent. It is noteworthy that, in the latter case, excitotoxic neuronal degeneration occurs even though the duration of exposure to an abnormal concentration of excitotoxin is only 1/6 as long as in the former case. It will be important to develop a better understanding of the delayed type of mechanism since many human neurological disorders entail the slow degeneration of neurons by a subacute or chronic mechanism. If excitotoxins play a role in such degenerative processes, having a wide time window for therapeutic intervention would be advantageous and, if the process is Ca^{2+} dependent, it is possible that Ca^{2+} channel blockers might be a useful addition to the therapeutic armamentarium.

Special features of the NMDA receptor

All three of the above mentioned EAA receptor subtypes are capable of mediating excitotoxic events. The most studied of these and reportedly the most abundant and widely distributed in the mammalian CNS, is the NMDA receptor (Fig. 2). Several features of the NMDA receptor (recently reviewed (TINS, 1987)) distinguish it from other subtypes of EAA receptor. This receptor is linked to a Na^+/Ca^{2+} ion channel which has a much higher Ca^{2+} conductance than ion channels associated with other EAA receptor subtypes, and the NMDA ion channel is subject to a voltage-dependent Mg^{2+} blockade. The NMDA receptor is closely associated with a strychnine-insensitive glycine receptor which facilitates opening of the NMDA ion channel and with phencyclidine receptors which are positioned within this channel permitting phencyclidine agonists to perform an open channel block. In addition, there is evidence that

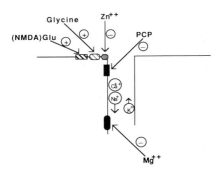

NMDA Multiceptor-ionophore complex

Fig. 2. A schematic depiction of the various components comprising the NMDA receptor – ionophore complex. Recent evidence (reviewed in TINS, 1987) suggests that endogenous transmitter (presumably Glu) released from pre-synaptic axon terminals activates NMDA receptors on post-synaptic dendrosomal membranes resulting in opening of a cation channel. Glycine, acting at strychnine insensitive receptors that are co-localized with NMDA receptors, facilitates opening of this channel, whereas PCP, Zn^{2+} and Mg^{2+}, each acting at a separate site, and presumably by separate mechanisms, are antagonists of channel function.

Zn^{2+}, acting at a separate site near the mouth of the NMDA ion channel, is an inhibitory modulator of channel function. Thus, as Fig. 2 illustrates, the NMDA receptor system is a remarkably complex entity, the normal function of which depends on a dynamic equilibrium among multiple facilitative and inhibitory factors. It follows that a pathological process adversely affecting any given factor might create an imbalance rendering the system hyperfunctional and prone to an expression of excitotoxicity.

Excitotoxins and neurodegenerative disorders

Given the abundance of excitotoxins in the environment, the high concentration of these agents in the CNS, their intrinsic neurotoxic potential and the several mechanisms by which such potential might be expressed, excitotoxins are logical candidates for complicity in neurodegenerative conditions. Over the past decade, evidence for such complicity has begun to accumulate. Neurodegenerative conditions in which EAA and an excitotoxic mechanism may be involved are grouped into several categories and discussed below.

Food excitotoxins

Glutamate/aspartate and neuroendocrinopathies

Glu, in the form of its sodium salt (monosodium glutamate, MSG) is one of the world's most widely and heavily used food additives. Aspartate, an excitotoxic analog of Glu, comprises 1/2 of the molecule of aspartame (Nutrasweet) which is used widely as a sweetener in foods and beverages. Currently, as in the past, the Food and Drug Administration sanctions the widespread use of excitotoxic food additives and fosters no program for educating against feeding excitotoxins to children. The wisdom of this policy has been questioned (Olney, 1984). Neurons vulnerable to destruction by oral intake of Glu or aspartate are those lying in certain brain regions that lack blood brain barriers, e.g., neuroendocrine regulatory neurons in the arcuate nucleus of the hypothalamus. Immature animals are much more sensitive than adults to the neurotoxic effects of Glu and aspartate. Oral intake in liquids (soups, beverages) poses the greatest risk since this ensures the most rapid and complete gastrointestinal absorption and, hence, the highest blood levels. Humans develop much higher blood Glu levels from a given oral dose of MSG than any known animal species. Although the issue has not been properly studied, the added MSG in a single bowl of certain commercially available soups is probably enough to cause blood Glu levels to rise as high in a human child as levels that predictably cause brain damage in immature animals. Since destruction of arcuate hypothalamic neurons in immature animals results in a complex delayed-onset neuroendocrine deficiency syndrome, the question arises whether feeding excitotoxins to young humans might have similar neuroendocrinopathic consequences (for more detailed information and supporting references see Olney, 1984, 1987).

BOAA and neurolathyrism

Neurolathyrism is a paralytic neurological disorder which occurs endemically in certain parts of the world where the legume, *lathyrus sativus,* is ingested in excess during periods of famine. The poisonous ingredient in *lathyrus sativus* is believed to be β-N-oxalylamino-L-alanine (BOAA, also sometimes abbreviated ODAP), an acidic amino acid with powerful excitotoxic properties (Olney et al., 1976; Spencer et al., 1984, 1986; Zeevalk et al., 1988). Spencer and coworkers (1986) have recently demonstrated that the paralytic symptoms of neurolathyrism can be reproduced in monkeys maintained chronically on a diet enriched in BOAA. The neurotoxic effects of BOAA in tissue culture are blocked by broad spectrum EAA antagonists (Ross et al., 1987; Zeevalk et al., 1988). Evidence linking exogenous excitotoxins to a paralytic disease such as neurolathyrism is of considerable interest since, if chronic exposure to exogenous excitotoxins can cause neuronal degeneration that develops gradually over a period of months or years, it may be possible for endogenous excitotoxins to cause neuronal degeneration on a similarly chronic basis (e.g., in Huntington's chorea, Alzheimer's dementia or Parkinsonism). Moreover, should research on neurolathyrism reveal a mechanism by which ingested exogenous excitotoxins can cause degeneration of neurons in parts of the CNS which are thought to be inaccessible to such agents, it will be necessary to reevaluate the possibility that exogenous excitotoxins, including those used as food additives, might contribute (in concert with endogenous excitotoxins) to a variety of chronic neurodegenerative conditions.

BMAA and ALS/Parkinsonism/dementia complex

Spencer and colleagues (1987) have postulated that a neurological disease endemic to certain south sea islands, especially Guam, which has combined features of amyotrophic lateral sclerosis (ALS), Parkinsonism and dementia may be caused by exposure to the seeds of a cycad plant which contain high concentrations of β-N-methylamino-

L-alanine (BMAA). It has been proposed that the gradual decrease in incidence of this disease in recent years can be attributed to a change in eating habits which has reduced the islanders' intake of BMAA (Spencer et al., 1987). While an excitotoxic mechanism has been suspected on the basis of in vitro studies showing that BMAA has neurotoxic properties that can be blocked by NMDA antagonists (Ross et al., 1987; Zeevalk et al., 1988), it is puzzling that the BMAA molecule lacks the omega acidic group which characterizes all other straight chain molecules with excitotoxic properties, including BOAA. Weiss and Choi (1988), having found that BMAA displays excitatory and neurotoxic activity only in the presence of physiological concentrations of bicarbonate, have proposed that bicarbonate interacts non-covalently with the positively charged beta-amino group of BMAA to produce a configuration appropriate for activation of Glu receptors. These studies provide an additional reminder that an investigation of mechanisms by which exogenous excitotoxins cause neurological diseases may eventually lead to a better understanding of mechanisms by which endogenous EAA, either alone or together with exogenous excitotoxins, can induce neurodegenerative processes.

Domoate poisoning

In 1987 there was an outbreak of food poisoning in northeastern Canada which affected 145 people, some of whom died and were found at autopsy to have disseminated acute lesions in the CNS (Hynie, 1989). Some of the survivors apparently sustained permanent brain damage as they were left with signs of mental confusion and profound memory impairment (anterograde amnesia). All of the afflicted individuals had eaten mussels from Prince Edward Island near Newfoundland. Analysis of these mussels by Canadian National Research Council scientists revealed high concentrations of domoic acid, an excitotoxic analog of Glu that interacts selectively and powerfully with the KA receptor (Debonnel et al., 1988). Some of the most severely affected individuals

were elderly. This provides a striking example of an acute excitotoxic neurodegenerative process being induced in human adults by accidental exposure to a food-born excitotoxic analog of Glu. The apparent hypersensitivity of elderly individuals to domoate poisoning is of particular interest as this suggests that the KA receptor is a potentially sensitive mediator of excitotoxic neuropathology in old age. In Fig. 1, the structural homology between Glu, KA and domoate is illustrated.

Metabolic disorders

Sulfite oxidase deficiency

The first human neurodegenerative condition to receive specific attention as a possible excitotoxin-mediated phenomenon was sulfite oxidase deficiency (Olney et al., 1975), a rare inherited disease in which an abnormal metabolite, cysteine-S-sulfate accumulates in body tissues and disseminated degeneration of CNS neurons occurs resulting in blindness, spastic quadriplegia and death in early infancy. It seems likely that cysteine-S-sulfate, acting by an excitotoxic mechanism, is responsible for neuronal degeneration in sulfite oxidase deficiency since cysteine-S-sulfate displays powerful excitotoxic activity when administered systemically to infant rats or microinjected into the adult rat brain (Olney et al., 1975).

Olivopontocerebellar degeneration

It has been shown (Plaitakis et al., 1980, 1982, 1984) that patients with the adult onset neurodegenerative disease, olivopontocerebellar degeneration (OPCD), have a deficiency of glutamic dehydrogenase enzyme activity which impairs their ability to metabolize Glu. Ingestion of Glu by such patients causes abnormally high levels of the amino acid in blood. Based on these findings, Plaitakis et al. (1982) have postulated a defect in CNS catabolism of Glu which may cause an excitotoxic build up of Glu at EAA receptors with consequent slow degeneration of CNS neurons.

Amyotrophic lateral sclerosis

Although individuals with amyotrophic lateral sclerosis (ALS) do not have a demonstrable deficiency of glutamic dehydrogenase, Plaitakis and Caroscio (1987) have shown that they resemble OPCD patients in developing abnormally high blood Glu levels following oral intake of Glu. Thus, a build up of Glu at CNS synapses on the basis of an unknown metabolic defect has been postulated to account for the degeneration of motor neurons in this disease. It should be borne in mind that if an exogenous excitotoxin such as BMAA can cause ALS-like degeneration of motor neuronal systems, it is possible that exogenous as well as endogenous excitotoxins might contribute to the development of the more classical form of ALS seen in the United States.

Epilepsy, hypoglycemia and hypoxia – ischemia

It has long been suspected that a common mechanism may underly brain damage associated with prolonged seizures, hypoglycemia and hypoxia – ischemia because the histopathology in each case has similar characteristics. Energy deficiency has been postulated as a common denominator although studies have not demonstrated an energy deficit at the site of injury in epilepsy-related brain damage. More recently, evidence implicating endogenous excitotoxins in the pathophysiology of each condition has provided a common denominator that may help clarify the situation. The most compelling evidence has been of three kinds. First, it is evident from both light and electron microscopic studies that similar cytopathological changes are induced in animal brain by each of these three conditions and that such changes are indistinguishable from those demonstrable in certain brain regions following subcutaneous administration of exogenous Glu (Fig. 3) (Auer et al., 1985; Olney et al., 1986a; Ikonomidou et al., 1989b). Second, there is evidence, especially in the case of hypoxia – ischemia (Benveniste et al., 1984), that these conditions trigger an outpouring of Glu and aspartate from the intra to extracellular compartment of brain which permits these agents to have prolonged contact with excitatory receptors through which they can exert excitotoxic effects. Third, it has been shown for each of these conditions that NMDA antagonists, such as MK-801, effectively protect against such damage (Rothman, 1984; Wieloch, 1985; Clifford et al., 1988; Olney et al., 1989). These three topics are more extensively reviewed elsewhere (Olney et al., 1986a; Rothman and Olney, 1986; Choi, 1988; Olney, 1989). A more detailed discussion of perinatal hypoxic – ischemic brain damage is given below.

CNS trauma

Brain and spinal cord injury

It is possible that CNS tissue injury may entail an outpouring of endogenous excitotoxins from the intra to extracellular compartment much as occurs under anoxic – ischemic conditions (Benveniste et al., 1984). If so, edematous swelling or other brain tissue pathology associated with trauma may be due, in part, to an excitotoxic action of endogenous EAA. Consistent with this interpretation, Katayama et al. (1988) recently demonstrated that concussive brain injury is associated with a 5-fold increase in extracellular Glu concentrations in the rat hippocampus. Other recent evidence suggests that behavioral morbidity associated with head trauma (Hayes et al., 1987) or spinal cord injury (Faden and Simon, 1987) is reduced by timely treatment with NMDA antagonists such as PCP and MK-801.

Dementia pugilistica

Dementia pugilistica is a dementing illness associated with professional boxing (Corsellis, 1978). If concussive brain injury is associated with elevated extracellular hippocampal concentrations of endogenous excitotoxins (Katayama et al., 1988), it is reasonable to propose that concussive blows delivered to the head in a boxing contest might cause a similar intra to extracellular translocation of excitotoxins. Conceivably, a series

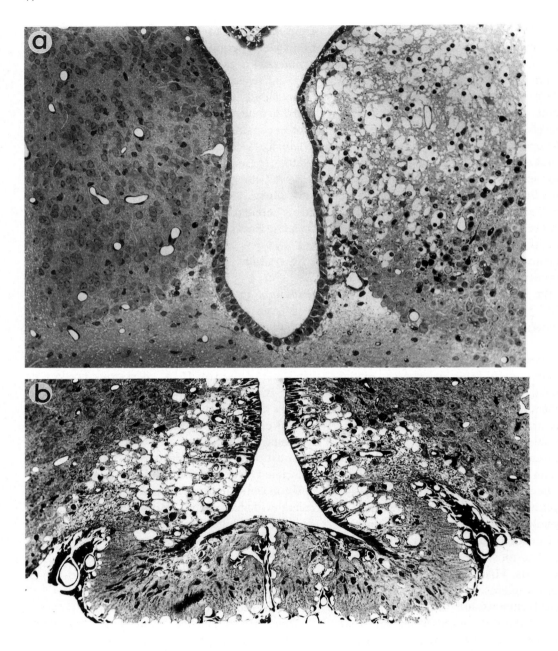

Fig. 3. *a* Depicts the medial habenular nucleus of a 10-day old rat subjected to unilateral carotid ligation and 75 min in a hypobaric chamber followed by 4 h recovery. The medial habenulum, a bilateral nucleus, exhibits damage unilaterally on the side ipsilateral to the carotid ligation. *b* Depicts the arcuate hypothalamic nucleus of a 21-day old mouse which had ingested a solution containing 10% monosodium Glu 4 h previously. Arcuate neurons are destroyed in a bilaterally symmetrical pattern. Note that the hypobaric/ischemic cytopathology (*a*) appears identical to that induced by exogenous Glu (*b*). Degenerating neurons in each case typically have swollen edematous cytoplasm and dark pyknotic nuclei. In this hypobaric/ischemic model neurons undergo this type of acute degeneration in numerous brain regions, including the dentate hippocampal gyrus, caudate nucleus, frontoparietal neocortex, olfactory tubercle, dorsal subiculum, islands of Calleja and several thalamic nuclei (magnification: 200 ×). (Adapted from Ikonomidou et al., 1989b.)

of initial concussive injuries and associated excitotoxin outpourings might sensitize hippocampal or other CNS neurons to an excitotoxic process rendering them hypervulnerable to eventual degeneration as subsequent concussive blows re-expose EAA receptors to abnormal concentrations of endogenous excitotoxins. It is noteworthy that neurofibrillary tangles (aggregates of paired helical filaments), which are prominently present in the brain in Alzheimer's disease, are found in great abundance in the brains of dementia pugilistica victims (Corsellis, 1978). This establishes a potential association between neurofibrillary tangles and repetitive exposure of EAA receptors to abnormal concentrations of endogenous excitotoxins. Reinforcing this association is the finding of De Boni and McLachlan (1985) that cultured human fetal spinal neurons develop paired helical filaments of the Alzheimer type when exposed to Glu or aspartate.

Other

Huntingtons disease

The demonstration that injection of excitotoxins, such as KA and ibotenic acid, into the rat striatum results in biochemical and pathomorphological changes resembling those in Huntington's disease (Coyle et al., 1978), provided a useful animal model for studying this neurodegenerative disease. More recent evidence that quinolinic acid, an excitotoxin found naturally in the brain, is more potent in destroying striatal than other CNS neurons (Schwarcz and Kohler, 1983; Beal et al., 1986) but selectively spares a population of aspiny striatal neurons (Martin et al., 1987) which are also spared in Huntington's disease (Ferrante et al., 1985), has raised hopes that the pathophysiology of neuronal degeneration in Huntington's disease might be traced to quinolinic acid or a similarly selective endogenous excitotoxin. A role for quinolinic acid itself is questionable in view of recent evidence that quinolinic acid concentrations in the striatum of individuals with Huntington's disease are not

elevated (Reynolds et al., 1988). However, this does not rule out the involvement of some other excitotoxic molecule with selective properties similar to those of quinolinic acid. It is thought that quinolinic acid acts predominantly at NMDA receptors and it has recently been shown that receptor loss in the striatum in Huntington's disease is disproportionately greater for NMDA than any other type of transmitter receptor (Young et al., 1988).

Alzheimer's disease

Several types of neurons, including cholinergic, somatostatinergic and noradrenergic, are known to degenerate in Alzheimer's disease (AD). Loss of basal forebrain cholinergic neurons that project to the cerebral cortex, hippocampus and amygdala is a striking feature of the neuropathology of AD which can be reproduced in experimental animals by injecting an excitotoxin into the basal forebrain region where these cells are located (Coyle et al., 1983). This has provided a useful animal model for studying the role of cholinergic neurons in the cognitive deficits associated with AD. The fact that excitotoxins are effective in destroying cholinergic neurons implies that these neurons have EAA receptors through which endogenous excitotoxins could act pathologically to destroy these neurons. Alternatively, it has been shown that topical application of an excitotoxin to the cerebral cortex causes retrograde degeneration of those basal forebrain cholinergic neurons that project to the cortex (Sofroniew and Pearson, 1985). Thus, an excitotoxic process can cause neuronal degeneration by either a direct or indirect mechanism and, since EAA receptors are present on many types of CNS neurons, an excitotoxic process, either direct or indirect, could explain the death of somatostatinergic and noradrenergic as well as cholinergic neurons.

Arendash et al. (1987) recently described late occurring pathological changes resembling neuritic plaques and neurofibrillary tangles in various limbic and neocortical regions of rat brain 14 months after injection of an excitotoxin into the basal forebrain to destroy cholinergic neurons. It will be important to determine whether this observation can be corroborated since, if it can, it becomes a tenable hypothesis that not only can the primary degeneration of various types of neurons in AD be explained by an excitotoxic process, but that other aspects of AD neuropathology (e.g., plaques and tangles) might arise as a delayed manifestation of or secondary reaction to this primary neurodegenerative process. Reinforcing this line of conjecture is the finding of De Boni and McLachlan (1985) that exposure of cultured human spinal neurons to abnormal concentrations of Glu or aspartate causes these neurons to produce paired helical filaments of the type that make up neurofibrillary tangles in AD. In addition, Procter and colleagues (1988) have presented evidence for a possible metabolic defect affecting glutamergic neurons in AD and Greenamyre et al. (1987) have described a striking loss of Glu receptors in the cerebral cortex and hippocampus of AD brains; however, the latter finding has been disputed (Cowburn et al., 1988). In summary, several lines of indirect evidence suggest that an excitotoxic mechanism could be involved in the pathophysiology of AD, but there is not enough direct evidence to establish the connection.

Parkinsonism

Although very little evidence has been presented to suggest a link between an excitotoxic mechanism and neuronal degeneration in Parkinsonism, Sonsalla et al. (1988) recently demonstrated that the neurotoxic action of methamphetamine against dopaminergic nigrostriatal neurons (a dopamine-dependent form of neurotoxicity) is blocked by MK-801. These authors suggest that methamphetamine neurotoxicity may resemble ischemic brain damage in the sense that oxidative stress and the unleashing of excitotoxic mechanisms may occur in both conditions. Since the neurons that degenerate selectively in Parkinsonism are dopaminergic nigrostriatal neurons, the demonstration that these neurons are vulnerable to excitotoxic injury triggered by a poorly understood

dopamine-linked mechanism provides a basis for postulating that an excitotoxic mechanism could play a role in Parkinsonian neuronal degeneration. Also of interest is the observation (Corsellis, 1978) that Parkinsonian symptoms and spontaneous degeneration of nigrostriatal neurons is a feature of the neuropathology in dementia pugilistica. Thus, it is possible that nigrostriatal neurons are sensitive to a pathological sequence in which either physical trauma or some toxic agent induces oxidative stress which unleashes the excitotoxic potential of endogenous EAA against these dopaminergic cells.

Excitotoxicity and the developing CNS

Perinatal hypoxia – ischemia and NMDA receptor hypersensitivity

Recently we have been exploring a new model for studying hypoxic – ischemic brain damage in which infant rats are subjected to unilateral carotid ligation followed by 75 min in a hypobaric chamber (225 mm Hg). We have shown (Ikonomidou et al., 1989b) that this approach results in patches of acute neuronal necrosis disseminated over many brain regions (frontoparietal neocortex, caudate/putamen, thalamus, hippocampus, medial habenulum, septum and olfactory tubercle) and that the acute neurodegenerative reaction is identical, both in time course and type of cytopathology, to that observed in the hypothalamus of immature rodents or monkeys treated systemically with Glu (Fig. 3) (Olney, 1971; Olney et al., 1972). We have also corroborated the observation of McDonald et al. (1988) that the infant rat is much more sensitive than the adult rat to the neurotoxic action of NMDA (Ikonomidou et al., 1989a). In fact, injection of nanomolar amounts of NMDA directly into the infant rat brain causes widespread neuronal degeneration that appears identical to hypobaric/ischemic neuronal degeneration, and the neuronal populations most sensitive to NMDA toxicity are the same as those most sensitive to hypobaric/ischemic degeneration (Ikonomidou et al., 1989a). Moreover, administration of the NMDA-specific antagonist, MK-801, provides excellent protection against either NMDA neurotoxicity or hypobaric/ischemic neuronal degeneration (Olney et al., 1989). These findings strongly implicate the NMDA receptor in perinatal hypoxic – ischemic brain damage.

Extending the above comparison further, we have found that sensitivity to either NMDA neurotoxicity or to hypobaric/ischemic brain damage increases during the first few days of life to reach peak sensitivity in the rat between postnatal days 6 – 10 and steadily declines thereafter (Ikonomidou et al., 1989a). This suggests that there is a period spanning approximately the first 2 weeks of neonatal life in the rat during which NMDA receptors may be hypersensitive to EAA stimulation. We propose that during this period, CNS neurons housing such receptors may be hypervulnerable to excitotoxic degeneration, i.e., only mild anoxia or oxidative stress may be sufficient to trigger neuronal degeneration. We also have observed that each neuronal group is governed by its own timetable for onset and duration of the period of peak sensitivity (Ikonomidou et al., 1989a). If the developing human is subject to a similar phenomenon, we propose that the period of NMDA receptor hypersensitivity in the human may span months rather than weeks and that different combinations of CNS neurons may be hypervulnerable at any given time during this period. Thus, a pathological process involving NMDA receptors might produce several different patterns of neuronal loss depending on the developmental stage in which the pathological event occurred. If so, the neuropsychiatric deficit syndrome resulting in later life might vary accordingly from cerebral palsy-like neurological disorders to schizophrenia-like psychiatric disturbances.

Necrobiosis

Recent studies (Aruffo et al., 1987; Pearce et al., 1987; Balazs et al., 1988) suggest that endogenous EAA may exert a neurotrophic action which the developing neuron depends upon for survival while it is establishing its functional connections with other neural CNS components. A process of necrobiosis is recognized whereby neurons which fail to establish appropriate connections (so called "redundant" neurons), are destroyed in the course of ontogenesis. It is possible that necrobiosis might be mediated by the simple termination of the neurotrophic influence of endogenous EAA at a time when a neuron that has not achieved its integrated status still needs neurotrophic assistance to survive. On the other hand, when neurons acquire the ability to excite other neurons by release of endogenous EAA, they presumably also acquire neurodestructive potential which must be held in check by various accessory mechanisms, such as EAA re-uptake transport processes and activation of Zn^{2+}, Mg^{2+} or PCP receptors. If substantial release of neuroexcitant should occur at NMDA receptors before these accessory mechanisms are in place to provide a counterbalancing action, excitotoxic destruction of the stimulated cell might occur. Conceivably this might be a mechanism built into the CNS for eliminating redundant neural units. While it is assumed that this is a benevolent process whereby only redundant components are eliminated, it is possible that the process might become aberrant and destroy many additional neurons that are not redundant; indeed, how do we know that any neurons are truly redundant?

Excitotoxicity and aging

In mid adult life it is believed that CNS neurons begin to die and that there is a steady attrition of neurons from that point unto death. Considering the several agonist and antagonist principles that constitute counterbalancing components of the NMDA/Gly/PCP/Zn^{2+}/Mg^{2+} receptor – ionophore complex, and evidence that this receptor – ionophore complex is widely distributed throughout the forebrain, it is not unreasonable to postulate an age-linked shift in the dynamic equilibrium of this system such that the agonist driving mechanisms overwhelm the antagonist forces in the micro-environment of a given neuron, the result being excitotoxic death of that neuron. Such a process could account for the "normal" death of a large number of CNS neurons as a function of age.

Whereas NMDA receptors are characteristically hypersensitive in early life and non-NMDA receptors are relatively hyposensitive, the opposite is true in adulthood. It is known, for example, that direct injection of KA into the rat brain causes a much more severe excitotoxic reaction in the adult than infant brain (Campochiaro and Coyle, 1978). Therefore, although we know less about non-NMDA receptors, it is reasonable to postulate that eventually they may prove at least as important as NMDA receptors in mediating neurodegenerative phenomena in the adult and aging brain. Considerable attention has been paid to the potential role of NMDA receptors in the mediation of long-term potentiation and memory, the implication being that these receptors are prime candidates for complicity in memory impairment disorders. However, the recent observation that domoate poisoning results in profound memory deficits in adult and aging humans suggests that excitotoxic mechanisms operating through non-NMDA EAA receptors can also give rise to memory disturbances in this critical age group.

In addition to the various components comprising the make up of post-synaptic EAA receptors and associated ion channels, there are pre-synaptic mechanisms governing the release and reuptake of EAA transmitters which must function optimally throughout life in order to maintain homeostatic balance and prevent the expression of an excitotoxic process. The high affinity uptake system that is responsible for removing synaptically released Glu from the receptor environment is an excellent case in point. Reduced efficiency of this system as a function of age or disease is a mechanism that could easily explain either a rapidly or slowly evolving neurodegenerative process. It is relevant to note that either hyper- or hypofunction of EAA receptor systems could lead to disturbances in cognition and memory. For example, excessive activation of EAA receptors can lead to an excitotoxic process that literally eliminates the EAA receptor-bearing neurons from neural networks subserving memory functions. However, hypofunction of EAA release mechanisms or hyposensitivity of EAA receptors would similarly reduce the capacity of EAA neurons to participate in the mediation of memory functions.

Summary

Here I have discussed current issues in excitotoxicology (neurotoxicity of Glu and related agents) with special emphasis on the NMDA receptor and its possible role in neuropsychiatric disorders. I have briefly described several classes of anti-excitotoxic agents which are currently under study for their ability to protect neurons against excitotoxin-mediated neuronal degeneration. There is growing interest in the possibility that such agents, especially NMDA antagonists, will prove useful in the clinical management of neurodegenerative disorders; however, neither their efficacy nor safety has been adequately established at present. With the plethora of new information about the NMDA receptor – ionophore complex, one tends to forget that non-NMDA receptors can also mediate excitotoxic events. Thus, although we know less about the physiology and make up of non-NMDA receptors, it seems likely that new information, as it becomes available, will reveal new links between endogenous excitotoxins and neuropsychiatric disease processes. In particular, since NMDA receptors are relatively more sensitive in early life and non-NMDA receptors more sensitive in adulthood, it is reasonable to postulate the greatest involvement of the former in developmental psychoneuropathology and the latter in neurodegenerative diseases of the elderly.

Acknowledgements

This work was supported in part by NIMH Research Scientist Award MH 38894 and HHS grants HD 24237, DA 05072 and AG 05681.

References

Arendash, G.W., Millard, W.J., Dunn, A.J. and Meyer, E.M. (1987) Long-term neuropathological and neurochemical effects of nucleus basalis lesions in the rat. *Science*, 238: 952 – 956.

Aruffo, C., Ferszi, R., Hildebrandt, A.G. and Cervos-Navarro, J. (1987) Low doses of L-monosodium glutamate promote neuronal growth and differentiation in vitro. *Dev. Neurosci.*, 9: 228 – 239.

Auer, R.N., Kalimo, H., Olsson, Y. and Wieloch, T. (1985) The dentate gyrus in hypoglycemia. Pathology implicating excitotoxin-mediated neuronal necrosis. *Acta Neuropathol. (Berl.)*, 67: 279 – 288.

Balazs, R., Hack, N. and Jorgensen, O.S. (1988) Stimulation of the N-methyl-D-aspartate receptor has a trophic effect on differentiating cerebellar granule cells. *Neurosci. Lett.*, 87: 80 – 86.

Beal, M.F., Kowall, N.W., Ellison, D.W., Mazurek, M.F., Swartz, K.J. and Martin, J.B. (1986) Replication of neurochemical characteristics of Huntington's disease by quinolinic acid. *Nature*, 321: 168 – 171.

Benveniste, H., Drejer, J., Schousboe, A. and Diemer, N.M. (1984) Elevation of the extracellular concentrations of glutamate and aspartate in rat hippocampus during transient cerebral ischemia monitored by intracerebral microdialysis. *J. Neurochem.*, 43: 1369 – 1374.

Campochiaro, P. and Coyle, J.T. (1978) Ontogenetic development of kainate neurotoxicity; correlates with glutamatergic innervation. *Proc. Natl. Acad. Sci. U.S.A.*, 75: 2025 – 2029.

Choi, D.W. (1985) Glutamate neurotoxicity in cortical cell culture is calcium dependent. *Neurosci. Lett.*, 58: 293 – 297.

Choi, D.W. (1988) Glutamate neurotoxicity and diseases of the nervous system. *Neuron*, 1: 623 – 634.

Choi, D.W., Koh, J. and Peters, S. (1988) Pharmacology of Glu neurotoxicity in cortical cell culture: attenuation by NMDA antagonists. *J. Neurosci.*, 8: 185 – 196.

Clifford, D.B., Benz, A., Olney, J.W. and Zorumski, C.F. (1988) MK-801 prevents seizure-related brain damage from pilocarpine and lithium – pilocarpine epidural well seizures. *Neurosci. Abstr.*, 14: 417.

Corsellis, J. (1978) Posttraumatic dementia. In: R.T. Katzman, R.D. Terry and K.L. Bick (Eds.), *Alzheimer's Disease: Senile Dementia and Related Disorders*, Raven Press, New York, pp. 125 – 133.

Cowburn, R., Hardy, J., Roberts, P. and Briggs, R. (1988) Presynaptic and postsynaptic glutamatergic function in Alzheimer's disease. *Neurosci. Lett.*, 86: 109 – 113.

Coyle, J.T., McGeer, E.F., McGeer, P.L. and Schwarcz, R. (1978) Neostriatal injections: a model for Huntington's chorea. In: E.G. McGeer, J.W. Olney and P.L. McGeer (Eds.), *Kainic Acid as a Tool in Neurobiology*, Raven Press, New York, pp. 139 – 159.

Coyle, J.T., Price, D.L. and De Long, M.A. (1983) Alzheimer's disease: a disorder of cortical cholinergic innervation. *Science*, 219: 1184 – 1190.

Curtis, D.R. and Watkins, J.C. (1963) Acidic amino acids with strong excitatory actions on mammalian neurons. *J. Physiol.*, 166: 1 – 14.

Debonnel, G., Teitelbaum, J., Carpenter, S.L., Beauchesne, L., Antel, J., Cashman, A.N. and De Montigny, C. (1988) The "mussel toxin", domoic acid, produces its neurotoxic effect through kainate receptor: clinical and electrophysiological studies. *Soc. Neurosci. Abstr.*, 14: 240.

De Boni, U. and McLachlan, D.R.C. (1985) Controlled induction of paired helical filaments of the Alzheimer type in cultured human neurons by Glu and aspartate. *J. Neurol. Sci.*, 68: 105 – 118.

Faden, A.I. and Simon, R.P. (1987) N-methyl-D-aspartate receptor antagonist MK-801 improves outcome following experimental spinal cord injury in rats. *Neurosci. Abstr.*, 13: 1031.

Ferrante, R.J., Kowall, N.W., Beal, M.F., Richardson, E.P., Jr., Bird, E.D. and Martin, J.B. (1985) Selective sparing of a class of striatal neurons in Huntington's Disease. *Science*, 230: 561 – 563.

Goldberg, M.P., Pham, P. and Choi, D.W. (1987) Dextrorphan and dextromethorphan attenuate hypoxic injury in neuronal culture. *Neurosci. Lett.*, 80: 11 – 15.

Greenamyre, T.J., Penny, J.B., D'Amato, C.J. and Young, A.B. (1987) Dementia of the Alzheimer's type: changes in hippocampal L-[^{3}H]Glu binding. *J. Neurochem.*, 48: 543 – 551.

Hayes, R.L., Chapouris, R., Lyeth, B.G., Jenkins, L., Robinson, S.E., Young, H.F. and Marmarou, A. (1987) Pretreatment with phencyclidine (PCP) attenuates long-term behavioral deficits following concussive brain injury in the rat. *Neurosci. Abstr.*, 13: 1254.

Honore, T., Davies, S.N., Drejer, J., Fletcher, E.J., Jacobsen, P., Lodge, D. and Nielsen, F.E. (1988) Quinoxalinediones: potent competitive non-NMDA Glu receptor antagonists. *Science*, 241: 701 – 703.

Hynie, I. (1989) *Proceedings of Symposium on Domoic Acid Toxicity held at the Health Protection Branch, Health and Welfare Canada, April 10 – 11, 1989* (in press).

Ikonomidou, C., Mosinger, J., Shahid Salles, K., Labruyere, J. and Olney, J.W. (1989a) Parallel patterns of hypersensitivity to NMDA toxicity and hypobaric/ischemic damage in developing rat brain. *Neurosci. Abstr.*, 14: 501.

Ikonomidou, C., Price, M.T., Mosinger, J.L., Frierdich, G.,

Labruyere, J., Shahid Salles, K. and Olney, J.W. (1989b) Hypobaric-ischemic conditions produce Glu-like cytopathology in infant rat brain. *J. Neurosci.* (in press).

Katayama, Y., Cheung, M.K., Gorman, L., Tamura, T. and Becker, D.P. (1988) Increase in extracellular Glu and associated massive ionic fluxes following concussive brain injury. *Neurosci. Abstr.,* 14: 1154.

Lodge, D. and Anis, N.A. (1982) Effects of phencyclidine on excitatory amino acid activation of spinal interneurons in the cat. *Eur. J. Pharmacol.,* 77: 203 – 204.

Lodge, D., Aram, J.A., Church, J. et al. (1987) Excitatory amino acids and phencyclidine-like drugs. In: T.P. Hicks, D. Lodge and H. McLennan (Eds.), *Excitatory Amino Acid Transmission,* Alan R. Liss, New York.

Lucas, D.R. and Newhouse, J.P. (1957) The toxic effect of sodium L-Glu on the inter layers of the retina. *AMA Arch. Ophthalmol.,* 58: 193 – 201.

Martin, J.B., Kowall, N.W., Ferrante, R.J., Cipolloni, P.B. and Beal, M.F. (1987) Differential sparing of NADPH-diaphorase neurons in quinolinic lesioned rat and primate striatum. *Neurosci. Abstr.,* 14: 1030.

McDonald, J.W., Silverstein, F.S. and Johnston, M.V. (1988) Neurotoxicity of N-methyl-D-aspartate is markedly enhanced in developing rat central nervous system. *Brain Res.,* 459: 200 – 203.

Olney, J.W. (1969a) Brain lesions, obesity and other disturbances in mice treated with monosodium Glu. *Science,* 164: 719 – 721.

Olney, J.W. (1969b) Glutamate-induced retinal degeneration in neonatal mice. Electron microscopy of the acutely evolving lesion. *J. Neuropathol. Exp. Neurol.,* 28: 455 – 474.

Olney, J.W. (1971) Glutamate-induced neuronal necrosis in the infant mouse hypothalamus: an electron microscopic study. *J. Neuropathol. Exp. Neurol.,* 30: 75 – 90.

Olney, J.W. (1984) Excitotoxic food additives – relevance of animal studies to human safety. *Neurobehav. Toxicol. Teratol.,* 6: 455 – 462.

Olney, J.W. (1987) Food additives, excitotoxic. In: G. Adelman (Ed.), *Encyclopedia of Neuroscience,* Birkhauser, Boston, MA, pp. 436 – 438.

Olney, J.W. (1989) Excitatory amino acids and neuro-psychiatric disorders. *Biol. Psychiatry* (in press).

Olney, J.W., Ho, O.L. and Rhee, V. (1971) Cytotoxic effects of acidic and sulphur-containing amino acids on the infant mouse central nervous system. *Exp. Brain Res.,* 14: 61 – 76.

Olney, J.W., Sharpe, L.G. and Feigin, R.D. (1972) Glutamate-induced brain damage in infant primates. *J. Neuropathol. Exp. Neurol.,* 31: 464 – 488.

Olney, J.W., Misra, C.H. and DeGubareff, T. (1975) Cysteine-S-sulfate: brain damaging metabolite in sulfite oxidase deficiency. *J. Neuropathol. Exp. Neurol.,* 34: 167 – 176.

Olney, J.W., Misra, C.H. and Rhee, V. (1976) Brain and retinal damage from the lathyrus excitotoxin, b-N-oxalyl-L-α β diaminopropionic acid (ODAP). *Nature,* 264: 659 – 661.

Olney, J.W., DeGubareff, T. and Labruyere, J. (1979) α-Aminoadipate blocks the neurotoxic action of N-methylaspartate. *Life Sci.,* 25: 537 – 540.

Olney, J.W., Labruyere, J., Collins, J.F. and Curry, K. (1981) D-Aminophosphonovalerate is 100-fold more powerful than D-alpha-aminoadipate in blocking N-methylaspartate neurotoxicity. *Brain Res.,* 221: 207 – 210.

Olney, J.W., Collins, R.C. and Sloviter, R.S. (1986a) Excitotoxic mechanisms of epileptic brain damage. In: A.V. Delgado-Escueta, A.A. Ward, D.M. Woodbury and R.J. Porter (Eds.), *Basic Mechanisms of the Epilepsies: Molecular and Cellular Approaches,* Raven Press, New York, pp. 857 – 878.

Olney, J.W., Price, M.T., Fuller, T.A., Labruyere, J., Samson, L., Carpenter, M. and Mahan, K. (1986b) The anti-excitotoxic effects of certain anesthetics, analgesics and sedative-hypnotics. *Neurosci. Lett.,* 68: 29 – 34.

Olney, J.W., Price, M.T., Samson, L. and Labruyere, J. (1986c) The role of specific ions in Glu neurotoxicity. *Neurosci. Lett.,* 65: 65 – 71.

Olney, J., Price, M., Shahid Salles, K., Labruyere, J. and Frierdich, G. (1987a) MK-801 powerfully protects against N-methyl aspartate neurotoxicity. *Eur. J. Pharmacol.,* 141: 357 – 361.

Olney, J.W., Price, M.T., Labruyere, J., Shahid Salles, K., Frierdich, G., Mueller, M. and Silverman, E. (1987b) Anti-parkinsonian agents are phencyclidine agonists and N-methyl aspartate antagonists. *Eur. J. Pharmacol.,* 142: 319 – 320.

Olney, J.W., Ikonomidou, C., Mosinger, J.L. and Frierdich, G. (1989) MK-801 prevents hypobaric-ischemic neuronal degeneration in infant rat brain. *J. Neurosci.* (in press).

Pearce, I.A., Cambray-Deakin, M.A. and Burgoyne, R.D. (1987) Glutamate acting on NMDA receptors stimulates neurite outgrowth from cerebellar granule cells. *FEBS Lett.,* 223: 143 – 147.

Plaitakis, A. and Caroscio, J.T. (1987) Abnormal Glu metabolism in amyotrophic lateral sclerosis. *Ann. Neurol.,* 22: 575 – 579.

Plaitakis, A., Nicklas, W.J. and Desnick, R.J. (1980) Glutamate dehydrogenase deficiency in three patients with spinocerebellar syndrome. *Ann. Neurol.,* 7: 297 – 303.

Plaitakis, A., Berl, S. and Yahr, M.D. (1982) Abnormal Glu metabolism in an adult-onset degenerative neurological disorder. *Science,* 216: 193 – 196.

Plaitakis, A., Berl, S. and Yahr, M. (1984) Neurological disorders associated with deficiency of Glu dehydrogenase. *Ann. Neurol.,* 15: 144 – 153.

Price, M.T., Honore, T., Mueller, M.E., Labruyere, J., Silverman, E. and Olney, J.W. (1988) CNQX potently and selectively blocks kainate excitotoxicity in the chick embryo retina. *Neurosci. Abstr.,* 14: 418.

Procter, A.W., Palmer, A.M., Francis, P.T., Lowe, S.L., Neary, D., Murphy, E., Doshi, R. and Bowen, D.M. (1988) Evidence of glutamergic denervation and possible abnormal metabolism in Alzheimer's disease. *J. Neurochem.,* 50: 790 – 801.

Reynolds, G.P., Pearson, S.J., Halket, J. and Sandler, M. (1988) Brain quinolinic acid in Huntington's disease. *J. Neurochem.,* 50: 1959 – 1960.

Robinson, M.B. and Coyle, J.T. (1987) Glutamate and related acidic excitatory neurotransmitters: from basic science to clinical application. *FASEB J.,* 1: 446 – 455.

Ross, S.M., Seelig, M. and Spencer, P.S. (1987) Specific antagonism of excitotoxic action of "uncommon" amino acids assayed in organotypic mouse cortical cultures. *Brain Res.,* 425: 120 – 127.

Rothman, S.M. (1984) Synaptic release of excitatory amino acid neurotransmitter mediates anoxic neuronal death. *J. Neurosci.,* 4: 1884 – 1891.

Rothman, S.M. (1985) Excitatory amino acid neurotoxicity is produced by passive chloride influx. *J. Neurosci.,* 6: 1483 – 1489.

Rothman, S.M. and Olney, J.W. (1986) Glutamate and the pathophysiology of hypoxic – ischemic brain damage. *Ann. Neurol.,* 19: 105 – 111.

Schwarcz, R. and Kohler, C. (1983) Differential vulnerability of central neurons of the rat to quinolinic acid. *Neurosci. Lett.,* 38: 85 – 90.

Sofroniew, M.V. and Pearson, R.C.A. (1985) Degeneration of cholinergic neurons in the basal nucleus following kainic or *N*-methyl-D-aspartic acid application to the cerebral cortex in the rat. *Brain Res.,* 339: 186 – 190.

Sonsalla, P.K., Nicklas, W.J. and Heikkila, R.E. (1988) (+)MK-801 protects against methamphetamine (METH)-induced, but not MPTP-induced, neurotoxicity in mice. *Neurosci. Abstr.,* 14: 1216.

Spencer, P.S., Schaumburg, H.H., Cohn, D.F. and Seth, P.K. (1984) Lathyrism: a useful model of primary lateral sclerosis. In: F.C. Rose (Ed.), *Research Progress in Motor Neurone Disease,* Pitman, London, pp. 312 – 327.

Spencer, P.S., Ludolph, A., Dwived, M.P., Roy, D.N., Hugon, J. and Schaumburg, H.H. (1986) Lathyrism: evidence for role of the neuroexcitatory amino acid BOAA. *Lancet,* 1066 – 1067.

Spencer, P.S., Nunn, P.B., Hugon, J., Ludolph, A.C., Ross, S.M., Roy, D.N. and Robertson, R.C. (1987) Guam amyotrophic lateral sclerosis – Parkinsonism – dementia linked to a plant excitant neurotoxin. *Science,* 237: 517 – 522.

TINS (1987) Excitatory amino acids in the brain − focus on NMDA receptors. *Trends Neurosci.,* 10: 263 – 302.

Watkins, J.C. (1978) Excitatory amino acids. In: E. McGeer, J.W. Olney and P. McGeer (Eds.), *Kainic Acid as a Tool in Neurobiology,* Raven Press, New York, pp. 37 – 69.

Watkins, J.C. and Evans, R.H. (1981) Excitatory amino acid transmitters. *Ann. Rev. Pharmacol. Toxicol.,* 21: 165 – 204.

Weiss, J.H. and Choi, D.W. (1988) Beta-*N*-methylamino-L-alanine neurotoxicity: requirement for bicarbonate as a cofactor. *Science,* 241: 973 – 975.

Wieloch, T. (1985) Hypoglycemia-induced neuronal damage prevented by an *N*-methyl-D-aspartate antagonist. *Science,* 230: 681 – 683.

Young, A.B., Greenamyre, J.T., Hollingsworth, Z., Albin, R., D'Amato, C., Shoulson, I. and Penney, J.B. (1988) NMDA receptor losses in putamen from patients with Huntington's disease. *Science,* 241: 981 – 983.

Zeevalk, G., Olynyk, S. and Nicklas, W. (1988) Excitotoxicity in chick retina caused by the unusual amino acids BOAA and BMAA: effects of MK-801 and DIDS. *Neurosci. Abstr.,* 14: 418.

SECTION III

Plasticity in Normal and Aging Systems and in AD

P. Coleman, G. Higgins and C. Phelps (Eds.)
Progress in Brain Research, Vol. 86
© 1990 Elsevier Science Publishers B.V. (Biomedical Division)

CHAPTER 5

Plasticity of excitatory amino acid receptors: implications for aging and Alzheimer's disease

Carl W. Cotman, James W. Geddes*, Jolanta Ulas and Martina Klein

*Department of Psychobiology, and * Division of Neurosurgery, University of California, Irvine, CA 92717, U.S.A.*

Introduction

Excitatory amino acid (EAA) pathways represent the major system responsible for information transduction in the telencephalic regions of the CNS. The endogenous EAAs L-glutamate, and possibly L-aspartate, act on at least five distinct receptors, each of which can be activated by a selective amino acid analog (Monaghan et al., 1989). The best understood receptor class is the NMDA (*N*-methyl-D-aspartate) type, which is a macromolecular complex consisting of glutamate binding site, an allosteric regulatory site, and an ion channel (see Cotman et al., 1988). More recently, it has become apparent that there are two distinct classes of NMDA receptors which differ in their anatomical distribution and in their pharmacological properties (Monaghan et al., 1988b). The other EAA receptor classes include the KA (kainic acid), QA/AMPA (quisqualate), L-AP4 (L-2-amino-4-phosphonobutyrate), and ACPD (trans-1-amino-cyclopentyl-1,3-dicarboxylic acid) sites (for further discussion see Monaghan et al., 1989).

NMDA receptors are particularly concentrated in brain areas such as hippocampal and cortical regions, where they appear to be involved in higher cognitive function (see Cotman and Iversen, 1987; Cotman et al., 1989). EAA synapses work through a dual receptor system: non-NMDA receptors, most probably the QA/AMPA type, serve fast-acting responses, while NMDA receptors both amplify the synaptic response and permit calcium entry if there is concurrent post-synaptic depolarization. Synapses that possess NMDA receptors display novel properties that are postulated to account for activity-dependent processes such as temporal integration and synaptic plasticity (Cotman et al., 1988). NMDA receptors may be part of a general mechanism common to both developmental plasticity and some forms of learning. These receptors may also play a pivotal role in the neuronal loss which results from epilepsy, ischemia and hypoglycemia (Meldrum, 1985), and it is often the large, pyramidal neurons which utilize EAA transmitters which appear to be particularly vulnerable in Alzheimer's disease (AD) (see Greenamyre et al., 1988).

In view of the critical role of the NMDA and other EAA receptors in higher brain function, it is essential to understand their properties in the developing, mature, aged, injured and diseased brain. We have developed radioligand binding techniques in order to examine the various receptor components of the EAA system. Our studies have largely focused on the hippocampus, in particular the hippocampal alterations that occur following the loss of the major cortical input to the hippocampus which originates in the entorhinal cortex. As will be discussed in more detail later, the entorhinal cortex is vulnerable in normal aging and in Alzheimer's disease, and lesions of the entorhinal cortex have been widely used as a model system in which to examine synaptic plasticity.

EAA receptors and development

NMDA receptors appear to play an important role in developmental plasticity. During development, fibers are guided to their proper targets and their synaptic position appears to be refined in an activity-dependent process. This fine tuning appears to involve NMDA receptor activation. In the kitten visual system (Singer, 1987), intracortical infusion of the NMDA antagonist AP5 during the critical period (2 – 3 months after birth) disrupted the formation of ocular dominance columns. Similarly, blockade of NMDA receptors in the neonatal rat interfered with olfactory learning and also blocked the enhanced uptake of 2-deoxyglucose normally observed after odor preference training (Lincoln et al., 1988). Recent evidence suggests that the increase in the activity of select glomeruli observed with early olfactory training is due to an increase (21%) in total neuronal number (Woo and Leon, 1989). This suggests that NMDA receptor activation may directly or indirectly affect neuronal number in select glomeruli.

Research with cultured neurons has suggested that glutamate, acting through NMDA receptors, may serve a trophic role on developing neurons. Enhancement of neurite outgrowth and cell survival in the presence of NMDA or glutamate, and blocked by AP5, has been demonstrated in cultured cerebellar granule cells (Balazs et al., 1989). In cultures of immature dentate gyrus granule cells NMDA stimulates neurite branching (Brewer and Cotman, 1989). Whether neurons in olfactory glomeruli are under similar influences is unknown at present.

Taken together, the above data suggest that the NMDA receptor may participate in both neurite elongation, branching, and the refinement of synaptic position during early development. In addition to serving synaptic transmission, NMDA receptors may serve a type of trophic function during reactive synaptogenesis.

EAA receptors and injury

Damage to the entorhinal cortex, a region sensitive to both age- and Alzheimer's disease related losses, has been used extensively as a model system to examine the compensatory mechanisms which strive to maintain the information conveyed by the EAA system. The perforant path, originating in the entorhinal cortex, represents the major cortical input to the hippocampus and utilizes glutamate as a transmitter. Entorhinal fibers terminate mainly on granule cell dendrites in the outer 2/3 of the molecular layer of the dentate gyrus. A second pathway, which is also thought to utilize glutamate as a transmitter, the commissural/associational (C/A) pathway, originates in the hilus and terminates in the inner 1/3 of the dentate gyrus molecular layer (see Cotman and Anderson, 1988 for review).

The excitatory amino acid receptors in the dentate gyrus molecular layer are distributed in accordance with the terminal zones of the afferent inputs, and this distribution is altered in association with the reorganization of the circuits which occurs following the loss of entorhinal input to this region.

In the rat and human hippocampus, there is a high density of kainic acid receptors in the inner 1/3 of the dentate gyrus molecular layer, corresponding to the terminal zone of the C/A system (Monaghan and Cotman, 1982; Geddes et al., 1985). In response to the loss of entorhinal neurons in rodents, the C/A terminal zone expands until it occupies the inner half of the molecular layer and this is accompanied by an expanded distribution of KA receptors (Geddes et al., 1985; Geddes and Cotman, 1986). Scatchard analysis revealed an increase in the B_{max} of both low and high affinity KA binding sites at 60 days post-lesion with no change in the Kd of either the low or high affinity sites (Ulas et al., 1990b).

The expansion of the C/A pathway is evident as early as 4 days post-lesion and synapse formation begins shortly thereafter, about 7 days post-lesion, yet the expanded distribution of KA receptors is not evident until post-lesion day 30 (Fig. 1; Ulas et

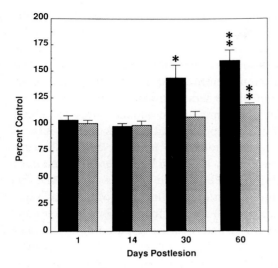

Fig. 1. Density of [³H] kainic acid binding sites in the rat inner and outer molecular layer of the dentate gyrus following lesions of the entorhinal cortex. The black bars represent values obtained from the outer 2/3, and the light bars represent binding densities observed in the inner 1/3 of the molecular layer of the dentate gyrus ipsilateral to the lesion. The results are expressed as percent of unoperated controls and represent the mean values (± S.E.M.) obtained from the dorsal and ventral blades; *P < 0.05; **P < 0.001. The results demonstrate that the increase in kainic acid receptor density in the outer 2/3 of the molecular layer is not apparent until approximately 30 days post-lesion (data obtained from Ulas et al., 1990b).

al., submitted). This time course suggests that synapse formation precedes the appearance of the additional KA acid receptors, and that the characteristics of the reinnervating afferent fibers help to determine the identity of the post-synaptic receptor systems.

The density of NMDA and QA receptors, which are more evenly distributed across the molecular layer, are also altered following entorhinal cortex lesions. A small transient decrease (15 – 20%) in the binding density of QA receptors was found in the deafferented molecular layer of the ipsilateral dentate gyrus 3 days post-lesion. At later post-lesion times (30 – 60 days), the density of both NMDA and QA receptors in the ipsilateral molecular layer was higher (15 – 50%) than in unoperated controls throughout the entire

molecular layer (Ulas et al., 1990a).

Contralateral to the lesion, the molecular layer of the dentate gyrus is only minimally denervated but exhibited a 10 – 15% increase in NMDA receptor density (relative to unoperated controls), with no change in the density of QA receptors. This increase was observed in both the partially denervated outer 2/3 and the non-denervated inner 1/3 of the molecular layer as early as 3 days post-lesion and remained through all post-lesion times examined (Ulas et al., 1990a). The appearance of the increased NMDA receptor density coincides with a period of intense synapse loss in the contralateral hippocampus and is indicative of an early compensatory plastic response of NMDA receptors by which transmission may be maintained despite a turnover of synapses. The bilateral response of NMDA receptors, in contrast to unilateral response of quisqualate receptors, suggests that NMDA receptors are in a position to play a special role in facilitating the overall functional balance of the system.

The increased KA receptor density would be predicted to enhance membrane depolarization, making it more probable that NMDA receptors would be activated. Overall, the greater receptor density might increase the ability of released glutamate to drive dentate granule cells, but the enhanced function may come at the expense of a heightened vulnerability to excitotoxicity. This would be particularly true in the aged brain where such changes may occur against changing EAA receptor properties.

EAA receptors and normal aging

In Fisher-344 rats, there are significant regional variations in NMDA receptor properties with age. In particular, there appears to be a selective loss of NMDA receptor density in the entorhinal cortex, striatum, and subiculum (Monaghan et al., 1988a). It is interesting that each of these regions is associated with age-related neuropathologies. Loss of striatal neurons occurs in Huntington's disease while Alzheimer's disease is associated with a loss of entorhinal and subicular neurons. In other rodents, the status of NMDA receptors appears to be dependent upon the brain region and the strain. There is a 45% loss in the NMDA receptor B_{max} in the Balb/c mouse whereas the loss in the C57/BL strain is only 17% (Peterson et al., 1989).

EAA receptors and AD

In Alzheimers's disease (AD) there is a striking pathology and significant loss of entorhinal neurons (Hyman et al., 1984) which in the molecular layer of the hippocampus appears to induce compensatory responses from the associational system and cholinergic septal afferents similar to those observed in the rat hippocampus after lesions of the entorhinal cortex (Geddes et al., 1985). Using [³H]KA as a ligand, the results observed following AD-associated entorhinal cell loss are very similar to those described above in the

rodent entorhinal lesion model. The zone of high-density KA binding sites, which is normally restricted to the inner 1/3 of the dentate molecular layer associated with the terminal zone of the associational pathway, expanded to occupy over one-half of the dentate molecular layer. Thus, the rodent entorhinal lesion model seems to mimic some of the hippocampal changes seen in AD.

A recent study by Ben-Ari and colleagues (Represa et al., 1988) did not observe a significant expansion of [³H]KA binding sites in the AD hippocampus. This may be the result of the small sample size (n = 3) and the fact that one of their control patients had significant pathology, but may also be due to the region of the hippocampus examined. The severity of AD pathology may not always be uniform throughout the rostral-caudal extent of the hippocampus (unpublished observations). In particular, the density of tangles in layer II of the parahippocampal gyrus neurons is most

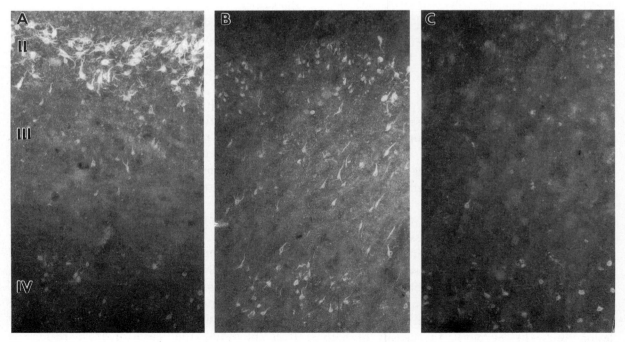

Fig. 2. Thioflavin S stained coronal sections of the parahippocampal gyrus obtained from a 83-year old Alzheimer's disease case. The photomicrograph shown in (A) was obtained from a section which included anterior (rostral) hippocampus, (B) a central region, and (C) a posterior (caudal) section of the hippocampal formation. The results demonstrate the shift in the distribution of pathology through the rostral-caudal extent of the parahippocampal gyrus in Alzheimer's disease.

prominent at the level of the anterior hippocampus, whereas layer IV parahippocampal gyrus pathology predominates at the level of the posterior hippocampus (Fig. 2).

An additional complicating factor is the 10-fold greater incidence of myoclonus in Alzheimer's disease victims as compared to the normal population (Hauser et al., 1986). An increased density of KA receptors in the inner molecular layer of the dentate gyrus has been observed in kindled rodents (Represa et al., 1989a) and KA receptors also are altered in the dentate gyrus in both temporal lobe epilepsy (Geddes et al., 1990a) and in childhood epilepsy where the hippocampus was histologically normal (Represa et al., 1989b). Thus, in the AD brain receptor properties may reflect not only denervation but also the activity-dependent state of the brain such as examplified by seizures. The relative contribution of these and other factors is as yet unknown but probably needs to be taken into account.

In contrast to the results obtained with the KA receptors, the intensification of acetylcholinesterase staining in the outer half of the molecular layer has been confirmed by Van Hoesen and colleagues (Hyman et al., 1987) and several other studies have provided evidence of hippocampal plasticity in AD (Gertz et al., 1987; Hamos et al., 1989).

The status of the NMDA receptor in AD is of importance considering the role of this receptor in learning and memory (see Cotman et al., 1988, 1989) and the suggestion that some of the cell loss observed in the hippocampus of AD patients may be mediated by NMDA receptors (Greenamyre et al., 1988). In support of this possibility is the correlation between NMDA receptor density and the predilection for AD neuropathology (see Geddes and Cotman, 1986; Geddes et al., 1986). In studies by our group (Monaghan et al., 1987) and by Young and colleagues (Maragos et al., 1987), using the ligand [^{3}H]N-(1-[2-thienyl]cyclohexyl)-piperidine ([^{3}H]TCP) which labels the ion channel associated with the NMDA receptor, there is no significant loss of [^{3}H]TCP binding site density in

the molecular layer of the dentate gyrus in AD. Thus, the severe pathology in the entorhinal cortex and the resultant loss of the projection to the dentate gyrus do not appear to alter the density of NMDA receptors.

In CA1, the results are less consistent. Some AD patients show levels of [^{3}H]TCP binding sites comparable to those found in elderly control cases, whereas in other AD individuals there are substantial losses (Monaghan et al., 1987). On average, the density of [^{3}H]TCP binding in CA1 is reduced (Maragos et al., 1987; Monaghan et al., 1987). Results obtained using [^{3}H]L-glutamate as the ligand, under conditions in which binding is displaceable by NMDA, also show considerable variability. When comparing cases in which both [^{3}H]TCP and [^{3}H]L-glutamate were used as ligands, the correlation between the results was 0.92. Both ligands demonstrate the maintenance of NMDA receptor density in the molecular layer of the dentate gyrus and, in most AD cases, in CA1. In contrast, initial results obtained by Greenamyre and coworkers (1985, 1987) reported a pronounced loss of NMDA receptors (75 – 87%) throughout the hippocampus and dentate gyrus in AD, with the most severe loss being observed in CA1. We have suggested that this discrepancy may be explained in part by the conditions of the binding assay used (Geddes et al., 1986) and Greenamyre, Young and colleagues recently commented that under their previous conditions (in the presence of quisqualate and CaCl$_2$), at least 50% of the [^{3}H]L-glutamate binding is not displaceable by NMDA (Young et al., 1988). Their more recent data, which do not use added ions in the buffer, suggest less severe losses occur (Young et al., 1989). However, it is still difficult to precisely determine the loss of NMDA-sensitive [^{3}H]L-glutamate binding from their results since 1 mM glutamate, not NMDA, was used to determine non-specific binding. Thus, based on the data available, it now appears that NMDA receptor number can be maintained, at least in select AD cases with only moderate cell loss. Overall, however, there still exists considerable variation in the data and caution needs to be exercised before the final answer is obtained. The next level of analysis of the NMDA receptor complex in Alzheimer's disease will need to take into account the exact status of the patient, but also will have to take into consideration not only NMDA receptor and neuronal density, but also the activation state of the NMDA receptor complex and the proportions of the two NMDA receptor subtypes. In addition, future studies will need to examine cell density in various regions of the hippocampus to determine the degree to which the heterogeneity in the distribution of the pathology is reflected in receptor density. Finally, the clinical history of the patient is of considerable importance since pre-mortem conditions such as pneumonia and myoclonus may influence both neuronal and receptor densities.

Conclusions

Given the critical role of the NMDA receptor in learning and memory, studies on these receptors are essential toward understanding the mechanisms underlying the cognitive deficits characteristic of aging and AD. As discussed in this chapter, NMDA receptors have been found to be important in the process of stabilizing appropriate synaptic contacts during development. In the adult brain no such role has been established but it is possible these receptors at least in part play some role in reactive synaptogenesis. Recently, we and others have proposed that the injury-induced sprouting response may result in a replay of select developmental mechanisms (Geddes et al., 1990b; Miller and Geddes, this volume). Thus, the increase in NMDA receptor density following injury- or disease-induced deafferentation may play a role similar to that described above during developmental plasticity.

The increase in KA and NMDA receptors after entorhinal lesions may facilitate synaptic transmission and enhance function. NMDA receptors, however, can also mediate excitotoxicity. Thus, following a partial loss of the entorhinal input, the hippocampus might be predicted to be more vulnerable to the excitotoxic actions of glutamate which may occur subsequent to seizures, ischemia or hypoglycemia.

EAA receptors represent a potential therapeutic target in AD. It is important, however, to consider not only the effects of therapy on the designated target, but also the potential for excitotoxic injury which could occur in a strongly overcompensated system.

References

Balazs, R., Hack, N., Jorgensen, O.S. and Cotman, C.W. (1989) N-methyl-D-aspartate promotes the survival of cerebellar granule cells: pharmacological characterization. *Neurosci. Lett.,* 101: 241–246.

Brewer, G.J. and Cotman, C.W. (1989) NMDA receptor regulation of neuronal morphology in cultured hippocampal neurons. *Neurosci. Lett.,* 99: 268–273.

Cotman, C.W. and Anderson, K.J. (1988) Synaptic plasticity and functional stabilization in the hippocampal formation: possible role in Alzheimer's disease. In: S. Waxman (Ed.), *Physiologic Basis for Functional Recovery in Neurological Disease,* Raven Press, New York, pp. 313–336.

Cotman, C.W. and Iversen, L.L. (1987) Excitatory amino acids in the brain — focus on NMDA. *Trends Neurosci.,* 10: 263–265.

Cotman, C.W., Monaghan, D.T. and Ganong, A.H. (1988) Excitatory amino acid neurotransmission: NMDA receptors and Hebb-type synaptic plasticity. *Ann. Rev. Neurosci.,* 11: 61–80.

Cotman, C.W., Bridges, R.J., Taube, J.S., Clark, A.S., Geddes, J.W. and Monaghan, D.T. (1989) The role of the NMDA receptor in central nervous system plasticity and pathology. *J. NIH Res.,* 1: 65–74.

Geddes, J.W. and Cotman, C.W. (1986) Plasticity in hippocampal excitatory amino acid receptors in Alzheimer's disease. *Neurosci. Res.,* 3: 672–678.

Geddes, J.W., Monaghan, D.T., Cotman, C.W., Lott, I.T., Kim, R.C. and Chui, H.C. (1985) Plasticity of hippocampal circuitry in Alzheimer's disease. *Science,* 230: 1179–1181.

Geddes, J.W., Chang-Chui, H., Cooper, S.M., Lott, I.T. and Cotman, C.W. (1986) Density and distribution of NMDA receptors in the human hippocampus in Alzheimer's disease. *Brain Res.,* 399: 156–161.

Geddes, J.W., Cahan, L.D., Cooper, S.M., Choi, B.H., Kim, R.C. and Cotman, C.W. (1990a) Altered distribution of excitatory amino acid receptors in temporal lobe epilepsy. *Exp. Neurol.,* 108: 214–220.

Geddes, J.W., Wong, J., Choi, B.H., Kim, R.C., Cotman, C.W. and Miller, F.D. (1990b) Increased expression of the embryonic form of a developmentally regulated mRNA in Alzheimer's disease. *Neurosci. Lett.,* 109: 54 – 61.

Gertz, H.J., Cervos-Navarro, J. and Ewald, V. (1987) The septo-hippocampal pathway in patients suffering from senile dementia of Alzheimer's type. Evidence for neuronal plasticity? *Neurosci. Lett.,* 76: 228 – 232.

Greenamyre, J.T., Olson, J.M., Penney, J.B., Young, A.B., D'Amato, C.J., Hicks, C.J. and Shoulson, I. (1985) Alterations in L-glutamate binding in Alzheimer's and Huntington's disease. *Science,* 227: 1496 – 1499.

Greenamyre, J.T., Penney, J.B., D'Amato, C.J. and Young, A.B. (1987) Dementia of the Alzheimer's type changes in hippocampal L-[^{3}H]-glutamate binding. *J. Neurochem.,* 48: 543 – 551.

Greenamyre, J.T., Maragos, W.F., Albin, R.L., Penney, J.B. and Young, A.B. (1988) Glutamate transmission and toxicity in Alzheimer's disease. *Prog. Neuropsychopharmacol. Biol. Psychiatry,* 12: 421 – 430.

Hamos, J.E., DeGennaro, L.J. and Drachman, D.A. (1989) Synaptic loss in Alzheimer's disease and other dementias. *Neurology,* 39: 355 – 361.

Hauser, W.A., Morris, M.L., Heston, L.L. and Anderson, V.E. (1986) Seizures and myoclonus in patients with Alzheimer's disease. *Neurology,* 36: 1226 – 1230.

Hyman, B.T., Van Hoesen, G.W., Damasio, A.R. and Barnes, C.L. (1984) Alzheimer's disease: cell-specific pathology isolates the hippocampal formation. *Science,* 225: 1168 – 1170.

Hyman, B.T., Kromer, L.J. and Van Hoesen, G.W. (1987) Reinnervation of the hippocampal perforant pathway zone in Alzheimer's disease. *Ann. Neurol.,* 21: 259 – 267.

Lincoln, J., Coopersmith, R., Harris, E.W., Cotman, C.W. and Leon, M. (1988) NMDA receptor activation and early olfactory learning. *Dev. Brain Res.,* 39: 309 – 312.

Maragos, W.F., Chu, D.C.M., Young, A.B., D'Amato, C.J. and Penney, J.B., Jr. (1987) Loss of hippocampal [^{3}H]TCP binding in Alzheimer's disease. *Neurosci. Lett.,* 74: 371 – 376.

Meldrum, B.S. (1985) Possible therapeutic applications of antagonists of excitatory amino acids. *Clin. Sci.,* 68: 113 – 122.

Monaghan, D.T. and Cotman, C.W. (1982) The distribution of [^{3}H] kainic acid binding sites in rat CNS as determined by autoradiography. *Brain Res.,* 252: 91 – 100.

Monaghan, D.T., Geddes, J.W., Yao, D., Chung, C. and Cotman, C.W. (1987) [^{3}H]TCP binding sites in Alzheimer's disease. *Neurosci. Lett.,* 73: 197 – 200.

Monaghan, D.T., Anderson, K.J., Peterson, C. and Cotman, C.W. (1988a) Age-dependent loss of NMDA receptors in rodent brain. *Soc. Neurosci. Abstr.,* 13: 486.

Monaghan, D.T., Olverman, H.J., Nguyen, L., Watkins, J.C. and Cotman, C.W. (1988b) Two classes of NMDA recognition sites: differential distribution and differential regulation by glycine. *Proc. Natl. Acad. Sci. U.S.A.,* 85: 9836 – 9840.

Monaghan, D.T., Bridges, R.J. and Cotman, C.W. (1989) The excitatory amino acid receptors: their classes, pharmacology, and distinct properties in the function of the central nervous system. *Ann. Rev. Pharmacol. Toxicol.,* 29: 365 – 402.

Peterson, C. and Cotman, C.W. (1989) Strain dependent decrease in glutamate binding to the NMDA receptor during aging. *Neurosci. Lett.,* 104: 309 – 313.

Represa, A., Duyckaerts, C., Tremblay, E., Hauw, J.J. and Ben-Ari, Y. (1988) Is senile dementia of the Alzheimer type associated with hippocampal plasticity? *Brain Res.,* 457: 355 – 359.

Represa, A., Le Gall La Salle, G. and Ben-Ari, Y. (1989a) Hippocampal plasticity in the kindling model of epilepsy in rats. *Neurosci. Lett.,* 99: 345 – 350.

Represa, A., Robain, O., Tremblay, E. and Ben-Ari, Y. (1989b) Hippocampal plasticity in childhood epilepsy. *Neurosci. Lett.,* 99: 351 – 355.

Singer, W. (1987) Activity-dependent self-organization of synaptic connections as a substrate of learning. *Life Sci. Res. Rep. Neural Mol. Mech. Learning,* 38: 301 – 335.

Ulas, J., Monaghan, D.T. and Cotman, C.W. (1990a) Plastic response of hippocampal excitatory amino acid receptors to deafferentation and reinnervation. *Neuroscience,* 34: 9 – 17.

Ulas, J., Monaghan, D.T. and Cotman, C.W. (1990b) Kainate receptors in the rat hippocampus: a distribution and time course of changes in response to unilateral lesions of the entorhinal cortex. *J. Neurosci.,* 10: 2352 – 2362.

Woo, C. and Leon, M. (1989) Early olfactory learning increases the number of neurons within enhanced 2-DG uptake foci. *Soc. Neurosci. Abstr.* (in press).

Young, A.B., Greenamyre, J.T., Hollingsworth, Z., Albin, R., D'Amato, C., Shoulson, I. and Penney, J.B. (1988) NMDA receptor losses in putamen from patients with Huntington's disease. *Science,* 241: 981 – 983.

Young, A.B., Cha, J.-H.J., Greenamyre, J.T., Maragos, W.F. and Penney, J.B. (1989) Distribution of PCP and glutamate receptors in normal and pathologic mammalian brain. In: E.A. Barnard and E. Costa (Eds.), *Allosteric Modulation of Amino Acid Receptors: Therapeutic Implications,* Raven Press, New York, pp. 357 – 375.

P. Coleman, G. Higgins and C. Phelps (Eds.)
Progress in Brain Research, Vol. 86
© 1990 Elsevier Science Publishers B.V. (Biomedical Division)

CHAPTER 6

Neurono-glial interactions and neural plasticity

Gustave Moonen, Bernard Rogister, Pierre Leprince, Jean-Michel Rigo, Paul Delrée, Philippe P. Lefebvre and Jean Schoenen

Service de Physiologie Humaine et de Physiopathologie, Institut Léon Frédéricq, University of Liège, Liège, Belgium

Introduction

Classical views of astroglia functions include (Fedoroff and Vernadakis, 1986): (i) a connective tissue-like function based upon the observation that astroglia cells invest and provide packing for other central nervous system components; (ii) ensheathment and hence isolation of synaptic complexes; (iii) regulation of local extracellular ionic concentrations and pH levels; (iv) uptake, metabolization and compartmentation of neurotransmitters; (v) control of blood-CNS exchanges through the astrocytic capillary investment; and (vi) control of developmental neuronal migration through neuronal guidance (this function is devoted to the radial glia, an "early subset" of astroglia). Other important functions of astrocytes are concerned with repair: after brain injury, astrocyte proliferation and hypertrophy occur, the latter phenomenon being due in part to a cytoplasmic accumulation of glycogen particles and of the glial fibrillary acidic protein and vimentin in the form of bundles of intermediate filaments (Eng, 1988). This so-called post-lesional gliosis has been considered as adaptive as well as maladaptive with regards to regeneration and nervous function recovery.

In this report, we will summarize recent data from our laboratory on intercellular messages that are exchanged between neurons and astroglia. Although in several instances these data have been obtained using embryonic or neonatal material, we believe that they are relevant to the understanding of brain reaction to injury and neuronal plasticity. Three aspects will be considered: (1) neuronal regulation of astroglia proliferation; (2) astroglial regulation of neuronal survival and death; and (3) glial modulation of neuronal neurotransmitter phenotype.

Neuronal regulation of astroglia proliferation

Fibrous and protoplasmic astrocytes have been classically considered as the opposite ends of a spectrum of the same cell type. More recently, however, Raff and colleagues (1984) have provided evidence that protoplasmic (type I) and fibrous (type II) astrocytes belong to different lineages, derived from different progenitors, the progenitor of type II astrocytes (O2A cells) also giving rise to the oligodendrocytes. The same group has also shown that type I astrocytes are generated earlier during ontogenesis and, through the release of diffusible factors, influence the fate of the O2A lineage (Hughes et al., 1988; Richardson et al., 1988).

During development, the bulk of astroglia proliferate at a rather late stage, roughly at a time during which neuronal differentiation is in progress. These simultaneous processes of neuronal dendritogenesis and astroglia proliferation end up with a nearly complete ensheathment of many neurons by protoplasmic astroglia processes, such as illustrated by the cerebellar Purkinje cells. Other neurons (very often late-generated microneurons), such as illustrated by the cerebellar granule cells, are "naked", that is nearly devoid of such an astroglial coverage. Thus, protoplasmic (type I) astrocyte proliferation ceases with the end of neuronal dendritic formation while some neuronal subsets are left unsheathed by glial processes. Two not mutually exclusive hypotheses can be proposed to explain these observations: (i) neurons (e.g., Purkinje cells) release a glial mitogen during their differentiation and stop releasing it once they have completed this process. Some neurons, however, do not release such a mitogen and hence remain associated with few protoplasmic astrocytes; and (ii) neurons begin to release a type I astrocyte proliferation inhibitor once they have completed their differentiation or at least their dendritogenesis. Some neurons (e.g., cerebellar granule cells) release such an inhibitor at an earlier stage of their differentiation. If we expand such a view to the glia proliferation that occurs in the adult nervous system, one would expect that, during post-lesional gliosis, neurons stop releasing the inhibitor and/or resume secretion of the mitogen. Also we should expect gliomas, in which proliferation is largely unregulated, to be insensitive or less sensitive to the proliferation inhibitor and/or to release an autocrine mitogen (Nister et al., 1984).

Neurons release an inhibitor of astroglia proliferation

Using an assay of type I astroglial proliferation that has a high signal-to-noise ratio, it is possible to demonstrate that medium conditioned by cultures enriched in cerebellar granule neurons inhibits, in a dose-dependent fashion, the proliferation of these astroglial cells (Rogister et al., 1990). The amount of proliferation inhibitory activity depends on the number of conditioning neurons (Fig. 1). A similar inhibitory activity is also released in some conditions by hippocampal neurons and various cell lines of neuronal origin, including the mouse neuroblastoma Neuro-2A. No such activity was found in media conditioned by primary

cultures of astroglia or by various glioma and fibroblastic cell lines. We have proposed the name astrostatine for this activity. As shown in Fig. 2, astrostatine acts only on primary astrocytes: other cells, including various malignant glial cell lines, are insensitive or much less sensitive to the inhibitory effect of astrostatine. Preliminary data suggest that astrostatine is active on type I but not

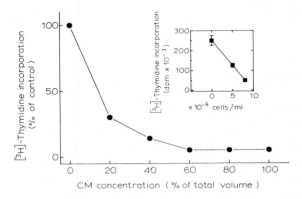

Fig. 1. Inhibition of the proliferation of astroglial cells in vitro by increasing concentrations of neuroblastoma cell conditioned medium. Neuro-2A cell CM was generated by incubating confluent (72 h subcultures) Neuro-2A cells for 24 h in serum-free DMEM supplemented with the N_1 components. Astrocytes were prepared from newborn rat cerebral cortex by the method of Booher and Sensenbrenner (1972). The dissociated cells were grown for 8 days in MEM supplemented with 10% FCS with medium changes every 48 h. These cultures contain more than 95% GFAP-positive cells showing the type I astrocyte morphology. For the proliferation assay, the astrocytes were trypsinized and plated at low density (125,000 cells/well) in the presence of 10% FCS and 2 μCi/ml [^{3}H]-thymidine, together with various dilutions of Neuro-2A cell CM. After 24 h, the cultures were washed with PBS, collected in 0.1 N NaOH and their content in tritium determined by scintillation counting. The values of [^{3}H]-thymidine incorporation in DPM (typically $3 \cdot 10^5 - 5 \cdot 10^5$ DPM per well for control cultures) are corrected for the quantity of protein in each culture. The results are expressed as percentage of the [^{3}H]-thymidine incorporated in the presence of 10% FCS alone. Inset: effect of granule cells density during conditioning on their release of astroglia proliferation inhibitor activity. Granule cells at the indicated density were used to generate conditioned media which were tested on astrocyte cultures as described above. Results are expressed as mean of triplicate determinations, plus or minus standard deviation, of total [^{3}H]-thymidine incorporation in astrocyte culture and are corrected for the content of protein in these cultures. (For abbreviations, see p. 72.)

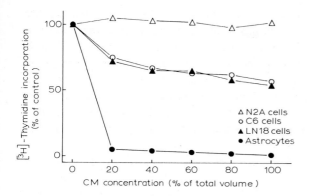

Fig. 2. Sensitivity of various cell lines to the astrostatine activity present in medium conditioned by Neuro-2A cells. Cultures of rat astrocytes, of the human glioblastoma cell line LN18, of the rat glioblastoma cell line C_6 and of the mouse neuroblastoma cell line Neuro-2A were used, as described in Fig. 1, in a proliferation assay in the presence of various concentrations of Neuro-2A cell CM. The results are expressed as described in Fig. 1.

on type II astrocytes. The astrostatine activity obtained from Neuro-2A has been further characterized: it is heat-labile, trypsin-sensitive, and retained on Affi-gel blue from which it can be eluted by increasing the NaCl concentration of the elution buffer. Gel filtration on Ultrogel AcA34 demonstrates a single peak of activity with a molecular weight around 17 kDa.

Several other points need also to be mentioned: the inhibition of astroglia proliferation has been documented using three different assay systems: [^{3}H]-thymidine incorporation and scintillation counting, bromodeoxyuridine (BrdU) incorporation followed by double-labeling using anti-BrdU and anti-GFAP (glial fibrillary acidic protein) antibodies and cell counting in fluorescence microscopy, and total DNA measurement of cultures treated for 3 days. Astrostatine does not act as the low molecular weight inhibitor of intracellular thymidine transport described by Aloisi et al. (1987). It is not gliotoxic and does not inhibit overall protein synthesis by astrocytes. Astrostatine is not immunologically or biologically related to various putative astroglia proliferation

inhibitors such as the epidermal growth factor receptor, TGFβ (transforming growth factor β), the interferons or the factors reported by Sharifi et al. (1986) and Kato et al. (1987). Hatten (1987) described an astroglia proliferation inhibitory activity involving a membrane-bound factor present on the surface of cerebellar granule neurons and able, through direct cell-to-cell contact, to inhibit the proliferation of cerebellar astrocytes. A relationship with astrostatine cannot be ruled out but seems unlikely since astrostatine is a secreted protein while the factor described by Hatten is membrane-bound. However, a relationship with a type I astrocyte proliferation inhibitor secreted by the rat neuroblastoma B104 remains possible (Bottenstein et al., 1988).

Injured neurons release an astroglia mitogen

If normal differentiated neurons release an astroglia proliferation inhibitor, the question arises whether the astroglial proliferation that follows neuronal injury results from the decreased production and release of this inhibitor and/or also from the release by injured neurons of a glial mitogen. We have tried to test this last hypothesis using in vitro techniques. Specific subsets of neurons can be selectively damaged using specific neuronotoxins such as the excitotoxins. We have compared the level of astroglia proliferation – using [^{3}H]-thymidine incorporation followed by scintillation counting, as well as BrdU incorporation followed by BrdU/GFAP double-immuno-labeling and cell counting – in newborn rat hippocampal and cerebellar microexplants. Kainic acid induces, in the first of these two preparations, a substantial neuronal death while in our culture conditions, it is virtually non-toxic in the cerebellar microexplants where most of the neurons are granule cells. After kainic acid treatment, significant stimulation of astroglia proliferation is observed only in the hippocampal cultures where neuronal death occurs (Fig. 3). When the experiments are made in a two compartment culture device in which hippocampal and cerebellar micro-

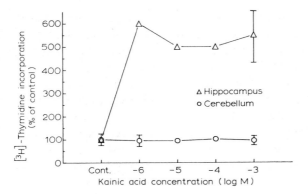

Fig. 3. Astroglial proliferation induced by neuronal cell death in rat hippocampal and cerebellar microexplants. Newborn rat hippocampal and cerebellar microexplants (20 microexplants per culture well) were incubated during 24 h in the presence of 2 μCi/ml [^{3}H]-thymidine together with the indicated concentrations of kainic acid. The microexplants were then washed in PBS, dissolved in 0.1 N NaOH and their tritium content was determined by scintillation counting. The results are expressed as described in Fig. 1.

explants are connected exclusively through the culture medium, kainate induces astroglia proliferation both in hippocampal and, although to a lesser degree, cerebellar microexplants. These data suggest that kainate is unable to directly stimulate astroglial proliferation and show that, when neuronal death is induced by kainate treatment, injured neurons release a diffusible glial mitogen. This system allows us to study not only the hyperplasic or proliferative aspect of post-lesional gliosis but also its hypertrophic aspect through, for instance, measurement of GFAP and GFAP-mRNA levels. This work is currently in progress in our laboratory.

Potential pathophysiological implications

The data reported in the previous sections illustrate part of the complexity of the neuronal regulation of astroglia proliferation. Such regulation might be relevant to problems of brain plasticity in aging and neurodegenerative disorders such as Alzheimer's disease and related disorders in which gliosis is a common neuropathological feature.

Various quantitative histological studies suggest that, in each area of CNS, a rather constant glia/neuron index is found which, however, varies for a given area such as cerebral cortex, from species to species (Pope, 1978). It is therefore possible that regulatory mechanisms maintain such an optimal fractional contribution of each cell type to cortical volume, during adulthood and even normal aging. If for any reason neuronal death occurs, local decrease of astroglial proliferation inhibitory activity and local increase of mitogenic activity would happen, leading to a new steady state characterized by an abnormally high glia/neuron index. If neuronal death becomes a chronic continuous process, the gliosis will also become continuous and contribute to a progressive worsening of brain function.

Astroglial regulation of neuronal number

In the restricted developmental sense, neuronotrophic factors or influences relate to agents and effects that are involved in the developmental regulation of neuronal number, that is in the mechanism which generates the correspondence between the size of the pool of innervating neurons and the target territory (Varon and Adler, 1981; Barde, 1988). Due in part to the seminal influence in that field of in vitro culture technique, an operational definition of neuronotrophic factors and influences can also be considered that does not necessarily imply a developmental meaning. A neuronotrophic effect can therefore be defined as an effect that promotes progressive or constructive neuronal behaviours such as survival, neuritogenesis and synthesis of neurotransmitters, as opposed to regressive behaviours such as cell death, axonal retraction or synaptolysis, for which we will use the term neuronotoxic effect.

In a previous study on the mechanisms of cell survival in cultured developing cerebellum, we found that both neuronotrophic and neuronotoxic activities were released (Grau-Wagemans et al., 1984). These activities were also found in medium conditioned by cultured astroglia cells. They could easily be separated from each other by a simple ultrafiltration step: the neuronotrophic activity being associated with the high molecular weight fraction (> 10 kDa) and the neuronotoxic activity with the low molecular weight fraction (< 1 kDa). Increased extracellular K^+ concentration occurs during regular neuronal activity and induces a depolarization of neighbouring astrocytes, a phenomenon that has also been observed in vitro. Spreading of that depolarization occurs through the astrocytic electrical syncytium. In acute pathological states, such as ischemia, hypoglycemia, trauma or status epilepticus, the increase of extracellular K^+ is much more important. We therefore investigated the effect of increasing K^+ concentration of the conditioning medium on the release by astroglia of both neuronotrophic and neuronotoxic activities (Lefebvre et al., 1987). The results demonstrated a clearcut difference in the regulation of the secretion by astroglia of neuronotoxic and neuronotrophic activities, the former being K^+-sensitive while the latter is not (Fig. 4). Furthermore, the astroglial release of neuronotoxic activity is independent of extracellular Ca^{2+} which is known to decrease in the above-mentioned pathological conditions. We have therefore proposed that part of the so-called secondary neuronal death is related to such an astroglia-derived neuronotoxic activity (Moonen et al., 1988; Leprince et al., 1990). Supporting (although not demonstrating) that view, was the finding of a similar activity in the cerebrospinal fluid of severely head-injured patients who, for therapeutic purposes, undergo a ventricular catheterization and drainage (Lefebvre et al., 1988).

It was important to look for similarities between the astroglia-derived neuronotoxic activity and excitatory amino acid-related neuronotoxins, since these have also been attributed a role in the pathophysiology of both acute and chronic neuronal damage. Recent data conclusively demonstrate that the astroglia-derived neuronotoxic activity does not belong to the family of the excitotoxins (Leprince et al., 1989b). The

arguments are: (i) several neuronal subsets are not sensitive to quisqualate, kainate, or N-methyl-D-aspartate while they are sensitive to the astroglia-derived neuronotoxic activity; (ii) the neuronal death induced by the astroglia-derived neuronotoxic activity cannot be prevented by manipulation of the ionic (including Ca^{2+}) com-

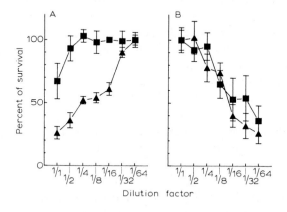

Fig. 4. Effect of K^+ concentration on the release by rat astrocytes of neuronotoxic and neuronotrophic activities. Astrocyte cultures were prepared as described in Fig. 1 and used, when reaching confluency (7 – 10 days in vitro) to generate serum-free CM in normal DMEM or in 50 mM K^+ DMEM in which K^+-concentration was increased and Na^+ decreased in equimolar amounts. These CMs were ultrafiltrated in two successive steps using Amicon PM10 and YM2 membranes (cut off: 10,000 and 1000 respectively). A. The neuronotoxic activity in the YM2 ultrafiltrates (low MW fraction) was measured on 7-day old rat cerebellar granule cells grown in DMEM-HS at a seeding density of 200,000 cells/well in laminin-coated 96-well microplates. Increasing dilutions of the experimental medium were added for 20 h after which cell survival was measured using a colorimetric microassay as described (Lefebvre et al., 1987). The relative survival (percentage of the survival measured in the corresponding unconditioned medium) has been plotted against medium dilution. B. The PM10 retentates (high MW fraction) were diluted to their original volumes with normal DMEM and their content in neuronotrophic activity was measured on non-self-supporting, low-density (50,000 cells/well) cultures of granule cells. Cell survival (percentage of the cell survival measured in the presence of 10% FCS) is plotted against PM10 retentates dilution and was measured using the colorimetric microassay. For both panels A and B, experimental media generated from normal K^+ containing CM are represented by filled squares while those generated from 50 mM K^+-containing CM are represented by filled triangles. Each point represents the mean of 5 samples ± standard deviation.

position of the extracellular medium; and (iii) antagonists of the three subclasses of glutamate receptors protect against the toxicity of the corresponding agonist but not against the astroglia-derived neuronotoxic activity. We have also investigated the possible mechanism of inactivation of that astroglia-derived neuronotoxic activity and found that astrocytes themselves are able to inactivate it, as illustrated in Fig. 5 (Leprince et al., 1989a). We are currently working on the molecular characterization of the astroglia-derived neuronotoxic activity using high performance liquid chromatography and mass spectrometry (Leprince et al., 1988).

Does neuronal survival depend on a balance between trophic and toxic activities?

Much emphasis has been given during the last few years on the possible involvement of neuronotrophic and neuronotoxic (either exogenous or endogenous) agents in the pathophysiology of various neurodegenerative disorders (Langston et al., 1983; Beal et al., 1986; Kurland, 1988; Tanner, 1989). Also, the potential therapeutic benefit of the administration of neuronotrophic factors is under investigation following the discovery that central subcortical cholinergic neurons are sensitive to nerve growth factor (NGF) (Hefti, 1986; Williams et al., 1986) and that NGF is synthetized in the hippocampus (Schwab et al., 1979; Korsching et al., 1985). Although astroglial cells are able to release both neuronotrophic and neuronotoxic activities, the regulation of these two releases, albeit only partly understood, is definitely different; since both activities can easily be separated and concentrated, we have looked for a possible interaction between glia-derived neuronotrophic and neuronotoxic activities. As illustrated in Fig. 6, neurons can be protected against the toxic activity by an excess of trophic activity.

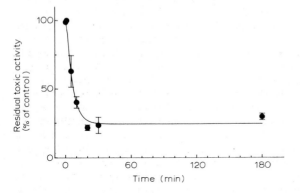

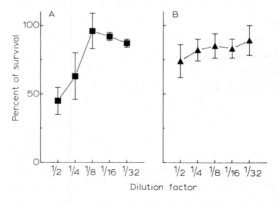

Fig. 5. Inactivation of astroglia-derived neuronotoxic activity by astrocytes in vitro. The low MW fraction of 50 mM K+-containing astrocyte CM was generated as described in Fig. 4. This fraction was extracted three times with isobutanol and the combined organic phases were evaporated under vacuum. The dry residue was rediluted in 1/5 of its original CM volume in normal DMEM and incubated for the time shown on confluent astrocyte cultures. The residual neuronotoxic activity in these media was then measured on low-density Neuro-2A cultures using the colorimetric assay described in Fig. 4. Control represents the toxic activity present after reconstitution of the isobutanol-extracted original astrocyte CM. Points represent the mean of 4 samples ± standard deviation.

Fig. 6. Protection against astroglia-derived neuronotoxic activity by astroglia-derived neuronotrophic activity. Astrocyte CM was generated using 50 mM K+-containing DMEM and was separated into a low MW fraction and a high MW fraction as described in Fig. 4. A represents the measurement of the neuronotoxic activity observed when 1 volume of progressive dilutions in unconditioned medium of the low MW fraction is mixed with 1 volume of unconditioned medium. B represents the measurement of the neuronotoxic activity observed when 1 volume of progressive dilutions in unconditioned medium of the low MW fraction is mixed with 1 volume of the high MW fraction. For both panels, cerebellar granule cells were used as target cells in the colorimetric cell survival assay mentioned in Fig. 4. Each point represents the mean of 5 samples ± standard deviation.

It is therefore possible that neuronal survival depends upon multiple influences, both positive (trophic) and negative (toxic), originating from various constituents of the neuronal environment (Moonen et al., 1988). Since, as proposed in the previous section, neuronal death induces gliosis through the release by injured neurons of diffusible factors, one might question whether the output of trophic and toxic factors by gliotic astrocytes is normal or not in such a condition. If gliotic astrocytes were unable or less able to secrete neuronotrophic factor(s) or to reuptake and further catabolize neuronotoxic factor(s), one could speculate that more gliosis will induce more neuronal death which in turn will induce more gliosis. Thus, a progressive speed-up of the sequence neuronal death – glia hyperplasia/hypertrophy – neuronal death could happen. The time constant of such a positive feedback loop might be a matter of months, compatible with the slowly progressive worsening of most neurodegenerative disorders.

Glial modulation of the neurotransmitter phenotype plasticity of adult rat dorsal root ganglion neurons

Neural crest cell derivatives from all levels of the neuraxis are endowed with a wide variety of developmental potentialities that they express after migration under the influence of developmental cues (Le Douarin, 1982). For instance, when sympathetic neurons are cultured in vitro — that is in conditions that dramatically alter the environment — their phenotypic expression of peptides is modified through increased levels of precursor mRNA (Roach et al., 1987). Dorsal root ganglion neurons also derive from the neural crest and their transmitter phenotype could also be influenced by cultivating them in vitro (Grothe and Unsicker, 1987; Lindsay and Harmar, 1989). Most of the results concerning their neurotransmitter plasticity have been obtained using embryonic or neonatal material (Mudge, 1981; Kessler et al., 1983). We have investigated the transmitter phenotype of

adult (3 – 6 month old) rat dorsal root ganglion neurons cultured in vitro (Delrée et al., 1989; Schoenen et al., 1989). Twenty-two antigens have been studied using immunocytochemical methods. The percentage of neurons positive for each antigen has been compared in two conditions: freshly dissociated (3 h in vitro) versus cultured (3 days in vitro) neurons. The medium in which these neurons have been cultured needs special mention since it has been conditioned for 24 h by C_6 glioma cells. Although C_6 cells are unusual as they possess differentiated properties of both astrocytes and oligodendrocytes, they definitely belong to the central nervous system glial lineages. When adult dorsal root ganglion neurons are cultured in such a medium, their environment is modified in at least three ways: (i) the neurons are deprived of their peripheral target field; (ii) they are also deprived of their central target field; and (iii) in spite of the presence of Schwann cells, the neuronal environment is abnormally "centralized", that is neurons are confronted to abnormally high concentrations of central glia-derived secretion products. Under such circumstances, several modifications of the expression of neurotransmitters happen (Fig. 7). For instance, some transmitters are expressed in a significantly higher proportion of cells in cultured versus freshly dissociated preparations. This was especially true for thyrotropin-releasing hormone (TRH, increase of positive neurons from 9 to 46%) or corticotropin-releasing factor (CRF, increase from 9 to 37%). Several transmitters, not hitherto described in vivo, are already present in some freshly dissociated neurons (3 h in vitro) and in a higher percentage of cultured neurons (3 days in vitro). 5-Hydroxytryptamine (5-HT) is not found in vivo in freshly dissociated neurons but is present in 45% of neurons cultured for 3 days. These data have been discussed in detail elsewhere (Schoenen et al., 1989). In the present context, it is worth mentioning results of recent experiments aimed at understanding the relative importance of the three modifications of the neuronal environment that have been cited above (Delrée et al., unpublished results). In these experiments, we have compared the percentage of neurons positive for various transmitters, in four conditions: freshly dissociated neurons (3 h in vitro) and neurons cultured for 3 days in media conditioned by primary cerebral cortex astroglia, Schwann cells (from sciatic nerves of new-born rats) or fibroblasts (from skin). Other experiments were made using feeder layers of these three cell types and led to similar conclusions. The results of such experiments for 4 transmitters, calcitonin-gene

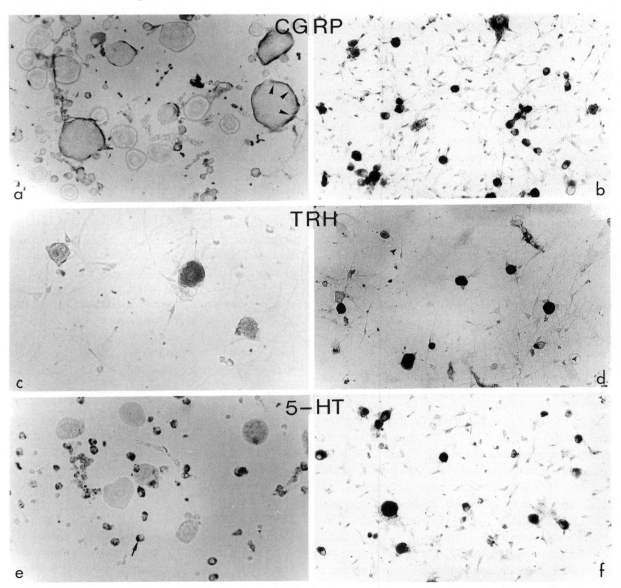

Fig. 7. Photomicrographs of neurons immunoreactive for CGRP, TRH and 5-HT in freshly dissociated preparations (*a, c, e*) and in 3-day old cultures in medium conditioned by C$_6$ glioma (*b, d, f*). Note circumferential cytoplasmic staining (arrow heads) for the CGRP antiserum in large and intermediate-sized freshly dissociated DRG neurons. Non-specific staining is seen in some non-neuronal cells (arrow). DRGs were dissected from 3-month old male Wistar rats. All preparations were processed with the avidin-peroxidase method. Microscopic magnification: × 440 in *a, c* and *e* and × 220 in *b, d* and *f* (data from Schoenen et al., 1989).

related peptide, vasoactive intestinal peptide, TRH and 5-HT, are illustrated in Fig. 8. They suggest that the nature of the non-neuronal environment modulates the neurotransmitter phenotype of these adult neurons. If we extrapolate to central adult neurons such data obtained on peripheral adult neurons, one can suggest that alteration of the glial environment could result in alteration of neurotransmitter (including neuropeptides) phenotype expression. This in turn could generate impairment of neuronal transmission through defective or abnormal release of neurotransmitters and neuromodulators. Furthermore, besides their role in neural communication, neuropeptides are likely to play other roles including trophic ones. Thus, modified neuronal peptidergic secretion might

result in defective neuronal trophic support, and hence in neuronal death.

Conclusions

The goal of the present contribution was obviously not to demonstrate, nor even to suggest, that some neurodegenerative disorders could result from a primary astroglial deficit. Rather, discussing some results of recent experiments performed in our laboratory, that are not primarily designed to study aging or degenerative dementias, we would like to point out possible involvement of glia-neuronal interactions at some steps of the pathophysiology of these disorders. The essential role of glial cells during development is now a

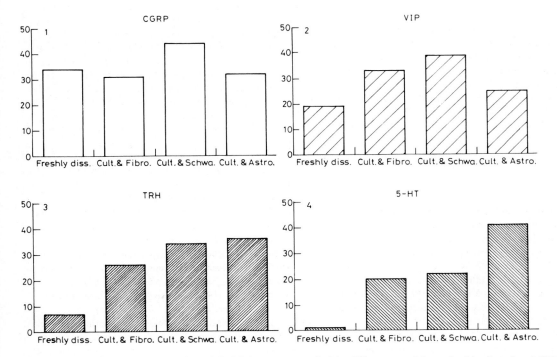

Fig. 8. Percentage of immunoreactive adult DRG neurons studied in different conditions: freshly dissociated DRG neurons and neurons cultured for 3 days in media conditioned by fibroblasts (Cult. and Fibro), Schwann cells (Cult. and Schwann) or C_6 glioma cells (Cult. and Astro). Four antigenes have been studied: CGRP, VIP, TRH and 5-HT. Note that the most dramatic changes are observed for 5-HT (4) and TRH (3). 5-HT positive neurons are absent in the freshly dissociated preparations; they represent 20% of all neurons after 3 days culturing in a medium conditioned by fibroblasts or Schwann cells; this percentage is doubled when the culture medium is conditioned by C_6 glioma. Percentages of CGRP (1) and VIP (2) positive neurons are highest in cultures conditioned by Schwann cells (data from Delrée et al., unpublished results).

widely accepted concept. There is no reason to believe that glial cells should not play similarly important roles during aging.

Acknowledgements

B.R. is Research Assistant and P.L. is Research Associate of the Belgian National Funds for Scientific Research. This study was supported by grants from the Fonds de la Recherche Scientifique Médicale, from the Fondation Médicale Reine Elisabeth (Belgium), and the Fonds de Recherches de la Faculté de Médecine de l'Université de Liège.

The authors would like to thank P. Ernst-Gengoux and A. Brose for their expert technical assistance.

Abbreviations

BrdU: bromodeoxyuridine; CGRP: calcitonin-gene related peptide; CM: conditioned medium; CNS: central nervous system; CRF: corticotropin-releasing-factor; DMEM: Dulbecco's modified eagle medium; FCS: fetal calf serum; GFAP; glial fibrillary acidic protein; HS: horse serum; 5-HT: 5-hydroxytryptamine; NGF: nerve growth factor; PBS: phosphate buffered saline; TGFβ: transforming growth factor β; TRH: thyrotropin-releasing hormone; VIP: vasoactive intestinal peptide.

References

Aloisi, F., Agresti, G. and Levi, G. (1987) Glial conditioned media inhibit the proliferation of cultured rat cerebellar astrocytes. *Neurochem. Res.,* 12: 189 – 195.

Barde, Y.-A. (1988) What, if anything, is a neuronotrophic factor? *Trends Neurosci.,* 11(8): 343 – 346.

Beal, F.M., Kowall, N.W., Ellison, D.W., Mazurek, M.F., Swartz, K.J. and Martin, J.B. (1986) Replication of the neurochemical characteristics of Huntington's disease by quinolinic acid. *Nature,* 321: 168 – 171.

Booher, J. and Sensenbrenner, M. (1972) Growth and cultivation of dissociated neurons and glial cells from embryonic chick, rat and human in flask culture. *Neurobiology,* 2: 97 – 105.

Bottenstein, J.E., Hunter, S.F. and Seidel, M. (1988) CNS neuronal cell line-derived factors regulate gliogenesis in neonatal rat brain cultures. *J. Neurosci. Res.,* 20: 291 – 303.

Delrée, P., Leprince, P., Schoenen, J. and Moonen, G. (1989) Purification and culture of adult rat dorsal root ganglia

neurons. *J. Neurosci. Res.,* 23: 198 – 206.

Eng, L. (1988) Regulation of glial intermediate filaments in astrogliosis. In: M.D. Norenberg, L. Hertz and A. Schousboe (Eds.), *Biochemical Pathology of Astrocytes,* A.R. Liss, New York, pp. 79 – 90.

Fedoroff, S. and Vernadakis, A. (1986) *Astrocytes, Vols. 1 – 3,* Academic Press, Orlando, FL.

Grau-Wagemans, M.-P., Selak, I., Lefebvre, P.P. and Moonen, G. (1984) Cerebellar macroneurons in serum-free cultures: evidence for intrinsic neuronotrophic and neuronotoxic activities. *Dev. Brain Res.,* 15: 11 – 19.

Grothe, C. and Unsicker, K. (1987) Neuron-enriched cultures of adult rat dorsal root ganglion: establishment, characterization, survival, and neuropeptide expression in response to trophic factors. *J. Neurosci. Res.,* 18: 539 – 550.

Hatten, M.E. (1987) Neuronal inhibition of astroglial cell proliferation is membrane mediated. *J. Cell Biol.,* 104: 1353 – 1360.

Hefti, F. (1986) Nerve growth factor promotes survival of septal cholinergic neurons after fimbrial transection. *J. Neurosci.,* 6: 2155 – 2162.

Hughes, S.M., Lilien, L.E., Raff, M.C., Rohrer, H. and Sendtner, M. (1988) Ciliary neurotrophic factor induces type-2 astrocyte differentiation in culture. *Nature,* 335: 70 – 73.

Kato, T., Ito, J. and Tanaka, R. (1987) Functional dissociation of dual activities of Glia Maturation Factor: inhibition of glial proliferation and preservation of differentiation by glial growth inhibiting factor. *Dev. Brain Res.,* 33: 153 – 156.

Kessler, J.A., Adler, J.E., Bell, W.O. and Black, I.B. (1983) Substance P and somatostatin metabolism in sympathetic and special sensory ganglia in vitro. *Neuroscience,* 9: 309 – 318.

Korsching, S., Auburger, G., Heumann, R., Scott, J. and Thoenen, H. (1985) Levels of nerve growth factor and its mRNA in the central nervous system of the rat correlate with cholinergic innervation. *EMBO J.,* 4: 1389 – 1393.

Kurland, L.T. (1988) Amyotrophic lateral sclerosis and Parkinson's disease complex on Guam linked to an environmental neurotoxin. *Trends Neurosci.,* 11(2): 51 – 54.

Langston, J.W., Ballard, P., Tetrud, J.W. and Irwin, I. (1983) Chronic Parkinsonism in humans due to a product of meperidine-analog synthesis. *Science,* 219: 979 – 980.

Le Douarin, N.M. (1982) *The Neural Crest,* Cambridge Univ. Press, Cambridge, 259 pp.

Lefebvre, P.P., Rogister, B., Delrée, P., Leprince, P., Selak, I. and Moonen, G. (1987) Potassium induced release of neuronotoxic activity by astrocytes. *Brain Res.,* 413: 120 – 128.

Lefebvre, P.P., Rigo, J.-M., Leprince, P., Rogister, B., Delrée, P., Hans, P., Born, J.D. and Moonen, G. (1988) Mise en évidence d'une activité neuronotoxique dans le liquide céphalorachidien de traumatisés crâniens graves. *Agressologie,* 29: 241 – 242.

Leprince, P., Lefebvre, P.P., Rigo, J.-M., Delrée, P., Rogister,

B. and Moonen, G. (1988) Astrocytic neuronotoxic activity: characterization and partial purification. *Neurochem. Int.,* 13(1): 143 (Abstract).

Leprince, P., Rigo, J.-M., Lefebvre, P.P., Rogister, B., Delrée, P. and Moonen, G. (1989a) In vitro kinetics of an astroglia-derived neuronotoxic activity. *Neurosci. Lett.,* 102: 268 – 272.

Leprince, P., Lefebvre, P.P., Rigo, J.-M., Delrée, P., Rogister, B. and Moonen, G. (1989b) Cultured astroglia release a neuronotoxic activity that is not related to the excitotoxins. *Brain Res.,* 502: 21 – 27.

Leprince, P., Rigo, J.-M., Rogister, B., Delrée, P., Lefebvre, P.P. and Moonen, G. (1990) Trophic and toxic influences on neurones. In: N. Osborne (Ed.), *Current Aspects of the Neurosciences, Vol. 1,* MacMillan, London, pp. 97 – 134.

Lindsay, R.M. and Harmar, A.J. (1989) Nerve growth factor regulates expression of neuropeptide genes in adult sensory neurons. *Nature,* 337: 362 – 364.

Moonen, G., Delrée, P., Leprince, P., Rigo, J.-M., Rogister, B. and Lefebvre, P.P. (1988) Developmental neurobiology and the physiopathology of brain injury. In: B. Sabel and D. Stein (Eds.), *Pharmacological Approach to the Treatment of Brain Injury and Spinal Cord Injury,* Plenum, New York, pp. 259 – 280.

Mudge, A.W. (1981) Effect of chemical environment on levels of substance P and somatostatin in cultured sensory neurones. *Nature,* 292: 764 – 767.

Nister, M., Heldin, C.-H., Wasteson, Å. and Westermark, B. (1984) A glioma-derived analog to platelet-derived growth factor: demonstration of receptor-competing activity and immunological cross-reactivity. *Proc. Natl. Acad. Sci. U.S.A.,* 81: 926 – 930.

Pope, A. (1978) Neuroglia: quantitative aspects. In: E. Schofeniels, G. Franck, D.B. Tower and L. Hertz (Eds.), *Dynamic Properties of Glia Cells,* Pergamon, Oxford, pp. 13 – 20.

Raff, M.C., Abney, E.R. and Miller, R.H. (1984) Two glial cell lineages diverge prenatally in rat optic nerve. *Dev. Biol.,* 106: 53 – 60.

Richardson, W.D., Pringle, N., Mosley, M., Westermark, B. and Dubois-Dalcq, M. (1988) A role for platelet-derived growth factor in normal gliogenesis in the central nervous system. *Cell,* 53: 309 – 319.

Roach, A., Adler, J.E. and Black, I.B. (1987) Depolarizing influences regulate preprotachykinin mRNA in sympathetic neurons. *Proc. Natl. Acad. Sci. U.S.A.,* 84: 5078 – 5081.

Rogister, B., Leprince, P., Bonhomme, V., Rigo, J.-M., Delrée, P., Colige, A. and Moonen, G. (1990) Cultured neurons release an inhibitor of astroglia proliferation (astrostatine). *J. Neurosci. Res.,* 25: 58 – 70.

Schoenen, J., Delrée, P., Leprince, P. and Moonen, G. (1989) Neurotransmitter phenotype plasticity in cultured dissociated adult rat dorsal root ganglia: an immunocytochemical study. *J. Neurosci. Res.,* 22: 473 – 487.

Schwab, M.E., Otten, U., Agid, Y. and Thoenen, H. (1979) Nerve growth factor (NGF) in the rat CNS: absence of specific retrograde axonal transport and tyrosine hydroxylase induction in locus coeruleus and substantia nigra. *Brain Res.,* 168: 473 – 483.

Sharifi, B.G., Johnson, J.C., Kuurana, V.K., Bascom, C.C., Fleenor, T.J. and Chou, H.H. (1986) Purification and characterization of a bovine cerebral cortex cell surface sialoglycopeptide that inhibits cell proliferation and metabolism. *J. Neurochem.,* 46(2): 461 – 469.

Tanner, C.M. (1989) The role of environmental toxins in the etiology of Parkinson's disease. *Trends Neurosci.,* 12(2): 49 – 54.

Varon, S. and Adler, R. (1981) Trophic and specifying factors directed to neuronal cells. *Adv. Cell. Neurobiol.,* 2: 115 – 163.

Williams, L.R., Varon, S., Peterson, G.M., Wictorin, K., Fischer, W., Björklund, A. and Gage, F.H. (1986) Continuous infusion of nerve growth factor prevents basal forebrain neuronal death after fimbria fornix transection. *Proc. Natl. Acad. Sci. U.S.A.,* 83: 9231 – 9235.

P. Coleman, G. Higgins and C. Phelps (Eds.)
Progress in Brain Research, Vol. 86
© 1990 Elsevier Science Publishers B.V. (Biomedical Division)

CHAPTER 7

Neuronal plasticity in normal aging and deficient plasticity in Alzheimer's disease: a proposed intercellular signal cascade

Paul D. Coleman[1], Kathryn E. Rogers[1] and Dorothy G. Flood[1,2]

Departments of [1] Neurobiology and Anatomy and [2] Neurology, University of Rochester Medical Center, Rochester, NY 14642, U.S.A.

Introduction

Alzheimer's disease (AD) is manifested behaviorally by deficits of memory and cognition, accompanied by personality (and other) changes. Neurobiologically the disease is associated with a veritable smorgasbord of changes which classically include excess loss of neurons in many (but not all) brain regions, deficits in some transmitter systems, excess in age-adjusted density of senile plaques, neurofibrillary tangles, vascular amyloid deposits, granulovacuolar degeneration and alterations in cytoskeletal proteins. The differences between the AD and control brain typically narrow with increasing age with respect to many of these parameters, except, perhaps in the hippocampus (e.g., Shefer, 1973; Ball, 1977; Hubbard and Anderson, 1985).

More recent additions to the list of changes in the AD brain include: decreased levels of APP 695 mRNA relative to APP 751 (Johnson et al., 1988, 1989), increased T-α-1 mRNA in some regions (Miller and Geddes, 1990), increased number of IL-1 positive cells (Griffin et al., 1989), decreased GAP-43 (see below), increased A-68 protein (Wolozin et al., 1986), decreased protein kinase C (Cole et al., 1988) and decreased levels of NGF receptor mRNA (Higgins and Mufson, 1989).

In spite of our extensive, but undoubtedly in-complete, catalog of alterations in the AD brain, we do not yet know how these changes are initiated, nor do we know how they may be linked to produce the cascade of pathologies that result in the brain failure of AD. Neither do we know how the brain pathologies of the disease lead to the extensive behavioral deterioration seen in AD. At this time it appears that earlier attempts to equate behavioral deterioration to single aspects of the disease such as plaque counts (Blessed et al., 1968) or even cholinergic deficits (summarized e.g., in Bartus et al., 1982) may have represented oversimplifications. The recognition of the necessity for age-adjusted criteria of plaque and tangle density for the neuropathological contribution to the definition of AD emphasizes that older non-demented individuals may have as high a density of plaques and tangles as younger demented persons (Katzman et al., 1988). Similarly, studies which have quantified aspects of the cholinergic system (typically ChAT activity) report data which, although showing statistically significant and often impressive decreases in cholinergic markers, also usually show some degree of overlap of values for AD and control cases (e.g., Bowen et al., 1979; Rossor et al., 1981). Although the evidence linking the cholinergic system to memory deficits in animals (e.g., Bartus et al., 1980; Gage et al., 1984) and in humans (e.g., Drachman and Leavitt, 1974;

Bartus et al., 1982) is appealing, the existence of overlap between AD and control populations in markers of the cholinergic system suggests that a deficit in this system may not be a singular cause of the behavioral devastation of AD. A similar argument applies to other measures. Certainly, it may be over-optimistic to emphasize one parameter in a disease that affects such a wide variety of structural, transmitter system, protein and molecular parameters.

If one argues that no one of the classical neurobiological or neuropathological deficits alone provides a full explanation of the cognitive, mnemonic and other behavioral changes of AD, then how may we relate the brain changes of AD to the devastation of the disease? One position is that a combination of morphological and neurochemical (in the broadest sense) deficits are responsible for the brain failure of AD. In other words, AD is a multivariate disease (Ball et al., 1988). This has been popularly known as the "rusty truck" hypothesis. In fact, we have obtained preliminary data in conjunction with our Rochester Alzheimer's Disease Program Project that a multivariate analysis separates AD and control cases in a multidimensional space when no single variable contributing to the analysis could do so (Hamill et al., 1987). Another position, not mutually exclusive with the first, is that there may be changes in other, less well studied, variables which are part of the pathophysiological cascade of AD and which better account for the brain failure of AD. Evidence exists suggesting that one of these "other" changing variables may be altered neuronal plasticity in AD, which results in decreased ability of neurons to change in response to demands of the external environment (to learn and remember) and to compensate for degenerative changes in the brain. Should this hypothesis prove correct, altered neuronal plasticity may be found to represent an eventual consequence of the cascade of multiple morphological, cytoskeletal, transmitter and other chemical defects and to provide a uniquely powerful relationship to the behavioral deficits of AD. On the other hand, it is possible that decreased neuronal plasticity in AD, if true, may be one more parameter affected by the disease (i.e., one more contribution to the defects of the rusty truck) but insufficient to alone account for the behavioral deficits. Both of the above suggestions are compatible with either a single initiating event in the etiology of AD or with a multivariate etiology.

In the paragraphs below we will examine the evidence for the hypothesis of neuronal plasticity in the normally aging brain and its decrease in AD and suggest a cascade of intercellular signals which may lead to plastic responses of surviving neurons to the death of their neighbors in normally aging brain and which may be affected by AD. We will focus initially on dendrites as markers of neuronal plasticity for reasons outlined below, but will also consider GAP-43 as a marker of plasticity of the axonal compartment of the neuropil.

Importance of dendrites, dendrites as markers of the axonal supply. The dendrites of many cell types constitute as much as 95% of the receptor surface that a neuron offers for contact with other neurons (Schade and Baxter, 1960). Dendrites, therefore, constitute important determinants of the ability of neuronal ensembles to receive and process information. Additionally, dendrites are among the more rapidly changeable elements of the neuronal light microscopic morphology in developing and adult nervous systems (e.g., Cowan et al., 1980; Purves and Hadley, 1985), as well as in mature brains as a response to lesions of afferent axons (e.g., Caceres and Steward, 1983), following learning (Greenough et al., 1979), and following alterations in environmental complexity (e.g., Uylings et al., 1978). Regression of dendrites after removal of a portion of their axonal input (see above; also e.g., Jones and Thomas, 1962) additionally indicates that dendritic extent is related to afferent axons and that changes of dendritic extent are a reflection of the axonal supply. This conclusion is strengthened by work showing that dendritic trees also expand in response to increased availability of afferent supply (Perry and Linden,

1982). Indeed, a Golgi-serial reconstruction electron microscopic study in our laboratory of tips of dendrites in rodent olfactory bulb, which show age-related proliferation and regression (Hinds and McNelly, 1977), demonstrates that as dendritic extent changes, the density of axonal contacts (synapses) in the tip region remains stable from 12 to 30 months (Carboni et al., 1985), implying sprouting and loss of axon terminals as dendrites change. Thus, growth, net stability and regression of dendrites and of axons appear to parallel each other.

Relation between plasticity and age-related dendritic changes.   Although the term "plasticity" is often applied to a neuronal response to an experimentally induced manipulation of the brain, we use this term in a manner that is more closely related to its use in studies of early development, the response of surviving neurons to age-related, naturally occurring, changes in the brain — such as loss of neighboring neurons, loss of afferent supply, alterations in transmitters, receptors and trophic factors, etc., thus, the adaptations of the brain to age-induced, rather than experimenter-induced, alterations of the brain. Static measures of dendritic extent in post-mortem tissue may then serve as markers of plastic dendritic response to age-related neuron loss, etc., when dendritic extent is examined in a range of ages that represent a range of age-associated lesion extent.

In normal aging dendritic extent increases in some brain regions that are also losing neurons. Such age-related increases in dendritic extent may be followed by dendritic regression in some regions.   Our previous quantitative Golgi studies suggest that neurons of the normally aging human brain are capable of plastic adaptations to some degenerative changes of normal aging. In several, but not all, regions of normally aging brain, the dendritic extent of surviving neurons is greater in older cases than in younger cases (Buell and Coleman, 1979, 1981; Flood et al., 1985, 1987; Flood and Coleman, 1990) (see Fig. 1). The regions in

which we found age-related increases in dendritic extent have been shown, or may be presumed, to lose neurons in normal aging (Brody, 1955; Mouritzen Dam, 1979; Henderson et al., 1980; Coleman and Flood, 1987, for review). Increased dendritic extent in the normally aging brain has also been found by others in rat (Hinds and McNelly, 1977) and macaque monkey (Cupp and Uemura, 1980; Uemura, 1985). The Hinds and McNelly (1977) and the Cupp and Uemura (1980) data were from regions showing age-related decreases in neuronal density (Hinds and McNelly, 1977; Brizzee et al., 1980). We interpret these age-related increases in dendritic extent as a dendritic proliferation which is a compensatory, plastic response of surviving neurons to the age-related death of their neighbors.

This age-related dendritic proliferation is not

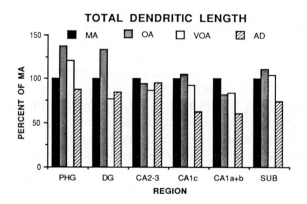

Fig. 1. Total dendritic length adjusted to a percent of that in the middle-aged group for each cell type studied in the hippocampal region. Age groups for neurologically and psychiatrically normal subjects are: middle-aged subjects (MA) with a mean age in the early fifties, old-aged subjects (OA) with a mean age in the early seventies, and very old-aged subjects (VOA) with a mean age in the early nineties. Subjects with clinically and neuropsychiatrically verified Alzheimer's disease (AD) averaged in their mid-seventies. Data are shown for apical trees of parahippocampal gyrus (PHG) layer II pyramidal cells, apical trees of dentate gyrus (DG) granule cells, basal trees of CA2 – 3 pyramidal cells, basal trees of CA1c pyramidal cells, basal trees of CA1a + b pyramidal cells, and apical trees of subiculum (SUB) layer III pyramidal cells. See Lorente de Nó (1934) for a description of the subdivisions of CA1 and of the layers of the subiculum. (Reprinted from Flood and Coleman, 1990.)

seen in all neuronal populations (see below). In addition, some populations that do exhibit such proliferation between middle age and old age show either reduced proliferation or regression in the "oldest old" (Fig. 1). Our data, as well as the monkey and rat data cited above, also show that in the oldest subjects, dendritic extent in some brain regions is less than at younger ages, suggesting dendritic regression in extreme old age. The reasons for this collapse are not known, but may be related to decreased compensatory capacity, regression antecedent to neuron death and/or regression consequent to increasing denervation due to death of input neurons and/or regression of afferent axons.

Dendritic extent does not increase in normal aging in brain regions that are not losing neurons. If normal age-related dendritic proliferation is a compensatory response to the loss of neighbor neurons, regions which do not lose neurons with age should show no age-related increase in dendritic extent. The absolute total number of neurons in barrel C3 of the cortical posteromedial barrel subfield of C57BL/6N mice was constant over six ages from 3 to 33 months (Curcio and Coleman, 1982). In this region with no age-related neuronal loss, the dendritic extent of single layer IV stellate neurons was unchanged between 4 and 45 months of age (Coleman et al., 1986).

Dendrites regress in normal aging in brain regions that are losing afferent supply. It is known that neurons respond to partial loss of afferent supply by regression of their dendritic trees (e.g., Jones and Thomas, 1962; Caceres and Steward, 1983). In most regions of aging brain it is difficult to distinguish dendritic regression that is antecedent to neuronal death from regression induced by deafferentation. However, the supraoptic nucleus (SON) of the rat hypothalamus does not lose neurons with age (Hsu and Peng, 1978). But this region does show significant loss of noradrenergic (NA) afferents in aging rat, and the remaining NA afferents shift dorsally in the nucleus, away from the ventrally directed dendrites of neurons in this nucleus (Sladek et al., 1980). Quantitative Golgi study of the SON of aging rats reveals a 34% regression of dendritic extent (Flood and Coleman, unpublished results). We suggest that whether dendrites regress, proliferate or show net stability in regions in which there is both death of neighboring neurons and partial deafferentation with age depends on the balance between these proliferative and regressive influences. When there is regression it may be limited to specific portions of the dendritic tree when afferent supplies are segregated on the tree (e.g., Globus and Scheibel, 1966).

Average dendritic extent does not increase with age in the AD brain, even in regions in which dendritic extent does increase in normal aging. In patients with clinically and neuropathologically confirmed AD we consistently find either (1) a failure of the age-related increase in dendritic extent found in normal human aging or (2) dendritic regression. Examples include: parahippocampal gyrus (Buell and Coleman, 1979, 1981), dentate gyrus (Flood et al., 1987), CA1 (Hanks and Flood, 1990) and subiculum (Flood, 1990). This suggestion of failure of neuronal plasticity in AD may seem to be at variance with the report of Geddes et al. (1985) of evidence for plasticity in AD in axons afferent to the dentate gyrus. However, our data on dendrites of dentate gyrus granule cells indicate a form of aborted plasticity in AD cases in that dendrites do show numbers of branches consistent with the increased branching seen in normally aging brain, but in AD this branching does not result in an increased dendritic extent because the dendritic segments are abnormally short compared to normal. This "abortive" branching is unique to the dentate gyrus of all regions we have examined. Other regions examined by us show no evidence of *net* increases in either dendritic branching or length in the AD brain. In addition, there have been recent reports of sprouting and regeneration in the AD brain using tau or MAP2 antibodies (e.g., Ihara, 1988; McKee et al., 1988). It is unclear from these qualitative reports how prevalent the sprouting and regeneration may be, as well as whether the antibodies used may be selective for epitopes which are more likely to be present in sprouting cells. However, such reports may not be inconsistent with our quantitative Golgi evidence, since we have seen similar phenomena, but base our reports on statistical averages. Thus, in AD sprouting or regeneration are, in our hands, much less frequent than degenerative phenomena. Nevertheless, the variety of results emphasizes the need for study of the prevalence of growth of neuronal processes in the AD brain through one of the more direct means currently available for human studies, such as quantification of the growth-associated protein, GAP-43, and its message, as well as studies of other markers of neurites such as tau and other MAPs. Although some of these MAP proteins may be subject to post-mortem degradation, their messages may remain reasonably intact in properly handled specimens.

In frontal association cortex growth-associated protein, GAP-43, message is decreased in normal aging but not in AD. In AD there may be defective posttranslational processing of the protein. Knowledge of protein correlates of plastic growth responses of neuronal processes offers the opportunity to use these proteins as markers of neuronal growth as an alternative to the Golgi method. Thus, the growth-associated protein, GAP-43/B50/F1/pp46, offers an alternative to morphological methods to test the hypothesis of failure of growth of neuronal processes in AD. GAP-43 is associated with plastic responses to injury of the nervous system (Benowitz et al., 1981; Skene and Willard, 1981; Ng et al., 1988). Both Skene and Virag (1989) and Van Hooff et al. (1989) have described a translocation of GAP-43 to the growth cone membrane, and suggest a role of this protein in neurite growth. It has been found to be enriched in growth cones and pre-synaptic nerve terminals (Oestreicher et al., 1981; De Graan et al., 1985; Meiri et al., 1986; Skene et al., 1986; Van Lookeren Campagne et al., 1989), and it is

abundant during early development, but continues to be expressed at significant levels in the adult (Jacobson et al., 1986; Basi et al., 1987). GAP-43 and its message have been described to occur preferentially in association regions of the brain, with less found in primary sensory and motor regions (Benowitz et al., 1988; Neve et al., 1988). It is traditionally considered to be localized to the axon, and as such offers the opportunity to examine potential plastic responses of the axonal compartment of the neuropil to complement data on dendritic extent. Recent data from our laboratory indicate that GAP-43 message is reduced in frontal association cortex (area 8/9) with increasing age. When AD cases are selected from equivalent age ranges, the level of GAP-43 message in this region of AD brain is not appreciably altered from normal (Fig. 2). Whether this reduced GAP-43 in normal aging is entirely at-

GAP-43 MESSAGE IN AREA 8/9 IN NORMAL AGING AND AD

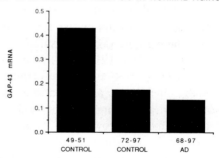

Fig. 2. Levels of GAP-43 message in frontal association cortex as a function of normal aging and AD. After determination of 260/280 ratios and Northern blotting to ensure the integrity of RNA from each sample, samples were slot-blotted with 4 serial dilutions for each case. Film densities were quantified with scanning densitometry. Adjusted levels of GAP-43 message are expressed with reference to values obtained with an oligo-dT probe of samples from each case. Note that there is an age-related decline in level of GAP-43 message which is most precipitous between about 50 years of age and the seventies. Although there may be a slight tendency for AD cases to yield less GAP-43 mRNA compared to comparably aged control cases, this tendency is small and not statistically significant. In addition, these data emphasize the importance of careful age matching of control and AD cases. AD = Alzheimer's disease cases. The numbers under each of the bars show the age range (years) of the cases represented.

tributable to age-related neuron loss remains to be determined. In addition, we have obtained preliminary data suggesting reduced levels of an acidic isoform of the GAP-43 protein in AD brain. This preliminary finding is consistent with the reduced isoform being a phosphorylated form of GAP-43. Since GAP-43 is a substrate for protein kinase C, this preliminary finding is, furthermore, consistent with the finding of reduced protein kinase C in AD (Cole et al., 1988). These protein data suggest that although normal levels of GAP-43 message may be present, there may be defective posttranslational processing of the protein in AD.

Dying neurons as sources of signals to glia. If selected classes of surviving neurons respond to the death of their neighbors it then becomes important to understand the inter- and intracellular signal cascade that leads to these responses. We will here deal only with the intercellular signals, starting with the dying neuron.

Since the work of Weigert and Nissl approximately 100 years ago it has been known that "any destruction of nervous tissue is compensated by a neuroglial neoplasm" (Cajal, 1913/1928). We now describe this "neuroglial neoplasm" as a complex response which includes accumulation of microglia, astrocytes, and other cells, as well as conversion of many astrocytes to reactive astrocytes. Some of the questions raised by these glial responses to injury have been: what is the nature of the signals that act on the glia to produce their responses? And, what are the cells of origin of these signals?

In the past "destruction of nervous tissue" has directly involved not only neurons, but also glial, vascular and meningeal elements, which has made it difficult to answer the latter question. Recently, Streit and Kreutzberg (1988) have used suicide transport of ricin to produce a lesion restricted to neurons of the rat facial nerve nucleus, and showed that the numbers of microglia and astrocytes in the nucleus of the facial nerve increased substantially after the lesion. A glial reaction remote from an injury site but in the field of axon termination

of damaged neurons has also been demonstrated (e.g., Gage et al., 1988). These data suggest that damage to non-neuronal cells is not required for the induction of a glial response.

Evidence that numbers of glia proliferate in aging human neocortex as neurons are lost is consistent with the hypothesis that neuron death may provide a signal for glial proliferation. Thus, Hansen et al. (1987) have shown that numbers of GFAP + astrocytes increase in aging human cerebral cortex, with the greatest increase apparently taking place in the age range between 70 and 80 years. Astrocyte hypertrophy accompanying neuron death has also been found in the normally aging rat hippocampus (Landfield et al., 1977). These data suggest that there are signals released into the microenvironment by normal age-related neuron death, or dying, that are mitogenic for glial cells. The nature of the signals acting on the glia has not been established. The possibilities include up or down regulation of proteins normally expressed by neurons (including neurotransmitters; see Vernadakis, 1988, pp. 167 – 174, for review), expression of de novo proteins, cellular breakdown products, release of cellular constituents by cell lysis, or altered ionic balance, all of which may regulate numbers and forms of glia, as well as their expression of neurotrophic/toxic/neurite-elongation factors. For example, excess potassium, which may be released by dying neurons, can alter the balance of glial expression of neurotrophic/toxic factors toward more neurotoxicity (Lefebvre et al., 1987).

It is now known that expression of a variety of messages and proteins (some of which appear to be de novo proteins) are associated with cell death. Cell types for which programmed cell death associated protein expression have been described include intersegmental muscles of the moth *Manduca sexta* (e.g., Schwartz and Kay, 1987; Wadewitz and Lockshin, 1988), and the rat ventral prostate gland (e.g., Buttyan et al., 1988). In the rat ventral prostate induction of cell death is accompanied by a sequential pattern of message expression in which the earliest known event is the induction of *c-fos* (Buttyan et al., 1988). This is followed by the expression of a variety of messages and proteins, some of which are not surprising (such as heat shock proteins), while others remain unique (e.g., Wadewitz and Lockshin, 1988). It appears that the expression of these cell death associated gene products may have a necessary role in cell death, since inhibiting message or protein synthesis has been shown to rescue cells ranging from *Manduca* cells (Fahrbach and Truman, 1987) to mammalian neurons (Martin et al., 1988) from their death fate. These proteins *may* provide the stimuli for the glial response to neuron death. However, since the toxic action of ricin is through inhibition of protein synthesis, the Streit and Kreutzberg (1988) study cited above suggests that we also consider the possibility that the signal for the glial response to neuron death may not be newly synthesized proteins, but rather the cessation of signal(s) normally expressed by uninjured neurons which inhibited the glial response or the release of signals consequent to cell lysis. Unfortunately, Streit and Kreutzberg (1988) did not establish the completeness. of inhibition of protein synthesis in their model. The alternatives of release from inhibition or positive stimulation of glial proliferation are not mutually exclusive and, indeed Moonen et al. (1990) have found a 17 kDa factor released by uninjured neurons, which they call "astrostatine", which inhibits astrocyte proliferation. In the same paper they also describe studies showing that injured neurons release glial mitogen(s). Glial proliferation in response to neuron death and reduced proliferation in the absence of neuron death may represent a shifting of the balance between proliferation stimulating and proliferation inhibiting signals.

The role of microglia and IL-1 in interactions with astrocytes. The glial cell type that may be acted on by signals of neuron death remains unclear. One potential route is action on phagocytic microglia, with the microglia then expressing protein(s) which act on astrocytes. IL-1 expressed by microglia may be a major signal for astrocyte pro-

liferation. Giulian and his co-workers (e.g., Giulian and Lachman, 1985; Giulian et al., 1986, 1988; Giulian, 1987) have indicated that: (1) brain IL-1 is increased by brain injury (confirmed by Nieto-Sampedro and Berman, 1987); (2) IL-1 is produced by ameboid microglia (Fontana, 1982; Merrill, 1987); (3) numbers of GFAP+ cells increase around the local site of an IL-1 intracerebral injection; and (4) IL-1 is mitogenic for astrocytes in vitro (confirmed by Nieto-Sampedro and Berman, 1987). IL-1 is not only expressed by microglia/macrophages, but also by astrocytes (e.g., Fontana et al., 1983), implying an autocrine mechanism in which injured or stimulated astrocytes may increase production of IL-1 to increase the numbers of astrocytes. It should be noted that some classes of neurons have receptors for IL-1 (e.g., Farrar et al., 1987) and that systemically or intraventricularly administered IL-1 can lead to a variety of actions on neurons, particularly in the hypothalamic region (e.g., Besedovsky and del Rey, 1987; Sapolsky et al., 1987; Hori et al., 1988). We have obtained evidence that IL-1β message levels show no age-related changes in normal aging and age-related *decreases* in AD (Fig. 3). Thus, the levels of IL-1β

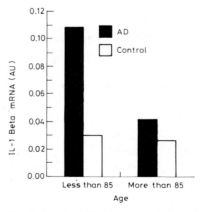

Fig. 3. Levels of IL-1β message in frontal association cortex as a function of age and AD. Data obtained as described for Fig. 2. Note that in normal brain there is no age-related change in levels of IL-1β message, while in AD brain there is an age-related *decrease* in IL-1β message. Thus, this aspect of the response to age and disease associated lesions is diminished in older AD cases.

message are higher in younger AD cases than in control cases (Griffin et al., 1989, have reported increased numbers of IL-1 positive cells in the AD brain). These data suggest that in young AD brain IL-1β production increases as a glial response is mounted to death of neurons. In older AD cases this aspect of the glial response to lesions appears to be reduced.

Astroglia as sources of neurotrophic, neurotoxic and neurite elongation factors. A variety of studies have shown that astrocytes provide factors that encourage the survival, death or neurite outgrowth of neurons. Due to space limitations, discussion will be limited to soluble factors at the expense of contact phenomena, even though the latter are also important to neuronal – glial interactions (e.g., Manthorpe et al., 1983; Grumet et al., 1984; Liesi et al., 1984; Fallon, 1985). (However, see Ard and Bunge, 1988.)

The production by cultured astrocytes of neurite proliferation factors has been reported by a number of laboratories (e.g., Banker, 1980; Müller et al., 1984; see Manthorpe et al., 1986 for a more comprehensive review of astrocytes as sources of neurotrophic and neurite elongation factors). It appears that there may be more than one neurite elongation factor expressed by astrocytes and released into serum-free conditioned medium (e.g., Beckh et al., 1987). Astrocytes support the survival of both NGF-sensitive and -insensitive neurons in vitro (e.g., Lindsay, 1979). One neuron-survival promoting factor may be pyruvate (e.g., Selak et al., 1985). The concentrations of both trophic and toxic factors have been reported to increase in injured brain (e.g., Nieto-Sampedro et al., 1982, for trophic and Whittemore et al., 1985, for toxic factors). (Lefebvre et al., 1987, have, in addition, described increased neurotoxic activity expressed by K$^+$ stimulated astrocytes.) The level of the neurotrophic factor of Nieto-Sampedro et al. is higher in aged than in neonatal rat brain, and its induction by injury is also greater in aged than in neonatal brain. Neurotoxic activity was also higher

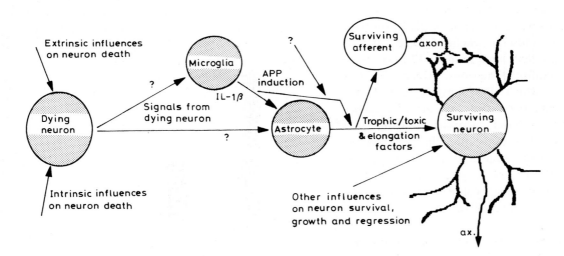

Fig. 4. Proposed model of an intercellular signal cascade through which surviving neurons may respond to the death of their neighbors. The model suggests that dying neurons release signals into the microenvironment that act on local glia to modulate glial numbers as well as their expression of neurotrophic/toxic and neurite elongation factors. These factors then act on surviving neurons to influence their responses to the death of their neighbors. Among the responses is proliferation of axons and dendrites of neurons in the local microenvironment. Whether the proposed cascade acts directly on axons of remote neurons that form part of the local neuropil or not remains an open question.

in aged than neonatal brain, and was not induced by injury (Whittemore et al., 1985). Both papers speculate that astrocytes may be the source of the trophic or toxic factor. Transplants of cultured astrocytes or Gelfoam presumed to contain astrocyte secretions will promote behavioral recovery after cortex ablation (Kesslak et al., 1986). For further review of astrocytes as sources of neurotrophic/toxic and neurite elongation factors and the modulation of expression of these factors by nervous system injury, see e.g., Lindsay (1986), Reier (1986) and Vernadakis (1988).

The above data lead us to suggest a model which is diagrammed in Fig. 4. The model proposed here provides a framework for studying selected aspects of the responses of surviving neurons to the death of their neighbors in normally aging brain and also for identifying potential AD-related lesion sites in the proposed intercellular signal cascade. It encompasses a number of hypotheses which are testable by in vitro and in vivo experimental methods. The model suggests a cascade of intercellular signals which is initiated by neuron death or dying and which results in plastic adaptations of surviving neurons to the death of their neighbors. Whether the signals emanating from dying neurons are ions or proteins (or both) is not defined. If proteins, it is not yet known whether the proteins are already existing proteins released by cell lysis or newly synthesized proteins. If newly synthesized proteins, it is not known whether they may relate to proteins whose expression has already been shown to be important to the death of neurons and other cells. In addition, the glial type(s) on which these ionic or protein signals first act is not yet known. Also unknown are the sequences and identities of many of the factors which are produced by glia following signals from dying neurons, as well as the mechanism of action of these factors on surviving neurons. Nevertheless, current techniques of cellular and molecular biology and protein chemistry offer the promise of identifying and defining these intercellular signals which seem to be required by the presently known facts regarding the responses of the brain to aging, injury and neurodegenerative disease.

Acknowledgements

The authors received support from National Institute on Aging grants AG 03644 and AG 01121 and Alzheimer's Disease and Related Disorders Grant IIRG-87-053.

References

Ard, M.D. and Bunge, R.P. (1988) Heparan sulfate proteoglycan and laminin immunoreactivity on cultured astrocytes: relationship to differentiation and neurite growth. *J. Neurosci.,* 8: 2844 – 2858.

Ball, M.J. (1977) Neuronal loss, neurofibrillary tangles and granulovacuolar degeneration in the hippocampus with ageing and dementia. *Acta Neuropathol. (Berl.),* 37: 111 – 118.

Ball, M.J., Griffin-Brooks, S., MacGregor, J.A., Nagy, B., Ojalvo-Rose, E. and Fewster, P.H. (1988) Neuropathological definition of Alzheimer disease: multivariate analyses in the morphometric distinction between Alzheimer dementia and normal aging. *Alzheimer Dis. Assoc. Dis.,* 2: 29 – 37.

Banker, G.A. (1980) Trophic interactions between astroglial cells and hippocampal neurons in culture. *Science,* 209: 809 – 810.

Bartus, R.T., Dean, R.L. and Beer, B. (1980) Memory deficits in aged *Cebus* monkeys and facilitation with central cholinomimetics. *Neurobiol. Aging,* 1: 145 – 152.

Bartus, R.T., Dean, R.L., III, Beer, B. and Lippa, A.S. (1982) The cholinergic hypothesis of geriatric memory dysfunction. *Science,* 217: 408 – 417.

Basi, G.S., Jacobson, R.D., Virag, I., Schilling, J. and Skene, J.H.P. (1987) Primary structure and transcriptional regulation of GAP-43, a protein associated with nerve growth. *Cell,* 49: 785 – 791.

Beckh, S., Müller, H. and Seifert, W. (1987) In: H.H. Althaus and W. Seifert (Eds.), *Glial-Neuronal Communication in Development and Regeneration,* Springer-Verlag, New York, pp. 385 – 406.

Benowitz, L.I., Shashoua, V. and Yoon, M. (1981) Specific changes in rapidly transported proteins during regeneration of the goldfish optic nerve. *J. Neurosci.,* 1: 300 – 307.

Benowitz, L.I., Apostolides, P.J., Perrone-Bizzozero, N., Finklestein, S.P. and Zwiers, H. (1988) Anatomical distribution of the growth-associated protein GAP-43/B-50 in the adult rat brain. *J. Neurosci.,* 8: 339 – 352.

Besedovsky, H. and del Rey, A. (1987) Neuroendocrine and metabolic responses induced by interleukin-1. *J. Neurosci. Res.,* 18: 172 – 178.

84

Blessed, G., Tomlinson, B.E. and Roth, M. (1968) The association between quantitative measures of dementia and of senile change in the cerebral grey matter of elderly subjects. *Brit. J. Psychiatry,* 114: 797 – 811.

Bowen, D.M., Spillane, J.A., Curzon, G., Meier-Ruge, W., White, P., Goodhardt, M.J., Iwangoff, P. and Davidson, A.N. (1979) Accelerated ageing or selective neuronal loss as an important cause of dementia? *Lancet,* i: 11 – 14.

Brizzee, K.R., Ordy, J.M. and Bartus, R.T. (1980) Localization of cellular changes within multimodal sensory regions in aged monkey brain: possible implications for age-related cognitive loss. *Neurobiol. Aging,* 1: 45 – 52.

Brody, H. (1955) Organization of the cerebral cortex. III. A study of aging in the human cerebral cortex. *J. Comp. Neurol.,* 102: 511 – 556.

Buell, S.J. and Coleman, P.D. (1979) Dendritic growth in the aged human brain and failure of growth in senile dementia. *Science,* 206: 854 – 856.

Buell, S.J. and Coleman, P.D. (1981) Quantitative evidence for selective dendritic growth in normal human aging but not in senile dementia. *Brain Res.,* 214: 23 – 41.

Buttyan, R., Zakeri, Z., Lockshin, R. and Wolgemuth, D. (1988) Cascade induction of *c-fos, c-myc,* and heat shock 70K transcripts during regression of the rat ventral prostate gland. *Mol. Endocrinol.,* 2: 650 – 657.

Caceres, A. and Steward, O. (1983) Dendritic reorganization in the denervated dentate gyrus of the rat following entorhinal cortical lesions: a Golgi and electron microscopic analysis. *J. Comp. Neurol.,* 214: 387 – 403.

Cajal, S. (1913/1928) *Degeneration and Regeneration of the Nervous System.* Hafner, New York.

Carboni, A.A., Jr., del Cerro, M. and Coleman, P.D. (1985) A combined Golgi high voltage-e.m. study of dendrite tips in olfactory bulb in aging Sprague-Dawley rat. *Neurosci. Abstr.,* 11: 896.

Cole, G., Dobkins, K.R., Hansen, L.A., Terry, R.D. and Saitoh, T. (1988) Decreased levels of protein kinase C in Alzheimer brain. *Brain Res.,* 452: 165 – 174.

Coleman, P.D. and Flood, D.G. (1987) Neuron numbers and dendritic extent in normal aging and Alzheimer's disease. *Neurobiol. Aging,* 8: 521 – 545.

Coleman, P.D., Buell, S.J., Magagna, L., Flood, D.G. and Curcio, C.A. (1986) Stability of dendrites in cortical barrels of C57Bl/6N mice between 4 and 45 months. *Neurobiol. Aging,* 7: 101 – 105.

Cowan, W.M., Stanfield, B.B. and Kishi, K. (1980) The development of the dentate gyrus. *Curr. Top. Dev. Biol.,* 15: 103 – 157.

Cupp, C.J. and Uemura, E. (1980) Age-related changes in prefrontal cortex of *Macaca mulatta:* quantitative analysis of dendritic branching patterns. *Exp. Neurol.,* 69: 143 – 163.

Curcio, C.A. and Coleman, P.D. (1982) Stability of neuron number in cortical barrels of aging mice. *J. Comp. Neurol.,* 212: 158 – 172.

De Graan, P.N.E., Van Hooff, C.O.M., Tilly, B.C., Oestreicher, A.B., Schotman, P. and Gispen, W.H. (1985) Phosphoprotein B-50 in nerve growth cones from fetal rat brain. *Neurosci. Lett.,* 61: 235 – 241.

Drachman, D.A. and Leavitt, J. (1974) Human memory and the cholinergic system. A relationship to aging? *Arch. Neurol.,* 30: 113 – 121.

Fahrbach, S.E. and Truman, J.W. (1987) Mechanisms for programmed cell death in the nervous system of a moth. *Selective Neuronal Death, Ciba Foundation Symposium,* 126: 65 – 81.

Farrar, W., Kilian, P., Ruff, M., Hill, J. and Pert, C. (1987) Visualization and characterization of interleukin-1 receptors in brain. *J. Immunol.,* 139: 459 – 463.

Fallon, J.R. (1985) Preferential outgrowth of central nervous system neurites on astrocytes and Schwann cells as compared with nonglial cells in vitro. *J. Cell Biol.,* 100: 198 – 207.

Flood, D.G. (1990) Region specific stability of dendritic extent in normal human aging and regression in Alzheimer's disease. II. Subiculum. *Brain Res.,* in press.

Flood, D.G. and Coleman, P.D. (1990) Hippocampal plasticity in normal aging and decreased plasticity in Alzheimer's disease. In: J. Storm-Mathisen, J. Zimmer and O.P. Ottersen (Eds.), *Understanding the Brain through the Hippocampus, Progress in Brain Research, Vol. 83,* Elsevier, Amsterdam, pp. 435 – 443.

Flood, D.G., Buell, S.J., DeFiore, C., Horwitz, G. and Coleman, P.D. (1985) Age-related dendritic growth in dentate gyrus of human brain is followed by regression in the "oldest old". *Brain Res.,* 345: 366 – 368.

Flood, D.G., Buell, S.J., Horwitz, G. and Coleman, P.D. (1987) Dendritic extent in human dentate gyrus granule cells in normal aging and senile dementia. *Brain Res.,* 402: 205 – 216.

Fontana, A. (1982) Astrocytes and lymphocytes: intercellular communication by growth factors. *J. Neurosci. Res.,* 8: 443 – 451.

Fontan, A., Weber, E., Grob, P., Lim, R. and Miller, J. (1983) Dual effect of glia maturation factor on astrocytes. *J. Neuroimmunol.,* 5: 261 – 269.

Gage, F.H., Bjorklund, A., Stenevi, U., Dunnett, S.B. and Kelly, P.A.T. (1984) Intrahippocampal septal grafts ameliorate learning impairments in aged rats. *Science,* 225: 533 – 536.

Gage, F.H., Olejniczak, P. and Armstrong, D.M. (1988) Astrocytes are important for sprouting in the septohippocampal circuit. *Exp. Neurol.,* 102: 2 – 13.

Geddes, J.W., Monaghan, D., Cotman, C., Lott, I., Kim, R. and Chui H. (1985) Plasticity of hippocampal circuitry in Alzheimer's disease. *Science,* 230: 1179 – 1181.

Giulian, D. (1987) Ameboid microglia as effectors of inflammation in the central nervous system. *J. Neurosci. Res.,* 18: 155 – 171.

Giulian, D. and Lachman, L. (1985) Interleukin-1 stimulation of astroglial proliferation after brain injury. *Science,* 228:

497 – 499.

Giulian, D., Baker, T., Shih, L.C. and Lachman, L. (1986) Interleukin-1 of the central nervous system is produced by ameboid microglia. *J. Exp. Med., 164*: 594 – 604.

Giulian, D., Young, D., Woodward, J., Brown, D. and Lachman, L. (1988) Interleukin-1 is an astroglial growth factor in the developing brain. *J. Neurosci., 8*: 709 – 714.

Globus, A. and Scheibel, A.B. (1966) Loss of dendrite spines as an index of pre-synaptic terminal patterns. *Nature, 212*: 463 – 465.

Greenough, W.T., Juraska, J.M. and Volkmar, F.R. (1979) Maze training effects on dendritic branching in occipital cortex of adult rats. *Behav. Neural Biol., 26*: 287 – 297.

Griffin, W.S.T., Stanley, L., Ling, C., White, L., MacLeod, V., Perrot, L., White, C.L., III and Araoz, C. (1989) Brain interleukin 1 and S-100 immunoreactivity are elevated in Down syndrome and Alzheimer disease. *Proc. Natl. Acad. Sci. U.S.A., 86*: 7611 – 7615.

Grumet, M., Hoffman, S. and Edelman, G.M. (1984) Two antigenically related neuronal cell adhesion molecules of different specificities mediate neuron – neuron and neuron – glia adhesion. *Proc. Natl. Acad. Sci. U.S.A., 81*: 267 – 271.

Hamill, R.W., Caine, E.D., Coleman, P.D., Eskin, T.A., Flood, D.G., Joynt, R.J., Lapham, L.W., McNeill, T.H. and Odoroff, C.L. (1987) Multiple morphological and biochemical measures completely distinguish patients with Alzheimer's disease. *Neurosci. Abstr., 13*: 442.

Hanks, S.D. and Flood, D.G. (1990) Region specific stability of dendritic extent in normal human aging and regression in Alzheimer's disease. I. CA1 of hippocampus. *Brain Res.,* in press.

Hansen, L.A., Armstrong, D.M. and Terry, R.D. (1987) An immunohistochemical quantification of fibrous astrocytes in the aging human cerebral cortex. *Neurobiol. Aging, 8*: 1 – 6.

Henderson, G., Tomlinson, B.E. and Gibson, P.H. (1980) Cell counts in human cerebral cortex in normal adults throughout life using an image analysing computer. *J. Neurol. Sci., 46*: 113 – 136.

Higgins, G.A. and Mufson, E.J. (1989) NGF receptor gene expression is decreased in the nucleus basalis in Alzheimer's disease. *Exp. Neurol., 106*: 222 – 236.

Hinds, J.W. and McNelly, N.A. (1977) Aging of the rat olfactory bulb: growth and atrophy of constituent layers and changes in size and number of mitral cells. *J. Comp. Neurol., 171*: 345 – 368.

Hori, T., Shibata, M., Nakashima, T., Yamasaki, M., Asami, A. and Koga, H. (1988) Effects of interleukin-1 and arachiodonate on the preoptic and anterior hypothalamic neurons. *Brain Res. Bull., 20*: 75 – 82.

Hsu, H.K. and Peng, M.T. (1978) Hypothalamic neuron number of old female rats. *Gerontology, 24*: 434 – 440.

Hubbard, B.M. and Anderson, J.M. (1985) Age-related variations in the neuron content of the cerebral cortex in senile dementia of Alzheimer type. *Neuropathol. Appl. Neurobiol., 11*: 369 – 382.

Ihara, Y. (1988) Massive somatodendritic sprouting of cortical neurons in Alzheimer's disease. *Brain Res., 459*: 138 – 144.

Jacobson, R.D., Virag, I. and Skene, J.H.P. (1986) A protein associated with axon growth, GAP-43, is widely distributed and developmentally regulated in rat CNS. *J. Neurosci., 6*: 1843 – 1855.

Johnson, S.A., Pasinetti, G.M., May, P.C., Ponte, P.A., Cordell, B. and Finch, C.E. (1988) Selective reduction of mRNA for the β-amyloid precursor protein that lacks a Kuntiz-type protease inhibitor motif in cortex from AD. *Exp. Neurol., 102*: 264 – 268.

Johnson, S.A., Rogers, J. and Finch, C.E. (1989) APP-695 transcript prevalence is selectively reduced during Alzheimer's disease in cortex and hippocampus but not in cerebellum. *Neurobiol. Aging, 10*: 267 – 272.

Jones, W.H. and Thomas, D.B. (1962) Changes in the dendritic organization of neurons in the cerebral cortex following deafferentation. *J. Anat., 96*: 375 – 381.

Katzman, R., Terry, R., DeTeresa, R., Brown, T., Davies, P., Fuld, P., Renbing, X. and Peck, A. (1988) Clinical, pathological, and neurochemical changes in dementia: a subgroup with preserved mental status and numerous neocortical plaques. *Ann. Neurol., 23*: 138 – 144.

Kesslak, J.P., Nieto-Sampedro, M., Globus, J. and Cotman, C.W. (1986) Transplants of purified astrocytes promote behavioral recovery after frontal cortex ablation. *Exp. Neurol., 92*: 377 – 390.

Landfield, P.W., Rose, G., Sandles, L., Wohlstadter, T. and Lynch, G. (1977) Patterns of astroglial hypertrophy and neuronal degeneration in the hippocampus of aged, memory-deficient rats. *J. Gerontol., 32*: 3 – 12.

Lefebvre, P.P., Rogister, B., Delree, P., Leprince, P., Selak, I. and Moonen, G. (1987) Potassium-induced release of neuronotoxic activity by astrocytes. *Brain Res., 413*: 120 – 128.

Liesi, P., Kaakkola, S., Dahl, D. and Vaheri, A. (1984) Laminin is induced in astrocytes of adult brain by injury. *EMBO J., 3*: 683 – 686.

Lindsay, R.M. (1979) Adult rat brain astrocytes support survival of both NGF-dependent and NGF-intensive neurones. *Nature, 282*: 80 – 82.

Lindsay, R.M. (1986) Reactive gliosis. In: S. Federoff and A. Vernadakis (Eds.), *Astrocytes, Vol. 3, Cell Biology and Pathology of Astrocytes,* Academic Press, Orlando, FL, pp. 231 – 262.

Lorente de Nó, R. (1934) Studies on the structure of the cerebral cortex. II. Continuation of the study of the ammonic system. *J. Psychol. Neurol., 46*: 113 – 177.

Manthorpe, M., Longo, F.M. and Varon, S. (1982) Comparative features of spinal neuronotrophic factors in fluids collected in vitro and in vivo. *J. Neurosci. Res., 8*: 241 – 250.

Manthorpe, M., Engvall, E., Ruoslahti, E., Longo, F.M.,

Davis, G.E. and Varon, S. (1983) Laminin promotes neuritic regeneration from cultured peripheral and central neurons. *J. Cell Biol.,* 97: 1882 – 1890.

Manthorpe, M., Rudge, J. and Varon, S. (1986) Astroglial cell contributions to neuronal survival and neuritic growth. In: S. Federoff and A. Vernadakis (Eds.), *Astrocytes, Vol. 2, Biochemistry, Physiology and Pharmacology of Astrocytes,* Academic Press, Orlando, FL, pp. 315 – 376.

Martin, D.P., Schmidt, R., DiStefano, P., Lowry, O., Carter, J. and Johnson, E.M., Jr. (1988) Inhibitors of protein synthesis and RNA synthesis prevent neuronal death caused by nerve growth factor deprivation. *J. Cell Biol.,* 106: 829 – 844.

McKee, A.C., Kowall, N. and Kosik, K.S. (1988) Microtubule disorganization and growth cone formation characterize degeneration and regeneration in Alzheimer's disease. *Neurosci. Abstr.,* 14: 155.

Meiri, K.F., Pfenninger, K.H. and Willard, M.B. (1986) Growth-associated protein, GAP-43, a polypeptide that is induced when neurons extend axons, is a component of growth cones and corresponds to pp46, a major polypeptide of a subcellular fraction enriched in growth cones. *Proc. Natl. Acad. Sci. U.S.A.,* 83: 3537 – 3541.

Merrill, J.E. (1987) Macroglia: neural cells responsive to lymphokines and growth factors. *Immunol. Today,* 8: 146 – 150.

Miller, F. and Geddes, J. (1990) Increased expression of the major embryonic alpha-tubulin mRNA, T-alpha-1, during neuronal regeneration, sprouting, and in Alzheimer's disease. (This volume).

Moonen, G., Rogister, B., Leprince, P., Rigo, J.-M., Delree, P., Lefebvre, P.P. and Schoenen, J. (1990) Neurono-glial interactions and neural plasticity. (This volume.)

Mouritzen Dam, A. (1979) The density of neurons in the human hippocampus. *Neuropathol. Appl. Neurobiol.,* 5: 249 – 264.

Müller, H.W. and Seifert, W. (1982) A neurotrophic factor (NTF) released from primary glial cultures supports survival and fiber outgrowth of cultured hippocampal neurons. *J. Neurosci. Res.,* 8: 195 – 204.

Müller, H.W., Beckh, S. and Seifert, W. (1984) Neurotrophic factor for central neurons. *Proc. Natl. Acad. Sci. U.S.A.,* 81: 1248 – 1252.

Neve, R.L., Finch, E.A., Bird, E.D. and Benowitz, L.I. (1988) Growth-associated protein GAP-43 is expressed selectively in associative regions of the adult human brain. *Proc. Natl. Acad. Sci. U.S.A.,* 85: 3638 – 3642.

Ng, S.-C., de la Monte, S.M., Conboy, G.L., Karns, L.R. and Fishman, M.C. (1988) Cloning of human GAP-43: growth association and ischemic resurgence. *Neuron,* 1: 133 – 139.

Nieto-Sampedro, M. and Berman, M. (1987) Interleukin-1-like activity in rat brain: sources, targets and effects of injury. *J. Neurosci. Res.,* 17: 214 – 219.

Nieto-Sampedro, M., Lewis, E.R., Cotman, C.W., Manthorpe, M., Skaper, S., Barbin, G., Longo, F.M. and Varon, S. (1982) Brain injury causes a time-dependent increase in

neuronotrophic activity at the lesion site. *Science,* 217: 860 – 861.

Oestreicher, A.B., Zwiers, H., Schotman, P. and Gispen, W.H. (1981) Immunohistochemical localization of a phosphoprotein (B-50) isolated from rat brain synaptosomal plasma membranes. *Brain Res. Bull.,* 6: 145 – 153.

Perry, V.H. and Linden, R. (1982) Evidence for dendritic competition in the developing retina. *Nature,* 297: 683 – 685.

Purves, D. and Hadley, R.D. (1985) Changes in the dendritic branching of adult mammalian neurons revealed by repeated imaging in situ. *Nature,* 315: 404 – 406.

Reier, P.J. (1986) Gliosis following CNS injury: the anatomy of astrocytic scars and their influences on axonal elongation. In: S. Federoff and A. Vernadakis (Eds.), *Astrocytes, Vol. 3, Cell Biology and Pathology of Astrocytes,* Academic Press, Orlando, FL, pp. 263 – 324.

Rogers, K.E., Wadhams, A.B. and Coleman, P.D. (1989) Interleukin 1-β message levels increase in Alzheimer's disease while GAP-43 message levels are diminished. *Neurosci. Abstr.,* 15: 844.

Rossor, M.N., Iversen, L.L., Johnson, A.J., Mountjoy, C.Q. and Roth, M. (1981) Cholinergic deficit in frontal cerebral cortex in Alzheimer's disease is age dependent. *Lancet,* ii: 1422.

Sapolsky, R., Rivier, C., Yamamoto, G., Plotsky, P. and Vale, W. (1987) Interleukin-1 stimulates the secretion of hypothalamic corticotropin-releasing factor. *Science,* 238: 522 – 524.

Schade, J.P. and Baxter, C.F. (1960) Changes during growth in the volume and surface area of cortical neurons in the rabbit. *Exp. Neurol.,* 2: 158 – 178.

Schwartz, L.M. and Kay, B.K. (1987) De novo transcription and translation of new genes is required for the programmed death of the intersegmental muscles of the tobacco hawkmoth, *Manduca sexta. Neurosci. Abstr.,* 13: 8.

Selak, I., Skaper, S.D. and Varon, S. (1985) Pyruvate participation in the low molecular weight trophic activity for central nervous system neurons in glia-conditioned media. *J. Neurosci.,* 5: 23 – 28.

Shefer, V.F. (1973) Absolute number of neurons and thickness of the cerebral cortex during aging, senile and vascular dementia, and Pick's and Alzheimer's diseases. *Neurosci. Behav. Physiol.,* 6: 319 – 324.

Skene, J.H.P., Jacobson, R.D., Snipes, G.J., McGuire, C.B., Norden, J.J. and Freeman, J.A. (1986) A protein induced during nerve growth (GAP-43) is a major component of growth-cone membranes. *Science,* 233: 783 – 786.

Skene, J.H.P. and Virag, I. (1989) Posttranslational membrane attachment and dynamic fatty acylation of a neuronal growth cone protein, GAP-43. *J. Cell Biol.,* 108: 613 – 624.

Skene, J.H.P. and Willard, M. (1981) Axonally transported proteins associated with growth in rabbit central and peripheral nervous system. *J. Cell Biol.,* 89: 96 – 103.

Sladek, J.R., Jr., Khachaturian, H., Hoffman, G.E. and

Scholer, J. (1980) Aging of central endocrine neurons and their aminergic afferents. *Peptides,* 1 (Suppl. 1): 141 – 157.

Streit, W.J. and Kreutzberg, G.W. (1988) Response of endogenous glial cells to motor neuron degeneration induced by toxic ricin. *J. Comp. Neurol.,* 268: 248 – 263.

Uemura, E. (1985) Age-related changes in the subiculum of *Macaca mulatta:* dendritic branching pattern. *Exp. Neurol.,* 87: 412 – 427.

Uylings, H.B.M., Kuypers, K., Diamond, M.C. and Veltman, W.A.M. (1978) Effects of differential environments on plasticity of dendrites of cortical pyramidal neurons in adult rats. *Exp. Neurol.,* 62: 658 – 677.

Van Hooff, C.O.M., Holthui, J.C.M., Oestreicher, A.B., Boonstra, J., De Graan, P.N.E. and Gispen, W.H. (1989) Nerve growth factor-induced changes in the intracellular localization of the protein kinase C substrate B-50 in pheochromocytoma PC12 cells. *J. Cell Biol.,* 108: 1115 – 1125.

Van Lookeren Campagne, M., Oestreicher, A., Van Bergen Henegouwen, P. and Gispen, W.H. (1989) Ultrastructural immunocytochemical localization of B-50/GAP43, a protein kinase C substrate, in isolated pre-synaptic nerve terminals and neuronal growth cones. *J. Neurocytol.,* 18: 479 – 489.

Vernadakis, A. (1988) Neuron-glia interrelations. *Int. Rev. Neurobiol.,* 30: 149 – 224.

Wadewitz, A.G. and Lockshin, R.A. (1988) Programmed cell death: dying cells synthesize a coordinated, unique set of proteins in two different episodes of cell death. *FEBS Lett.,* 241: 19 – 23.

Whittemore, S.R., Nieto-Sampedro, M., Needels, D. and Cotman, C.W. (1985) Neuronotrophic factor for mammalian brain neurons: injury induction in neonatal, adult and aged rat brain. *Dev. Brain Res.,* 20: 169 – 178.

Wolozin, B.L., Pruchnicki, A., Dickson, D.W. and Davies, P. (1986) A neuronal antigen in the brains of Alzheimer patients. *Science,* 232: 648 – 650.

P. Coleman, G. Higgins and C. Phelps (Eds.)
Progress in Brain Research, Vol. 86
© 1990 Elsevier Science Publishers B.V. (Biomedical Division)

CHAPTER 8

Effects of aging on the dynamics of information processing and synaptic weight changes in the mammalian hippocampus

C.A. Barnes

Department of Psychology, University of Colorado, Boulder, CO 80309, U.S.A.

Introduction

One of the most interesting forms of plasticity to be discovered in the mammalian central nervous system is the persistent increase in cellular communication that can be recorded following convergent, patterned activation of inputs to certain neuronal cell groups. This increase in synaptic strength can be induced, for example, in the hippocampal formation of species as diverse as rabbits, rats (e.g., Bliss and Lømo, 1973; Douglas and Goddard, 1975) and humans (Haas, 1987). Moreover, a number of its properties suggests that it may reflect the processes normally involved in information storage in the brain. For these reasons it has been important to develop an understanding of how this form of neuronal plasticity might change with age, and to examine its potential contribution to cognitive changes observed in aged organisms.

The following is an overview of this long-lasting form of neuronal plasticity as it is observed in the fascia dentata (FD) and in the CA1 region of the hippocampus, primarily in the rat. This is not to imply that such changes do not occur in other cortical or subcortical regions (in fact there is evidence that it can be induced elsewhere, e.g., Lee, 1983; Racine et al., 1983) nor does this imply that other types of plastic change (such as that found in the

specialized mossy fiber boutons in the CA3 region of the hippocampus, e.g., Harris and Cotman, 1986) will not turn out to be equally important to our overall understanding of information processing in the brain. Rather, the synaptic change that can be induced in the granule cells of FD and pyramidal cells of CA1 is the point of focus here because evoked potentials and intracellular records in these regions are easily measured and interpreted. Therefore, most of the work on the underlying mechanisms and potential relation to behavior has been described in these regions. This emphasis is simply meant to facilitate the illustration of how associative memories might be represented as changes in the synaptic weight distributions among populations of neurons. The idea that, under specific conditions, lasting cellular changes could be induced that would act as an associative information storage device was outlined by Hebb in his book *The Organization of Behavior* (1949), although the notion that brain elements should be capable of modification through experience certainly has a much older history (c.f., the excerpt from Thomas Reid's (1710 – 1796) *The Essays on the Intellectual Powers of Man: Essay III. Concerning Memory* (1969)): ". . . Aristotle imputes the shortness of memory in children to this cause, that their brain is too moist and soft to retain impressions made upon it: and the defect of memory in old men he imputes, on the contrary, to the hardness and rigidity of the brain, which hinders its receiving any durable impression.''

Other reviews of the long-lasting change that can be artificially induced at synapses in the central nervous system of mammals have organized the material differently from the way it is presented here (cf., Teyler and Discenna, 1984; Andersen, 1987; Baudry et al., 1988; Bliss and Lynch, 1988; Lynch et al., 1988; Nicoll et al., 1988). The goal of the present review is to describe the characteristics of this form of plasticity that make it particularly interesting as a potential associative memory mechanism and to discuss the possible contributions to age-related memory deficits made by alterations in this plastic process.

In 1966 Lømo obtained the first evidence that it was possible to change synaptic efficacy for time periods outlasting the classically defined mechanisms of post-tetanic potentiation (PTP) described originally in the neuromuscular junction (Lloyd, 1949). Bliss joined Lømo in Oslo to further characterize this phenomenon, and the first complete manuscripts describing these changes in anesthetized and awake animals were published in 1973 (Bliss and Gardner-Medwin, 1973; Bliss and Lømo, 1973). They called this durable form of synaptic plasticity ''long-lasting potentiation,'' because they initially believed that it represented a more durable form of PTP known to be due to an increase in the probability of transmitter release (Landau et al., 1973; Magleby, 1973). Douglas and Goddard (1975) subsequently called this phenomenon ''long-term potentiation.'' Because the requirements for induction of the synaptic change were different from those that produced PTP, McNaughton et al. (1978) later called it ''long-term enhancement'' (LTE). LTE will be used to refer to this phenomenon in the following, because McNaughton (1982) clearly demonstrated that the probability of transmitter release (as measured by paired-pulse facilitation) before and after LTE induction remains constant. The mechanism of this long-lasting change is, therefore, clearly different

from the potentiation observed at the neuromuscular junction. The shorter-lasting processes of depression, facilitation, augmentation and potentiation (Magleby and Zengel, 1975, 1976a, b) also occur at these hippocampal synapses (McNaughton, 1980, 1982). The central nervous system, however, appears to have an additional process (LTE) that is strikingly durable.

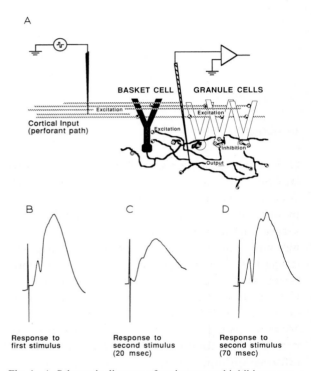

Fig. 1. A. Schematic diagram of excitatory and inhibitory connections in the fascia dentata, and of the typical stimulation and recording configuration used to obtain evoked field potentials from the activation of entorhinal cortical afferents (perforant path fibers). B. Typical field potential recorded from an electrode positioned approximately as shown in A. The rising phase of the response reflects the summed depolarization of the granule cells or ''field EPSP'' (excitatory post-synaptic potentials), and the negative deflection reflects the compound action potentials of the granule cells or ''population spike.'' C. Field potential recorded to a second stimulus following the first (as in B) by 20 msec. The dramatic inhibition of the population spike in this response is due to the recurrent inhibitory pathway from the inhibitory interneurons (basket cells, as shown in A). D. At longer inter-stimulus intervals, the population spike is actually increased over the first (in B), due to a prolonged depression of the inhibitory circuit.

Induction of LTE

LTE was first discovered in the synaptic connection between entorhinal cortical afferents (via the perforant pathway) and the granule cells in the FD of the hippocampus (see Fig. 1A). The afferent fibers from cortex contact not only the granule cells but also the inhibitory interneurons in the area (the basket cells) that feed forward inhibition onto the granule cells. These basket cells also feed back inhibition onto the granule cells through a recurrent inhibitory loop. As shown in Fig. 1A, this loop involves granule cell axon collaterals that contact basket cells, and the axons of these inhibitory cells that subsequently contact the granule cell bodies. Thus, the response that is recorded following stimulation of the perforant path fibers is actually a combination of both excitatory (EPSP) and inhibitory (IPSP) processes. The synaptic component of either the field potential or the intracellular record following afferent stimulation is typically measured to monitor the baseline response amplitude and the changes that are produced following patterned high-frequency activation. The population excitatory post-synaptic potential (field EPSP, see Fig. 1B) has been emphasized as the proper measure of the extracellular records because the interest in LTE revolves around making inferences concerning synaptic events. This is especially important in view of the fact that the population spike (which reflects synchronous action potential discharge of the recorded cells, Fig. 1B) can vary independently of the field EPSP, partly as a result of extrinsic modulation of the inhibitory interneurons. Therefore, one cannot be certain that a synaptic change has taken place if only the spike component is measured (e.g., Andersen et al., 1980; Bliss and Lynch, 1988).

The stimulation parameters first used by Bliss and Lømo (1973) to induce LTE consisted of hundreds of pulses delivered at frequencies of approximately 15 Hz (see Fig. 2A). The stimulation parameters that are the most effective in artificially generating LTE in hippocampal synapses, how-

ever, involve shorter bursts of high-frequency stimulation (Douglas, 1977; see Fig. 2B). Furthermore, it has recently been shown that if a single "priming" stimulus is given shortly preceding such a burst of stimulation, then these parameters are particularly conducive to generating enduring LTE (Larson et al., 1986; Rose and Dunwiddie, 1986; Diamond et al., 1988). The optimal interval between the prime stimulus and the burst corresponds approximately to the time of one cycle (200 msec) of the EEG "theta" rhythm that characterizes the hippocampus of actively moving animals (Green and Arduini, 1954; Vanderwolf, 1969).

The effect of this prime stimulus now appears to be due to a peculiar characteristic of the inhibitory

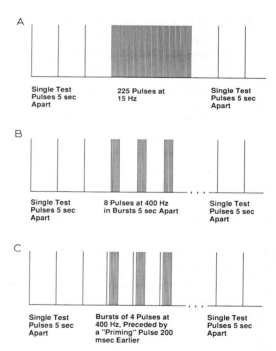

Fig. 2. Schematic representation of different parameters of electrical activation used to induce LTE. The parameters shown in A were used by Bliss and Lømo (1973) in their initial demonstration of LTE. Brief bursts of stimuli (shown in B) were found to be more effective (Douglas, 1977) in inducing LTE than those shown in A. The most effective parameters for LTE induction are shown in C, and involve a single pulse ("priming stimulus") followed 200 msec later by short bursts of stimulation (Larson et al., 1986; Rose and Dunwiddie, 1986).

circuitry in the hippocampus. When the perforant path fibers are activated, there is direct excitation of both the principal cells and the inhibitory cells (see Fig. 1A). The onset of the IPSP that results from activation of the inhibitory cells is fast enough that, in fact, a significant proportion of the principal cells are prevented from firing. If the perforant path is stimulated a second time, shortly afterwards (as shown in Fig. 1C), the combination of the feedforward and feedback inhibition induced by the first stimulus can block discharge in the principal cells. Although the underlying IPSP decays in about 50 msec, for reasons that are not yet completely understood, the inhibitory system exhibits a rather prolonged period of post-activation depression or "refractoriness." During this period, which lasts about 200 msec (see example in Fig. 1D), the feedforward inhibition is less effective, and therefore more depolarization and post-synaptic discharge is observed than when the system is not "primed" (Larson et al., 1986). This increased depolarization for an equivalent excitatory input at the long inter-stimulus intervals (as in Fig. 1D) appears to account for the increased efficacy of "primed burst" stimulation for the induction of LTE.

Repetition, saturation, and persistence

One interesting feature of LTE induction is that, if the patterned stimulus is repeated, the synaptic strength can be increased up to some maximum level (e.g., Bliss and Gardner-Medwin, 1973; Barnes, 1979; see Fig. 3) and can be shown to be very durable following such stimulation. This property finds an analogy in the behavioral literature, as practice (repetition) is known to improve retention. There comes a point in time, however, where LTE does not increase further, or is "saturated" (see Figs. 3, 4). On the other hand, the short-lasting processes of facilitation, augmentation, and potentiation can be repeatedly elicited and decay relatively rapidly back to baseline (McNaughton, 1982; see Fig. 3), even when the LTE mechanism is saturated. Several groups have suggested

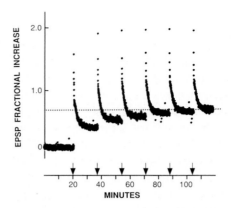

Fig. 3. Synaptic strength (represented here as the fractional increase in the field EPSP amplitude in the fascia dentata) can be increased to some maximum level by repeating the LTE-inducing burst stimulation. The arrows point to the times when a brief burst of high-frequency stimulation was delivered to the perforant path fibers. All other stimulations were delivered at much lower frequency (0.5 Hz). Notice that LTE can be "saturated" to some level (dotted line) by such repetition, while the short-lasting process of PTP continues to be observed (McNaughton, 1982).

that a long-lasting form of depression may also be induced at these synapses (Dunwiddie and Lynch, 1978; Levy and Steward, 1983). However, to date, this has never been studied in chronically prepared animals over the time courses necessary to directly compare it to the LTE phenomenon, and it appears that some of its properties may be different from those of LTE.

Depending on the parameters of stimulation, including number of repetitions and the synapses in question, the time constant of decay of this process can vary in chronically prepared animals from under 1 h to over a month (Bliss and Gardner-Medwin, 1973; Douglas and Goddard, 1975; Barnes, 1979; Racine et al., 1983; Staubli and Lynch, 1987; Castro et al., 1989). The approximately exponential decay of LTE over days in FD appears to be a true decay of synaptic strength rather than an artifact of the chronic recording situation. At least two lines of evidence support this conclusion. First of all, the decay appears to return to some constant baseline level over days in chronically prepared animals (Barnes, 1979;

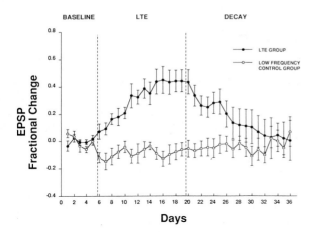

Fig. 4. Data from Castro et al. (1989) illustrating saturation and the persistence of LTE. The fractional change in the field EPSP is plotted as a function of days. All responses are collected at "low frequency" of 0.1 Hz (test stimulation). Baseline responses are shown for the control group (low-frequency stimulation only; open circles) and the LTE group (closed circles). Beginning at day 6 the LTE group received daily high-frequency stimulation for 2 weeks (through day 20). The responses to test stimulation were measured 24 h after the LTE-inducing stimulation. On days 20 – 36 only test stimulation was given to both groups. Note that the magnitude of the EPSP decayed back towards baseline during this time period in the LTE group, and that the control group did not differ significantly from baseline levels over this time period.

Racine et al., 1983; Castro et al., 1989), and, along the same line of argument, pharmacological treatments that reversibly block LTE after its induction also bring the synaptic response down to a "baseline" level (Lovinger et al., 1987; Madison et al., 1989). Furthermore low-frequency stimulated control animals, that are tested over the same time period as rats in which LTE is induced, show stable records over this time period (Castro et al., 1989; see Fig. 4). This suggests that, under the right conditions, these responses can be stable for intervals outlasting the necessary recording time period.

Selectivity

One important requirement of a mechanism of information storage is the necessity for the modification to occur only in the elements involved in the initial encoding of the event and not on synapses that were not involved in the high-frequency event. This condition of specificity has been met for both "post-synaptic" and "pre-synaptic" cases in the hippocampus and is illustrated in Fig. 5. The post-synaptic example is taken from McNaughton and Barnes (1977), where it was shown that induction of LTE on the lateral perforant path fibers (located on distal granule cell dendrites) did not induce LTE in the medial perforant path fibers (more proximally located, see Fig. 5A). Importantly, this was demonstrated under conditions where the lateral and medial perforant path fibers were shown to converge onto the same granule cells.

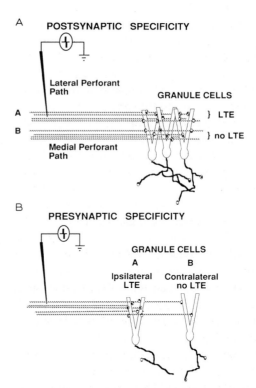

Fig. 5. A. Diagram illustrating "post-synaptic specificity" of the LTE process in the fascia dentata (McNaughton and Barnes, 1977). Induction of LTE on one set of inputs (A) does not cause enhancement of unstimulated inputs (B) to the same cells. B. Diagram illustrating "pre-synaptic specificity" of the LTE process in the fascia dentata (Levy and Steward, 1979). Induction of LTE on one set of inputs (A), does not cause enhancement of non-convergent connections from the same axons (B).

94

This principle also holds for LTE in CA1 (Andersen et al., 1977; Dunwiddie and Lynch, 1978). The pre-synaptic example is taken from Levy and Steward (1979) who demonstrated that the induction of LTE *ipsilaterally* on one set of convergent synapses did not change the sparse *contralateral* synapses that were stimulated and were from the same axon collaterals (see Fig. 5B). Therefore, LTE is only induced on synapses that are both stimulated and convergently active.

Cooperativity

Probably the most exciting property that LTE possesses in terms of its relation to learning and memory is the fact that it is an associative process. The first clear demonstration that this was the case was made by McNaughton et al. (1978) in FD, and this finding was confirmed (Levy and Steward, 1979) and extended to observations in CA1 by others (Schwartzkroin and Wester, 1975; Andersen et al., 1977; Dunwiddie and Lynch, 1978; Barrionuevo and Brown, 1983). As shown in Fig. 6A, LTE requires the convergent activation of multiple inputs onto the post-synaptic neuron for its induction. That is, LTE cannot normally be produced if the stimulus intensity is very low, thereby activating too few fibers at high frequency. Under conditions of sparse fiber activation, only PTP can be elicited at these synapses (McNaughton, 1982).

More recently, however, it has been demonstrated that LTE can be induced with a sparse input under certain conditions of stimulation. This is illustrated in Fig. 6B. If the level of depolarization of the cell is increased directly by intracellular current injection, then LTE can be induced on only a small number of fibers (Wigström et al., 1986; Gustafsson et al., 1987). Therefore, it appears that the level of depolarization of the post-synaptic neuron is a critical variable controlling the initial induction of LTE and explains the initial observation that there is a certain level of convergence of inputs necessary to produce the effect (cooperativity). Other methods that have been used to induce LTE-like increases in the synaptic response, in the

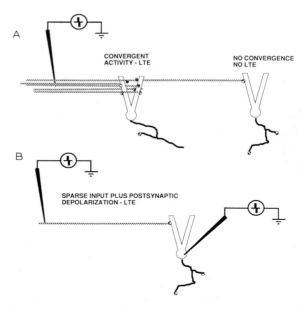

Fig. 6. *A*. Illustration of the associative property of "cooperativity" of the LTE process as first described by McNaughton et al. (1978). Unlike PTP, LTE cannot normally occur on a single fiber; it requires cooperation among multiple convergent inputs. *B*. LTE can, however, be induced with sparse inputs, if these inputs are paired with depolarization of the post-synaptic cell (Wigström et al., 1986). This associative property therefore appears to be controlled by the level of depolarization of the post-synaptic cell.

absence of convergent fiber input, include iontophoresis of glutamate or NMDA (Collingridge et al., 1983; Kauer et al., 1988) and the quisqualate receptor agonist AMPA (Davies et al., 1989), or the direct intracellular injection of protein kinase C into the post-synaptic cell (Hu et al., 1987). While these latter treatments are likely to act through several different mechanisms, they support the point that a critical feature in the induction process is a certain form of activation of the post-synaptic cell.

Glutamate and the NMDA and non-NMDA receptors

There is considerable evidence that the main neurotransmitter released by the perforant path synapses onto the granule cells of the fascia dentata, and from the Schaffer collateral synapses onto CA1, is L-glutamate (and to a lesser extent L-aspartate). Although a number of different forms of glutamate receptors are thought to exist in the hippocampus (see Cotman, this volume), the three main subtypes include the N-methyl-D-aspartate (NMDA), quisqualate, and kainate types (Watkins and Evans, 1981; Foster and Fagg, 1984). Of these, only the NMDA receptor can be selectively blocked by competitive antagonists such as AP5 (Davies et al., 1981) or non-competitive antagonists such as MK-801 (Wong et al., 1986). Because of the difficulty of pharmacologically separating the other receptor types, the glutamate receptors will be referred to as either NMDA or non-NMDA types in the following.

While the work in this area is rapidly evolving at present, the current understanding of glutamate receptor involvement in LTE is that the non-NMDA receptors mediate normal synaptic transmission ("fast EPSPs") in granule and CA1 pyramidal cells (see Fig. 7A), while the voltage-dependent NMDA receptors contribute to a slower component of the EPSP (see Fig. 7B; Collingridge et al., 1988a, b). NMDA receptor activation is clearly necessary for LTE induction, because, if the NMDA antagonist AP5 is applied, then it is not possible to produce LTE (Collingridge et al., 1983; Harris et al., 1984; Wigström and Gustafsson, 1984). The special voltage-dependent property of this receptor therefore explains why there must be a certain level of depolarization or convergent afferent input (cooperativity) before LTE can be induced. Furthermore, Worley, Cole, Saffen and Baraban (this volume) have shown that LTE induction produces activation of genes that encode transcription factors, the "immediate early genes." LTE was shown to selectively activate messenger RNA for at least one type of these genes, $zif/268$ (and not the protooncogene c-fos, see Douglas et al., 1988), and MK-801 was found to block $zif/268$ induction after such LTE-inducing stimulation. It

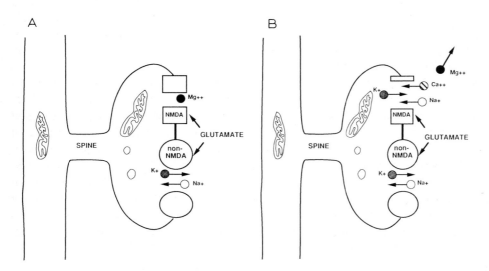

Normal synaptic transmission through non-NMDA receptors -important for EXPRESSION of LTE

Depolarization through convergent input releases Mg++ block on NMDA allowing Ca++ to enter - important for INDUCTION of LTE

Fig. 7. *A*. Illustration of normal synaptic transmission in CA1 and fascia dentata of hippocampus occurring through non-NMDA receptors. The longer lasting change in synaptic conductance is probably expressed through these receptors. *B*. Illustration of the activation of the NMDA receptors following depolarization of the post-synaptic cell. The initial induction of LTE is normally dependent on NMDA receptor activation.

is possible, therefore, that the processes involved in NMDA receptor activation may lead to some form of gene expression.

The mechanisms involved in the long-lasting expression of LTE are less well understood, although a rather good case is being constructed for non-NMDA involvement in the persistent increases in conductance observed following LTE-inducing stimulation. It appears, for example, that iontophoresis of NMDA agonists onto hippocampal slices produces increases in the EPSP that are far too short to account for the full expression of LTE (Kauer et al., 1988). Furthermore, if the AP5-sensitive and AP5-insensitive components are measured following LTE, then the latter (non-NMDA) post-synaptic component shows a persistent increase in strength, whereas the NMDA component does not (Muller and Lynch, 1988). More support for non-NMDA involvement in the lasting expression of LTE was provided in a very recent report by Davies et al. (1989), where iontophoretic application of quisqualate receptor agonists following LTE-inducing stimulation was shown to lead to a slowly developing, but very durable, increase in sensitivity to the agonist (at least 3 h). Because protein kinase C (PKC) activators can prolong LTE (Malenka et al., 1986; Routtenberg et al., 1986; Linden et al., 1987; Lovinger and Routtenberg, 1988), and LTE in the presence of PKC inhibitors has a time course comparable to the NMDA-mediated changes in synaptic strength, it is possible that the changes produced in non-NMDA-mediated synaptic transmission may involve the prolonged action of PKC (Lovinger et al., 1987; Madison et al., 1989). Taken together, these findings suggest that the more durable synaptic changes may occur through non-NMDA rather than the NMDA receptor-mediated mechanisms, although the latter appears to be required for the initial induction of the complete chain of events.

Maintenance of LTE

There is general agreement that the entry of calcium, both through the pre-synaptic terminal and during the release of the magnesium block on the NMDA receptor on the post-synaptic neuron, is critical for the mechanisms underlying LTE (e.g., Dingledine, 1983). There is as yet, however, no clear consensus on how calcium might trigger changes in synaptic strength and perhaps the morphological alteration of hippocampal pyramidal and granule cell spines on which the majority of synaptic contacts are formed. There are at least two major theoretical positions concerning changes in either the pre-synaptic terminal or post-synaptic cell that have accumulated a good deal of support. It should be noted that there are other variations of these hypotheses that may be equally plausible. However, for the sake of illustration, only two of these positions will be presented here.

The first possibility is that LTE leads to an increased pre-synaptic transmitter release. As mentioned earlier, there is clear evidence that the probability of transmitter release does not change following LTE induction (McNaughton, 1982), however, transmitter release can be influenced by other parameters of the quantal release equation. Evidence for an increase in release of endogenous glutamate in vivo and an increase in potassium-stimulated glutamate release in vitro has been found in the fascia dentata following LTE-induction (Bliss et al., 1986; Feasey et al., 1986; but also see Aniksztejn et al., 1989). This increase in release could be prevented by application of AP5 during the high-frequency stimulation event (Errington et al., 1987). Consistent with the finding of a change in the pre-synaptic mechanism of release are a variety of results from Routtenberg's laboratory over the past decade (e.g., Routtenberg, 1986). The phosphorylation of the pre-synaptically-located PKC substrate protein F1 (GAP-43/-48/B50/pp46) has been implicated in the mechanisms underlying the maintenance of LTE in the hippocampus (Lovinger et al., 1985, 1986; Akers et al., 1986; Schrama et al., 1986), and possibly of plasticity in a number of other synaptic types (e.g., Benowitz and Routtenberg, 1987). Of interest here is the observation that there is a translocation of PKC from the cytosol to the membrane following LTE induction and that the degree of phosphorylation of the F1 protein is correlated with the durability of LTE measured in chronically prepared animals. Furthermore, PKC inhibitors block the induction of LTE (Lovinger et al., 1987; Madison et al., 1989) and can even reverse the effect of high-frequency stimulation if LTE has been induced before the application of the blocker H-7 (Madison et al., 1989). It thus appears that this calcium-dependent kinase is normally required for the long-lasting expression of LTE. These post-translational changes in a substrate protein such as F1 could potentially lead to pre-synaptic terminal growth or other alterations. Such a membrane change could be responsible for the greater transmitter release observed by Bliss and his colleagues, possibly involving an increase in the number of release sites.

Another major theoretical position has been proposed by Lynch and his colleagues and involves a post-synaptic mechanism as an explanation for the long-lasting changes that accompany LTE. In this view (Baudry et al., 1988; Lynch et al., 1988) calcium entry into the post-synaptic neuron may initiate a process whereby the proteolytic enzyme calpain becomes activated. This could result in at least two possible outcomes: calpain could lead to post-synaptic membrane modifications or changes in the distribution of proteins in the membrane that result in the enduring conductance changes observed following LTE; in addition, calpain could degrade major cytoskeletal proteins in the spine (brain spectrin). This could lead to spine shape changes that also have been observed following LTE (Lee et al., 1980; Fifková and Anderson, 1981; Chang and Greenough, 1984). The influx of calcium through NMDA channels into spines may thus raise the concentration of calcium in the spine heads sufficiently to induce a cascade of changes that are ultimately responsible for the enduring change in synaptic strength.

The problem that is raised by the present hypotheses is how to reconcile the pre-synaptic and post-synaptic findings into a consistent and complementary explanation for the persistent changes observed in cellular communication found following LTE induction. Unanswered questions for the proponents of pre-synaptic hypotheses include why the calcium blocker EGTA injected into a single post-synaptic neuron can block LTE in the synapses on that cell (Lynch et al., 1983) and why there is a persistent change in sensitivity to non-NMDA receptor agonists. A crucial question for the proponents of post-synaptic hypotheses is why there is an increase in glutamate release. Furthermore, while the assumption has been that NMDA receptors reside on spines (as shown here in Fig. 7) and some theoretical arguments specifically rely on high levels of calcium in the spine through these channels, there is no direct evidence that this is the case. They could reside on dendritic shafts. The resolution of this debate will most likely involve hypotheses that propose reciprocal interactions between the pre- and post-synaptic sites that are more complex than have been hitherto assumed. In fact it is possible that the modifications that occur both in the pre-synaptic terminal and in the post-synaptic spine might both be required for the full expression of LTE. Investigators are now beginning to speculate on how pre-synaptic factors might influence post-synaptic sites or whether there might be post-synaptic release of a factor that can influence pre-synaptic sites (e.g., Bliss and Lynch, 1988; Davies et al., 1989). In summary, the only hypothesis that is consistent with all of the data is that the expression of LTE involves both an increase in number of sites for transmitter release and a complementary change in post-synaptic responsiveness. Such an hypothesis begins to sound like the formation of an entirely new synapse or the simultaneous formation of release and receptor complexes at existing synapses.

LTE and behavior

The arguments concerning LTE's role in information processing ultimately must consider more direct tests of this physiological mechanism in relation to behavior. Although it does not seem highly probable that the nervous system would have evolved a mechanism with many of the characteristics that might be desired for associative memory, without actually utilizing it, a certain amount of uncertainty as to the role of LTE in memory remains. It must be noted at the outset that the kinds of experiments that attempt to implicate LTE in associative operations are necessarily correlational in nature and therefore cannot provide evidence for causal relationships. What must also be kept in mind, however, is the fact that many of these experiments were designed in such a way that the outcome could have strongly argued either for or against a role for LTE in associative processes. What is striking in the experiments presented below, is that no data have been collected that argue against LTE's role in learning. This is not to say that there will never be data that contradict the conclusion that LTE and learning operations are related but rather that the growing body of positive evidence makes it increasingly unlikely.

It is well accepted now that one of the most striking behavioral deficits that result from damage to the hippocampal formation in rats is the inability to navigate in space (e.g., O'Keefe and Nadel, 1978). The first evidence that a relationship existed between spatial memory and hippocampal LTE was provided by a study that compared the performance of young and old rats on the circular platform task (in which the object is to remember the location in space of a dark escape chamber), with the ability of the same rats to maintain elevated synaptic strength following LTE-inducing stimulation (Barnes, 1979). The age differences will be described in the next section. The important point regarding LTE was that there was a statistically significant positive correlation between an individual rat's memory for the location of the escape chamber in the circular platform task and the rate of decay of LTE.

One of the potential mechanisms of LTE's involvement in associative learning is the idea that information is stored as a specific distribution of synaptic weights of modifiable synapses and that LTE acts selectively to change this weight distribution. If, in fact, the specific distribution of synaptic weights in a population of neurons is critical to normal information processing, then the disruption of that distribution through saturating the LTE mechanism should lead to a disruption in the ability to acquire new information of the sort normally stored in that system. An experiment addressing this question in relation to spatial memory was performed by McNaughton et al. (1986). LTE was induced bilaterally in chronically prepared rats to saturation levels (see Fig. 4) at various points during the acquisition of the circular platform task. If the saturating stimulation was given before training began, it prevented the animals from learning the spatial location of the hidden escape chamber. Furthermore, if the animals were first allowed to learn the location of the escape chamber, then given stimulation leading to LTE saturation, and finally tested on their ability to learn a change in the goal location, these rats were impaired.

An extension of this kind of experiment has recently been performed by Castro et al. (1989). The electrophysiological data from animals in the low-frequency control group and the high-frequency LTE saturation group can be seen in Fig. 4. At day 20 (after LTE saturation in the experimental group) the rat's spatial memory was tested using the Morris water task (Morris, 1981), where animals must find a submerged platform using distal visual cues. In direct support of the results of McNaughton et al. (1986), the LTE group could not learn this spatial problem. They had no difficulty, however, in learning to escape to a visible platform. The additional question addressed by this experiment, however, was whether spatial learning ability would recover following the decay of LTE back to baseline levels. When the animals were retested following LTE decay (at day 36 in Fig. 4), there were no longer any spatial learning impairments. This evidence therefore supports the overall notion that selective LTE plays a crucial role in the ability to acquire new spatial information.

Another approach to the question of whether associative memory takes place at hippocampal synapses through an LTE-like mechanism is to utilize agents that block the induction of LTE. That is, treatments that block LTE in the hippocampus should by logical inference also block spatial learning. This was demonstrated by Morris et al. (1986) where they gave doses of APV (the NMDA receptor antagonist) that would normally block LTE, and tested the rat's behavior in the Morris water task. These investigators found that the APV treatment blocked the rat's ability to learn the spatial version of this problem, but it did not influence their ability to learn the non-spatial version. These data therefore provide additional support that LTE at hippocampal synapses may be important for the normal acquisition of spatial information.

If hippocampal synapses are modified, through a process such as LTE, while an animal is acquiring novel spatial information, then under some conditions one might expect to see a strengthening in the synaptic response recorded from these animals after such information storage has occurred. These changes, of course, would be expected to be relatively small or short-lived over the population of cells studied, because under normal conditions such "environmentally-induced" LTE should not lead to saturation levels that are actually detrimental to learning. Sharp et al. (1985) have examined this question and have been able to record a spontaneous growth in the field response when animals were exposed to a novel, complex environment consisting of a large room with numerous ramps and other objects. These data, again, are consistent with the hypothesis that changes in the strength of hippocampal synapses may underlie acquisition and storage of information that is important for effective navigation within an environment.

Other evidence that supports the notion that the processes involved in LTE may form the basis of information storage in the brain includes those treatments where either learning is known to be improved (therefore LTE would be expected to be improved under the same conditions) or states where learning is not thought to be possible (and

therefore LTE would not be expected to occur). Two examples that bear on these issues involve stimulation of the mesencephalic reticular formation and slow-wave sleep, respectively. Bloch and Laroche (1985) were able to show that the same type of stimulation of the reticular formation that produces reliable improvement in memory of rats also produces an extension of the decay time constant of LTE. Furthermore, Jones Leonard et al. (1987) were able to show that it was not possible to induce LTE in rats if they were in slow-wave sleep, although LTE could be induced immediately upon waking. This is clearly an active blockade of LTE induction, because LTE can be induced easily in anesthetized animals.

In summary, while this is not a comprehensive review of all experiments that favor the idea that LTE may be related to associative memory processes, it does provide an overview of the kinds of experiments that have been conducted to examine this issue. Again, the author is not aware of any experiments that have been done where the outcome favored the hypothesis that LTE is not used by the nervous system to store information through the strengthening of synapses.

Age-related changes in LTE

The study of LTE in old animals is of particular interest with regard to the known learning and memory changes that occur, even in the healthiest old humans, primates and rodents (c.f., Barnes, 1990). In fact the study that initially found a positive correlation between LTE and behavior (described above) was a comparison of young and old rats' behavior and synaptic plasticity (Landfield et al., 1978; Barnes, 1979). The hypothesis tested in Barnes' (1979) experiment was that if LTE represents the underlying mechanism of spatial information storage, then spatial memory-deficient old rats should show an altered ability for either the induction or maintenance of LTE at hippocampal synapses. The results showed that if LTE was induced to saturation levels, then the absolute magnitude of the synaptic change reached by the old rats was the same as that for the young rats. However, there was a striking difference between groups in the decay of LTE back towards baseline levels (Barnes, 1979; Barnes and McNaughton, 1980, 1985; De Toledo-Morrell and Morrell, 1985). That is, the old perforant path synapses showed a decay time constant of about 16 days compared with a decay time constant of about 37 days for young rats. Because the LTE-inducing stimulation was only given once per day and LTE was essentially allowed to decay a certain amount each day between high-frequency stimulation sessions, the older animals took longer to actually reach saturation levels of LTE than did the young animals (Barnes and McNaughton, 1980). Nevertheless, it appears that the induction process is intact in the old animals. One prediction of this outcome, then, is that the NMDA receptor mechanisms involved in induction should be reasonably intact in the old rats. Evidence in support of this idea comes from Cotman's laboratory (see this volume), where levels of NMDA receptors were found to be similar in the fascia dentata of young and old Fischer-344 rats.

As mentioned in the previous section, when the performance of young and old rats on the circular platform spatial memory task was compared with the decay of LTE in hippocampal synapses, there was a significant correlation between the durability of LTE and the rat's performance. In other words, the old animals showing the poorest behavior on the spatial task also showed the fastest decaying synaptic enhancement. Furthermore, when the rates of forgetting of the spatial task were compared with the rates of decay of LTE in groups of young and old rats, the young/old ratio for forgetting rate was virtually the same as the young/old ratio of decay of LTE (Barnes and McNaughton, 1985). Moreover, when young and old animals were compared on their ability to show the "environmentally-induced" enhancement in the field response, this response showed a differential decay in a manner very similar to electrically-induced LTE in the two age groups (Sharp et al., 1987). Taken together, this evidence favors the

hypothesis that the faster forgetting in old animals may be partly due to the faster decay of LTE.

Because it has been shown that the phosphorylation of the F1 (GAP-43/-48/B50/pp46) substrate protein was correlated with the maintenance of LTE (Lovinger et al., 1985), it was important to investigate whether F1 might be involved in the age-related changes in this form of plasticity. In fact, evidence was found for a 46% decline in the F1 substrate protein in the hippocampus of old rats using gel electrophoretic methods (Barnes et al., 1988). A converging line of evidence was also reported from Gispen's group, who used radio-immunoassay procedures. In their experiment, B-50 content was found to be lower in the hippocampus of old than of young rats (Oestreicher et al., 1986). Furthermore, Coleman's group (this volume) has found reduced levels of message for this protein in very old normal aged humans and those with Alzheimer's disease. The loss of this protein may be part of the explanation for the faster decay of this hippocampal plasticity. On the other hand, it may simply be a reflection of a loss of incoming terminals rather than a reduction in the content of this phosphoprotein per neuron. This issue needs to be resolved in future experiments.

Summary

It is clear that the properties of LTE make it a plausible mechanism for associative information storage at some synapses in the central nervous system. While many of the factors that regulate LTE's induction and expression have been discovered and a strong case is being developed for its role in learning and memory processes, until we understand more clearly the mechanisms underlying both the expression and maintenance of LTE, an understanding of its change with age will be difficult. Judging by the progress that has been made over the past several years in uncovering some of the molecular events that are critical for LTE's expression, one may be optimistic that answers will be forthcoming reasonably soon. Of particular importance to aging mammals, such answers may provide insights into why older organisms show faster forgetting. This may have a profound impact on therapeutic strategies for memory disorders in both normal and pathological conditions of aging.

Acknowledgements

I am grateful to the organizers of the NIA Conference for their efforts and to the participants for their stimulating interactions that led to modifications and additions to this chapter. I thank B. McNaughton, T. Foster, and G. Rao for comments on the manuscript and to B. McNaughton, C. Castro, G. Rao, and E.J. Green for their contributions to the figures. Manuscript preparation was supported by AG-03376 and AG-00243.

References

Akers, R.F., Lovinger, D.M., Colley, P.A., Linden, D.J. and Routtenberg, A. (1986) Translocation of protein kinase C activity may mediate hippocampal long-term potentiation. *Science*, 231: 587 – 589.

Andersen, P.O. (1987) Properties of hippocampal synapses of importance for integration and memory. In: G.M. Edelman, W.E. Gall and W.M. Cowan (Eds.), *Synaptic Function*, Wiley, New York, pp. 403 – 429.

Andersen, P., Sundberg, S.H., Sveen, O. and Wigström, H. (1977) Specific long-lasting potentiation of synaptic transmission in hippocampal slices. *Nature*, 266: 736 – 737.

Andersen, P., Sundberg, S.H., Sveen, O., Swann, J.W. and Wigström, H. (1980) Possible mechanisms of long-lasting potentiation of synaptic transmission in hippocampal slices from guinea pigs. *J. Physiol. (Lond.)*, 302: 463 – 482.

Aniksztejn, L., Roisin, M.P., Amsellem, R. and Ben-Ari, Y. (1989) Long-term potentiation in the hippocampus of the anaesthetized rat is not associated with a sustained enhanced release of endogenous excitatory amino acids. *Neuroscience*, 28: 387 – 392.

Barnes, C.A. (1979) Memory deficits associated with senescence: a neurophysiological and behavioral study in the rat. *J. Comp. Physiol. Psychol.*, 93: 74 – 104.

Barnes, C.A. (1990) Animal models of age-related cognitive decline. In: F. Boller and J. Grafman (Eds.), *Handbook of Neuropsychology*, Elsevier, Amsterdam, pp. 169 – 196.

Barnes, C.A. and McNaughton, B.L. (1980) Spatial memory and hippocampal synaptic plasticity in senescent and middle-aged rats. In: D. Stein (Ed.), *Psychobiology of Aging: Problems and Perspectives*, Elsevier, Amsterdam, pp. 253 – 272.

Barnes, C.A. and McNaughton, B.L. (1985) An age comparison of the rates of acquisition and forgetting of spatial information in relation to long-term enhancement of hippocampal synapses. *Behav. Neurosci.*, 99: 1040 – 1048.

Barnes, C.A., Mizumori, S.J.Y., Lovinger, D.M., Sheu, F.-S., Murakami, K., Chan, S.Y., Linden, D.J., Nelson, R.B. and Routtenberg, A. (1988) Selective decline in protein F1 phosphorylation in hippocampus of senescent rats. *Neurobiol. Aging*, 9: 393 – 398.

Barrionuevo, G. and Brown, T.H. (1983) Associative long-term synaptic potentiation in the hippocampal slice. *Proc. Natl. Acad. Sci. U.S.A.*, 80: 7347 – 7351.

Baudry, M., Larson, J. and Lynch, G. (1988) Long-term changes in synaptic efficacy: potential mechanisms and implications. In: P.W. Landfield and S.A. Deadwyler (Eds.), *Long-Term Potentiation: From Biophysics to Behavior*, Alan R. Liss, New York, pp. 109 – 136.

Benowitz, L.I. and Routtenberg, A. (1987) A membrane phosphoprotein associated with neural development, axonal regeneration, phospholipid metabolism, and synaptic plasticity. *Trends Neurosci.*, 10: 527 – 531.

Bliss, T.V.P. and Gardner-Medwin, A.R. (1973) Long-lasting potentiation of synaptic transmission in the dentate area of the unanaesthetized rabbit following stimulation of the perforant path. *J. Physiol. (Lond.)*, 232: 357 – 371.

Bliss, T.V.P. and Lømo, T. (1973) Long-lasting potentiation of synaptic transmission in the dentate area of the anaesthetized rabbit following stimulation of the perforant path. *J. Physiol. (Lond.)*, 232: 331 – 356.

Bliss, T.V.P. and Lynch, M.A. (1988) Long-term potentiation of synaptic transmission in the hippocampus: properties and mechanisms. In: P.W. Landfield and S.A. Deadwyler (Eds.), *Long-Term Potentiation: From Biophysics to Behavior*, Alan R. Liss, New York, pp. 3 – 72.

Bliss, T.V.P., Douglas, R.M., Errington, M.L. and Lynch, M.A. (1986) Correlation between long-term potentiation and release of endogenous amino acids from dentate gyrus of anaesthetized rats. *J. Physiol. (Lond.)*, 377: 391 – 408.

Bloch, V. and Laroche, S. (1985) Enhancement of long-term potentiation in the rat dentate gyrus by post-trial stimulation of the reticular formation. *J. Physiol. (Lond.)*, 360: 215 – 231.

Castro, C.A., Silbert, L.H., McNaughton, B.L. and Barnes, C.A. (1989) Recovery of spatial learning following decay of electrically-induced synaptic enhancement in the hippocampus. *Nature*, 342: 545 – 548.

Chang, F.L.F. and Greenough, W.T. (1984) Transient and enduring morphological correlates of synaptic activity and efficacy changes in the rat hippocampal slice. *Brain Res.*, 309: 35 – 46.

Collingridge, G.L., Kehl, S.J. and McLennan, H. (1983) Excitatory amino acids in synaptic transmission in the Schaffer collateral-commissural pathway of the rat hippocampus. *J. Physiol. (Lond.)*, 334: 33 – 46.

Collingridge, G.L., Heron, C.E. and Lester, R.A.J. (1988a) Synaptic activation of N-methyl-D-aspartate receptors in the Schaffer collateral-commissural pathway of rat hippocampus. *J. Physiol. (Lond.),* 399: 283 – 300.

Collingridge, G.L., Heron, C.E. and Lester, R.A.J. (1988b) Frequency-dependent N-methyl-D-aspartate receptor-mediated synaptic transmission in rat hippocampus. *J. Physiol. (Lond.),* 399: 301 – 312.

Davies, J., Francis, A.A., Jones, A.W. and Watkins, J.C. (1981) 2-amino-5-phosphonovalerate (2APV), a potent and selective antagonist of amino acid-induced and synaptic excitation. *Neurosci. Lett.,* 21: 77 – 81.

Davies, S.N., Lester, R.A., Reymann, K.G. and Collingridge, G.L. (1989) Temporally distinct pre- and post-synaptic mechanisms maintain long-term potentiation. *Nature,* 338: 500 – 503.

De Toledo-Morrell, L. and Morrell, F. (1985) Electrophysiological markers of aging and memory loss in rats. *Ann. N.Y. Acad. Sci.,* 444: 296 – 311.

Diamond, D.M., Dunwiddie, T.V. and Rose, B.M. (1988) Characteristics of hippocampal primed burst potentiation in vitro and in the awake rat. *J. Neurosci.,* 8: 4079 – 4088.

Dingledine, R. (1983) Excitatory amino acids: modes of action on hippocampal pyramidal cells. *Fed. Proc.,* 42: 2881 – 2885.

Douglas, R.M. (1977) Long lasting synaptic potentiation in the rat dentate gyrus following brief high frequency stimulation. *Brain Res.,* 126: 361 – 365.

Douglas, R.M. and Goddard, G.V. (1975) Long-term potentiation of the perforant path – granule cell synapse in the rat hippocampus. *Brain Res.,* 86: 205 – 215.

Douglas, R.M., Dragunow, M. and Robertson, H.A. (1988) High-frequency discharge of dentate granule cells, but not long-term potentiation, induces c-fos protein. *Mol. Brain Res.,* 4: 259 – 262.

Dunwiddie, T. and Lynch, G. (1978) Long-term potentiation and depression of synaptic reponses in the hippocampus: localization and frequency dependency. *J. Physiol. (Lond.),* 276: 353 – 361.

Errington, M.L., Lynch, M.A. and Bliss, T.V.P. (1987) Long-term potentiation in the dentate gyrus: induction and increased glutamate release are blocked by D-amino-phosphonovalerate. *Neuroscience,* 20: 279 – 284.

Feasey, K.J., Lynch, M.A. and Bliss, T.V.P. (1986) Long-term potentiation is associated with an increase in calcium-dependent, potassium-stimulated release of [14C] glutamate from hippocampal slices: an ex vivo study in the rat. *Brain Res.,* 364: 39 – 44.

Fifková, E. and Anderson, C.L. (1981) Stimulation-induced changes in dimensions of stalks of dendritic spines in the dentate molecular layer. *Exp. Neurol.,* 74: 621 – 627.

Foster, A.C. and Fagg, G.E. (1984) Acidic amino acid binding sites in mammalian neuronal membranes: their characteristics and relationship to synaptic receptors. *Brain Res. Rev.,* 7: 103 – 164.

Green, J.D. and Arduini, A.A. (1954) Hippocampal electrical activity in arousal. *J. Neurophysiol.,* 17: 533 – 557.

Gustafsson, B.H., Wigström, W.C., Abraham, W.C. and Huang, Y.-Y. (1987) Long-term potentiation in the hippocampus using depolarizing current pulses as the conditioning stimulus to single volley synaptic potentials. *J. Neurosci.,* 7: 774 – 780.

Haas, H. (1987) Recording from human hippocampus in vitro. *Neurosci. Lett. (Suppl.),* 29: S13.

Harris, E.W. and Cotman, C.W. (1986) Long-term potentiation of guinea-pig mossy fiber responses is not blocked by N-methyl-D-aspartate receptor antagonists. *Neurosci. Lett.,* 70: 132 – 137.

Harris, E.W., Ganong, A.H. and Cotman, C.W. (1984) Long-term potentiation in the hippocampus involves activation of N-methyl-D-aspartate receptors. *Brain Res.,* 323: 132 – 137.

Hebb, D.O. (1949) *The Organization of Behavior,* Wiley, New York.

Hu, G.-Y., Hvalby, O., Walaas, S.I., Albert, K.A., Skejflo, P., Andersen, P. and Greengard, P. (1987) Protein kinase C injection into hippocampal pyramidal cells elicits features of long-term potentiation. *Nature,* 328: 426 – 429.

Jones Leonard, B., McNaughton, B.L. and Barnes, C.A. (1987) Suppression of hippocampal synaptic plasticity during slow-wave sleep. *Brain Res.,* 425: 174 – 177.

Kauer, J.A., Malenka, R.C. and Nicoll, R.A. (1988) NMDA application potentiates synaptic transmission in the hippocampus. *Nature,* 334: 250 – 252.

Landau, E.M., Smolinsky, A. and Lass, Y. (1973) Post-tetanic potentiation and facilitation do not share a common calcium-dependent mechanism. *Nature,* 244: 155 – 157.

Landfield, P.W., McGaugh, J.L. and Lynch, G. (1978) Impaired synaptic potentiation processes in the hippocampus of aged, memory-deficient rats. *Brain Res.,* 150: 85 – 101.

Larson, J., Wong, D. and Lynch, G. (1986) Patterned stimulation at the theta frequency is optimal for the induction of hippocampal long-term potentiation. *Brain Res.,* 368: 347 – 350.

Lee, K.S. (1983) Sustained modification of neuronal activity in the hippocampus and neocortex. In: W. Seifert (Ed.), *Neurobiology of the Hippocampus,* Academic Press, New York, pp. 265 – 272.

Lee, K., Schottler, G., Oliver, M. and Lynch, G. (1980) Brief bursts of high-frequency stimulation produce two types of structural change in rat hippocampus. *J. Neurophysiol.,* 44: 247 – 258.

Levy, W.B. and Steward, O. (1979) Synapses as associative memory elements in the hippocampal formation. *Brain Res.,* 175: 233 – 245.

Levy, W.B. and Steward, O. (1983) Temporal contiguity requirements for long-term associative potentiation/depression in the hippocampus. *Neuroscience,* 8: 791 – 797.

Linden, D.J., Sheu, R.-S., Murakami, K. and Routtenberg, A. (1987) Enhancement of long-term potentiation by cis-unsaturated fatty acid: relation to protein kinase C and phospholipase A2. *J. Neurosci.*, 7: 3783–3792.

Lloyd, D.P.C. (1949) Post-tetanic potentiation of response in monosynaptic reflex pathways of the spinal cord. *J. Gen. Physiol.*, 33: 147–170.

Lømo, T. (1966) Frequency potentiation of excitatory synaptic activity in the dentate area of the hippocampal formation. *Acta Physiol. Scand. (Suppl.)*, 68: 128.

Lovinger, D.M. and Routtenberg, A. (1988) Synapse-specific protein kinase C activation enhances maintenance of long-term potentiation in rat hippocampus. *J. Physiol. (Lond.)*, 400: 321–333.

Lovinger, D.M., Akers, R.F., Nelson, R.B., Barnes, C.A., McNaughton, B.L. and Routtenberg, A.W. (1985) A selective increase in the phosphorylation of protein F1, a protein kinase C substrate, directly related to three day growth of long-term synaptic enhancement. *Brain Res.*, 343: 137–143.

Lovinger, D.M., Colley, P.A., Akers, R.F., Nelson, R.B. and Routtenberg, A. (1986) Direct relation of long-term synaptic potentiation of synaptic transmission in the hippocampus of the rat: effect of calmodulin and oleoyl-acetyl-glycerol on release of [^{3}H]glutamate. *Neurosci. Lett.*, 65: 171–176.

Lovinger, D.M., Wong, K., Murakami, K. and Routtenberg, A. (1987) Protein kinase C inhibitors eliminate hippocampal long-term potentiation. *Brain Res.*, 436: 177–183.

Lynch, C., Larson, J., Kelso, S., Barrionuevo, G. and Schottler, F. (1983) Intracellular injections of EGTA block the induction of hippocampal long-term potentiation. *Nature*, 305: 719–721.

Lynch, G., Muller, D., Seubert, P. and Larson, J. (1988) Long-term potentiation: persisting problems and recent results. *Brain Res. Bull.*, 21: 363–372.

Madison, D.V., Malinow, R. and Tsien, R.W. (1989) Inhibitors of protein kinase C block long-term potentiation in rat hippocampus. *J. Physiol. (Lond.)*, in press.

Magleby, K.L. (1973) The effect of tetanic and post-tetanic potentiation on facilitation of transmitter release at the frog neuromuscular junction. *J. Physiol. (Lond.)*, 234: 353–371.

Magleby, K.L. and Zengel, J.E. (1975) A quantitative description of tetanic and post-tetanic potentiation of transmitter release at the frog neuromuscular junction. *J. Physiol. (Lond.)*, 245: 183–208.

Magleby, K.L. and Zengel, J.E. (1976a) Augmentation: a process that acts to increase transmitter release at the frog neuromuscular junction. *J. Physiol. (Lond.)*, 257: 449–470.

Magleby, K.L. and Zengel, J.E. (1976b) Long-term changes in augmentation, potentiation and depression of transmitter release as a function of repeated synaptic activity at the frog neuromuscular junction. *J. Physiol. (Lond.)*, 257: 471–494.

Malenka, R.C., Madison, D.V. and Nicoll, R.A. (1986) Potentiation of synaptic transmission in the hippocampus by phorbol esters. *Nature*, 321: 175–177.

McNaughton, B.L. (1980) Evidence for two physiologically distinct perforant pathways to the fascia dentata. *Brain Res.*, 199: 1–20.

McNaughton, B.L. (1982) Long-term synaptic enhancement and short-term potentiation in rat fascia dentata act through different mechanisms. *J. Physiol. (Lond.)*, 324: 249–262.

McNaughton, B.L. and Barnes, C.A. (1977) Physiological identification and analysis of dentate granule cell responses to stimulation of the medial and lateral perforant pathways in the rat. *J. Comp. Neurol.*, 175: 439–454.

McNaughton, B.L., Douglas, R.M. and Goddard, G.V. (1978) Synaptic enhancement in fascia dentata: co-operativity among coactive afferents. *Brain Res.*, 157: 277–293.

McNaughton, B.L., Barnes, C.A., Rao, G., Baldwin, J. and Rasmussen, M. (1986) Long-term enhancement of hippocampal synaptic transmission and the acquisition of spatial information. *J. Neurosci.*, 6: 563–571.

Morris, R.G.M. (1981) Spatial localization does not require the presence of local cues. *Learn. Motiv.*, 12: 239–260.

Morris, R.G.M., Anderson, E., Lynch, G.S. and Baudry, M. (1986) Selective impairment of learning and blockade of long-term potentiation by an N-methyl-D-aspartate receptor antagonist, AP5. *Nature*, 319: 774–776.

Muller, D. and Lynch, G. (1988) Long-term potentiation differentially affects two components of synaptic responses in hippocampus. *Proc. Natl. Acad. Sci. U.S.A.*, 85: 9346–9350.

Nicoll, R.A., Kauer, J.A. and Malenka, R.C. (1988) The current excitement in long-term potentiation. *Neuron*, 1: 97–103.

O'Keefe, J. and Nadel, L. (1978) *The Hippocampus as a Cognitive Map*, Clarendon Press, Oxford.

Oestreicher, A.B., De Graan, P.N.E. and Gispen, W.H. (1986) Neuronal cell membranes and brain aging. In: D.F. Swaab, E. Fliers, M. Mirmiran, W.A. Van Gool and F. Van Gaaren (Eds.), *Progress in Brain Research, Vol. 70*, Elsevier, Amsterdam, pp. 239–253.

Racine, R.J., Milgram, N.W. and Hafner, S. (1983) Long-term potentiation phenomena in the rat limbic forebrain. *Brain Res.*, 260: 217–231.

Reid, T. (1969) *The Essays on the Intellectual Powers of Man*, M.I.T. Press, Cambridge.

Rose, G.M. and Dunwiddie, T.V. (1986) Induction of hippocampal long-term potentiation using physiologically patterned stimulation. *Neurosci. Lett.*, 69: 244–248.

Routtenberg, A. (1986) Synaptic plasticity and protein kinase C. In: W.H. Gispen and A. Routtenberg (Eds.), *Phosphoproteins in Neuronal Function, Progress in Brain Research, Vol. 69*, Elsevier, Amsterdam, pp. 411–435.

Routtenberg, A., Colley, P.A., Linden, D.J., Lovinger, D., Murakami, K. and Sheu, F.-S. (1986) Phorbol ester promotes growth of synaptic plasticity. *Brain Res.*, 378: 374–378.

Schrama, L., De Graan, P.N.E., Wadman, W.J., Lopes da Silva, F.H. and Gispen, W.H. (1986) Long-term potentiation and 4-aminopyridine-induced changes in protein and lipid phosphorylation in the hippocampal slice. In: W.H. Gispen and A. Routtenberg (Eds.), *Phosphoproteins in Neuronal Function, Progress in Brain Research, Vol. 69,* Elsevier, Amsterdam, pp. 245 – 258.

Schwartzkroin, P.A. and Wester, K. (1975) Long-lasting facilitation of a synaptic potential following tetanization in the in vitro hippocampal slice. *Brain Res.,* 89: 107 – 119.

Sharp, P.E., McNaughton, B.L. and Barnes, C.A. (1985) Enhancement of hippocampal field potentials in rats exposed to a novel, complex environment. *Brain Res.,* 339: 361 – 365.

Sharp, P.E., Barnes, C.A. and McNaughton, B.L. (1987) Effects of aging on environmental modulation of hippocampal evoked responses. *Behav. Neurosci.,* 101: 170 – 178.

Staubli, U. and Lynch, G. (1987) Stable hippocampal long-term potentiation elicited by "theta" pattern stimulation. *Brain Res.,* 435: 227 – 234.

Teyler, T.J. and Discenna, P. (1984) Long-term potentiation as a candidate mnemonic device. *Brain Res. Rev.,* 7: 15 – 28.

Vanderwolf, C.H. (1969) Hippocampal electrical activity and voluntary movement in the rat. *Electroenceph. clin. Neurophysiol.,* 26: 407 – 418.

Watkins, J.C. and Evans, R.H. (1981) Excitatory amino acid transmitters. *Ann. Rev. Pharmacol. Toxicol.,* 21: 165 – 204.

Wigström, H. and Gustafsson, B. (1984) A possible correlate of the post-synaptic condition for long-lasting potentiation in the guinea pig hippocampus in vitro. *Neurosci. Lett.,* 44: 327 – 332.

Wigström, H., Gustafsson, B., Huang, Y.-Y. and Abraham, W.C. (1986) Hippocampal long-term potentiation is induced by pairing single afferent volleys with intracellularly injected depolarizing current pulses. *Acta Physiol. Scand.,* 126: 317 – 319.

Wong, E.H.F., Kemp, J.A., Priestley, T., Knight, A.R., Woodrugg, G.N. and Iversen, L.L. (1986) The anticonvulsant MK-801 is a potent *N*-methyl-D-aspartate antagonist. *Proc. Natl. Acad. Sci. U.S.A.,* 83: 7104 – 7108.

P. Coleman, G. Higgins and C. Phelps (Eds.)
Progress in Brain Research, Vol. 86
© 1990 Elsevier Science Publishers B.V. (Biomedical Division)

CHAPTER 9

Synaptic plasticity and behavioral modifications in the marine mollusk *Aplysia*

Vincent F. Castellucci[1] and Samuel Schacher[2]

[1] *Laboratory of Neurobiology and Behavior, Clinical Research Institute of Montreal, Montreal, Canada, and* [2] *Center for Neurobiology and Behavior, Columbia University, New York, NY, U.S.A.*

Introduction

A key idea to emerge in neurobiology during the last few decades is the realization that the adult nervous system is surprisingly modifiable. By analogy to the developmental processes mediating growth and differentiation of the immature nervous system scientists have suggested that many of them may be at work in the adult system. This hypothesis is not novel, neuroscientists like Cajal (1911) or Tanzi (1893) have speculated that mechanisms related to growth and differentiation may be involved in creating the physical substratum underlying memory traces or engrams in the adult nervous system. The results of many current investigations support this idea (Martinez and Kesner, 1986; Greenough and Bailey, 1988; Matthies, 1989). The key question though is to identify the signals and the mechanisms that lead to these specialized forms of growth and differentiation.

Since in aging brain there is difficulty to encode new information, it is conceivable that the processes mentioned above may be impaired with age (Terry and Gershon, 1976). By comparing the same nervous system at different stages of its development and maturation, it may be possible to capture the crucial elements that are varying with its changing adaptability. To look at this plasticity at the cellular and molecular level we have studied elementary forms of learning and memory in the marine mollusk *Aplysia*. Biophysical, pharmacological and biochemical determinations can be carried out in this animal at the level of identified neurons which in turn can be related to specific modifiable reflexes (Kandel et al., 1987).

In the adult *Aplysia* the cellular basis of several reflexes have already been studied such as feeding and satiation (Kupfermann, 1974), gill and siphon withdrawal (Byrne et al., 1978; Perlman, 1979), tail withdrawal (Walters et al., 1983), egg laying (Strumwasser, 1988), copulation (Painter et al., 1989), circadian behavior (Yeung and Eskin, 1988) and locomotion (Jahan-Parwar and Fredman, 1978). Simple forms of learning like habituation, dishabituation and sensitization have been studied together with more complex forms of learning like classical conditioning, operant conditioning, differential conditioning and fear conditioning (Hawkins et al., 1986). Finally some of these behavioral modifications have also been studied in young *Aplysias* (Rankin et al., 1987) or old ones (Papka et al., 1981; Rattan and Peretz, 1981).

An important set of questions in the study of long-term memory is to find the signals involved in triggering the transition between short-term and longer term forms of memory. A second set of questions is to ask if there are many intermediate forms of memory and what are the mechanisms that maintain them. We have started to investigate these issues in *Aplysia*. In one approach, we have analyzed short lasting behavioral modifications and longer lasting ones in adult animals; in the second approach we have compared young *Aplysias* in which good mnemonic traces can be established and older ones in which various types of memory impairments are present. A better understanding of these differences may be helpful in defining critical components in more complex systems.

In this paper we will review some studies we have done on the relationships of short-term and long-term depression (habituation) and facilitation (dishabituation or sensitization) of the gill and siphon withdrawal reflex in intact adult animals, in isolated reflex preparations and in dissociated cell culture systems. These studies indicate that the transition between short-term (minutes to hours) and long-term effects (days and weeks) may be dependent on synthesis of new proteins. Since this relationship had been observed before in vertebrates (Davis and Squire, 1984) the studies in *Aplysia* may be of value to people interested in the mechanisms of long-term memory.

The monosynaptic connection between sensory mechanoreceptor neurons and their follower cells is a critical site for plasticity during short-term facilitation and depression of the gill and siphon withdrawal reflex

Tactile stimulation of the siphon skin or the mantle shelf evokes a withdrawal of the siphon, the gill and the parapodia of *Aplysia*. If the same tactile stimulation is repeated, the reflex habituates or decreases in amplitude. The reflex can be restored with a period of rest or immediately when a strong tactile or noxious stimulus is delivered to the same region or to a different region of the animal such as the head or the tail (Pinsker et al., 1970). Since many of the sensory neurons, motor neurons and interneurons mediating this reflex have been identified, it is possible to determine where in the neuronal network key physiological changes occur when the amplitude of the reflex is modified by a training protocol (Kupfermann et al., 1974; Byrne et al., 1978).

One critical site of plasticity or change in synaptic efficacy that occurs during depression and facilitation of the reflex is the monosynaptic connection between the sensory neurons and their follower neurons (motor neurons and interneurons) (Castellucci et al., 1970). Other sites have been identified as well but they will not be discussed in this paper (Jacklet and Rine, 1977; Frost et al., 1988).

During habituation of the reflex, there is a synaptic depression at the junction between the sensory neurons and their followers. This change is pre-synaptic and it is due to a decrease in the probability of transmitter release (Castellucci and Kandel, 1974). During facilitation of the reflex the same EPSP is increased in amplitude due to the activation of some interneurons. Some of them have been characterized but their transmitter is still unknown (Hawkins et al., 1981). This synaptic facilitation is also pre-synaptic (Castellucci and Kandel, 1976). It is possible to simulate the effect of the facilitating stimulation on the reflex or at the monosynaptic junction with serotonin and two small peptides SCPa and SCPb (Abrams et al., 1984).

This important synapse can be studied in restrained and intact animals, in isolated reflexes and in dissociated cell cultures. When this monosynaptic junction is reconstituted in vitro, it shows essentially the properties found in the intact ganglion. As in the intact ganglion, the synapse is depressed with repeated activation of the sensory neuron and its efficacy can be restored with rest or exposure to a facilitating transmitter like serotonin or the peptides SCPa and SCPb (Rayport and Schacher, 1986; Fig. 1).

One proposed sequence of events leading to the facilitation of the monosynaptic connection is that facilitating transmitters activate receptors on the membrane of the sensory neuron which are coupled to an adenylate cyclase (Castellucci et al., 1980; Klein and Kandel, 1980). The resulting rise in cyclic AMP content activates a cyclic AMP-dependent protein kinase which phosphorylates some substrate proteins. The identification of

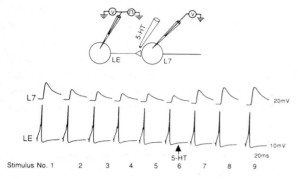

Fig. 1. Short-term synaptic depression and facilitation in a dissociated cells culture system. One sensory mechanoreceptor neuron (LE cell) and one major gill and siphon motor neuron (L7) were cocultured (see Schacher, 1985 for details). The sensory neuron was depolarized intracellularly every 20 sec and the evoked excitatory post-synaptic potentials were recorded in L7. There was a gradual synaptic depression with repetition of the stimulus; after the sixth stimulus, a brief pulse of 5-HT was ejected from a nearby extracellular pipette. Subsequent excitatory potentials were larger in amplitude and duration.

these phosphoproteins is currently under investigation (Sweatt and Kandel, 1988). One of the effects of this phosphorylation is a reduction of a potassium current (S-K) which contributes significantly to the repolarization of the action potential in the sensory neuron (Schuster et al., 1985). The reduction of this potassium current in turn slows down the repolarization of the action potential; this results in an action potential of longer duration and the activation of calcium currents for a longer amount of time. Thus, in the facilitated state, a longer action potential is accompanied by a larger calcium current and a greater release of transmitter. Similar findings have been reported for the connection between the tail mechanoreceptor neurons and motor neurons of *Aplysia* (Walters et al., 1983; Ocorr et al., 1985). The increased duration of the action potential is not the only mechanism involved in the facilitation at this synaptic junction; there is evidence that another process may be present (Hochner et al., 1986).

Long-term facilitation of the withdrawal reflex

We want to identify the signals neurons use to distinguish between an information which is to remain transient and another one that should be kept for a longer time. We took advantage of the gill and siphon withdrawal reflex which shows short- and long-lasting changes to begin our analysis.

First, we wanted to know if the monosynaptic connection between the sensory neurons and their follower cells, which changes during short-term depression and facilitation of the reflex, changes also when the reflex is altered for longer period of time (days or weeks). We therefore used a protocol that induces long-term effects in intact animals and sampled the connection between the mechanoreceptor neurons of the siphon skin (LE cells) and an identified major gill motor neuron, L7 (Frost et al., 1985). We found that the connection in the abdominal ganglia of facilitated animals was twice as large as the one from the abdominal ganglia of control animals. In addition, Bailey and Chen (1983, 1988) found that in the terminals of sensory neurons of the abdominal ganglia from trained animals the number of varicosities and the number and area of active sites per varicosity were increased. These data suggest that some kind of growth and differentiation may accompany long-term behavioral changes in *Aplysia*. This idea is also supported by recent data that indicate a change of labeling in some proteins [^{35}S]methionine in abdominal ganglia of animals that were long-term facilitated when compared to the labeling from ganglia of control animals; protein labeling was measured by using a quantitative analysis of two-dimensional gels (Castellucci et al., 1988). Two of these protein candidates have been partially sequenced (Kennedy et al., 1988); this information should help in determining their cellular localization, their function and their relation to long-term memory of this simple reflex. In addition, it will be important to verify if similar proteins could be detected in other invertebrate or vertebrate systems.

We were able also to show that long-lasting

facilitation was possible in a reduced preparation which offers technical advantages for intracellular recordings and drug applications over intact animals (Castellucci et al., 1989). This preparation consists of an isolated abdominal ganglion connected to the gill by a branchial nerve, to the siphon skin by the siphon nerve and to the tail skin by the tail nerves. The results obtained in this preparation were another indication that the abdominal ganglion which contains the cell bodies of the mechanoreceptor neurons and of several motor neurons and interneurons of the reflex is indeed a key structure in which long-lasting changes can be established.

Finally a third type of preparation was used for the analysis of long-term effects, the coculture of neurons that form the monosynaptic junction of the reflex (Fig. 1). In this system, the amplitude of the connections can be measured on one day and remeasured on subsequent days. By substituting the facilitating transmitter serotonin to the facilitating stimulus applied to the head or the tail in intact animals or in the isolated reflex one can obtain a long-lasting facilitation (Montarolo et al., 1986). Dale et al. (1988) have shown that, as in short-term facilitation, the amplitude is due to a pre-synaptic change; the probability of transmitter release is increased in a sustained manner. Dale et al. (1987) also found another pre-synaptic effect: the excitability of the sensory neuron was changed and this was probably due to a sustained reduction of a potassium current (see also Scholz and Byrne, 1987). Finally, Schacher et al. (1988) substituted an analog of cyclic AMP to serotonin and found that, like in short-term effect, the second messenger cyclic AMP had a role in the long-lasting facilitation of the monosynaptic connection between the sensory neurons and the motor neuron L7.

The role of kinase A in long-term effect is also suggested by the experiment of Greenberg et al. (1987). They found that the relative amount of regulatory subunits of the kinase to its catalytic subunits was reduced in intact long-term trained animals. This change in ratio should free more catalytic subunits for the same content of cAMP in the sensory neurons at any time, consequently the level of phosphorylation may be higher in trained animals. This could result in key physiological states being modified more permanently such as a larger proportion of S-K channels being closed which could lead in turn to greater synaptic transmission and greater excitability in the sensory neurons.

Sensitivity of long-term effects to protein synthesis inhibitors

If there are growth and differentiation processes at work during consolidation of long-term memory, one would like to know if there are any stages during which a dependence of new protein synthesis exists. In the affirmative, it may be possible to

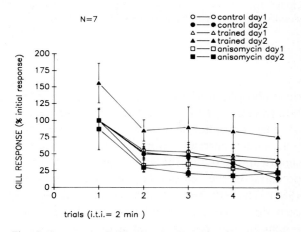

Fig. 2. Long-term facilitation in the isolated reflex and its blockade by the protein synthesis inhibitor anisomycin. Three groups of animals were compared, a control group (○ – ○), a group that received repeated tail shocks on day 1 (trained, △ – △) and a group that received repeated tail shocks on day 1 in presence of the protein synthesis inhibitor (anisomycin, □ – □). The gill responses were normalized to the first evoked response of day 1. For each group, the first five evoked responses of day 1 are compared to the first five responses of day 2. There was a significant increase in gill response amplitudes for the trained group only (▲ – ▲), the control group (● – ●) and the trained group in presence of anisomycin (anisomycin, ■ – ■) were not changed. The data are expressed as means and standard errors of the means, n = 7 for each group; initial gill response was about 35% of maximum gill contraction in each case.

block the consolidation of short-term memory into long-term memory by blocking the synthesis of new proteins at some crucial time as was shown in vertebrate studies (Davis and Squire, 1984). Studies in vertebrates where protein or RNA synthesis were blocked were at times ambiguous due to serious side effects of the drugs and the difficulty to identify the neural centers directly involved in a given learning task. In our isolated reflex preparation and dissociated cell culture we could exclude systemic effects by applying the drugs to the critical neurons involved in the reflex; the properties of these neurons could be monitored directly before, during and after any of the protocols we used. We found that we could block the long-term effect (Fig. 2) while leaving the short-term effect intact (Castellucci et al., 1989; Fig. 3; Table I).

A more extensive set of observations was carried out in our dissociated cell system and here again protein or RNA synthesis inhibitors blocked the long-term EPSP facilitation or the excitability change of the sensory neurons without affecting any short-term changes (Montarolo et al., 1986; Dale et al., 1987, 1988; Schacher et al., 1988; Table I). More importantly, as in verebrate systems, the inhibitors needed to be present only during exposure to the facilitating stimulus (tail shock) or facilitating transmitter (serotonin) in order to be effective (Montarolo et al., 1986). Recently Barzilai et al. (1988) and Sweatt and Kandel (1988) have focussed on this important time window to identify key proteins that could mediate early signals for the induction of long-term effect.

It is conceivable that different training protocols may have different or more than one sensitive periods for protein synthesis inhibition; this has been reported in the hippocampus (Grecksch and Matthies, 1980; Frey et al., 1988), and may be pre-

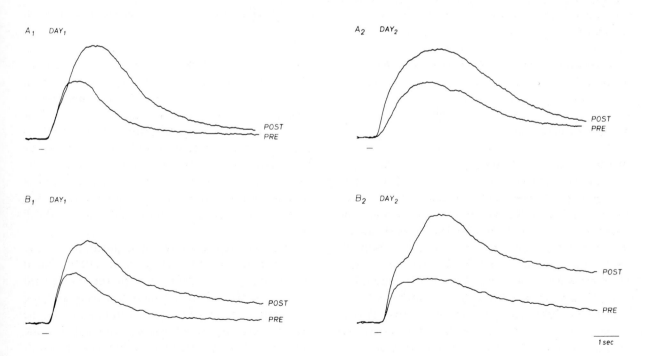

Fig. 3. Short-term facilitation of the reflex, unlike long-term facilitation, is not blocked by anisomycin. The facilitation was determined by comparing the amplitudes of the gill contraction evoked by siphon stimulation at 2-min intervals before and after tail shocks were applied to enhance the reflex. Short-term effects on day 1 and 2 are similar for the trained group (A) and trained and anisomycin group (B). These are representative gill responses on day 1 and day 2 before (pre) and after (post) tail shocks.

TABLE I

Sensitivity of long-term effects to macromolecular synthesis

	Drug[1]	Treatment	n	Percent change
Dissociated cells culture	–	–	8	-14 ± 12
(1)	–	5HT	9	$+71 \pm 31$*
	anisomycin	5HT	7	-16 ± 14
	emetine	5HT	5	-21 ± 10
	actinomycin D	5HT	7	$+3 \pm 18$
	amanitin	5HT	7	$+11 \pm 9$
	–	–	5	-8 ± 4
(2)	–	8-Benzylthio-cAMP	5	$+52 \pm 5$*
	anisomycin	8-Benzylthio-cAMP	5	-8 ± 7
	–	–	7	$+14 \pm 10$
(3)	–	FMRFamide	7	-28 ± 5*
	anisomycin	FMRFamide	7	$+12 \pm 12$
Isolated reflex	–	–	7	-10 ± 11
(4)	–	tail shock	7	$+78 \pm 30$*
	anisomycin	tail shock	7	-8 ± 24

[1] Drug dosages: anisomycin 10 or 20 μM, emetine 100 μM, actinomycin D 50 μg/ml, amanitin 2 μg/ml.
* Groups that are significantly different: (1) Montarolo et al., 1986; (2) Schacher et al., 1988; (3) Montarolo et al., 1988; (4) Castellucci et al., 1989.

sent in *Aplysia* as well (Barzilai et al., 1988). The relationship between these various time windows remains to be investigated.

Long-term habituation

When tactile stimuli are repeated over days, one can observe habituation or depression of the reflex lasting weeks (Carew et al., 1972). Castellucci et al. (1978) have sampled the connections between the sensory neurons and the identified motor neuron L7 in ganglia from long-term habituated animals and control animals. They found that the number of detectable connections was greatly reduced in long-term habituated animals. Subsequently Bailey and Chen (1983), using the same habituating protocol, observed that there were fewer varicosities and active sites in the sensory neuron terminals and that the areas of the remaining active sites were smaller. These observations are like a mirror image of those for facilitation of the reflex. In both cases, there is a short-term form and a long-term form of

the changes. In both cases, there are some morphological changes in the sensory neurons which are associated with long-term effects. Because of these similarities, one would like to know if it is possible to dissociate a short-term form of habituation from a long-term form by using protein or RNA synthesis inhibitors as was possible in the case of the facilitation of the reflex. There are no complete data on the isolated reflex yet but a first analysis has been carried out in the dissociated cell system.

As a first step to study the acquisition of long-term habituation, Montarolo et al. (1988) found that homosynaptic depression in the dissociated cell system may not be the main process underlying long-term habituation; repeated stimulation of the sensory neurons did not lead to sustained synaptic depression. On the other hand, since two transmitters, dopamine and the small peptide FMRFamide, simulate short-term heterosynaptic depression in the intact ganglion (Abrams et al., 1984; Mackey et al., 1987) they use dopamine or FMRFamide in a protocol similar to the one with serotonin. Even if both transmitters seem to use the same biochemical cascade which involves metabolites of arachidonic acid (Belardetti and Siegelbaum, 1988), they found that only FMRFamide produced a significant long-term effect (Fig. 4). They found also that this effect, like in the case of long-term EPSP facilitation with serotonin or a cAMP analog, was blocked by anisomycin, a reversible inhibitor of protein synthesis (Table I). Preliminary evidences suggest that arachidonic acid itself may play a role in long-term depression.

It would be interesting indeed to check if some of the phosphoproteins that may be involved in the onset of long-term facilitation are also involved in the onset of long-term depression or if some of the proteins whose labeling [^{35}S]methionine changes during long-term facilitation also change in this protocol. Preliminary evidences suggest that this may be the case (Sweatt and Kandel, 1988).

Effects of aging

Is it possible to detect differences in the acquisition or retention of long-term memory of the withdrawal reflex if one compares young and older *Aplysias*? To answer this question, we took advantage of the short life span of *Aplysia* (less than two years) to compare processes mediating long-term memory in the same organism. We found to our surprise (Bailey et al., 1983) that very large and presumably old animals did not facilitate their reflex at all (Fig. 5). Equally interesting was the observation that the acquisition for long-term habituation in intact animals was normal in old animals but the retention was much shorter than for younger animals (Fig. 6). A protocol that induced a habituation lasting for more than a week in young animals did not maintain the habituation in older animals for more than a few days. By tracking the proteins that may play a role in long-term effects, one may be in a position to determine the essential ones for the onset or the maintenance of long-term memory. Finally these proteins or

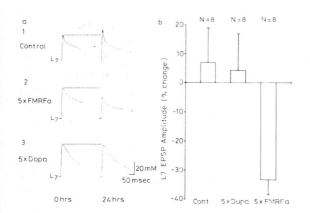

Fig. 4. Long-term heterosynaptic inhibition in dissociated cell culture. Repeated applications of FMRFamide evokes depression of sensory-L7 connections lasting 24 h. *a*. The first evoked EPSP in the L7 motor neuron (0 h column) is compared to the first evoked EPSP for the same connection 24 h later (24 h column). Whereas control or dopamine treatments resulted in slight changes, FMRFamide applications evoked a significant depression in the amplitude of the EPSP. *b*. Summary of long-term depression induced by FMRFamide. The height for each bar is the mean ± S.E.M. of the percent change in the amplitude of the EPSP retested 24 h after treatment. Only the FMRFamide treatment produced a significant effect (from Montarolo et al., 1988).

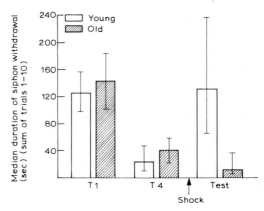

Fig. 5. Facilitation of the withdrawal reflex in young (n = 14) and old (n = 19) intact animals. Both groups of animals exhibited significant acquisition of habituation. The protocol was four blocks (T1 – T4) of ten stimulations (jet of sea water) presented at 30-sec intervals, each block separated by 1.5 h. After the fourth block a facilitating stimulus (shocks to the tail) was applied to each group; the reflex of the young animals was facilitated, but not in the older animals (from Bailey et al., 1983).

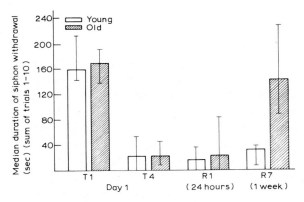

Fig. 6. Retention of habituation in young and old animals. Behavioral scores of young (n = 12) and old animals (n = 15) are shown on blocks 1 (T1) and 4 (T4) of habituation training (ten tactile stimuli per block) on day 1. Retention of habituation was tested 24 h (R1) and 1 week (R7) after training. Both groups of animals showed significant acquisition of habituation by block 4 of day 1 and significant retention of habituation 24 h later. One week later young animals still exhibited significant retention of habituation whereas old animals did not. Data are expressed as medians ± interquartiles ranges (from Bailey et al., 1983).

some members of their family may be searched for in other organisms, including vertebrates, to find general mechanisms involved in encoding permanent information.

Discussion

Several phenomena in neurobiology are observed in practically all species of animals. It is our belief that by comparing several systems in vertebrates or invertebrates we could begin to unravel general and important common mechanisms, be it that there may be different ways to achieve this goal.

A first generalization that can be made is that modifications of existing proteins can lead to transient or short-lasting behavioral changes. The studies of the gill and siphon withdrawal reflex or the tail withdrawal reflex in *Aplysia* suggest that a behavioral modification of short duration, lasting minutes or up to 1 h may be due to modifications of existing proteins which could change the properties of some enzymes or the properties of some

ionic channels in key neurons. The group of Levitan (Kramer et al., 1988) in the study of cell R15 of *Aplysia*, of Kazcmarek (1988) in the study of the peptidergic neurons involved in egg-laying in *Aplysia* and of Alkon in the studies of behavior in the mollusc *Hermissenda* (Alkon, 1984; Naito et al., 1988) have gathered data showing the role of phosphorylation in changing neuronal properties. This is also true in vertebrates (Akers and Routtenberg, 1987; Malenka et al., 1988; Malinow et al., 1988).

Another common generalization that is emerging from recent studies in vertebrates or invertebrates is the idea of cotransmission and the idea of transmitters and neuropeptides acting on common targets (Hokfelt et al., 1986). In the case of the gill and siphon withdrawal reflex, we have noticed an interesting symmetry. Serotonin and the peptides SCPa and SCPb can facilitate the monosynaptic connection between the sensory neurons and their followers. The action of these transmitters leads to the modulation of the same potassium channel through a common pathway, the cyclic AMP cascade (Abrams et al., 1984). On the other hand, dopamine and FMRFamide can depress the same monosynaptic connection and affect the same potassium channel. In this case the two transmitters share another biochemical cascade which involves arachidonic acid (Piomelli et al., 1987; Yaari, 1988). Despite the fact that there is an overlap in the mechanism involved for short-term synaptic depression, there is a suggestion that these substances may have different long-term effects since only FMRFamide can have a prolonged action (Montarolo et al., 1988; Fig. 4). In addition, FMRFamide which depresses the monosynaptic connection of the withdrawal reflex has a facilitatory action on the peripheral system; it seems to act directly on the gill muscle or on local peripheral neurons (Cawthorpe et al., 1988). It will be important to analyze further the extent of overlap and the functional meaning of modulators affecting a reflex, an identified synapse or a specific channel.

Another general principle that seems common to

both vertebrates and invertebrates is that the consolidation of short-term memory to longer term memory is dependent on the synthesis of new proteins (see Lisman (1985) for an alternative point of view). For example, we have found in the isolated withdrawal reflex, where monosynaptic and polysynaptic pathways are involved (Castellucci et al., 1989) or in the dissociated cell culture system (Montarolo et al., 1986, 1988) where only the monosynaptic connection is present, that long-term effects were blocked if protein or RNA synthesis was inhibited at a crucial time. Similar findings have been reported in *Hermissenda* (Crow, 1988) and in vertebrate systems (Davis and Squire, 1984).

The identification of macromolecules that could be important in any one system will be useful to the study of other organisms if one assumes that similar encoding mechanisms may have been retained across different classes of animals (Goelet et al., 1986).

Finally, it seems that lowly invertebrates do not escape the problems of aging. Our preliminary results in aging *Aplysias* show that old animals have difficulty to facilitate their withdrawal reflex and, more importantly, they retain poorly newly acquired information. This difficulty may exist in many other reflexes since we have observed already that a component of food arousal is impaired in older animals (Bailey et al., 1983). These results which have parallels in vertebrates indicate that we could compare systematically various biochemical cascades and macromolecules thought to be necessary for the onset and maintenance of memory in vertebrates and invertebrates.

References

Abrams, T.W., Castellucci, V.F., Camardo, J.S., Kandel, E.R. and Lloyd, P.E. (1984) Two endogenous neuropeptides modulate the gill and siphon withdrawal reflex in *Aplysia* by pre-synaptic facilitation involving cAMP-dependent closure of a serotonin-sensitive potassium channel. *Proc. Natl. Acad. Sci. U.S.A.,* 81: 7956–7960.

Akers, R.F. and Routtenberg, A. (1987) Calcium-promoted translocation of protein kinase C to synaptic membranes: relation to the phosphorylation of an endogenous substrate (protein F1) involved in synaptic plasticity. *J. Neurosci.,* 7: 3976–3983.

Alkon, D.L. (1984) Calcium-mediated reduction of ionic current: a biophysical memory trace. *Science,* 26: 1037–1045.

Bailey, C.H. and Chen, M. (1983) Morphological basis of long-term habituation and sensitization in *Aplysia. Science,* 220: 91–93.

Bailey, C.H. and Chen, M. (1988) Long-term memory in *Aplysia* modulates the total number of varicosities of single identified sensory neurons. *Proc. Natl. Acad. Sci. U.S.A.,* 85: 2373–2377.

Bailey, C.H., Castellucci, V.F., Koester, J. and Chen, M. (1983) Behavioral changes in aging *Aplysia*: a model system for studying the cellular basis of age-impaired learning, memory and arousal. *Behav. Neural Biol.,* 38: 70–81.

Barzilai, A., Kennedy, T.E., Kandel, E.R. and Sweatt, J.D. (1988) Serotonin (5HT) causes changes in protein synthesis in pleural sensory neurons from *Aplysia. Soc. Neurosci. Abstr.,* 14: 909.

Belardetti, F. and Siegelbaum, S.A. (1988) Up- and down-modulation of single K^+ channel function by distinct second messengers. *Trends Neurosci.,* 11: 232–238.

Byrne, J.H., Castellucci, V.F. and Kandel, E.R. (1978) Contribution of individual mechanoreceptor sensory neurons to the defensive gill-withdrawal reflex in *Aplysia. J. Neurophysiol.,* 41: 418–431.

Cajal, S.R. (1911) *Histologie du Système Nerveux de l'Homme et des Vertébrés,* Maloine, Paris.

Carew, T.J., Pinsker, H. and Kandel, E.R. (1972) Long-term habituation of a defensive withdrawal reflex in *Aplysia. Science,* 175: 451–454.

Castellucci, V.F. and Kandel, E.R. (1974) A quantal analysis of the synaptic depression underlying habituation of the gill-withdrawal reflex in *Aplysia. Proc. Natl. Acad. Sci. U.S.A.,* 71: 5004–5008.

Castellucci, V.F. and Kandel, E.R. (1976) Pre-synaptic facilitation as a mechanism for behavioral sensitization in *Aplysia. Science,* 194: 1176–1178.

Castellucci, V.F., Pinsker, H., Kupfermann, I. and Kandel, E.R. (1970) Neuronal mechanisms of habituation and dishabituation of the gill-withdrawal reflex in *Aplysia. Science,* 167: 1745–1748.

Castellucci, V.F., Carew, T.J. and Kandel, E.R. (1978) Cellular analysis of long-term habituation of the gill-withdrawal reflex of *Aplysia californica. Science,* 202: 1306–1308.

Castellucci, V.F., Kandel, E.R., Schwartz, J.H., Wilson, F.D., Nairn, A.C. and Greengard, P. (1980) Intracellular injection of the catalytic subunit of cyclic AMP-dependent protein kinase stimulates facilitation of transmitter release underlying behavioral sensitization in *Aplysia. Proc. Natl. Acad. Sci. U.S.A.,* 77: 7492–7496.

Castellucci, V.F., Kennedy, T.E., Kandel, E.R. and Goelet, P. (1988) A quantitative analysis of 2-D gels identifies proteins whose labeling is increased following long-term sensitization in *Aplysia. Neuron,* 1: 321 – 328.

Castellucci, V.F., Blumenfeld, H., Goelet, P. and Kandel, E.R. (1989) Inhibitor of protein synthesis blocks long-term behavioral sensitization in the isolated gill-withdrawal reflex in *Aplysia. J. Neurobiol.,* 20: 1 – 9.

Cawthorpe, D., Higgins, A. and Lukowiak, K. (1988) FMRFamide prevents habituation and potentiates the gill-withdrawal reflex in the isolated gill preparation of *Aplysia. Regul. Pept.,* 22: 227 – 236.

Crow, T. (1988) Cellular and molecular analysis of associative learning and memory in *Hermissenda. Trends Neurosci.,* 11: 136 – 142.

Dale, N., Kandel, E.R. and Schacher, S. (1987) Serotonin produces long-term changes in the excitability of *Aplysia* sensory neurons in culture that depends on new protein synthesis. *J. Neurosci.,* 7: 2232 – 2238.

Dale, N., Schacher, S. and Kandel, E.R. (1988) Long-term facilitation in *Aplysia* involves increase in transmitter release. *Science,* 239: 282 – 285.

Davis, H.P. and Squire, L.R. (1984) Protein synthesis and memory: a review. *Psychol. Bull.,* 96: 518 – 559.

Frey, U., Krug, M., Reymann, K.G. and Matthies, H. (1988) Anisomycin, an inhibitor of protein synthesis, blocks late phases of LTP phenomena in the hippocampal CA1 region in vitro. *Brain Res.,* 452: 57 – 65.

Frost, W.N., Castellucci, V.F., Hawkins, R.D. and Kandel, E.R. (1985) Monosynaptic connections made by the sensory neurons of the gill- and siphon-withdrawal reflex in *Aplysia* participate in the storage of long-term memory for sensitization. *Proc. Natl. Acad. Sci. U.S.A.,* 82: 8266 – 8269.

Frost, W.N., Clark, G.A. and Kandel, E.R. (1988) Parallel processing of short-term memory for sensitization in *Aplysia. J. Neurobiol.,* 19: 297 – 334.

Goelet, P., Castellucci, V.F., Schacher, S. and Kandel, E.R. (1986) The long and short of long-term memory. A molecular framework. *Nature,* 322: 419 – 422.

Grecksch, G. and Matthies, H. (1980) Two sensitive periods for the amnesic effect of anisomycin. *Pharmacol. Biochem. Behav.,* 12: 663 – 665.

Greenberg, S.M., Castellucci, V.F., Bayley, H. and Schwartz, J.H. (1987) A molecular mechanism for long-term sensitization in *Aplysia. Nature,* 329: 62 – 65.

Greenough, W.T. and Bailey, C.H. (1988) The anatomy of a memory: convergence of results across a diversity of tests. *Trends Neurosci.,* 11: 142 – 147.

Hawkins, R.H., Castellucci, V.F. and Kandel, E.R. (1981) Interneurons involved in mediation and modulation of the gill-withdrawal reflex in *Aplysia.* II. Identified neurons produce heterosynaptic facilitation contributing to behavioral sensitization. *J. Neurophysiol.,* 45: 315 – 326.

Hawkins, R.H., Clark, G. and Kandel, E.R. (1986) Cell biological studies of learning in simple vertebrate and invertebrate systems. *Handbook of Physiology. The Nervous*

System. Higher Functions of the Brain, Vol. 6, American Physiological Society, Bethesda, MD, Sect. 1, Chapt. 2, pp. 25 – 83.

Hochner, B., Klein, M., Schacher, S. and Kandel, E.R. (1986) Additional component in the cellular mechanism of pre-synaptic facilitation contributes to behavioral dishabituation in *Aplysia. Proc. Natl. Acad. Sci. U.S.A.,* 83: 8794 – 8798.

Hokfelt, T., Fuxe, K. and Pernow, B. (Eds.) (1986) Coexistence of neuronal messengers: a new principle in chemical transmission. *Progress in Brain Reseach, Vol. 68,* Elsevier, Amsterdam, 411 pp.

Jacklet, J.W. and Rine, J. (1977) Facilitation at neuromuscular junctions: contribution to habituation and dishabituation of the *Aplysia* gill-withdrawal reflex. *Proc. Natl. Acad. Sci. U.S.A.,* 74: 1267 – 1271.

Jahan-Parwar, B. and Fredman, S.M. (1978) Control of pedal and parapodial movements in *Aplysia.* I. Proprioceptive and tactile reflexes. *J. Neurophysiol.,* 41: 600 – 608.

Kaczmarek, L.K. (1988) The regulation of neuronal calcium and potassium channels by protein phosphorylation. *Adv. Sec. Messenger Phosphoprotein Res.,* 22: 113 – 138.

Kandel, E.R., Klein, M., Hochner, B., Schuster, M., Siegelbaum, S.A., Hawkins, R.D., Glanzmann, D.L., Castellucci, V.F. and Abrams, T.W. (1987) Synaptic modulation and learning: new insights into synaptic transmission from the study of behavior. In: G.N. Edelman, W.E. Gall and W.M. Cowan (Eds.), *Synaptic Function,* Wiley, New York, pp. 471 – 518.

Kennedy, T.E., Gawinowicz, M.A., Barzilai, A., Kandel, E.R. and Sweatt, J.D. (1988) Sequencing of proteins from two-dimensional gels using in situ digestion and transfer of peptides to polyvinylidene difluoride membranes: application to proteins associated with sensitization in *Aplysia. Proc. Natl. Acad. Sci. U.S.A.,* 85: 7008 – 7012.

Klein, M. and Kandel, E.R. (1980) Mechanism of calcium current modulation underlying pre-synaptic facilitation and behavioral sensitization in *Aplysia. Proc. Natl. Acad. Sci. U.S.A.,* 77: 6912 – 6916.

Kramer, R.H., Levitan, E.S., Wilson, M.P. and Levitan, I.B. (1988) Mechanisms of calcium-dependent inactivation of a potassium current in *Aplysia* neuron R15: interaction between calcium and cyclic AMP. *J. Neurosci.,* 8: 1804 – 1813.

Kupfermann, I. (1974) Feeding behavior in *Aplysia:* a simple system for the study of motivation. *Behav. Biol.,* 10: 1 – 26.

Kupfermann, I., Carew, T.J. and Kandel, E.R. (1974) Local, reflex, and central commands controlling gill and siphon movements in *Aplysia. J. Neurophysiol.,* 37: 996 – 1019.

Lisman, J.E. (1985) A mechanism for memory storage insensitive to molecular turnover: a bistable autophosphorylating kinase. *Proc. Natl. Acad. Sci. U.S.A.,* 82: 3055 – 3057.

Mackey, S.L., Glanzman, D.L., Small, S.A., Dyke, A.M., Kandel, E.R. and Hawkins, R.D. (1987) Tail shock produces inhibition as well as sensitization of the siphon-withdrawal reflex of *Aplysia:* possible behavioral role for pre-synaptic inhibition mediated by the peptide Phe-Met-Arg-Phe-NH$_2$. *Proc. Natl. Acad. Sci. U.S.A.,* 84: 8730 – 8734.

Malenka, R.C., Kauer, J.A., Zucker, R.S. and Nicoll, R.A. (1988) Post-synaptic calcium is sufficient for potentiation of hippocampal synaptic transmission. *Science,* 242: 81 – 84.

Malinow, R., Madison, D.V. and Tsien, R.W. (1988) Persistent protein kinase activity underlying long-term potentiation. *Nature,* 335: 820 – 824.

Martinez, J.L., Jr. and Kesner, R.P. (1986) *Learning and Memory. A Biological View,* Academic Press, New York, 452 pp.

Matthies, H. (1989) Neurobiological aspects of learning and memory. *Ann. Rev. Psychol.,* 40: 381 – 404.

Montarolo, P.G., Goelet, P., Castellucci, V.F., Morgan, J., Kandel, E.R. and Schacher, S. (1986) A critical period for macromolecular synthesis in long-term heterosynaptic facilitation in *Aplysia. Science,* 234: 1249 – 1254.

Montarolo, P.G., Kandel, E.R. and Schacher, S. (1988) Long-term heterosynaptic inhibition in *Aplysia. Nature,* 333: 171 – 174.

Naito, S., Bank, B. and Alkon, D.A. (1988) Transient and persistent depolarization-induced changes of protein phosphorylation in a molluscan nervous system. *J. Neurochem.,* 50: 704 – 711.

Ocorr, K.A., Walters, E.T. and Byrne, J.H. (1985) Associative conditioning analog selectively increases cAMP levels of tail sensory neurons in *Aplysia. Proc. Natl. Acad. Sci. U.S.A.,* 82: 2548 – 2555.

Painter, S.D., Gustavson, A.R., Kalman, V.K., Nagle, G.T. and Blankenship, J.E. (1989) Induction of copulatory behavior in *Aplysia*: atrial gland factors mimic the excitatory effects of freshly deposited egg cordons. *Behav. Neural Biol.,* 51: 222 – 236.

Papka, R., Peretz B., Tudor, J. and Becker, J. (1981) Age-dependent anatomical changes in an identified neuron in the CNS of *Aplysia californica. J. Neurobiol.,* 12: 455 – 468.

Perlman, A.J. (1979) Central and peripheral control of siphon-withdrawal reflex in *Aplysia californica. J. Neurophysiol.,* 42: 510 – 529.

Pinsker, H., Kupfermann, I., Castellucci, V.F. and Kandel, E. (1970) Habituation and dishabituation of the gill-withdrawal reflex in *Aplysia. Science,* 167: 1740 – 1744.

Piomelli, D., Volterra, A., Dale, N., Siegelbaum, S.A., Kandel, E.R., Schwartz, J.H. and Belardetti, F. (1987) Lipoxygenase metabolites of arachidonic acid as second messengers for pre-synaptic inhibition of *Aplysia* sensory cells. *Nature,* 328: 38 – 45.

Rankin, C.H., Stopfer, M., Marcus, E.A. and Carew, T.J. (1987) Development of learning and memory in *Aplysia*: functional assembly of gill and siphon withdrawal. *J. Neurosci.,* 7: 120 – 132.

Rattan, K.S. and Peretz, B. (1981) Age-dependent behavioral changes and physiological changes in identified neurons in *Aplysia californica. J. Neurobiol.,* 12: 469 – 478.

Rayport, S.G. and Schacher, S. (1986) Synaptic plasticity in vitro: cell culture of identified *Aplysia* neurons mediating short-term habituation and sensitization. *J. Neurosci.,* 6: 759 – 763.

Schacher, S. (1985) Differential synapse formation and neurite outgrowth at two branches of the metacerebral cell of *Aplysia* in dissociated cell culture. *J. Neurosci.,* 5: 2028 – 2034.

Schacher, S., Castellucci, V.F. and Kandel, E.R. (1988) cAMP evokes long-term facilitation in *Aplysia* sensory neurons that requires new protein synthesis. *Science,* 240: 1667 – 1669.

Scholz, K.P. and Byrne, J.H. (1987) Long-term sensitization in *Aplysia*: biophysical correlates in tail sensory neurons. *Science,* 233: 685 – 687.

Schuster, M.J., Camardo, J.S., Siegelbaum, S.A. and Kandel, E.R. (1985) Cyclic AMP-dependent protein kinase closes the serotonin-sensitive K$^+$ channels of *Aplysia* sensory neurones in cell-free membrane patches. *Nature,* 313: 392 – 395.

Strumwasser, F. (1988) The bag cell neuroendocrine system of *Aplysia. Curr. Top. Neuroendocr.,* 9: 105 – 125.

Sweatt, J.D. and Kandel, E.R. (1988) Serotonin (5-HT) causes a persistent increase in protein phosphorylation that is transcription-dependent: a molecular mechanism contributing to long-term sensitization in *Aplysia* sensory neurons. *Soc. Neurosci. Abstr.,* 14: 909.

Tanzi, E. (1893) I fatti e le induzioni nell'odierna istologia dell sistema nervoso. *Riv. Sper. Freniat. Med. Leg. Alien. Ment.,* 19: 419 – 472.

Terry, R.D. and Gershon, S. (Eds.) (1976) *Aging, Vol. 3: Neurobiology of Aging,* Raven Press, New York.

Walters, E.T., Byrne, J.H., Carew, T.J. and Kandel, E.R. (1983) Mechanoafferent neurons innervating tail of *Aplysia*. II. Modulation by sensitizing stimulation. *J. Neurophysiol.,* 50: 1543 – 1559.

Yaari, Y. (1988) Evidence that lipoxygenase metabolites link dopamine D2 receptors to potassium S-channel in *Aplysia* sensory neurons. *Soc. Neurosci. Abstr.,* 14: 1205.

Yeung, S.J. and Eskin, A. (1988) Responses of the circadian system in the *Aplysia* eye to inhibitors of protein synthesis. *J. Biol. Rhythms,* 3: 225 – 236.

P. Coleman, G. Higgins and C. Phelps (Eds.)
Progress in Brain Research, Vol. 86
© 1990 Elsevier Science Publishers B.V. (Biomedical Division)

CHAPTER 10

Integration by the neuronal growth cone: a continuum from neuroplasticity to neuropathology

S.B. Kater, P.B. Guthrie and L.R. Mills

Program in Neuronal Growth and Development, and Department of Anatomy and Neurobiology, Colorado State University, Ft. Collins, CO 80523, U.S.A.

Introduction

This paper forwards the hypothesis that the neuronal growth cone is a primary locus for control of neuroplasticity. We will describe several forms that the growth cone can manifest, ranging from the classical form characteristic of pioneering nerve fibers to the form recognized as the presynaptic terminal. We will develop the idea that all of these forms should be regarded as *transition states* of a highly dynamic structure rather than as final structures in some specific temporal blueprint. In this sense, we regard the growth cone as the key morphological substrate of neuroplasticity. The same characteristics which endow this structure with a high degree of both morphological and functional plasticity also make it more labile for morphological changes that extend beyond the normal range of function and into the range of pathological degeneration. In this view, we regard the growth cone and associated terminal structures as the primary potential locus of both neuroplasticity and neurodegeneration.

In addition to developing a dynamic view of the neuronal growth cone, this review will propose that a major determinant of the status of a tip of a given neurite lies in specific intracellular calcium levels. Intracellular calcium has long been known to be one of the most precisely regulated commodities within the complex machinery of the ner-

vous system. We will develop evidence that indicates that intracellular calcium levels set the growth status of the tip of a neurite and can determine which of the many possible morphologies these tips will take.

In developing these ideas, we will begin to view the growth cone as an integrator of complex environmental information. This integration, under normal conditions, provides a delicate balance, a balance which, as we will demonstrate, depends upon the intricate mechanisms of calcium homeostasis. Finally, we will consider whether changes in one or more components of calcium homeostasis might, in fact, be responsible in the discrete transition between elongating growth cones and functional synaptic terminals.

Forms of the neuronal growth cone

The last decade has seen monumental changes in our view of the neuronal growth cone (see Kater and Letourneau, 1985). Our first image of the growth cone was that of a "living battering ram" (Ramon y Cajal, 1890), and many of our subsequent views of neuronal growth cones were formed as static snapshots from fixed preparations. What is becoming more evident, however, is that the growth cone can change its form in response to appropriate stimuli. Within a given system we know that similar neurons can give rise to growth cones with quite different forms. For instance, Macagno and collaborators (Lopresti et al., 1973) demonstrated that the growth cones of pioneering fibers were quite different from the growth cones of following fibers. The pioneering fibers had the characteristic broadened lamellipodium and multiple long filopodia that seems to be characteristic of pioneer fibers throughout the animal kingdom (c.f., in insect limb: Bentley and Toroian-Raymond, 1986; or developing tadpole: Roberts and Patton, 1985). In contrast, fibers which followed the pioneer and fasciculated upon it had quite different morphologies. Namely, there were few, if any, filopodia and essentially no lamellipodium. It seems reasonably to suggest that these diverse and divergent morphologies develop as a consequence of encounters with very specific sets of environmental cues.

Growth cones can be experimentally made to go through a variety of transitions. Fig. 1 demonstrates that growth cones from the snail *Helisoma* go through a characteristic transition when viewed over time in cell culture (Hadley et al., 1985). Neurons grow for up to 5 days, and then reach a stable state. Concomitant with these two conditions are very different growth cone morphologies. The growing growth cone is characteristic of that pioneering fiber growth cone seen by Macagno and others. The stable state growth cone, on the other hand, is no longer motile and quite different in that there are no filopodia and essentially no lamellipodium. This may, in fact, represent the presumptive pre-synaptic terminal. In addition to

spontaneously obtaining this stable state, we have found a variety of naturally occurring stimuli (such as the neurotransmitters to be discussed below) which can totally inhibit neurite outgrowth and produce stable state growth cones indistinguishable from those which occur spontaneously.

Stable state growth cones, whatever their origin, are actually not fixed and static but rather are dormant. Under appropriate experimental conditions, regrowth and reactivation can occur. For instance, in Fig. 1*B*, the application of serum factor(s) from *Helisoma* can reliably "reawaken" stable state growth cones to an actively growing state indistinguishable from that seen during initial outgrowth (Grega and Kater, 1987). The transitions that we have described are key to the concept that the tips of growing neurites are dynamic structures capable of displaying a variety of forms and functions under appropriate environmental conditions. Of course, the corollary to this is that, under inappropriate conditions, these terminal ends are probably also extremely labile.

The growth cone as an integrator

In many systems, including molluscan and mammalian neurons, we have now found that a variety of signals which impinge upon neuronal growth cone can determine its behavior. For example, we know that classical neurotransmitters can act as important signals for the guidance of growth cones. Growth cones·from a subset of *Helisoma*

Fig. 1. Neuronal growth cones exist in morphologically distinguishable forms representing specific activity states. In culture, growth cones of *Helisoma* actively grow for several days, then spontaneously progress to stable state. They can also be induced to assume this stable state, and they can be re-awakened from this stable, dormant condition. *A*. Neurons of *Helisoma* display continuous outgrowth for periods up to 5 days in culture. During this time, the growth cones display numerous filopodia and a large lamellipodium. With time, these growth cones mature to the stable state form which is characterized by a lack of filopodia and lamellipodium, and a club-shaped appearance. Such growth cones will remain in stable state or dormant unless they receive specific environmental signals. *B*. Growing growth cones can be prematurely induced to assume stable state form by a variety of agents. Here, the neurotransmitter serotonin converts a growing neuron B19 growth cone (*B*) to its stable state form (*B'*). Without further perturbation, this growth cone would have remained in this form for the remainder of its time in culture. However, prior to the photomicrograph in the third panel, *Helisoma* serum was added to the medium. This resulted in a re-awakening of the dormant growth cone to an active growing branching state (*B''*). In cell culture, this treatment can result in up to a 100% increase in total neurite outgrowth. Such reactivation could well occur in situ under neuroplastic conditions.

119

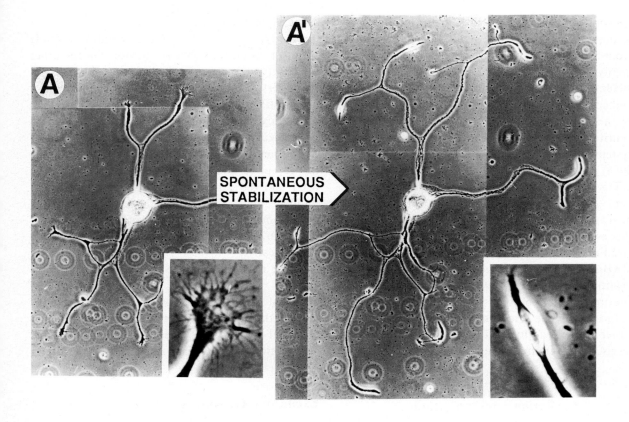

SPONTANEOUS STABILIZATION

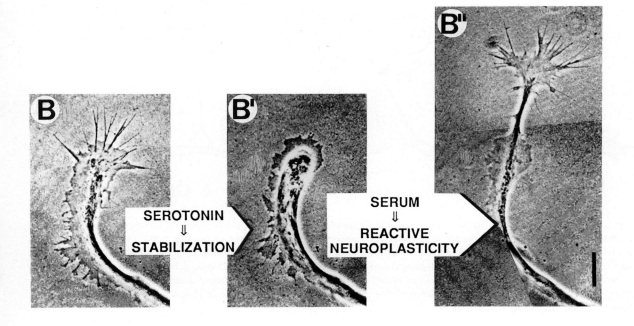

SEROTONIN ⇓ STABILIZATION

SERUM ⇓ REACTIVE NEUROPLASTICITY

120

neurons will cease elongation in the presence of serotonin (Haydon et al., 1987). Growth cones from hippocampal pyramidal neuron dendrites are highly sensitive to glutamate (Mattson et al., 1988a). Glutamate can inhibit neurite outgrowth and actually result in the regression, or "pruning", of a dendrite. Neurotransmitter regulation of neurite elongation has now been seen in many systems (Lankford et al., 1988; Lipton et al., 1988).

Fig. 2 is a schematic selection from our extensive data demonstrating how the presence of one neurotransmitter can have significant effects on the response of a neuron to another neurotransmitter. For example, the inhibitory neurotransmitter GABA can retard the glutamate pruning effect (Mattson and Kater, 1989). Thus, a balance of excitation and inhibition is conducive to dendritic outgrowth while excitatory imbalance, imposed either by excess glutamate or insufficient GABA levels, results in modification of growth cones and

a subsequent dendritic regression.

Clearly, the growth cone integrates multiple stimuli to produce a given behavior. On the other hand, growth cones from different neurons can react very differently to the same stimulus (e.g., neuron B5 is unaffected by serotonin while B19 is dramatically inhibited by serotonin). Fig. 3 generalizes this interpretation. Thus, the behavior of the neuronal growth cone is the composite of the receptive characteristics of the growth cone itself and the complex environmental cues which impinge upon it. It must be emphasized that throughout the time course of the life of an organism, both of these components may change dramatically.

There may, in fact, be hierarchies of responsiveness to information impinging upon the neuronal growth cone. For example, Fig. 4 summarizes data on *Helisoma* neurons. Stimulation of electrical activity in any neuron reversibly inhibits neurite elongation (Cohan et al., 1987). Serotonin

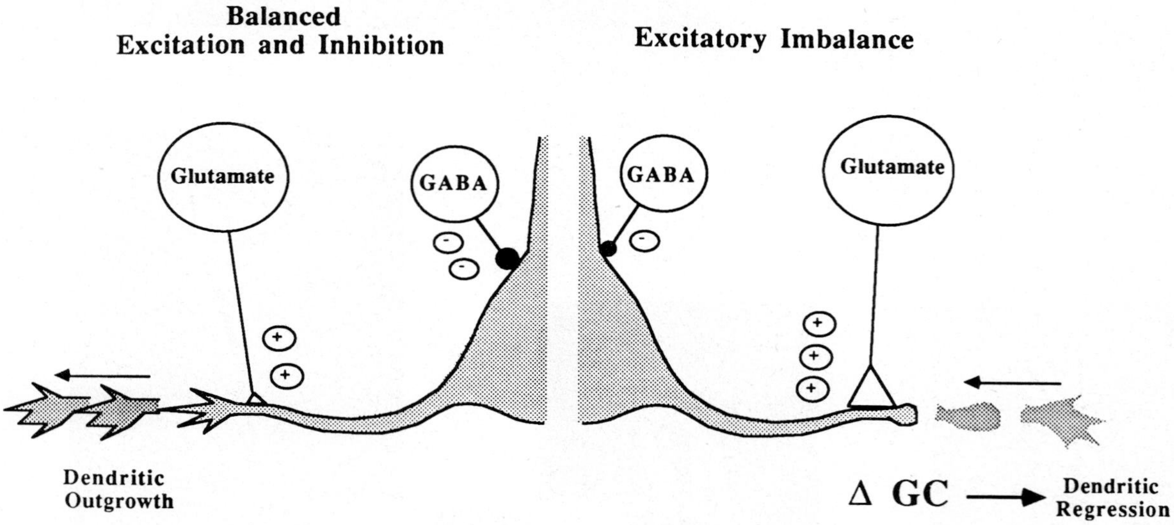

Balanced Excitation and Inhibition

Excitatory Imbalance

Fig. 2. A balance of excitation and inhibition is required for normal neurite outgrowth to proceed. Hippocampal pyramidal neurons react to the presence of moderate levels of glutamate by a selective effect on the dendritic growth cones. Dendritic growth cones are inhibited from additional outgrowth and actually regress. Interestingly, not all pyramidal neuronal growth cones are the same since axonal growth cones are relatively immune to effects of glutamate. This inhibitory effect on dendritic outgrowth can be negated by the inhibitory transmitter GABA (and its potentiator diazepam). Therefore, in a balanced condition, outgrowth occurs. When there is excitatory imbalance, as would be the case from either too little GABA, or too much glutamate, dendritic regression occurs (modified from Mattson and Kater, 1989).

inhibits the outgrowth of the growth cones of specific neurons (e.g., buccal neuron B19; Haydon et al., 1985). Acetylcholine alone has no effects on such neurons. But, when acetylcholine is present along with serotonin, the serotonin inhibiting effects on the growth cone are negated (McCobb et al., 1988). Even in the presence of both acetylcholine and serotonin, however (the condition where outgrowth should have continued), the generation of action potentials prevents further outgrowth. This integration of three different kinds of information by the neuronal growth cone represents but a small fraction of the environmental cues that must be seen by the growth cones during normal development. The result of the integra-

tion determines which of the repertoire of morphologies the growth cone will exhibit.

This integration is highly reminiscent of signal processing within the mature nervous system. In fact, there is now extensive evidence to indicate that these outgrowth regulating effects are integrated at the level of membrane potential. The neurotransmitters which inhibit outgrowth also produce sustained depolarizations in those neurons; conversely, these neurotransmitters have no significant effect on neurons whose outgrowth is unaffected (McCobb and Kater, 1988a, b). In addition, it has been possible to experimentally counteract the effects of excitatory neurotransmitters with direct injection of hyperpolarizing current. Under these conditions, both the prolonged

A GROWTH CONE INTEGRATES MULTIPLE STUMULATION TO PRODUCE A GIVEN BEHAVIOR:

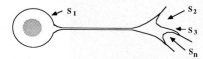

GROWTH CONES FROM DIFFERENT NEURONS CAN RESPOND DIFFERENTLY TO A GIVEN STIMULUS:

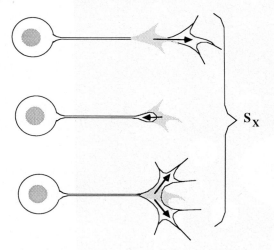

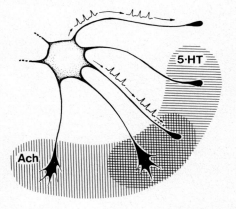

Fig. 4. A potential hierarchy of effects of stimuli on the neuronal growth cone. Neuronal growth cones can be influenced to change their form by a variety of agents. Generation of action potentials inhibits neurite outgrowth and produces stable state growth cones (uppermost growth cone). Application of serotonin to a specific subset of neurons (e.g., neuron B19) inhibits neurite outgrowth in a similar fashion (second growth cone from the top). Application of acetylcholine alone has no effect on behavior of a B19 growth cone (bottom growth cone). However, the presence of acetylcholine can negate the serotonin growth cone inhibitory effects (second growth cone from the bottom). Finally, it should be noted that even though a growth cone would elongate and remain motile in the presence of acetylcholine and serotonin, the generation of action potentials will abruptly terminate motility and convert a growing growth cone to its non-motile form. These results suggest that many additional environmental cues may be integrated in this system to affect the final behavior displayed by a growth cone.

Fig. 3. The growth cone is an integrator of complex environmental information. *A*. Stimuli may impinge upon the cell body or on the growth cone proper and ultimately are integrated into a final common path to affect the decisions that the growth cone will take. *B*. The growth cones of different neurons can react to the same stimulus in very different ways. A good example is the selective effect of serotonin on the outgrowth of B19 neurons, while B5 neurons are unaffected.

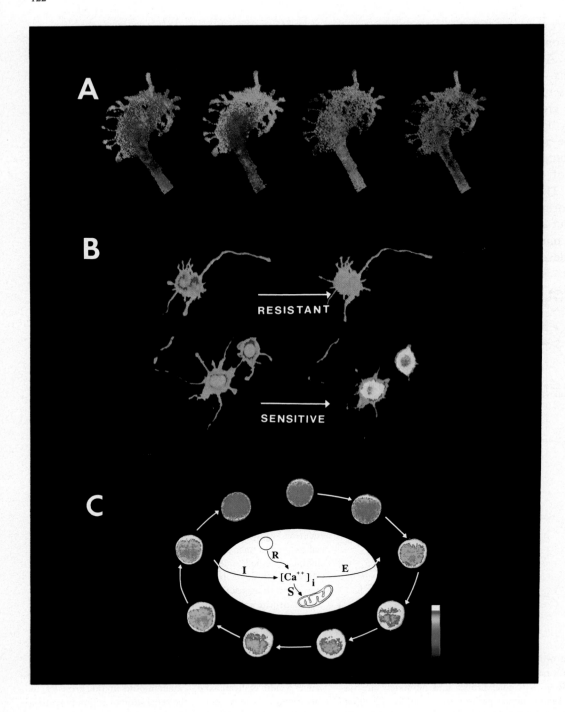

depolarization and the outgrowth inhibiting effects of serotonin are abolished. Finally, electrical activity of the neuron itself can modify the behavior of the growth cone. Generation of action potentials can totally, and reversibly, inhibit growth cone behavior and neurite extension.

The behavioral integration that we have observed can be interpreted as indicating that each of the complex stimuli which can impinge upon the growth cone acts at the level of a final common path. To some extent, we know that this path involves membrane potential in the same way as classical neuronal integration. But as shown below, one further step toward a common path resides at the level of intracellular calcium.

Intracellular calcium as a regulator of growth cone form and function

The agents known to affect neuronal growth cone behavior are now all known to evoke predictable effects on the concentrations of intracellular calcium within the neuronal growth cone (Kater et al., 1988a, b; Mills et al., 1988). The generation of action potentials, which stops outgrowth, significantly raises intracellular calcium (Cohan et al., 1987; Fig. 5A). The application of neurotransmitters, which also stops outgrowth, significantly raises intracellular calcium (Cohan et al., 1987; Fig. 5B). Similarly, blocking transmembrane calcium fluxes by using either medium containing no calcium, or medium containing inorganic calcium channel blockers, negates the inhibitory effects of both transmitters and action potentials (Cohan et al., 1987; Mattson and Kater, 1987; Mattson et al., 1988a). It has become clear through a variety of data that massive influxes of calcium are causally related to the inhibiton of neuronal growth cone behavior. In fact, a comprehensive picture is emerging that indicates that intracellular calcium play a major role in regulating the behavior of the neuronal growth cone.

Fig. 5. Calcium concentrations in *Helisoma* and hippocampal neurons measured with the fluorescent calcium indicator fura-2. Neurons were loaded with fura-2 in the AM (acetoxymethylester) form (Cohan et al., 1987). Pairs of images were captured (using 350 ± 10 nm and 380 ± 10 nm excitation filters with a 505 nm long-pass emission filter) using a Quantex QX7 image data acquisition system. The ratio of the two images is converted to calcium concentration according to the equation $[Ca^{2+}] = K_D^* ((R - R_{min})/(R_{max} - R))^*F_O/F_S$ (Grynkiewicz et al., 1985). Calcium concentration is represented as color on the calcium maps with blue being low calcium and red being high calcium. The calibration bar in the middle represents calcium concentration for each panel: *A*: 0 – 800 nM; *B*: 0 – 1000 nM; *C*: 0 – 600 nM. *A*. Stimulation of action potentials in the cell body causes calcium levels to rise in growth cones. First (left) panel: rest calcium levels in the growth cone. The neuron was then stimulated with a microelectrode to fire 8 action potentials at 4/sec. Calcium concentrations increased throughout the growth cone, but particularly at the leading edge of the main body of the growth cone (second panel; $t = 2$ sec). The calcium concentrations decreased following cessation of the stimulation (third panel: $t = 15$ sec; fourth panel: $t = 45$ sec). *B*. Neurotransmitters selectively affect neurite outgrowth via intracellular calcium levels. In the hippocampus, a majority (ca. 80%) of neurons are pruned and/or die in response to the addition of glutamate. The same percentage of neurons are found to respond to glutamate by the rise in intracellular calcium. The upper pair of cells shows neurons whose calcium levels become elevated in response to glutamate (100 μM; $t = 30$ min). These neurons would have had dendrites pruned or, depending upon the dose, been selectively killed. The bottom images display neurons which are resistant to high levels of extracellular glutamate and show no responses of intracellular calcium; neither the behavior nor survival of these neurons would have been affected by the glutamate. *C*. Calcium homeostasis requires a balance between those components affecting rises in intracellular calcium and those components affecting decreases in intracellular calcium. There are several factors involved in determining calcium levels. Calcium concentrations are increased by influx (I) and release (R) from intracellular stores; levels are decreased by efflux (E; pumping) and sequestration (S; uptake into internal stores or buffering). Each of the components of the calcium homeostasis appears to be balanced with the others in order to produce steady state levels. Perturbation of calcium concentrations is usually followed by compensatory changes in one or several of the components of calcium homeostasis. In this example, application of the calcium ionophore A23187 results in predictable changes in a *Helisoma* neuron B5 cell body. Following the addition of A23187 ($2.5 \cdot 10^{-7}$ M) is an initial rise in intracellular calcium. Within approximately 20 min, calcium levels start returning towards their original set point. Even in the continued presence of A23187, calcium levels return to normal. The experimentally increased influx is compensated for by what must be an increase in sequestering and/or efflux mechanisms.

124

Specific intracellular calcium levels are now seen as regulating specific neuronal growth cone behaviors (Fig. 6). Extremely high levels of calcium, as evoked by the ionophore A23187, the generation of action potentials, or specific neurotransmitters, all stop outgrowth. Similarly, low levels of calcium intracellularly in the growth cone, as occur during spontaneous stabilization of outgrowth or in the presence of ion channel blockers, also result in cessation of outgrowth. Within the outgrowth permissive range of intracellular calcium concentrations, we envision not just one form of growing growth cone, but potentially the wide array of morphologies associated previously with different growth cone behaviors.

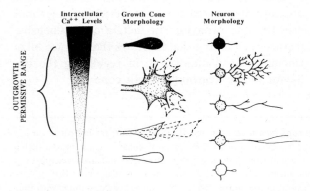

Fig. 6. Our present view of the calcium hypothesis of the control of neurite outgrowth considers that there is an outgrowth permissive range for neurite outgrowth. This range may indeed be different for individual classes of neurons. Elevation of intracellular calcium in excess of that range (as would occur with the generation of action potentials or with excitatory neurotransmitters), inhibits neurite outgrowth. Decreasing intracellular calcium below that range (as occurs during the spontaneous transition to stable state morphology and/or with the addition of high levels of calcium channel blockers), also results in inhibition of outgrowth. Within the outgrowth permissive range, however, many additional morphologies can be observed. At the low extreme, neuronal growth cones have no filopodia or lamellipodium, never branch and have very high rates of outgrowth. At the upper end of the outgrowth permissive range, growth cones have numerous filopodia and a large lamellipodium and rather slow rates of highly branched outgrowth. Thus the intracellular calcium set point can determine not just whether or not a neuron grows, but also the form of the growth cone.

By employing low levels of calcium channel blockers and reducing the intracellular calcium levels, growth cones are formed which have no filopodia and very abbreviated lamellipodia, elongate at comparatively high rates and essentially never or rarely branch (Mattson and Kater, 1987). On the other hand, at the normal rest level, numerous filopodia and extensive lamellipodial surfaces are seen. Branching is common and outgrowth rates are somewhat reduced. Preliminary data suggest that somewhat higher levels than the normal set point result in more extensive branching and even more reduced outgrowth rates. Thus, according to the present "Calcium Hypothesis" of control of the neuronal growth cone, we envision that the form taken at any given neurite tip can be dictated precisely by a given level of intracellular calcium with respect to the particular set point of that neuron (Kater et al., 1988a, b).

The absolute values of high and low are, however, quite neuron-specific. We now regard each neuron as having a unique "set point" such that what is high for one neuron may in fact be within the outgrowth permissive range of another. This understanding greatly clarifies a large amount of previously contradictory data. In fact, the observation that different cell types in fact have different "setpoints" (Guthrie et al., 1988) suggests that cells actively establish different rest intracellular calcium concentrations. This conclusion necessitates an examination of the factors controlling calcium concentrations within the neuronal growth cone.

Calcium homeostasis as a key to growth cone function

All cells possess significant degrees of calcium homeostasis (McBurney and Neeting, 1987), as can be demonstrated experimentally with a wide range of perturbations. One example of calcium homeostasis is shown in Fig. 5C. A rise in intracellular calcium can occur over a period of a few minutes in response to addition of the calcium ionophore

A23187 to the medium. When the increase in calcium is small, such a rise is compensated for and intracellular calcium levels return to their former set point (Kater et al., 1988a, b). Since calcium concentrations return towards the rest levels despite the continued influx into the cell (due to the continued presence of the ionophore), there must be a compensatory increase in calcium efflux. In fact, our preliminary data indicate that a sodium-dependent mechanism (presumably the Na^+/Ca^{2+} exchanger) is responsible for this restoration.

When larger doses of A23187 are used to generate larger calcium transients, different classes of neurons are seen: those with high regulating capacity and those with considerably lower regulating capacity (Fig. 7). Those cells with high regulating capacities survive large calcium influxes extremely well. Those cells with low regulating capacity, on the other hand, do not readily survive the ionophore-induced calcium challenges, where levels might reach in excess of 3,000 nM from their

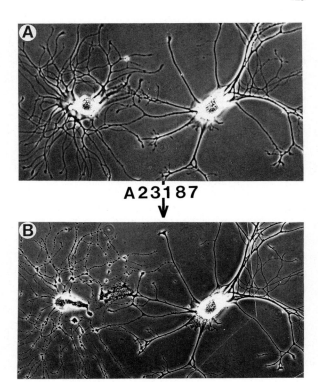

Fig. 8. Neurons with different calcium homeostatic capability can be selectively removed from circuit connections through selective neuronal death. This figure provides examples of weakly and strongly calcium regulating neurons. Application of A23187 ($2 \cdot 10^{-7}$ M) to this pair of neurons resulted in neuron B5 (right) regulating its calcium concentration. Thus, there is no apparent change in its morphology. On the other hand, neuron B19, known to be a weakly regulating neuron, was unable to compensate for this calcium load and degenerated in a matter of 30 min.

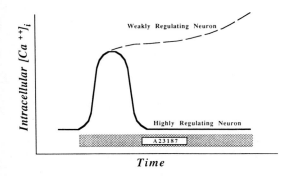

Fig. 7. Calcium homeostasis is an important function for the generation, maintenance and modification of neuronal architecture as well as neuronal survival. Individual neurons fall into two basic ranges, those which have strong reactive capacities and those which have weak reactive capacities to perturbations of intracellular calcium. This figure schematically represents these two classes and their responses to the continuous presence of the ionophore A23187. The strongly regulating forms of neurons show discrete rises in intracellular calcium which restore back to rest levels. On the other hand, weakly regulating forms frequently show rises which explosively exceed lethal calcium levels. Thus neurons with different calcium homeostatic capabilities will respond quite differently to the same stimulus.

original set points of the order of 100 nM. Again, preliminary data suggest that a sodium-dependent mechanism (presumably the Na^+/Ca^{2+} exchanger) is at least partly responsible for the distinction between these two classes.

Fig. 8 demonstrates that particular identified neurons in *Helisoma* have different calcium homeostatic capability. B5 neurons are extremely good calcium regulators. Even very high doses of A23187, which result in calcium concentrations transiently reaching micromolar levels, are compensated for; calcium levels come down and the neuron survives. B19 neurons on the other hand, can not tolerate such large increases in intracellular

126

calcium; ultimately, even within a few minutes, such neurons will die. Such mechanisms may function normally in bringing about the physiological cell death that characterizes development (Oppenheim, 1985). On the other hand, such mechanisms may represent the underpinnings of gross pathological neurodegeneration. When the cell can no longer regulate its intracellular calcium levels, death may ensue.

We now know that a variety of agents, ranging from action potentials, neurotransmitters, depolarization and a variety of growth-associated factors, can all change intracellular calcium levels. Small changes can result in changes of outgrowth both in rate and pattern. On the other hand, large changes can result in cell death (Fig. 9). The final outgrowth pattern is generated by integration of a variety of signals at the growth cone. While there are many other second messenger systems which might affect the behavior of growth cones (Matt-

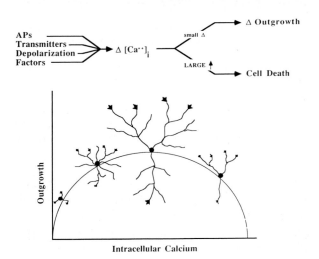

Fig. 9. A continuum of effects of changes in intracellular calcium. Intracellular calcium can be changed by a variety of agents ranging from action potentials to growth factors. Integration of these diverse environmental signals by the growth cone results in net changes in intracellular calcium levels. Small changes in intracellular calcium can result in changes in outgrowth rates; large changes can result in cell death. Thus, there is a continuum of responses that a neuron can display in response to a gradation in changes in intracellular calcium.

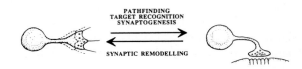

GROWTH CONE	CHARACTERISTIC FEATURE	PRESYNAPTIC TERMINAL
✓	RESOURCES TRANSPORTED FROM CELL BODY	✓
✓	VESICLES INTEGRAL TO FUNCTION	✓
✓	MITOCHONDRIA CONCENTRATED	✓
✓	RELEASE NEUROTRANSMITTERS	✓
✓	FEEDBACK SIGNALS FROM TARGET	✓
✓	NEUROTRANSMITTER RECEPTORS PRESENT	✓
✓	ACTION POTENTIALS TRANSMIT INFORMATION FROM CELL BODY	✓
✓	MEMBRANE IS EXCITABLE	✓
✓	CALCIUM REGULATES PRIME FUNCTION	✓

Fig. 10. The striking relationship between characteristics to the neuronal growth cone in the pre-synaptic terminal. Both growth cones and pre-synaptic terminals share many features including active membrane properties, ultrastructural features and control systems. These shared features raise the question as to the potential relationship of these structures. In fact, it is most plausible to assume that the pre-synaptic terminal and the growth cone are but two of a wide range of interconvertible morphologies seen at the tips of neurites under different conditions.

son et al., 1988b), calcium is a major locus for the final integration.

Plasticity and the neuronal growth cone

Fig. 10 outlines a striking set of characteristics shared by the neuronal growth cone and the pre-synaptic terminal. It also illustrates one of the most challenging questions in neurosciences. To what extent is there an interconvertibility between the growth cone (with its pathfinding, target recognition and synaptogenic capabilities) and the neuronal pre-synaptic terminal (with its characteristic integrative properties?) Available evidence supports the hypothesis that the growth cone could well become a pre-synaptic terminal. Obviously, contact, which is initially made by the growth cone, is a necessary prerequisite for the establishment of a functional synapse. In addition, the growth cone has excitable membrane (Guthrie et al., 1989), and is capable of performing the primary function of the pre-synaptic terminal, namely releasing neurotransmitter (Hume et al., 1983; Young and Poo, 1983). The question of whether the growth cone itself becomes a pre-synaptic terminal, or whether it proceeds beyond the post-synaptic site, leaving the following neurite to become the pre-synaptic terminal will require detailed study. In fact, without an extremely narrow, and perhaps artificial, definition of the difference between the growth cone and the pre-synaptic terminal, this question may not be answerable.

Available evidence also leads us to the speculation that the same terminal, under appropriate conditions, can be re-awakened and converted to a growth cone capable of traversing out new terrain to seek out and establishing new connections. Surely, the pre-synaptic terminal must become motile during the synaptic remodeling that has been observed by many researchers (Levine and Truman, 1982; Purves et al., 1986; Bailey and Chen, 1988; Wigston, 1989). Again, whether the pre-synaptic terminal itself becomes motile, or whether it is resorbed in the process of generating a new growth cone, will require detailed study. With such a dramatic range of remodeling capabilities built in to this system, it is not surprising that even minor dysfunctions might result in major pathological conditions. What is more astonishing, in fact, is the tremendous degree of regulatory capabilities that exists in these systems that allows them to assume their appropriate form and function under the wide range of stimuli which impinge upon them.

References

Bailey, C.H. and Chen, M. (1988) Long-term memory in *Aplysia* modulates the total number of varicosities of single identified sensory neurons. *Proc. Natl. Acad. Sci. U.S.A.,* 85: 2373 – 2377.

Bentley, D. and Toroian-Raymond, A. (1986) Disoriented pathfinding by pioneer neurone growth cones deprived of filopodia by cytochalasin treatment. *Nature,* 323: 712 – 715.

Cohan, C.S. and Kater, S.B. (1986) Suppression of neurite elongation and growth cone motility by electrical activity. *Science,* 232: 1638 – 1640.

Cohan, C.S., Connor, J.A. and Kater, S.B. (1987) Electrically and chemically mediated increases in intracellular calcium in neuronal growth cones. *J. Neurosci.,* 7: 3588 – 3599.

Grega, D.S. and Kater, S.B. (1987) Reinitiation of outgrowth from dormant neurons in cell culture. *Soc. Neurosci. Abstr.,* 13: 167.

Grynkiewicz, G.M., Poenie, M. and Tsien, R. (1985) A new generation of Ca^{2+} indicators with greatly improved fluorescence properties. *J. Biol. Chem.,* 260: 3440 – 3450.

Guthrie, P.B., Mattson, M.P., Mills, L.R. and Kater, S.B. (1988) Calcium homeostasis in molluscan and mammalian neurons: neuron-selective set-point of calcium rest concentration. *Soc. Neurosci. Abstr.,* 14: 582.

Guthrie, P.B., Lee, R.E. and Kater, S.B. (1989) A comparison of neuronal growth cone and cell body membrane: electrophysiological and ultrastructural properties. *J. Neurosci.,* 9: 3596 – 3605.

Hadley, R.D., Bodnar, D.A. and Kater, S.B. (1985) Formation of electrical synapses between isolated, cultured *Helisoma* neurons requires mutual neurite elongation. *J. Neurosci.,* 5: 3145 – 3153.

Haydon, P.G., Cohan, C.S., McCobb, D.P., Miller, H.R. and Kater, S.B. (1985) Neuron-specific growth cone properties as seen in identified neurons of *Helisoma. J. Neurosci. Res.,* 13: 135 – 147.

Haydon, P.G., McCobb, D.P. and Kater, S.B. (1987) The regulation of neurite outgrowth, growth cone motility, and electrical synaptogenesis by serotonin. *J. Neurobiol.,* 18: 197 – 215.

Hume, R.L., Role, L. and Fischbach, G.D. (1983) Acetylcholine release from growth cone detected by patches of acetylcholine receptor-rich membrane. *Nature,* 305: 632 – 634.

Kater, S.B. and Letourneau, P. (Eds.) (1985) *The Biology of the Neuronal Growth Cone,* Alan R. Liss, New York.

Kater, S.B., Guthrie, P.B., Mattson, M.P., Mills, L.R. and Zucker, R.S. (1988a) Calcium homeostasis in molluscan and mammalian neurons: dynamics of calcium regulation. *Soc. Neurosci. Abstr.,* 14: 582.

Kater, S.B., Mattson, M.P., Cohan, C. and Connor, J. (1988b) Calcium regulation of the neuronal growth cone. *Trends Neurosci.,* 11: 315 – 321.

Lankford, K.L., DeMello, F.G. and Klein, W.L. (1988) D1 dopamine receptors inhibit growth cone motility in cultured retinal neurons; evidence that neurotransmitters act as morphogenetic growth regulators in the developing nervous system. *Proc. Natl. Acad. Sci. U.S.A.,* 85: 4567 – 4571.

Levine, R.B. and Truman, J.W. (1982) Metamorphosis of the insect nervous system: changes in the morphology and synaptic interactions of identified cells. *Nature,* 299: 250 – 252.

Lipton, S.A., Frosch, M.P., Phillips, M.D., Tauck, D.L. and

Aizenman, E. (1988) Nicotinic agonists enhance process outgrowth by retinal ganglion cells in culture. *Science,* 239: 1293 – 1296.

Lopresti, V., Macagno, E.R. and Levinthal, C. (1973) Structure and development of neuronal connections in isogenic organisms: cellular interactions in the development of the optic lamina of *Daphnia. Proc. Natl. Acad. Sci. U.S.A.,* 70: 433 – 437.

Mattson, M.P. and Kater, S.B. (1987) Calcium regulation of neurite elongation and growth cone motility. *J. Neurosci.,* 7: 4034 – 4043.

Mattson, M.P. and Kater, S.B. (1989) Excitatory and inhibitory neurotransmitters in the generation and degeneration of hippocampal neuroarchitecture. *Brain Res.,* 478: 337 – 348.

Mattson, M.P., Dou, P. and Kater, S.B. (1988a) Outgrowth-regulating actions of glutamate in isolated hippocampal pyramidal neurons. *J. Neurosci.,* 8: 2087 – 2100.

Mattson, M.P., Taylor-Hunter, A. and Kater, S.B. (1988b) Neurite outgrowth in individual neurons of a neuronal population is differentially regulated by calcium and cyclic AMP. *J. Neurosci.,* 8: 1704 – 1711.

Mattson, M.P., Guthrie, P.B. and Kater, S.B. (1989) Intracellular messengers in the generation and degeneration of hippocampal neuroarchitecture. *J. Neurosci. Res.,* 21: 447 – 464.

McBurney, R.N. and Neeting, R. (1987) Neuronal calcium homeostasis. *Trends Neurosci.,* 10: 164 – 169.

McCobb, D.P. and Kater, S.B. (1988a) Dopamine and serotonin inhibition of neurite elongation of different iden-tified neurons. *J. Neurosci. Res.,* 19: 19 – 26.

McCobb, D.P. and Kater, S.B. (1988b) Membrane voltage and neurotransmitter regulation of neuronal growth cone motility. *Dev. Biol.,* 130: 599 – 609.

McCobb, D.P., Cohan, C.S., Connor, J.A. and Kater, S.B. (1988) Interactive effects of serotonin and acetylcholine on neurite elongation. *Neuron,* 1: 377 – 385.

Mills, L.R., Murrain, M., Guthrie, P.B. and Kater, S.B. (1988) Intracellular calcium concentrations in neuronal growth cones change with induced turning and branching behavior. *Soc. Neurosci. Abstr.,* 14: 583.

Oppenheim, R.W. (1985) Naturally occurring cell death during neural development. *Trends Neurosci.,* 8: 487 – 493.

Purves, D., Hadley, R.D. and Voyvodic, J.T. (1986) Dynamic changes in the dendritic morphology of individual neurons visualized over periods of up to three months in the superior cervical ganglion of living mice. *J. Neurosci.,* 6: 1051 – 1060.

Ramon y Cajal, S. (1890) A quelle époque apparaissent les expansions des cellules nerveuses de la moelle epinière du poulet. *Anat. Anz.,* 5: 609 – 613; 631 – 639.

Roberts, A. and Patton, D.T. (1985) Growth cones and the formation of central and peripheral neurites by sensory neurones in amphibian embryos. *J. Neurosci. Res.,* 13: 23 – 38.

Wigston, D.J. (1989) Remodeling of neuromuscular junctions in adult mouse soleus. *J. Neurosci.,* 9: 639 – 647.

Young, S.H. and Poo, M. (1983) Spontaneous release of transmitter from growth cones of embryonic neurones. *Nature,* 305: 634 – 637.

P. Coleman, G. Higgins and C. Phelps (Eds.)
Progress in Brain Research, Vol. 86
© 1990 Elsevier Science Publishers B.V. (Biomedical Division)

CHAPTER 11

Intracortical processes regulating the integration of sensory information

Ford F. Ebner[1] and Michael A. Armstrong-James[2]

[1]*Neurobiology Section and Center for Neural Science, Brown University, Providence, RI 02912, U.S.A., and* [2]*Neuroscience Group, The London Hospital Medical College, University of London, London E1 2AD, U.K.*

The mechanisms that link sensory inputs in spatially separated regions of cortex can be elucidated by analyzing the mechanisms that generate receptive field properties in cortical neurons under conditions that mimic the waking state; a state when learning, memory and the modification of synaptic strength can be most readily demonstrated. Important advances in understanding receptive field mechanisms in sensory cortex have arisen from studying the precise relationship between the mystacial vibrissae or "whiskers" and their neural representation in separate cortical domains or "barrels". The anatomical precision of whisker projections to barrels permits a unique delineation of thalamocortical and intracortical components of cortical cell responses based on latency and security of response to peripheral receptor stimulation. When recorded in awake animals or even under very light anesthesia, cortical neurons show two components to their response to whisker movement. Neurons in layer IV of a whisker's primary projection zone respond with short latency (7 – 10 msec) and a high response magnitude (two or more action potentials (spikes) per stimulus). This "Center Receptive Field" (CRF) for layer IV cells is generated in large part by sensory fiber inputs from the thalamus. The CRF is restricted to 1.4 whiskers on average and is the only response detectable when cortical responses are depressed by deep anesthesia. In the "waking state" the same neuron often will respond to deflection of 4 – 6 surrounding whiskers, but only at longer latency (15 – 40 msec) and with fewer spikes per stimulus. These more labile responses form an excitatory surround receptive field (SRF). Sensory information that is transduced by individual whiskers and that generates the SRF of a cortical neuron achieves this added response complexity through intracortical mechanisms. The control of the mechanisms that determine the dissemination of sensory information within cortex include: (1) regulating the level of GABAergic inhibition; and (2) potentiation or depression of the response level generated by repeated sensory experience. State-dependent "modulatory" inputs to cortex, such as the noradrenergic and cholinergic fiber systems, could regulate the degree of horizontal spread of a sensory input, in part through global changes in the level of inhibition and/or regulating the amplitude of cortical responses, thereby determining the level of associative interactions between sensory inputs.

Introduction

Throughout life, information must be represented, stored and accessed in the central nervous system by the integrated action of neuronal networks. The cerebral cortex is the region of the brain that is necessary for processing and storing many features of sensory information. The neocortex is uniquely identified with the conscious appreciation of sensory information and it is therefore a logical structure to analyze in order to understand mechanisms that regulate the associative and integrative processes of sensation.

In somatic sensory areas of cortex the representation of the body surface is spread out topographically as layered sheets of cells which receive modulatory as well as sensory inputs in an orderly array. Because of this anatomical arrangement each point on the body is associated with its own sensory and modulatory circuitry within a vertical cortical module; neurons located within different modules maintain cooperative interactions through horizontal cortical circuitry. The association of two sensory stimuli at the cortical level is

130

dependent upon cellular mechanisms that link the activity generated by the two inputs when they arrive in separated regions of the cortex. The problem of associating the activity generated by two separate sensory inputs to cortex is illustrated in Fig. 1.

One of the most characteristic features of cortical integration is that the response of cortical neurons to a sensory stimulus is influenced by the recent history of sensory experience (Merzenich et al., 1988). The change in cortical response as a function of sensory experience may underlie the plasticity associated with learning of sensory-motor tasks, and we will argue that a key component of cortical response is the extent to which a spatially restricted afferent volley is allowed to propagate horizontally within cortex. Under certain conditions, two simultaneous sensory volleys will each activate a restricted cortical zone. Under different conditions, presumably mediated by

ascending modulatory systems, the same thalamic volleys will each activate widespread cortical regions. Indeed, the activated cortical zones may overlap, such that a given cell is driven by both inputs; in that case the synaptic connections between neurons within the activated cortical regions will be strengthened, according to the rules of Hebbian synaptic modification that have been the object of much recent speculation (Bear et al., 1987). The changes in synaptic efficacy induced by paired inputs to cortex are not generalized; they are specific to the active inputs. The problem of great interest is to identify the cellular mechanisms that mediate and regulate the horizontal spread of activity in cortex.

Cortical integration of sensory information is altered dramatically by the state of alert wakefulness or sleep. In the waking state the extent of intracortical spread of activity around the active zone is more widespread than during deep sleep. The mechanism that "gates" synaptic modification may be closely linked with the mechanisms that set the level of overall or regional cortical excitability. Regulation of cortical excitability is usually assigned to ascending subcortical projections, both those arising in the thalamus and outside the thalamus, that project in a topographically organized, but not point-to-point, manner over the entire neocortex. Within the somatic sensory system one would expect experience-dependent cortical modification to cause neurons, that had not responded at any level of stimulus intensity prior to potentiation, to be easily driven afterwards. The same mechanisms could come into play to keep a cortical map continuously in register with the status of the sensory periphery.

Our challenge, then, is to identify the mechanisms that regulate the strength of synapses within cortex and to determine how synaptic changes are reflected in cortical receptive fields, the commonly applied measure of cortical cell properties. We will explore these issues using what is known about the properties of rodent "barrel field cortex" as a single case from which to generalize to other species and to other cortical areas.

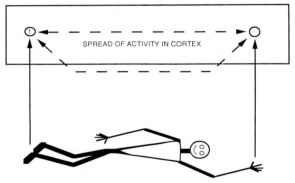

Fig. 1. Diagram of the problem posed by the need for sensory inputs that arrive in different regions of the cerebral cortex to be associated by altering the activity in a common pool of neurons. In this hypothetical case the sensory activity generated by receptors in the hand and foot would arrive many millimeters apart in the hand and foot regions of the postcentral gyrus. Initially cell 1 would respond only to stimulation of receptors in the foot. However, after repeated, temporally linked, paired stimulation of the hand and foot sites, cell 1 may respond to stimulation of either input alone. The problem is to define mechanisms that support this type of associative process.

Receptive field organization in barrel field cortex

The barrel field cortex of rodents provides a unique model system in which to study the intracortical spread of activity generated by sensory inputs because each whisker is a distinctly circumscribed receptor assembly that projects through a small number of synapses (usually 2) to an anatomically localized zone in the contralateral cortex (Woolsey and Van der Loos, 1970; Welker, 1971). Therefore, the inputs from each whisker activate cortical neurons in the contralateral hemisphere at a known distance from one another. The total whisker representation in SI occupies a substantial 2 × 4 mm region on the lateral surface of the hemisphere in the rat.

Anatomy of the sensory pathways to barrel field cortex

The anatomy of the pathway from the large whiskers or "mystacial vibrissae" to the somatic sensory cortex in the rat has been reviewed in detail several times recently (Killackey, 1983) and a current understanding of the system can be roughly

sketched as follows (see Fig. 3): each mystacial vibrissa is innervated by around 200 trigeminal nerve fibers. The central processes of these trigeminal ganglion cell axons terminate in two subdivisions of the trigeminal nuclear complex; the principal trigeminal nucleus (PrV) in the pons and the interpolaris portion of the spinal trigeminal nucleus (SpVi) in the medulla. Both PrV and SpVi project to both the ventral posteromedial thalamic nucleus (VPM) and the posterior nucleus (PO); the PrV – VPM pathway appears dominant in the sense that their properties are imposed on cells in cortex that receive direct VPM inputs. While the SpVi projects to VPM and PO, and PrV also pro-

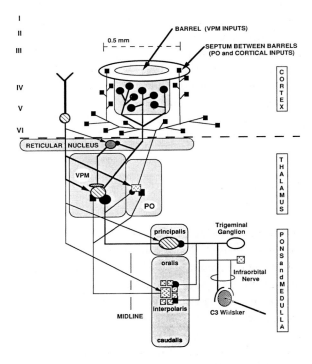

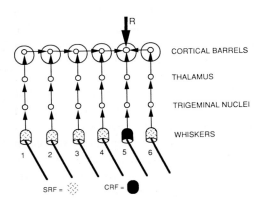

Fig. 2. Diagram of the information flow that generates the center receptive field (CRF = solid black whisker 5 follicle) and the surround receptive field (SRF = cross-hatched whisker 1, 2, 3, 4 and 6 follicles) in rat barrel field neurons. The arrows represent the synaptic relays between the whiskers and the barrel field cortex. The inputs from each whisker is strongly channeled to its respective cortical barrel. The intracortical connections allow many whiskers to influence cortical neurons.

Fig. 3. Drawing of the pathways from the whiskers to the barrel field cortex. The oval cell bodies and the similar shaped black axon terminals in the principal nucleus of the trigeminal complex and in the VPM nucleus of the thalamus form relays directly to the cortical barrels. The square cell bodies and their axon terminals represent the "parallel pathway" to cortex, which in the rat trigeminal system is not exclusively parallel in the subcortical relay nuclei.

jects to PO, the function of these separate pathways to the thalamus remains to be elucidated. VPM and PO give rise to interdigitating terminal fields in the posteromedial barrel subfield region (BF) of SI cortex; VPM fibers give rise to collaterals in layer VI and then terminate in high density in the layer IV barrel, while PO fibers terminate in a continuous horizontal band in layers V, III and I. In layer IV PO axons form a discontinuous band as they synapse only in the "septal zones" that surround the individual barrels (Lin et al., 1987; Koralek, 1988), but avoid the barrel centers. The most posterior part of PO also projects to a second somatic sensory area lateral to SI (called SII cortex; Spreafico and Rustioni, 1987). Finally, two additional thalamic nuclei, not known to receive sensory afferent fibers, project to the barrel field cortex; the ventral medial nucleus (VM) which projects nearly exclusively to layer I and the central lateral nucleus (CL) which projects mainly to layers V and I (Herkenham, 1980). The outline given above provides a hint of the inputs to cortex, but the sequence of activation of cortical neurons following the arrival of afferent volleys in layer IV can be specified only by physiological analysis.

Response of barrel field neurons to stimulation of the whiskers

In awake, sleeping and anesthetized animals very discrete whisker deflections lasting only a few milliseconds, inevitably lead to cell responses in the brain stem PrV + SpVi nuclei, the thalamic VPM + PO nuclei and their cortical target cells. The physiological record of these responses becomes the window through which one can observe and characterize the distribution of activity generated in cortex by whisker movement. Two main techniques have been employed in conjunction with the extracellular microelectrode method to analyze cortical cell responses to cutaneous stimuli; the technique in widest use is to characterize the relation of a single cell to the periphery (the receptive field method). This is often accomplished by measuring the number and the latency of action potentials produced by a single cortical neuron in response to movement of each of the whiskers in turn. The other method is to characterize the relation of a single site in the periphery to the entire cortex. This may be done by mapping the total area of barrel field cortex that contains neurons responsive to the movement of a single whisker (the cortical domain method).

The initial receptive field analyses of rat barrel field neurons led to the conclusion that each layer IV barrel neuron responds almost exclusively to a single vibrissa. This conclusion, based on studies carried out under deep nembutal anesthesia, established the idea that one whisker, called the principal whisker, provides the dominant input to one cortical zone (corresponding to a single barrel) labeled by the row and rank of the principal whisker (Welker, 1971, 1976). Cells in the radial cylinder of neurons located above and below the layer IV barrel responded to more than one whisker and thus had larger receptive fields.

Following whisker deflection, a characteristic post-stimulus response is recorded extracellularly from cortical neurons with an onset latency never shorter than 6 msec. The response typically consists of: (1) a burst of action potentials lasting about 5 – 10 msec; (2) a silent period of variable length; and (3) a prolonged period of up to 200 msec when there may be more or less activity depending on variables such as the depth of anesthesia (Fig. 4). The silent period suggests that inhibitory as well as excitatory events are initiated by whisker inputs. Inhibitory interactions between whisker initiated events have been demonstrated in cortex directly by moving two whiskers in close succession ($\sim$ 10 – 20 msec apart) in lightly anesthetized or unanesthetized animals. The response to whisker 2 is diminished if the volley initiated by moving whisker 2 is timed so that it arrives during the inhibitory period generated by the whisker 1 input (Simons, 1985).

Another dimension to barrel field receptive fields was added in 1987 when Armstrong-James and Fox reported a detailed analysis of cortical cell

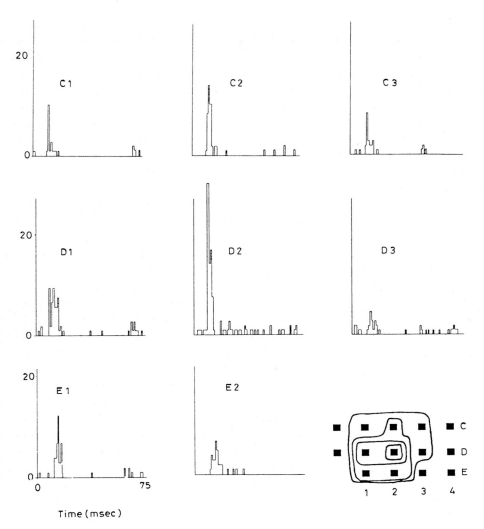

Time (msec)

Fig. 4. Histograms showing the number of spikes (ordinate) recorded from a single cortical neuron in layer IV of barrel field cortex in response to 50 repeated 200 μm deflections of the 8 whiskers that could activate the cell (C1-3, D1-3 and E1-2). Clearly, all whiskers do not drive the cell with equal vigor; the cell is located in the D2 barrel and the D2 whisker elicits the greatest number of spikes at the shortest latency from the neuron. Other whiskers produce a lesser magnitude of response at a longer latency: in descending order, the D1 whisker is next best, the E1-2 and C2 whiskers are equally less effective and finally C1-3 and D3 are least effective as illustrated in the pictogram of the whisker rows in the lower right corner. For this cortical neuron the D2 whisker forms the CRF and the other 7 whiskers form the SRF (modified from Armstrong-James and Fox, 1987).

responses to whisker stimulation. They grouped cortical neurons in urethane-anesthetized rats into 4 classes based on their relative response magnitude and correlated these classes with response latency. The comparison of latencies and levels of synaptic drive in cells located in each cor-

tical layer led to the conclusion that the greatest number of neurons, as high as 50% of the cells in layer IV, respond to whisker movement with short latency (in the range of 6 – 10 msec) and with an average of 2 or more spikes per stimulus (50 trials were presented at 1 Hz). This "best response" defines the Center Receptive Field (CRF); the CRF typically consists of only 1–2 whiskers (1.4 on average). Neurons in other layers of barrel field cortex also exhibit a CRF, but their best response usually has a longer latency and a lower magnitude (1 or fewer spikes/stimulus) to movement of the same whisker. Cortical cells in lightly anesthetized or awake animals typically respond to movement of several whiskers, but only at a longer latency and a lower average number of spikes per stimulus. The additional whiskers that drive a cortical

neuron at longer latency constitute the excitatory surround receptive field (SRF). The SRF could be generated either by mechanisms operating in the sensory pathways at subcortical levels or, alternatively, by spread of activity through intracortical connections or both. Recent studies by Armstrong-James et al. (1989a) showed that after a single barrel is damaged, neurons in other barrels have diminished responsiveness to the principal whisker of the damaged barrel. The loss of responsiveness is in direct proportion to the percent destruction of the barrel: when 95% of one barrel was destroyed, neurons in other barrels retained no response to the principal whisker of the damaged barrel. These results indicate that the main lemniscal pathway through VPM carries somatic sensory information from each whisker to a restricted zone of cortex (i.e., 1 barrel), after which corticocortical connections disperse the activity horizontally to neighboring barrels. To summarize: the response of cortical neurons to sensory inputs beyond the principal whisker is mediated mainly by intracortical connections coursing vertically between layers near the site of entry and horizontally within layers (Fig. 5).

A characteristic feature of the SRF is its variable size under different conditions and at different times. What are some of the conditions that change the horizontal spread of activity responsible for the SRF in the intact cerebral cortex?

Conditions that change the size of the SRF in barrel field cortex

Condition 1: sensory deprivation

There is only one report of changes in cortical RFs produced by trimming the whiskers during the early postnatal period in the rat (Simons and Land, 1987). Trimming all but one row of whiskers for 53 days after birth and then allowing the cortex to receive normal sensory inputs for an additional 3 months led to substantial changes in the RFs of neurons in barrel field cortex. The RFs of cells in cortical barrels corresponding to the trimmed whiskers were larger than normal, the response of the cells to directional movement werre less selec-

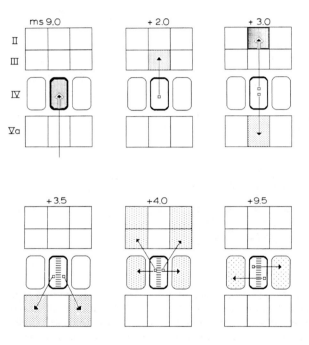

Fig. 5. Illustration of the time required to activate neurons in various layers of the barrel field cortex. The average latency for the arrival of a sensory volley from the whiskers in cortical layer IV is 9 msec (upper left panel). The average increase in latency for the cells in layer III of the same cortical column is 2 msec (upper middle panel) and 3 msec for both layers II and V (upper right panel). The responses produced by whisker movement in adjacent columns always occur at a longer latency than the column of the corresponding barrel (lower 3 panels). II, III, IV and Va identify cortical layers. The density of stippling in the projection zones is proportional to the intensity of the response (redrawn from Armstrong-James et al., 1989b).

tive than normal and the levels of spontaneous activity remained higher than normal. All of these alterations could be explained by a deficiency in the ability of inhibitory cells to develop their usual effectiveness. Subsequent studies from the same group (Akhtar and Land, 1987) support the notion that this set of altered properties results from the failure of cortical GABAergic neurons to adjust to new levels of sensory activity. The cellular and molecular bases for the effects of sensory deprivation have been speculated on (Bear et al., 1987), but remain to be clarified.

Condition 2: repeated paired stimulation

In normal, awake, adult rats stimulation of sets of whiskers in a fixed temporal sequence changes the response of cortical neurons in a predictable way. Using 500 msec interstimulus intervals (longer than the immediate 200 msec synaptic events; Simons, 1985), cortical neurons can be induced to increase their responses to one or both sets of stimulated whiskers. The enlarged SRF consists of either (1) a new response to whiskers that were ineffective before the pairing, (2) an enhancement of the response to one set of whiskers, or (3) the appearance of action potentials during the period that previously constituted the post-excitatory "inhibitory trough" (Delacour et al., 1987) These increased responses to paired stimuli constitute a type of change in cortical neuronal response that depends upon increasing the overall excitability of the cortex in the regions receiving the two inputs and/or upon relaxing the inhibitory constraints on horizontal spread of activity in cortex. Importantly, in contrast to the excitation – inhibition – excitation (E – I – E) response sequence observed in cortical neurons in the absence of conditioning (see Simons, 1985), this conditioned response emerges as a purely excitatory augmentation that progressively increases in magnitude with repetitive stimulation at 1 Hz. The potentiated response was observed for at least 20 min and presumably would have remained for a more extended time period had the experiments continued.

Condition 3: injury to the peripheral and central nervous system

The response of the CNS to peripheral or central injury includes reorganization of sensory pathways that extends several synapses beyond the lesioned neurons and their processes. Injury of the periphery can induce the representation of the body surface in mature somatic sensory cortex to shift in a predictable manner (see Merzenich et al., 1988 for review). For example, transection of a peripheral nerve leads to a progressive expansion of the body surface representation innervated by remaining intact nerves (Wall and Cusick, 1984). Map expansion generally has a limit of less than 1 mm, and in an area as extensive as the barrel field several square millimeters of cortex can be rendered unresponsive to sensory stimulation for at least 3 months if a peripheral nerve is cut and not allowed to regenerate (Waite, 1984). When the area deprived of its sensory inputs is less extensive, the expansion of cortical representation after peripheral nerve injury or digit amputation appears as a type of competitive interaction in which the active inputs are able to dominate the responses of cells in the periphery of their cortical domain. The problem with generalizing these phenomena from the barrel field cortex to other modalities and species is that the responses of cortical neurons have not been characterized in a similar manner in other systems. However, a strong prediction for explaining the map rearrangement seen after amputation of a single digit in monkeys is that the loss of the sensory inputs forming the SRF in a cortical region allows the area to become dominated by the intracortical connections normally forming the SRF. The net result is an increased horizontal extent of cortical activity generated by the inputs from the remaining digits; the original cortical territory is retrieved partially, but not completely, by the original inputs when the damaged nerve regenerates.

Fig. 6 illustrates two features of the somatic sensory pathways that could have a potentially strong impact on RF size, but are not normally detectable unless one of the two pathways is lesioned. The

136

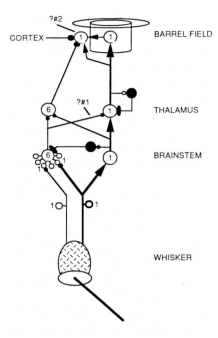

CORTEX

?#2

BARREL FIELD

?#1

6

1

1

THALAMUS

6

1

1

BRAINSTEM

1

1

WHISKER

Fig. 6. Simplified schema of the parallel pathways from a whisker to the barrel field indicating the synapses in the brain stem trigeminal nuclei and the thalamus before the sensory information reaches barrel field cortex. The numbered open circles represent the excitatory neurons and the average number of whiskers that activate them. The arrows indicate the dominant normal (lemniscal) pathway to cortex. Two questions are particularly puzzling: ? # 1 raises the question of why the anatomically demonstrated spinal V inputs to VPM are not reflected in the RF properties of VPM cells unless the principal trigeminal nucleus in the brain stem is destroyed (Rhoades et al., 1987). ? # 2 queries why the layer IV cells in the septal regions of the barrel field have the same sized RF as the barrel cells themselves. See text for discussion.

issue, simply stated, is that as a group, neurons in the two parallel sensory pathways to cortex have different RF sizes. Cells in the PrV – VPM pathway typically respond to only 1 whisker whereas cells in the SpVi – PO pathway respond to about 6 whiskers. Both the 1-whisker and the 6-whisker cell groups in the brain stem project to both the 1-whisker and the 6-whisker cell group in the next relay in the thalamus; given this fact, why don't 6 whiskers, on average, drive both cell groups in thalamus ("? # 1" in Fig. 6)? Is the 1-

whisker RF an artifact of anesthesia? Recent studies have shown that the larger RF of thalamic VB neurons can be revealed if the precise inputs to VPM are eliminated by ablation of PrV (Rhoades et al., 1987). A similar paradox exists in cortex as illustrated by "? #2" in Fig. 6. These results imply that inputs to cortex from PO, under some conditions, may have the capacity to modulate RF size in the alert, exploring animal.

Cellular processes that alter horizontal spread in cerebral cortex

The effect of GABAergic inhibition on horizontal spread of activity in neocortex

One consistent morphological correlate of the abnormal activity seen in epileptic seizure discharge is a reduction in the number of GABAergic cells and processes around the epileptic focus, both in clinical cases and in animal models (Ribak et al., 1979). Whether the decrease in GABAergic activity is a cause of seizure activity, or a result of it has been difficult to establish because the primary etiology remains elusive. However, a recent investigation of the GABAergic control of horizontal spread of activity in in vitro cortical slices provides direct evidence that GABAergic inhibition is one mechanism controlling the horizontal spread of activity in cortex (Chagnac-Amitai and Connors, 1989). These results clearly demonstrate that graded concentrations of bicuculline, an effective $GABA_A$ receptor antagonist, progressively increase the horizontal spread of activity from a narrow zone around the stimulated site up to several millimeters away from the site of stimulation. The implication of these results is that a control system which modulates the amount of GABAergic cell activity could also have more wide-ranging effects; in addition to regulating the local level of inhibition, more global modulation of inhibition could influence the horizontal cortical domain over which sensory inputs can spread. GABAergic neurons are strongly activated by acetylcholine through muscarinic receptors (McCormick and Prince, 1986). Is it possible that the role of the demonstrated modulators of developmental "cortical plasticity" (Bear and Singer, 1986) persists in the adult, where they regulate the size of the SRF and hence the level of associative interactions between sensory inputs? If so, the same modulators would dictate the extent of "representation" of any sensory input to cortex as well as the configuration of the cortical map.

The effect of LTP on horizontal spread of activity in neocortex

A second type of regulation of horizontal spread of activity could be achieved through the selective increase in amplitude or "potentiation" of cortical responses to sensory inputs, especially if the potentiation persists for periods of time measured in hours or days. Enhancement of the response to single test inputs to neocortex usually requires repeated sensory stimulation or, if induced by electrical stimulation, a train of conditioning stimuli. In a recent study of LTP in neocortical slice preparations from adult rats, Lee et al. (1989) showed that the horizontal spread of evoked responses can be increased markedly by the simple expedient of lowering the concentration of Mg^{2+} in the bathing medium from the normal 2 mM to $100-500$ μM. When conditioning stimuli are presented to layer VI at 2 Hz for 80 sec under low $[Mg^{2+}]$ conditions, the responses in layers II/III are potentiated for over 2 h across wide areas of the slice. This apparently transsynaptic LTP identifies another mechanism that could influence the horizontal propagation of sensory information, although the phenomenon has not, as yet, been demonstrated in cortex in vivo. The important question about GABAergic and other regulators of horizontal spread of activity induced by sensory inputs remains open: how are they controlled in the normal, awake, adult animal.

Non-sensory projections control cortical excitability and may influence the horizontal spread of sensory activity

Brain stem influences were assigned a key role in the control of cortical excitability long before the demonstration that noradrenergic neurons in the pons and cholinergic neurons in the basal forebrain project directly to cortex. The idea of brain stem regulated changes in cortical excitability has its origins in the discovery of the cortical activating system by Moruzzi and Magoun (1949), who showed that desynchronization of the cortical EEG could be produced by electrical stimulation of the midbrain or the pontomedullary reticular formation. This initial concept assumed that a multisynaptic ascending midbrain reticular core extended without interruption through the midline and intralaminar thalamic nuclei; these nuclei, in turn, controlled the cortical state through nonspecific (and non-sensory) inputs to cortex. Sleep (characterized by low frequency synchronous discharges or "slow waves") resulted from the absence of active ascending reticular inputs. The awake state was characterized by a high-frequency, low-amplitude EEG, and in the waking condition cortex was supposed to be in an optimal state to analyze sensory inputs. Recent evidence suggests that the origin of the delta waves characteristic of slow wave sleep is in the intralaminar region of the thalamus, specifically the central lateral nucleus for the barrel field cortex (delta waves are to be distinguished from "spindling" activity which will not be discussed here; see Steriade and Llinas, 1988, for a recent review). These synchronized bursts of action potentials appear to be mediated in part through the N-methyl-D-aspartate (NMDA) type of glutamate receptors since the application of 2-amino-5-phosphonovaleric acid (APV) is able to block the generation of burst-pause (delta wave) activity in cortex (Armstrong-James and Fox, 1987).

The overall excitability state of the cortex when it receives specific sensory information is greatly influenced by the inputs from the parallel PO sensory pathway (Ebner et al., 1989) as well as the non-sensory inputs that arise from both thalamic and extrathalamic subcortical cell groups (Singer and Rauschecker, 1982). Much of the current interest in "non-specific" inputs to cortex arises from the belief that non-specific systems modulate or "gate" neural transmission and thus determine when learning, memory and cortical plasticity in all its manifestations are permitted (Bear and Singer, 1986). This gating process could regulate Hebbian-type synaptic modifications that occur as a result of repeated sensory experience even in the adult cortex. Often a dual cooperativity is mandatory for the associative process to occur; one input requiring paired activation with another input in a fixed temporal relationship. It is not yet clear whether one of the coactive inputs can be "nonspecific" and could thus depend more upon the behavioral state of the animal than on the specific sensory information.

Most of the direct tests of sensory interactions on cortical response properties have been carried out on the developing brain during the early postnatal period when sensory experience occurs for the first time and when nearly all cortical operations are still immature by anatomical, physiological and biochemical criteria. The development of normal responsiveness of neurons in sensory cortex depends upon a period of adjustment by sensory experience when sensory systems first become functional. This period of synaptic modification by any pattern of sensory inputs ends at the age of a few weeks or months; afterwards changes in cortical cell responses and the synaptic modification upon which they depend become harder to elicit. Since the initial demonstration by Kasamatsu and Pettigrew (1976) that depletion of norepinephrine (NE) interferes with the cortical ocular dominance shift normally induced by monocular deprivation in kittens, a whole literature has emerged in the search for the mechanisms through which NE can gate or enhance synaptic modification. The search has not been without controversy (Daw et al., 1985). Much more recently it has been argued that the effects of acetylcholine (ACh) are coupled with those of NE as promotors of synaptic plasticity; some types of synaptic modification that could not be blocked by NE or ACh depletion alone, could be blocked when NE and ACh were depleted simultaneously in cortex (Bear and Singer, 1986). Most current views of cortical plasticity in adult cortex, therefore, incorporate the idea that the mechanisms controlling experience-dependent synaptic modification in the developing brain persist to subserve analogous functions in the mature cortex, such as learning and memory. The crucial premise is that throughout life synapses continue to be modified by use so that the response of cortical neurons to new sensory information remains dynamic. This hypothesis has led to a search for a model of cortical plasticity that can be reproducibly analyzed with combined anatomical, physiological and pharmacological techniques in the mature mammalian neocortex (Fox et al., 1988). Insights from such a model would form a basis for understanding synaptic modification which must occur during elaborate perceptual and cognitive functions (Hyvarinen et al., 1980).

The state-dependent control of sensory information processing becomes an issue of central importance in the control of learning from sensory experience. The most fundamental and easily defined change in cortical state is from the awake, alert state to deep sleep. Pioneering single unit studies were carried out independently by Evarts and Hubel in 1959 when they documented changes in the patterned activity of cortical neurons when an awake animal fell asleep. The awake state is characterized by pseudo-random single cortical cell firing, whereas sleep is characterized by a coherent burst-pause cortical firing pattern. During the awake state the dependence of *spontaneous activity* on NMDA receptors decreases, and cortical activity becomes uncorrelated with discharge patterns in the thalamic intralaminar nuclei (Armstrong-James and Fox, 1986). What global modulators could regulate the spread of horizontal activity in the normal, awake, mature neocortex of an alert mammal? Hobson (1984) has suggested that both ACh and NE are found at high levels in cortex in the awake state. During sleep ACh also is high, but NE falls to very low levels in the brain at this time. Simultaneous release of NE and ACh could be a characteristic of alert cortex, a time when synaptic plasticity is required. How do NE and ACh influence receptive field properties of cortical neurons?

NE influences on cortical receptive field properties

Among the earliest studies on monoamine influences on cortex were carried out by Jouvet and his coworkers to test early theories on ascending activating systems. On the basis of complex neuropharmacological and central lesion studies, they concluded that noradrenergic neurons in the locus coeruleus (LC) were the final common path for "cortical activation" (Jouvet, 1972). More recent results support a number of these early conclusions. For example, brief (1 min) iontophoresis of norepinephrine onto cortical neurons, was found to change neuronal activity from a slow wave sleep burst pattern to an awake pattern for periods exceeding 1 h (Armstrong-James and Fox, 1983). The noradrenergic actions appear to operate through second messenger systems, since prolonged effects of this type are not easily explained in terms of transient membrane ion gate actions.

A small number of studies have examined the effect of released NE on the responses of cortical neurons to somatic sensory stimulation. For example, Waterhouse and Woodward (1980) showed that NE enhanced both excitatory and inhibitory responses in lightly halothane-anesthetized rats in all layers of cortex. Either the level of response to peripheral stimulation or spontaneous discharge or both could be affected by NE, but the net effect in many cases appeared to be a greater signal-to-noise ratio that might enhance detection of a sensory event. These and similar studies implicating neurotransmitter-specific systems in cortical modulation depend upon work in anesthetized preparations. Such animals are already in a defined cortical "state" in which some or all systems that normally maintain sensory-perceptual functions, in essence, are eliminated. Therefore, the goal in the future must be to understand the role of modulatory inputs acting in an animal receptive to and learning from interactions with its environment.

Acetylcholine (ACh) influences on cortical excitability and receptive field properties

More recently the basal forebrain cholinergic system has been strongly implicated in initiating and perhaps maintaining the waking cortical state (Buzsaki et al., 1988). Damage to the cholinergic neurons in the nucleus basalis (NB) that project directly to cortex resulted in a dramatic increase of slow delta waves on the side of the lesion, mimicking the effect of scopolamine administration. One interpretation of these results is that the NB plays a key role in arousal and cortical activation through suppression of the spindle-type spontaneous discharge generated by the reticular nucleus – thalamocortical circuitry. However, the effect of ACh on somatic sensory receptive fields is more complicated. Donoghue and Carroll (1987) showed that neurons in all layers of rat SI barrel field cortex respond to whisker stimulation and can be influenced by ACh application. Response enhancement was usually found in the supragranular layers and the infragranular layers, while the most common response in layer IV was response suppression. Lamour et al. (1988) reported that 34% of the cells in rat SI cortex were influenced by the local application of ACh with a bewildering array of modifications; some neurons respond when no driven response was detectable before ACh was applied, some by an increased number of spikes per stimulus, some by an increased size of RF and some by a change in the most effective stimulus modality. The effect on RF size fell between that caused by bicuculline and the lesser effect of applied glutamate. The probability of finding a cell influenced by ACh was highest in layers VI and V under their conditions, although some affected cells were located in all layers.

Thus, the net effect of modulatory influences on cortical cell responses is complex and different for different neurons. Often the effect mimics that of changing the level of GABAergic inhibition or of inducing long-term potentiation of responses in vitro. The human brain is in its most awesome state when we are quietly "free-associating" elements of our past experience with a task at hand. When we gain insight into the regulation of normal sensory information processing needed to achieve learning and memory, the goal of understanding the pathogenesis of dementia will be much closer.

Acknowledgements

We are endebted to Dr. Mathew Diamond for critical reading and suggested improvements to earlier drafts of this manuscript. This study was supported by NIH grants NS-13031 and NS-25907.

References

Akhtar, N.D. and Land, P.W. (1987) The effects of sensory deprivation on glutamic acid decarboxylase immunoreactivity in the rat SmI barrel cortex. *Neurosci. Abstr.*, 13: 77.

Armstrong-James, M. (1975) The functional status and columnar organization of single cells responding to cutaneous stimulation in neonatal rat somatosensory cortex. *J. Physiol. (Lond.)*, 246: 501–538.

Armstrong-James, M. and Callahan, C.A. (1990) Spatiotemporal convergence in the thalamic ventroposterior medial nucleus (VPm) of the rat. *J. Comp. Neurol.*, in press.

Armstrong-James, M. and Fox, K. (1986) The role of the anterior intralaminar nuclei and NMDA receptors in the generation of spontaneous bursts in rat neocortical neurones. *Exp. Brain Res.*, 63: 505–518.

Armstrong-James, M. and Fox, K. (1987) Spatiotemporal convergence and divergence in the rat SI "barrel" cortex. *J. Comp. Neurol.*, 263: 265–281.

Armstrong-James, M., Callahan, C.A. and Friedman, M.A. (1989a) Intracortical origins of surround receptive fields in rat SI barrel field cortex. *J. Comp. Neurol.*, in press.

Armstrong-James, M., Das-Gupta, A. and Fox, K. (1989b) Laminar latency analysis of centre and surround receptive fields in the rat SI barrel field cortex. *J. Comp. Neurol.*, in press.

Artola, A. and Singer, W. (1987) Long-term potentiation and NMDA receptors in rat visual cortex. *Nature*, 330: 649–652.

Bear, M.F. and Singer, W. (1986) Modulation of visual cortical plasticity by acetylcholine and noradrenaline. *Nature*, 320: 172–176.

Bear, M.F., Cooper, L.N. and Ebner, F.F. (1987) A physiological basis for a theory of synapse modification. *Science*, 237: 42–48.

Bear, M.F., Kleinschmidt, A. and Singer, W. (1988) Experience-dependent modifications of kitten striate cortex are not prevented by thalamic lesions that include the in-

tralaminar nuclei. *Exp. Brain Res.*, 70: 627–631.

Buzsaki, G., Bickford, R.G., Ponomareff, G., Thal, L.J., Mandel, R. and Gage, F.H. (1988) Nucleus basalis and thalamic control of neocortical activity in the freely moving rat. *J. Neurosci.*, 8: 4007–4026.

Chagnac-Amitai, Y. and Connors, B.W. (1989) Horizontal spread of synchronized activity in neocortex, and its control by GABA-mediated inhibition. *J. Neurophysiol.*, 61: 747–758.

Chapin, J.K. and Lin, C.S. (1984) Mapping the body representation in the SI cortex of anesthetized and awake rats. *J. Comp. Neurol.*, 229: 199–213.

Daw, N.W., Videen, T.O., Robertson, T and Rader, R.K. (1985) An evaluation of the hypothesis that noradrenaline affects plasticity in the developing visual cortex. In: A. Fein (Ed.), *The Visual System*, Alan Liss, New York, pp. 133–144.

Delacour, J., Houcine, O. and Talbi, B. (1987) "Learned" changes in the responses of the rat barrel field neurons. *Neuroscience*, 23: 63–71.

Donoghue, J.P. and Carroll, K.L. (1987) Cholinergic modulation of sensory responses in rat primary somatic sensory cortex. *Brain Res.*, 408: 367–371.

Ebner, F.F., Armstrong-James, M. and Diamond, M. (1989) Changes in receptive field properties of rat barrel field neurons following thalamic lesions. *Neurosci. Abstr.*, 15: 1222.

Fox, K., Sato, H. and Daw, N.W. (1988) The location and function of NMDA receptors in cat and kitten visual cortex. *Neurosci. Abstr.*, 14: 744.

Herkenham, M. (1980) Laminar organization of thalamic projections to rat neocortex. *Science*, 207: 532–534.

Hobson, J.A. (1984) How does the cortex know when to do what? A neurobiological theory of state control. In: *Dynamic Aspects of Neocortical Function*, Neuroscience Institute Publications, Chapter 8, pp. 219–257.

Hyvarinen, J., Poranen, A. and Jokinen, Y. (1980) Influence of attentive behavior on neuronal responses to vibration in somatosensory cortex of the monkey. *J. Neurophysiol.*, 43: 870–882.

Jouvet, M. (1972) The role of monoamines and acetylcholine containing neurons in the regulation of the sleep–waking cycle. *Ergeb. Physiol.*, 64: 166–307.

Kasamatsu, T. and Pettigrew, J.D. (1976) Depletion of brain catecholamines: failure of ocular dominance shift after monocular occlusion in kittens. *Science*, 194: 206–209.

Killackey, H.P. (1983) The somatosensory cortex of the rodent. *Trends Neurosci.*, 6: 425–429.

Koralek, K.-A., Jensen, K.F. and Killackey, H.P. (1988) Evidence for two complementary patterns of thalamic input to the rat somatosensory cortex. *Brain Res.*, 463: 346–351.

Lamour, Y., Dutar, P., Jobert, A. and Dykes, R.W. (1988) An iontophoretic study of single somatosensory neurons in rat granular cortex serving the limbs: a laminar analysis of glutamate and acetylcholine effects on receptive field properties. *J. Neurophysiol.,* 60: 725 – 750.

Lee, S.M., Weisskopf, M.G. and Ebner, F.F. (1989) Horizontal long-term potentiation of responses in rat somatosensory cortex. *Brain Res.* (in press).

Lin, C.-S., Lu, S.M. and Yamawaki, R.M. (1987) Laminar and synaptic organization of terminals from the ventrobasal and posterior thalamic nuclei in the rat barrel cortex. *Neurosci. Abstr.,* 13: 248.

McCormick, D.A. and Prince, D.A. (1986) Mechanisms of action of acetylcholine in the guinea-pig cerebral cortex in vitro. *J. Physiol. (Lond.),* 375: 169 – 194.

Merzenich, M.M., Recanzone, G., Jenkins, W.M., Allard, T.T. and Nudo, R.J. (1988) Cortical representational plasticity. In: P. Rakic and W. Singer (Eds.), *Neurobiology of Neocortex,* Wiley, New York, pp. 41 – 67.

Moruzzi, G. and Magoun, H.W. (1949) Brain stem reticular formation and activation of the EEG. *Electroenceph. Clin. Neurophysiol.,* 1: 455 – 473.

Rhoades, R.W., Belford, G.R. and Killackey, H.P. (1987) Receptive field properties of rat ventral posterior medial neurons before and after selective kainic acid lesions of the trigeminal brain stem complex. *J. Neurophysiol.,* 57: 1577 – 1600.

Ribak, C.E., Harris, A.B., Bankan, J.E. and Roberts, E. (1979) Inhibitory, GABAergic nerve terminals decrease at sites of focal epilepsy. *Science,* 205: 211 – 214.

Simons, D.J. (1985) Temporal and spatial integration in the rat SI vibrissa cortex. *J. Neurophysiol.,* 54: 615 – 635.

Simons, D.J. and Land, P.W. (1987) Early experience of tactile stimulation influences organization of somatic sensory cortex. *Nature,* 326: 694 – 697.

Singer, W. and Rauschecker, J.P. (1982) Central core control of developmental plasticity in the kitten visual cortex. II. Electrical activation of mesencephalic and diencephalic projections. *Exp. Brain Res.,* 41: 199 – 215.

Spreafico, M. and Rustioni, A. (1987) SII-projecting neurons in rat thalamus: a single- and double-retrograde tracing study. *Somatosens. Res.,* 4: 359 – 375.

Steriade, M. and Llinas, R.R. (1988) The functional states of the thalamus and the associated neuronal interplay. *Physiol. Rev.,* 68: 649 – 742.

Waite, P.M.E. (1984) Rearrangement of neuronal responses in the trigeminal system of the rat following peripheral nerve section. *J. Physiol. (Lond.),* 352: 425 – 455.

Wall, J.T. and Cusick, C.G. (1984) Cutaneous responsiveness in primary somatosensory (SI) hindpaw cortex before and after partial hindpaw deafferentation in adult rats. *J. Neurosci.,* 4: 1499 – 1515.

Waterhouse, B.D. and Woodward, D.J. (1980) Interaction of norepinephrine with cerebrocortical activity evoked by stimulation of somatosensory afferent pathways in the rat. *Exp. Neurol.,* 67: 11 – 34.

Welker, C. (1971) Microelectrode delineation of the fine grain somatotopic organization of SmI cerebral neocortex in albino rat. *Brain Res.,* 26: 259 – 275.

Welker, C. (1976) Receptive fields of barrels in the somatosensory neocortex of the rat. *J. Comp. Neurol.,* 166: 173 – 190.

Woolsey, T.A. and Van der Loos, H. (1970) The structural organization of layer IV in the somatosensory region (SI) of mouse cerebral cortex. The description of a cortical field composed of discrete cytoarchitectural units. *Brain Res.,* 17: 205 – 232.

Intercellular Mechanisms: Growth Factors and their Receptors

P. Coleman, G. Higgins and C. Phelps (Eds.)
Progress in Brain Research, Vol. 86
© 1990 Elsevier Science Publishers B.V. (Biomedical Division)

CHAPTER 12

Selective and non-selective trophic actions on central cholinergic and dopaminergic neurons in vitro

Franz Hefti, Beat Knusel and Patrick P. Michel

Andrus Gerontology Center, University of Southern California, Los Angeles, CA 90089-0191, U.S.A.

Introduction

It is widely believed that for a given neuron or neural connection to survive during development, proper contact with the projection area has to be established. The known biology of nerve growth factor (NGF) supports the concept, that such neuron – target interactions are based on the production and release of specific trophic molecules by the target area which are required by the innervating neurons (for review, see Thoenen and Edgar, 1985; Purves, 1986; Thoenen et al., 1987). Besides NGF, several other substances or factors have been characterized which are able to support survival or differentiation of neurons. Ciliary neurotrophic factors (CNTF) have been isolated from chick eye (Barbin et al., 1984), rat sciatic nerve (Manthorpe et al., 1986) and from bovine heart (Watters and Hendry, 1987) based on their ability to provide survival of chick embryonic ciliary ganglion cells in culture. A brain derived neurotrophic factor (BDNF) was purified from pig brain and promotes survival and fiber outgrowth of embryonic chick sensory neurons and rat retinal cells (Johnson et al., 1986; Barde et al., 1987; Kalcheim et al., 1987; Hofer and Barde, 1988). Furthermore, substances which were previously known for their effects on non-neuronal tissues, have recently been recognized to display neurotrophic effects when tested in cell culture assays. Among these molecules are basic fibroblast

growth factor (bFGF), insulin, the insulin-like growth factors I and II (IGF-I, IGF-II) and epidermal growth factor (EGF). bFGF has been shown to promote survival and fiber outgrowth of dissociated mouse and rat fetal neurons (Morrison et al., 1986; Walicke et al., 1986; Unsicker et al., 1987; Walicke, 1988) and to stimulate neurite formation in PC12 cells (Togari et al., 1985; Rydel and Greene, 1987). Insulin, IGF-I and IGF-II have only recently been suggested to possess physiological functions for the central nervous system (review: Baskin et al., 1988). EGF is primarily known as a potent mitogen for several cell types including astrocytes (Schlesinger et al., 1983; Avola et al., 1988) but, similar to bFGF, has been shown to promote neuronal survival and neurite outgrowth of dissociated neonatal rat brain cells in serum-free medium (Morrison et al., 1987, 1988).

The concept of NGF as an instrument of target-controlled neuronal survival has been established in the peripheral nervous system. The exact role of NGF in the central nervous system remains to be fully elucidated. Presently, actions of NGF on the cholinergic neurons of the basal forebrain and the corpus striatum are well characterized (reviews: Thoenen et al., 1987; Whittemore and Seiger, 1987; Hefti et al., 1989) and distribution and developmental changes of NGF and its receptor in the CNS have been extensively investigated (for recent studies see Ayer-LeLievre et al., 1988; Buck et al., 1988; Ernfors et al., 1988; Hefti and Mash,

1988; Kiss et al., 1988; Schatteman et al., 1988; Yan and Johnson, 1988). All data are compatible with the view that NGF serves as a target-derived survival factor for basal forebrain neurons. However, it is still not known, whether there is neural cell death during the development of the basal forebrain or striatal cholinergic system and whether the availability of NGF regulates the number of cholinergic neurons. Furthermore, the selectivity of the action of NGF in the central nervous system remains one of the principal unresolved questions. While the distributions of NGF and its receptor suggest actions of NGF on neurons other than the cholinergic ones (Buck et al., 1988; Ernfors et al., 1988; Schatteman et al., 1988; Yan and Johnson, 1988; Large et al., 1989), no other NGF-responsive central populations have been identified with certainty yet. Far less is known about the other neurotrophic factors and their functions in the central nervous system.

In an attempt to clarify the degree of selectivity of the actions of various neurotrophic substances we used previously established cell culture models of fetal rat septum, pons and ventral mesencephalon (Hartikka and Hefti, 1988; Knusel and Hefti, 1988; Michel et al., 1989). Septal cholinergic cells in culture respond to NGF in various ways, among them by increasing the activity of the enzyme choline acetyltransferase (ChAT; Hefti et al., 1985; Hartikka and Hefti, 1988; Hatanaka et al., 1988). Pontine cholinergic neurons, located in the pedunculopontine and dorsolateral tegmental nuclei share some of the morphological characteristics of basal forebrain cholinergic neurons and have medium to large sized cell bodies and long centrally ascending axons (Woolf and Butcher, 1986; Rye et al., 1987; Goldsmith and van der Kooy, 1988). However, this cell group has been shown in vitro not to respond to NGF (Knusel and Hefti, 1988). Cultures of the ventral mesencephalon were used to test for effects of trophic factors on dopaminergic cells of the substantia nigra. Trophic actions on septal and pontine cholinergic neurons and mesencephalic dopaminergic neurons were examined for bFGF, insulin, IGF-I, IGF-II, EGF and NGF.

Results

Cell culture methods used in these studies have been described in detail elsewhere (Hartikka and Hefti, 1988; Knusel and Hefti, 1988; Michel et al., 1989). NGF was purified from mouse salivary glands. Bovine insulin and mouse submaxillary gland EGF were purchased from Sigma (St. Louis, MO). Human recombinant bFGF was provided by Synergen (Boulder, CO). Human recombinant IGF-I and IGF-II were obtained from Eli Lilly Laboratories (Indianapolis, IN).

In cultures of septal cells, the activity of the cholinergic marker enzyme, ChAT, was elevated by bFGF, insulin, IGF-I and IGF-II in a similar way as earlier shown for NGF. The dose – response relationship was established for each of the compounds (Fig. 1). NGF was most potent in stimulating ChAT activity. When measured 7 days after plating, the various factors were approximately equally effective in producing elevation of ChAT activity but concentrations of approximately 1 ng/ml NGF, 1 μg/ml IGF-I, IGF-II and bFGF, and 5 μg/ml insulin had to be used to produce maximal responses. EGF at concentrations between 1 and 500 ng/ml was ineffective.

In marked contrast to the situation in septal cultures, NGF did not enhance ChAT activity in pontine cultures and failed to elevate dopamine uptake in mesencephalic cultures. In contrast, insulin, IGF-I and IGF-II markedly increased transmitter-specific differentiation in both systems. Effective concentrations of the three factors in pontine and mesencephalic cultures were similar to those observed in septal cultures and the rank order of potency, in all three culture systems was IGF-I > IGF-II > insulin. bFGF did not enhance ChAT activity in pontine cultures but elevated dopamine uptake in mesencephalic cultures, although to a smaller degree than the insulin family of growth factors. As in septal cultures, EGF failed to increase ChAT activity in pedunculopontine cultures, however, in mesencephalic cultures EGF resulted in a modest increase of dopamine uptake.

bFGF which is a potent mitogen for various cell

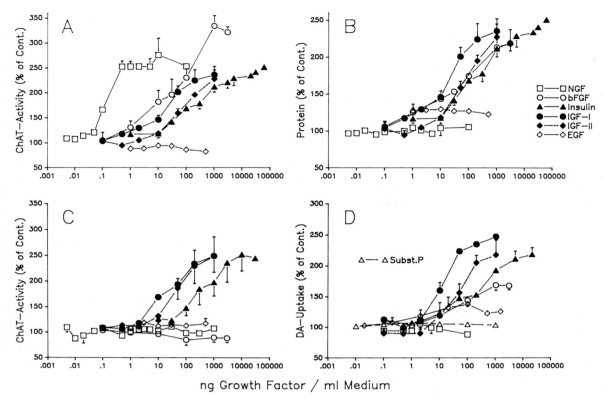

Fig. 1. Dose – response curves for effects of growth factors on fetal rat brain cultures. Cultures of dissociated fetal rat brain cells (E16/E17) were prepared as described in detail elsewhere (Hartikka and Hefti, 1988; Knusel and Hefti, 1988). They were grown in modified L-15 medium with serum for 1 week in the presence of growth factors as indicated in the graphs. Plating density was $0.8 \cdot 10^6$/16-mm well. For each factor data were pooled from 2 or 3 experiments. Each symbol represents the mean of 4 – 8 individual cultures. Bars represent S.E.M., they were omitted where they would have appeared smaller than the symbol. Note order of potency in all four graphs: IGF-I > IGF-II > insulin. A. ChAT activity per well in septal cultures. Note high potency of NGF, but absence of effect in graphs B, C and D. B. Protein content per well in septal cultures. C. ChAT activity per well in cultures of pons. D. Dopamine uptake per well in cultures of ventral mesencephalon. Note limited effects of bFGF, EGF and absence of effect of substance P.

populations stimulated cell proliferation in our cultures which was reflected by a dose-dependent increase in protein mass in all three culture systems used (Fig. 1B). The presence of insulin, IGF-I or IGF-II resulted in cell proliferation and a similar maximal protein increase as bFGF. NGF, as shown previously (Hartikka and Hefti, 1988; Knusel and Hefti, 1988) did not influence the protein content in septal, pontine, or mesencephalic cells. Growth factors which stimulated both transmitter-specific differentiation and cellular proliferation, always showed very similar concentration requirements

for these effects.

The actions of IGF-I, IGF-II and insulin on septal cultures were not additive. Combining maximally effective concentrations of these substances did not elevate ChAT activity or protein content above the level which was attained by either of the three factors alone (Table I). Given these findings further studies were limited to insulin which served as a representative for this family of growth factors.

Despite the similarities of the effects of bFGF, insulin and NGF on cultured septal cholinergic neurons, there were pronounced differences among these factors with regard to the time course of their action on ChAT activity (Fig. 2). During the first week in vitro, ChAT activity was highest in bFGF-treated cultures. After one week bFGF produced no further increase in ChAT activity but continued to stimulate proliferation of non-

TABLE I

Effects on insulin, IGF-I and IGF-II of septal cultures

Growth factors	ChAT/well (pmol/min)	Protein/well (µg)
Control	82.55 ± 2.85	146.22 ± 3.58
IGF-I	167.58 ± 4.08	282.68 ± 10.92
IGF-II	153.02 ± 9.06	251.81 ± 5.37
Insulin	148.97 ± 3.01	253.14 ± 2.90
IGF-I + IGF-II	163.27 ± 6.42	278.90 ± 6.00
IGF-I + insulin	153.12 ± 6.97	263.96 ± 7.60
IGF-II + insulin	159.25 ± 8.31	257.98 ± 13.51

Cultures were prepared and grown as described in the legend of Fig. 1. Concentrations: IGF-I and IGF-II 1 µg/ml; insulin 30 µg/ml. Values are mean ± S.E.M.; n = 4–8. All differences to control are statistically significant ($P < 0.001$; Student's t test).

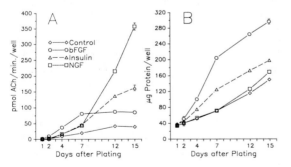

Fig. 2. Time course of action of NGF, bFGF and insulin on ChAT activity and protein content in septal cultures. At day 0 $0.6 \cdot 10^6$ fetal (E16) rat septal cells were plated per 16-mm well. Growth factors were added immediately after plating and with every medium change. Four cultures per treatment group were taken for ChAT and protein assays at the indicated times. The rate of increase of ChAT activity in bFGF-treated cultures was initially highest but leveled off after 7 days. In contrast, the rate of NGF-mediated increase continued to rise throughout the culture time.

neuronal cells as reflected by a continuous rise of the protein content. In contrast, the most pronounced increase of ChAT activity in NGF-treated cultures was observed after more than 1 week in culture. Similarly, in the presence of insulin the ChAT increase was more pronounced after 1 week in vitro but, in contrast to NGF-treated cultures, started to level off thereafter. Final levels of ChAT activity which were measured after 2 weeks in vitro were 909% of control in NGF-treated cultures, 413% in cultures treated with insulin, and 216% in cultures treated with bFGF.

Since bFGF and insulin strongly promoted the growth of non-neuronal cells and may affect other neuronal populations besides the cholinergic cells in our septal cultures, their stimulatory actions on these neurons could be indirect and secondary to an action on receptors located on other cells. In particular, in septal cultures bFGF or insulin could stimulate production and release of NGF. Anti-NGF antibodies, at a sufficient concentration to completely block the NGF mediated increase of ChAT activity failed to abolish the bFGF or insulin mediated elevations (data not shown). This experiment does not completely rule out the possibility that the antibodies failed to penetrate to the sites of synthesis and action of endogenously produced NGF. However, the effects of maximally effective concentrations of bFGF, insulin and NGF on ChAT activity and protein content were additive (Table II), suggesting that NGF, bFGF and insulin each stimulate different cellular mechanisms.

To test whether the effects of bFGF and insulin on cultured cholinergic neurons were mediated by glial cells, cell proliferation was inhibited by the addition of cytosine arabinoside (ara-C, 1.8 µM) to the medium (Table III). We have earlier shown that adding ara-C to our septal cultures reduces the number of astrocytes to less than 5% of the number counted in control cultures without affecting the number of neurons (Hartikka and Hefti, 1988). In confirmation of our earlier results NGF was found to elevate ChAT activity in septal cultures in presence or absence of glial cells.

Similarly, bFGF produced similar relative increases in ChAT activity in septal cultures, and insulin in septal, pontine and mesencephalic cultures with or without ara-C, suggesting that the action of neither factor in these cultures depends on the presence of glial cells. In contrast, in mesencephalic cultures, the stimulatory actions of bFGF and EGF on dopamine uptake was abolished by the presence of ara-C in the medium.

Discussion

Basic fibroblast growth factor which was originally purified from brain and pituitary based on its mitogenic activity for Balb/c 3T3 cells is a potent mitogen for many cells (see Gospodarowicz, 1984). Recently, this molecule has been shown in vitro to support survival and neurite outgrowth of neurons from various brain regions (Morrison et al., 1986; Walicke et al., 1986; Unsicker et al., 1987; Hatten et al., 1988; Walicke, 1988) and to promote neuronal differentiation of PC12 cells (Rydel and Greene 1987; Schubert et al., 1987). Intracerebral administration of bFGF prevents degenerative changes of lesioned cholinergic neurons of the basal forebrain (Anderson et al., 1988; Otto et al., 1989). Although bFGF stimulates proliferation and influences the morphology of astrocytes in culture (Kniss and Burry, 1988; Perraud et al., 1988), its actions on neurons are believed not to be mediated by glial cells (Morrison et al., 1986; Walicke and Baird, 1988). In support of a possible

TABLE II

Additivity of the increases in ChAT activity produced by bFGF, insulin and NGF in septal cultures

Growth factors	ChAT/well (pmol/min)	Protein/well (μg)
Control	20.22 ± 0.33	76.16 ± 4.94
bFGF	64.99 ± 4.11	212.58 ± 15.13
Insulin	47.11 ± 8.55	162.63 ± 21.98
NGF	43.30 ± 7.44	70.62 ± 3.74
NGF + bFGF	85.57 ± 12.04*	194.92 ± 25.79
NGF + insulin	97.94 ± 6.49*	148.99 ± 7.38
bFGF + insulin	83.52 ± 3.11*	348.67 ± 8.24*
NGF + bFGF + insulin	117.64 ± 2.21*	348.05 ± 12.17*

Cultures were grown for 6 days. Concentrations of factors: NGF 50 ng/ml; bFGF 1 μg/ml; insulin 30 μg/ml. Values are mean ± S.E.M.; n = 4. Values of all treated groups are higher than those of control group, $P < 0.01$. *Higher than value obtained in culture grown with one the growth factors only, $P < 0.05$.

TABLE III

Preventing cell proliferation abolishes effects of bFGF and EGF in mesencephalic cultures but does not prevent the action of bFGF and NGF in septal cultures and of insulin in all culture types

		No ara-C	Ara-C (1.8 μM)
Septal cultures (pmol ACh/min/well)	Control	114.4 ± 7.5	82.1 ± 7.3
	bFGF	251.3 ± 26.4**	217.4 ± 17.7***
	Insulin	180.9 ± 20.4*	120.4 ± 12.9*
	NGF	370.0 ± 28.6***	179.1 ± 18.1**
Pontine cultures (pmol ACh/min/well)	Control	17.2 ± 0.2	20.1 ± 1.3
	bFGF	14.7 ± 0.5**	19.9 ± 0.7
	Insulin	32.6 ± 2.2***	35.8 ± 1.9***
Mesencephalic cultures (fmol DA/min/well)	Control	55.3 ± 2.3	57.5 ± 2.7
	bFGF	86.4 ± 5.9**	60.7 ± 4.2
	Insulin	106.3 ± 8.3**	92.2 ± 5.7**
	EGF	70.0 ± 5.0*	58.6 ± 3.3

Cultures were grown for 8 days. Concentrations of factors as in Table II. Values are mean ± S.E.M.; n = 4 − 6. Values higher than corresponding control: *$P < 0.05$; **$P < 0.01$; ***$P < 0.001$ (Student's t test).

function of bFGF in the CNS, bFGF activity and immunoreactivity, and receptor for bFGF have been found in the brain (Presta et al., 1988). A neuronal bFGF receptor with properties distinct from the mesenchymal receptor has recently been characterized (Walicke et al., 1989). Suggestive of many different roles of this molecule in the mammalian organism is the fact that as many as 15 previously characterized growth factors are probably similar or identical to bFGF (Gospodarowicz et al., 1986).

Our experiments demonstrate a profound trophic action of bFGF on septal cholinergic neurons which is independent of cell proliferation. The bFGF-mediated elevation of ChAT activity, at least at early times in vitro when this effect is particularly pronounced, does not seem to reflect a general effect of bFGF on survival of dissociated neurons in culture as could be expected from the above mentioned data (Morrison et al., 1986; Walicke et al., 1986), since, under our culture conditions, bFGF did not increase the total number of cells in septal cultures up to 2 days after plating, whereas ChAT activity in bFGF-treated cultures at this time was enhanced to approximately three times control levels (data not shown). The concentrations of bFGF which were required to stimulate cholinergic differentiation in our septal cultures were higher than those found to promote survival and neurite outgrowth of freshly plated neurons. Reported concentrations producing 50% of maximal neuron survival range from 15 pg/ml to 1 ng/ml (Morrison et al.,1986; Walicke et al., 1986; Unsicker et al., 1987; Walicke, 1988). Concentrations of bFGF stimulating half maximal proliferation of various non-neuronal cells have been found to be approximately 50 pg/ml (Esch et al., 1985; Ferrara et al., 1988). Walicke et al. (1989) recently characterized a neuronal bFGF receptor with an affinity ten times lower than that of mesenchymal bFGF receptors, suggesting that neuronal cells respond to higher concentrations of bFGF. Possibly, at least part of the difference might be due to differences in plating densities of the cells, since, under our culture conditions the effectiveness of

bFGF receptors, suggesting that neuronal cells respond to higher concentrations of bFGF. Possibly, at least part of the difference might be due to differences in plating densities of the cells, since, under our culture conditions the effectiveness of bFGF seemed to be negatively correlated with plating density. It has indeed been shown for a non-transformed cell line that with increasing cell density the number of surface bFGF receptors decreases (Veomett et al., 1989). It seems also possible that the added bFGF is more rapidly removed from the medium at higher cell density by specific and non-specific binding or other mechanisms and that the effective concentration of bFGF in the medium may decline very quickly.

Insulin, IGF-I and IGF-II and their mRNA have been reported to occur and to be heterogeneously distributed in the adult mammalian brain (Dorn et al., 1982; Rotwein et al., 1988). Similarly, receptors for all three factors appear to be heterogeneously distributed throughout the brain (Sara et al., 1982; Hill et al., 1986; Mendelsohn, 1987; Bohannon et al., 1988). In cultures of brain cells insulin, IGF-I and IGF-II promote neuronal survival, neurite extension, and expression of neuronal enzymes and, in astrocytes but possibly also in neurons, DNA synthesis (Bothwell, 1982; Bhat, 1983; Lenoir and Honegger, 1983; Mill et al., 1985; Recio-Pinto et al., 1986; Aizenman and DeVellis, 1987; Kyriakis et al., 1987; Avola et al., 1988; CiCicco-Bloom and Black, 1988). In our cultures, insulin, IGF-I and IGF-II promoted transmitter-specific development in all three culture systems to a similar extent. Maximal concentrations of the three factors, when applied to septal cultures, were equally effective in increasing ChAT activity and combinations of the factors did not result in additive effects, suggesting that insulin, IGF-I and IGF-II acted via the same receptors. In all three systems the potency of IGF-I was highest, followed by IGF-II and insulin. This rank order is in accordance with the relative affinities of the factors for a recently characterized neuronal IGF-I receptor (Burgess et al., 1987).

None of the areas used for our cell cultures or

the target regions of the neuronal populations studied have been recognized as being rich in insulin or IGF receptors in the abovementioned studies. Thus, it seems surprising that insulin, IGF-I and IGF-II act similarly and profoundly on cholinergic neurons of the septal and pontine areas as well as on dopaminergic neurons of the substantia nigra in culture. However, it has been shown that the expression of insulin and IGFs and of their receptors is developmentally regulated. In rats the binding capacity for insulin and IGF-I is high at birth and decreases until postnatal day 15 after which it remains stable (Pomerance et al., 1988). mRNA levels for IGF-I and IGF-II are highest at embryonic day 14 and decline by a factor of 3 – 4 at birth to levels similar to those in the adult brain (Rotwein et al., 1988). In the chick embryonic brain binding of IGF-I and IGF-II shows a sharp increase during early development followed by a gradual fall during the second and third weeks of ontogeny (Bassas et al., 1985). In the same study it was found that IGF receptors develop earlier than insulin receptors. The regional distributions of receptors for insulin and IGFs or mRNAs coding for receptor proteins in the embryonic brain are not known. It is conceivable that insulin and, in particular, the IGFs play a different and more widespread role during early neuronal development than in the adult brain.

Many recent studies on neurotrophic actions have been based on the concept of target-derived survival factors as it is suggested by the well known biology of nerve growth factor (for reviews see Thoenen and Edgar, 1985; Purves, 1986; Thoenen et al., 1987). This concept does not exclude that a multitude of different factors is required at specific ontogenetic stages for a neuron to develop properly and to maintain its structural integrity and function during adult life. Different roles for bFGF, insulin, IGFs, and NGF in neural development are suggested by the observed time courses of their stimulatory action on ChAT activity in septal cultures. A reduced late effect of bFGF could be explained by the presence of endogenous bFGF in the control cultures at later culture times. An alter-native interpretation to an intrinsic, timed modulation of responsiveness to bFGF is suggested by a possible role of bFGF in repair processes (Finklestein et al., 1988). The mechanical trituration of the tissue which is used to dissociate embryonic cells in the preparation of the cell cultures severs existing neurites and may also disrupt cell body membranes. During the initial culture period, stimulation of repair processes may lead to similar measurable effects as enhancement of developmental processes. It can be speculated that the relatively larger effect of bFGF during the initial culture period demonstrates an active role of this substance in healing and regeneration, whereas NGF, which exerts its most significant influence on ChAT-activity during later stages, promotes the differentiation of the cholinergic cells. While attractive, this hypothesis is not supported by our finding that bFGF did not enhance ChAT activity in pontine cultures, where, because of the more advanced development, the dissociation inflicts more cell damage than in septal cells (Knusel and Hefti, 1988).

We believe that part of the importance of the present study lies in the comparison of effects of several known trophic substances on different neuronal populations studied under identical conditions. The exact roles and importance of neurotrophic factors in CNS development are poorly understood. While there is strong evidence that NGF serves as a target-derived neurotrophic factor for cholinergic neurons of the basal forebrain and promotes their differentiation, it is still unclear whether, similar to the situation in the peripheral sympathetic system, NGF controls the developmental survival of these cells. No comparable target-derived neurotrophic factors for other central neuronal populations have been identified with certainty. It is not known whether most or all central neuronal populations depend on target-derived factors for development and survival and, if they do, whether there exists a multitude of population-specific factors or only a small number of factors with a precise developmental regulation of their mechanisms.

152

Our results emphasize the relative selectivity of the action of NGF on the basal forebrain cholinergic neurons despite recent reports of a more widespread localization of NGF and NGF receptors in developing than in adult brain (Buck et al., 1988; Ernfors et al., 1988; Schatteman et al., 1988; Yan and Johnson, 1988; Large et al., 1989). bFGF, similar to NGF, strongly stimulates ChAT activity in septal cholinergic neurons. Considering the antero-posterior gradient in brain development, a developmentally short-lasting influence of bFGF on neuronal development could explain the lack of effect on pontine cholinergic, the relatively minor effect on mesencephalic dopaminergic and the pronounced early effect on septal cholinergic cells. However, the action of bFGF on dopaminergic cells of the mesencephalic cultures, contrasting to its effect on the cholinergic neurons of the septal cultures, depends on cell proliferation. It is likely, therefore, that the effect of bFGF on the dopaminergic cells is mediated by glia cells and that its only direct effect on neurons in our cultures is on the septal cholinergic cells. The stimulatory actions of insulin and the IGFs on neural development and differentiation are most likely very widespread. These growth factors therefore seem unlikely candidates for target-derived, neuron population-specific neurotrophic factors. Nevertheless, their time- and site-specific presence could be required during development and their function during this time might be different from later, more general, stimulating influences on many biochemical parameters.

Our finding that NGF and bFGF directly influence cholinergic neurons of the basal forebrain, but not the other studied neuronal populations, invites an interpretation which seems interesting in another context than that discussed so far. It can be speculated that septal cholinergic neurons have a higher intrinsic plasticity than pontine cholinergic or mesencephalic dopaminergic neurons and therefore can respond with changes in morphology and biochemistry to different trophic or specifying factors (Varon and Adler, 1980). This possibility seems particularly interesting,

since central cholinergic mechanisms have long been recognized to be instrumental in memory processes (see Squire and Davis, 1981; Singh et al., 1985).

Conclusions

It is well established that developmental growth and differentiation of septal forebrain cholinergic neurons are stimulated by NGF. Our studies suggest that bFGF, insulin and the insulin-like growth factors, but not EGF exert similar actions. While the magnitude of the cholinergic enhancement, reflected by an increased activity of the cholinergic marker enzyme ChAT after 1 week in culture, was similar with all effective molecules, NGF was more potent than the other factors. The actions of NGF, bFGF and insulin on septal cholinergic neurons were additive and appear to be mediated by different mechanisms, whereas insulin, IGF-I and IGF-II probably act via the same receptors. Development of pontine cholinergic neurons in vitro was stimulated by insulin and IGFs, but not by NGF, bFGF or EGF. In vitro development of mesencephalic dopaminergic neurons was stimulated by insulin, IGFs, and, to a smaller degree by bFGF and EGF. In all three culture systems, proliferation of non-neuronal cells was increased by insulin, IGFs, bFGF, and EGF but not NGF. Our results suggest different degrees of selectivity of neurotrophic molecules. They are compatible with the view that, in the CNS, neuronal survival and differentiation upon proper contact with the target area are regulated by a large number of different, population-specific neurotrophic factors, or alternatively, that there is only a small number of neurotrophic factors, which may be precisely regulated during development.

Acknowledgements

This study was supported by NIH grant NS22933 and NSF grant BNS-8708049 and a grant from the National Parkinson Foundation, Miami.

References

Aizenman, Y. and DeVellis, J. (1987) Brain neurons develop in a serum and glial free environment: effects of transferrin, insulin, insulin-like growth factor-I and thyroid hormone on neuronal survival, growth and differentiation. *Brain Res.,* 406: 32 – 42.

Anderson, K.J., Dam, D., Lee, S. and Cotman, C.W. (1988) Basic fibroblast growth factor prevents death of lesioned cholinergic neurons in vivo. *Nature,* 332: 360 – 362.

Avola, R., Condorelli, D.F., Surrentino, S., Turpeenoja, L., Costa, A. and Giuffrida Stella, A.M. (1988) Effect of epidermal growth factor, and insulin on DNA, RNA, and cytoskeletal protein labeling in primary rat astroglial cell cultures. *J. Neurosci. Res.,* 19: 230 – 238.

Ayer-LeLievre, C., Olson, L., Ebendal, T., Seiger, A. and Persson, H. (1988) Expression of the beta-nerve growth factor gene in hippocampal neurons. *Science,* 240: 1339 – 1341.

Barbin, G., Manthorpe, M. and Varon, S. (1984) Purification of the chick eye ciliary neurotrophic factor. *J. Neurochem.,* 43: 1468 – 1478.

Barde, Y-A., Davies, A.M., Johnson, J.E., Lindsay, R.M. and Thoenen, H. (1987) Brain-derived neurotrophic factor. *Prog. Brain Res.,* 71: 185 – 189.

Baskin, D.G., Wilcox, B.J., Figlewicz, D.P. and Dorsa, D.M. (1988) Insulin and insulin-like growth factors in the CNS. *Trends Neurosci.,* 11: 107 – 111.

Bassas, L., De Pablo, F., Lesniak, M.A. and Roth, J. (1985) Ontogeny of receptors for insulin-like peptide in chick embryo tissues: early dominance of insulin-like growth factor over insulin receptors in brain. *Endocrinology,* 117: 2321 – 2329.

Bhat, N. (1983) Insulin-dependent neurite outgrowth in cultured embryonic mouse brain cells. *Dev. Brain Res.,* 11: 315 – 318.

Bohannon, N.J., Corp, E.S., Wilcox, B.J., Figlewicz, D.P., Dorsa, D.M. and Baskin, D.G. (1988) Localization of binding sites for insulin-like growth factor I (IGF-I) in the rat brain by quantitative autoradiography. *Brain Res.,* 444: 205 – 213.

Bothwell, M. (1982) Insulin and somatemedin MSA promote nerve growth factor-independent neurite formation by cultured chick dorsal root ganglionic sensory neurons. *J. Neurosci. Res.,* 8: 225 – 231.

Buck, C.R., Martinez, H.J., Chao, M.V. and Black, I. (1988) Differential expression of the nerve growth factor receptor gene in multiple brain areas. *Dev. Brain Res.,* 44: 259 – 268.

Burgess, S.K., Jacobs, S., Cuatrecasas, P. and Sahyoun, N. (1987) Characterization of a neuronal subtype of insulin-like growth factor I receptor. *J. Biol. Chem.,* 262: 1618 – 1622.

CiCicco-Bloom, E. and Black, I. (1988) Insulin growth factors regulate the mitotic cycle in cultured rat sympathetic neuroblasts. *Proc. Natl. Acad. Sci. U.S.A.,* 85: 4066 – 4070.

Dorn, A., Bernstein, H.G., Rinne, A., Hahn, H.J. and Ziegler, M. (1982) Insulin-like immunoreactivity in the human brain. *Histochemistry,* 74: 293 – 300.

Ernfors, P., Hallbook, F., Ebendal, T., Shooter, E.M., Radeke, M.J., Misko, T.P. and Persson, H. (1988) Developmental and regional expression of β-nerve growth factor receptor mRNA in the chick and rat. *Neuron,* 1: 983 – 996.

Esch, F., Baird, A., Ling, N., Ueno, N., Hill, F., Denoroy, L., Klepper, R., Gospodarowics, D., Bohlen, P. and Guillemin, R. (1985) Primary structure of bovine pituitary basic fibroblast growth factor (FGF) and comparison with the amino-terminal sequence of bovine brain acidic FGF. *Proc. Natl. Acad. Sci. U.S.A.,* 82: 6507 – 6511.

Ferrara, N., Ousley, F. and Gospodarowicz, D. (1988) Bovine brain astrocytes express basic fibroblast growth factor, a neurotropic and angiogenic mitogen. *Brain Res.,* 462: 223 – 232.

Finklestein, S.P., Apostolides, P.J., Caday, C.G., Prosser, J., Philips, M.F. and Klagsbrun, M. (1988) Increased basic fibroblast growth factor (bFGF) immunoreactivity at the site of focal brain wounds. *Brain Res.,* 460: 253 – 259.

Goldsmith, M. and van der Kooy, D. (1988) Separate non-cholinergic descending and cholinergic ascending projections from the nucleus tegmenti pedunculopontinus. *Brain Res.,* 445: 386 – 391.

Gospodarowicz, D. (1984) Brain and pituitary fibroblast growth factors. In: C.H. Li (Ed.), *Hormonal Proteins and Peptides, Vol. XII,* Academic Press, New York, pp. 205 – 230.

Gospodarowicz, D., Neufeld, G. and Schweigerer, L. (1986) Molecular and biological characterization of fibroblast growth factor, an angiogenic factor which also controls the proliferation and differentiation of mesoderm and neuroectoderm derived cells. *Cell Differ.,* 19: 1 – 17.

Hartikka, J. and Hefti, F. (1988) Development of septal cholinergic neurons in culture: plating density and glial cells modulate effects of NGF on survival, fiber growth, and expression of transmitter-specific enzymes. *J. Neurosci.,* 8: 2967 – 2985.

Hatanaka, H., Tsukui, H. and Nihonmatsu, I. (1988) Developmental change in the nerve growth factor action from induction of choline acetyltransferase to promotion of cell survival in cultured basal forebrain cholinergic neurons from postnatal rats. *Dev. Brain Res.,* 39: 88 – 95.

Hatten, M.E., Lynch, M., Rydel, R.E., Sanchez, J., Joseph-Silverstein, J., Moscatelli, D. and Rifkin D. (1988) In vitro neurite extension by granule neurons is dependent upon astroglial-derived fibroblast growth factor. *Dev. Biol.,* 125: 280 – 289.

Hefti, F. and Mash, D.C. (1988) Localization of nerve growth factor receptors in the human brain. In: E.G. Jones (Ed.), *Molecular Biology of the Human Brain. UCLA Symposia on Molecular and Cellular Biology,* Vol. 72, A.R. Liss, New York, pp. 119 – 132.

154

Hefti, F., Hartikka, J., Eckenstein, F., Gnahn, H., Heumann, R. and Schwab, M. (1985) Nerve growth factor (NGF) increases choline acetyltransferase but not survival or fiber outgrowth of cultured fetal septal cholinergic neurons. *Neuroscience,* 14: 55 – 68.

Hefti, F., Hartikka, J. and Knusel, B. (1989) Function of neurotrophic factors in the adult and aging brain and their possible use in the treatment of neurodegenerative diseases. *Neurobiol. Aging,* in press.

Hill, J.M., Lesniak, M.A., Pert, C.B. and Roth, J. (1986) Autoradiographic localization of insulin receptors in rat brain: prominence in olfactory and limbic areas. *Neuroscience,* 17: 1127 – 1138.

Hofer, M.M. and Barde, Y.A. (1988) Brain-derived neurotrophic factor prevents neuronal death in vivo. *Nature,* 331: 261 – 262.

Johnston, J.E., Barde, Y.A., Schwab, M. and Thoenen, H. (1986) Brain-derived neurotrophic factor supports the survival of cultured rat retinal ganglion cells. *J. Neurosci.,* 6: 3031 – 3038.

Kalcheim, C., Barde, Y.A., Thoenen, H. and LeDouarin, N.M. (1987) In vivo effect of brain-derived neurotrophic factor on the survival of developing dorsal root ganglion cells. *EMBO J.,* 6: 2811 – 2813.

Kiss, J., McGovern, J. and Patel, A.J. (1988) Immunohistochemical localization of cells containing nerve growth factor receptors in the different regions of the adult rat forebrain. *Neuroscience,* 27: 731 – 748.

Kniss, D.A. and Burry, R.W. (1988) Serum and fibroblast growth factor stimulate quiescent astrocytes to re-enter the cell cycle. *Brain Res.,* 439: 281 – 288.

Knusel, B. and Hefti, F. (1988) Nerve growth factor promotes development of rat forebrain but not pedunculopontine cholinergic neurons in vitro; lack of effect of ciliary neuronotrophic factor and retinoic acid. *J. Neurosci. Res.,* 21: 365 – 375.

Kyriakis, J.M., Hausman, R.E. and Peterson, S.W. (1987) Insulin stimulates choline acetyltransferase activity in cultured embryonic chicken retina neurons. *Proc. Natl. Acad. Sci. U.S.A.,* 84: 7463 – 7467.

Large, T.H., Weskamp, G., Helder, J.C., Radeke, M.J., Misko T.P., Shooter, E.M. and Reichardt, L.F. (1989) Structure and developmental expression of the nerve growth factor receptor in the chicken central nervous system. *Neuron,* 2: 1123 – 1134.

Lenoir, D. and Honegger, P. (1983) Insulin-like growth factor I (IGF-I) stimulates DNA synthesis in fetal rat brain cell cultures. *Dev. Brain Res.,* 7: 205 – 213.

Manthorpe, M., Skaper, S.D., Williams, L.R. and Varon, S. (1986) Purification of adult rat sciatic nerve ciliary neuronotrophic factor. *Brain Res.,* 367: 282 – 286.

Mendelsohn, L.G. (1987) Visualization of IGF-II receptors in rat brain. In: M.K. Raizada, M.I. Phillips and D. LeRoith (Eds.), *Insulin, Insulin-like Growth Factors and their Receptors in the Central Nervous System,* Plenum, New York, pp. 269 – 275.

Michel, P.P., Dandapani, B.K., Sanchez-Ramos, J., Efange, S., Pressman, B.C. and Hefti, F. (1989) Toxic effects of potential environmental neurotoxins related to 1-methyl-4-phenylpyridinium on cultured rat dopaminergic neurons. *J. Pharmacol. Exp. Ther.,* 248: 842 – 850.

Mill, J.F., Chao, M.V. and Ishii, D.N. (1985) Insulin, insulin-like growth factor II, and nerve growth factor effects on tubulin mRNA levels and neurite formation. *Proc. Natl. Acad. Sci. U.S.A.,* 82: 7126 – 7130.

Morrison, R.S., Sharma, A., DeVellis, J. and Bradshaw, R.A. (1986) Basic fibroblast growth factor supports the survival of cerebral cortical neurons in primary culture. *Proc. Natl. Acad. Sci. U.S.A.,* 83: 7537 – 7541.

Morrison, R.S., Kornblum, H.I., Leslie, F.M. and Bradshaw, R.A. (1987) Trophic stimulation of cultured neurons from neonatal rat brain by epidermal growth factor. *Science,* 238: 72 – 75.

Morrison, R.S., Keating, R.F. and Moskal, J.R. (1988) Basic fibroblast growth factor and epidermal growth factor exert differential trophic effects on CNS neurons. *J. Neurosci. Res.,* 21: 71 – 79.

Otto, D, Frotscher, M. and Unsicker, K. (1989) Basic fibroblast growth factor and nerve growth factor administered in gel foam rescue medial septal neurons after fimbria fornix transection. *J. Neurosci. Res.,* 22: 83 – 91.

Perraud, F., Labourdette, G., Miehe, M., Loret, C. and Sensenbrenner, M. (1988) Comparison of the morphological effects of acidic and basic fibroblast growth factors on rat astroblasts in culture. *J. Neurosci. Res.,* 20: 1 – 11.

Pettman, B., Labourdette, G., Weibel, M. and Sensenbrenner, M. (1986) The brain fibroblast growth factor (FGF) is localized in neurons. *Neurosci. Lett.,* 68: 175 – 180.

Presta, M., Foiani, M., Rusnati, M., Joseph-Silverstein, J., Maier, J.A.M. and Ragnotti, G. (1988) High molecular weight immunoreactive basic fibroblast growth factor-like proteins in rat pituitary and brain. *Neurosci. Lett.,* 90: 308 – 313.

Purves, D. (1986) The trophic theory of neural connections. *Trends Neurosci.,* 9: 486 – 489.

Recio-Pinto, E., Rechter, M.M. and Ishii, D.N. (1986) Effects of insulin, insulin-like growth factor-II and nerve growth factor on neurite formation and survival in cultured sympathetic and sensory neurons. *J. Neurosci.,* 6: 1211 – 1219.

Rotwein, P., Burgess, S.K., Milbrandt, J.D. and Krause, J.E. (1988) Differential expression of insulin-like growth factor genes in rat central nervous system. *Proc. Natl. Acad. Sci. U.S.A.,* 85: 265 – 269.

Rydel, R.E. and Greene, L.A. (1987) Acidic and basic fibroblast growth factors promote stable neurite outgrowth and neuronal differentiation in cultures of PC12 cells. *J. Neurosci.,* 7: 3639 – 3653.

Rye, D.B., Saper, C.B., Lee, H.J. and Wainer, B.H. (1987)

Pedunculopontine tegmental nucleus of the rat: cytoarchitecture, cytochemistry, and some extrapyramidal connections of the mesopontine tegmentum. *J. Comp. Neurol.,* 259: 483 – 528.

Sara, V.R., Hall, K., von Holtz, H., Humber, R., Sjogren, B. and Wetterberg, L. (1982) Evidence for the presence of specific receptors for insulin-like growth factors 1 (IGF-1) and 2 (IGF-2) and insulin throughout the adult human brain. *Neurosci. Lett.,* 34: 39 – 44.

Schatteman, G.C., Gibbs, L., Lanahan, A.A., Claude, P. and Bothwell, M. (1988) Expression of NGF receptor in the developing and adult primate central nervous system. *J. Neurosci.,* 8: 860 – 873.

Schlesinger, J., Schreiber, A.B., Levi, A., Lax, I., Libermann, T. and Yarden, Y. (1983) Regulation of cell proliferation by epidermal growth factor. *CRC Crit. Rev. Biochem.,* 14: 93 – 111.

Schubert, D., Ling, N. and Baird, A. (1987) Multiple influences of a heparin-binding growth factor on neuronal development. *J. Cell Biol.,* 104: 635 – 643.

Singh, M.M., Warburton, D.M. and Lal, H. (1985) *Central Cholinergic Mechanisms and Adaptive Dysfunctions,* Plenum, New York.

Squire, L.R. and Davis, H.P. (1981) The pharmacology of memory: a neurobiological perspective. *Annu. Rev. Pharmacol. Toxicol.,* 21: 323 – 356.

Thoenen, H. and Edgar, D. (1985) Neurotrophic factors. *Science,* 229: 238 – 242.

Thoenen, H., Bandtlow, C. and Heumann, R. (1987) The physiological function of nerve growth factor in the central nervous system: comparison with the periphery. *Rev. Physiol. Biochem. Pharmacol.,* 109: 145 – 178.

Togari, A., Dickens, G., Kuzuya, J. and Guroff, G. (1985) The effect of fibroblast growth factor on PC12 cells. *J. Neurosci.,* 5: 307 – 316.

Unsicker, K., Reichert-Preibsch, H., Schmidt, R., Pettmann, B., Labourdette, G. and Sensenbrenner, M. (1987) Astroglial and fibroblast growth factors have neurotrophic functions for cultured peripheral and central nervous system neurons. *Proc. Natl. Acad. Sci. U.S.A.,* 84: 5459 – 5463.

Varon, S. and Adler, R. (1980) Nerve growth factors and control of nerve growth. *Curr. Top. Dev. Biol.,* 16: 207 – 252.

Veomet, G., Kuszynski, C., Kazakoff, P. and Rizzino, A. (1989) Cell density regulates the number of cell surface receptors for fibroblast growth factor. *Biochem. Biophys. Res. Comm.,* 159: 694 – 700.

Walicke, P.A. (1988) Basic and acidic fibroblast growth factors have trophic effects on neurons from multiple CNS regions. *J. Neurosci.,* 8: 2618 – 2627.

Walicke, P.A. and Baird, A. (1988) Neurotrophic effects of basic and acidic fibroblast growth factors are not mediated through glial cells. *Dev. Brain Res.,* 40: 71 – 79.

Walicke, P., Cowan, W.M., Ueno, N., Baird, A. and Guillemin, R. (1986) Fibroblast growth factor promotes survival of dissociated hippocampal neurons and enhances neurite extension. *Proc. Natl. Acad. Sci. U.S.A.,* 83: 3012 – 3016.

Walicke, P.A., Feige, J.-J. and Baird, A. (1989) Characterization of the neuronal receptor for basic fibroblast growth factor and comparison to receptors in mesenchymal cells. *J. Biol. Chem.,* 264: 4120 – 4126.

Watters, D.J. and Hendry, I.A. (1987) Purification of ciliary neurotrophic factor from bovine heart. *J. Neurochem.,* 49: 705 – 713.

Whittemore, S.R. and Seiger, A. (1987) The expression, localization and functional significance of beta-nerve growth factor in the central nervous system. *Brain Res. Rev.,* 12: 439 – 464.

Woolf, N.J. and Butcher, L.L. (1986) Cholinergic systems in the rat brain. III. Projections from the pontomesencephalic tegmentum to the thalamus, tectum, basal ganglia, and basal forebrain. *Brain Res. Bull.,* 16: 603 – 637.

Yan, Q. and Johnson, E.M. (1988) An immunohistochemical study of the nerve growth factor receptor in developing rats. *J. Neurosci.,* 8: 3481 – 3498.

P. Coleman, G. Higgins and C. Phelps (Eds.)
Progress in Brain Research, Vol. 86
© 1990 Elsevier Science Publishers B.V. (Biomedical Division)

CHAPTER 13

Neurotrophic factors in the CNS: biosynthetic processing and functional responses

Ralph A. Bradshaw[1], Joseph G. Altin[1], Michael Blaber[1], Kathleen P. Cavanaugh[1], David D. Eveleth[1], Harley I. Kornblum[2], Francis M. Leslie[2], and Simona Raffioni[1]

Departments of [1]Biological Chemistry and [2]Pharmacology, College of Medicine, University of California, Irvine, CA 92717, U.S.A.

Introduction

It has become a popular model in neurobiology, based primarily on studies on the action of nerve growth factor (NGF) in the peripheral nervous system (Greene and Shooter, 1980; Levi-Montalcini, 1987), that neurons throughout higher vertebrates, and possibly lower organisms as well, interact with and depend upon neurotrophic factors (NTFs) elaborated in neuronal target cells. Complexes formed between NTFs and specific receptors on pre-synaptic membranes lead to signal transduction and receptor-mediated endocytosis followed by retrograde axonal transport to the perikaryon. Either or both events are required for the full manifestation of response (maintenance of viability and under some conditions neurite proliferation). The model has been useful in explaining many observations, particularly during development, but remains substantially unproven in a rigorous sense, particularly in the CNS. Nonetheless, it has provided highly attractive hypotheses regarding the etiology of various neurodegenerative pathologies and the possibilities for the development of effective therapeutics. A distinct problem in applying the neurotrophic hypothesis broadly has been the identification of additional suitable candidates. The discovery of new NTFs, based on specific neuronal assays, has

been a distinctly barren process, particularly in the central nervous system (Perez-Polo and DeVellis, 1982). Among the more disappointing efforts have been the failure to identify factors effective with motor neurons that might be of value in treating spinal cord injury. The brightest area has been the recognition of neurotrophic activities of previously identified factors, including NGF, for CNS neurons. The NGF responsive cells seem to be substantially limited to the principal cholinergic tracts in marked distinction to the types of neurons responsive in the PNS. Several other factors, already well known as polypeptide growth factors, i.e., they act as mitogens on non-neuronal cells, have now been shown to also act on both neuronal and glial elements of the CNS, producing, at least in culture, responses reminiscent of those well characterized for NGF by PNS neurons (Bradshaw et al., 1988; Walicke, 1989). Tables I and II list well-characterized growth factors that can apparently act as NTFs on neurons and glial cells, respectively. It may be reasonably expected that both lists will be further extended in the near future.

Effect of epidermal growth factor and the fibroblast growth factors on CNS neurons

Several studies suggest that both basic and acidic

FGF may be involved in regulating CNS function (Morrison et al., 1986, 1987; Walicke et al., 1986; Anderson et al., 1988). Brain, in fact, is a very rich source of both FGFs along with pituitary (Esch et al., 1985a, b; Baird et al., 1986) and is commonly used as starting material for preparation of the naturally occurring forms. Basic FGF is widely distributed; the localization of acidic FGF is much more proscribed. Both are also found outside the CNS. Importantly, receptors for the FGFs are also found in brain tissue (Walicke and Baird, 1988b).

The ability of bFGF to supply trophic support to brain neurons was first demonstrated using primary cultures of hippocampal and cortical rat neurons (Morrison et al., 1986; Walicke et al., 1986). In these studies, when neurons derived from fetal hippocampus or postnatal cortex were grown in serum-free media, they exhibited limited neurite outgrowth and most cells died after a few days in culture. However, adding bFGF to the culture media resulted in a significant improvement in cell survival, increasing the number of cells surviving 1 week in culture by 5 – 10 fold. Treatment with bFGF also caused a pronounced stimulation of neurite extension among the surviving cells. The concentrations of bFGF required to produce these effects were extremely low. Survival of hippocampal neurons was enhanced by as little as 1 pM bFGF (15 pg/ml), while higher concentrations supported process extension from hippocampal neurons and stimulated neuronal survival and neurite elaboration in cortical cultures. In addition to promoting neurite extension, treatment with bFGF increased the average number of primary

TABLE I

Polypeptide growth factors that act on peripheral and central neurons

Factor[1]	Effect	Reference
bFGF, aFGF	Neuronal survival Neurite extension PC12 cells (+)	Anderson et al. (1988) Morrison et al. (1986) Walicke et al. (1986) Rydel and Greene (1987)
EGF, TGF-alpha	Neuronal survival Neurite extension PC12 cells (−)	Morrison et al. (1987)
IGF-I	Neuronal survival (PNS and CNS)	I. Black (personal communication)
IGF-II	Neuronal survival Neurite extension	Recio-Pinto and Ishii (1988)
NGF	Neuronal survival (CNS and PNS) Neurite extension (PNS) PC12 cells (+)	Levi-Montalcini (1987) Greene and Tischler (1982) Yankner and Shooter (1982)
IL-6	PC12 cells (+)	Satoh et al. (1988)
BDNF	Neurite extension Neuronal survival (PNS)	Lindsay et al. (1985)

[1]For explanation of the abbreviations, see p. 164.

TABLE II

Polypeptide growth factors that act on glial cells

Factor	Effect	Reference
bFGF, aFGF	Glial mitogen Angiogenic factor	Morrison and DeVellis (1981)
EGF, TGF-alpha	Glial mitogen	Simpson et al. (1982) Westermark (1976)
IGF-1	Glial mitogen Inhibits GH and PRL release	McMorris et al. (1986)
IGF-2	Glial mitogen Inhibits GH and PRL release	Lim et al. (1985)
Insulin	Glial mitogen	Lim et al. (1985) Aizenman and DeVellis (1987)
PDGF	Glial mitogen	Heldin et al. (1977)
IL-1	Glial mitogen	Guilian and Lachman (1985)
Il-2	Glial mitogen	Benveniste and Merril (1986)
IFN-alpha, IFN-beta, IFN-gamma	Glial mitogen	Erkman et al. (1989)

[1]For explanation of the abbreviations, see p. 164.

processes elaborated by neurons and increased the extent of process branching in neuronal cultures derived from cortical and subneocortical telencephalic regions of postnatal rat brain (Kornblum et al., 1986, 1989). The concentrations of bFGF required to support such a multipolar, highly branched neuronal morphology were similar to those that promoted cell survival and neurite extension.

The studies described above were performed using cultures comprising predominantly neurons, with only a small percentage (less than 10%) nonneuronal cells such as glia and meningeal cells. Since such non-neuronal cells are known to secrete neurotrophic factors, it is possible that bFGF may not act directly on neurons but may produce its neurotrophic effects by stimulating the release of an unidentified neurotrophic factor from the contaminating non-neuronal cells. The results of several studies argue against this. First, the neurotrophic effects of bFGF on cultured cortical neurons are observed under conditions where non-neuronal cells represent as little as 3% of the cell population (Morrison et al., 1986). Secondly, bFGF enhances survival and neurite outgrowth in hippocampal cultures that do not contain a single identifiable astrocyte (Walicke and Baird, 1988a). Finally, cultured hippocampal neurons specifically bind and internalize ^{125}I-bFGF (Walicke and Baird, 1988b). Similar arguments apply to the EGF responses described below.

Recent studies have shown that a broad spectrum of brain neurons respond to FGF in culture. These responsive cells include hippocampal pyramidal and dentate gyrus neurons, cerebellar granule neurons, and neurons from striatum, septum, thalamus, as well as neurons from the entorhinal, frontal, parietal and occipital cortices (Morrison et al., 1986; Hatten et al., 1988; Needels and Cotman, 1988; Walicke, 1988). However, discrete subpopulations of FGF-responsive neurons may exist within these different brain regions.

For example, the proportion of responsive neurons varies considerably from one region to another, ranging from 12% (in septum) to 60% (in hippocampus). This is also supported by data showing that distribution patterns of neurite outgrowth are qualitatively dissimilar between different regions (Walicke, 1988) and by the shape of dose – response curves representing neuronal survival in response to varying amounts of bFGF.

In most instances, neurons from different regions display a high degree of similarity both in their sensitivity to FGF and in the qualitative manner in which they respond. In general, both neuronal survival and neurite extension were stimulated by concentrations of bFGF ranging from 1 to 20 pM. Interestingly, certain neuronal populations did not follow this pattern. For example, striatal neurons were less sensitive to bFGF compared to most other neuronal types and required about 3-fold higher concentrations of bFGF to survive. Also, bFGF did not stimulate neurite outgrowth from striatal neurons (Walicke, 1988). Cerebellar granule neurons also appear to require significantly higher concentrations of bFGF (from 1 to 25 ng/ml) to support survival and neurite outgrowth (Hatten et al., 1988).

Acidic FGF exerts qualitatively similar neurotrophic actions as bFGF, enhancing both survival and process outgrowth from neurons derived from several brain regions. As is the case in other biological systems, about 100-fold greater concentrations of aFGF, compared to bFGF are required to achieve equivalent responses. Like bFGF, aFGF stimulates survival of neurons derived from hippocampus, striatum, and the entorhinal and parietal cortices. However, whereas bFGF is unable to promote the survival of subiculum neurons, aFGF produces significant increase in cell survival (Walicke, 1988). This suggests the possibility that in some instances bFGF and aFGF may have functions in the CNS distinct from one another.

The ability of EGF to support cultured brain neurons was first described using cells derived from subneocortical telencephalic regions of neonatal rat brain (Morrison et al., 1987). EGF supports both survival and neurite outgrowth in cultured brain neurons at concentrations of about 100 pg/ml. Similar concentrations of EGF are also effective in supporting neuronal survival and neurite outgrowth in cultures of cortical and cerebellar neurons (Morrison et al., 1987, 1988). Since the cultures of cerebellar neurons were prepared from brain prior to the generation of basket, stellate and granule cells, it can be inferred that the neurons responding to EGF were most likely either Purkinje or Golgi cells. As well as stimulating process outgrowth, treatment of cortical and subneocortical telencephalic neurons with EGF increased both the average number of processes elaborated by neurons and the degree of neurite branching. EGF does not, however, seem to be as efficient as bFGF in this regard. Although some brain regions contain neurons that respond to both EGF and FGF, there are other regions that may contain neurons that respond to only one factor. Indeed, postnatal rat cortex is composed of three types of responsive neurons: those that respond only to EGF, others that respond only to FGF, and a third population that requires the presence of both EGF and bFGF to survive in culture (Kornblum et al., 1989). In contrast, although fetal hippocampal neurons clearly responded to FGF, they were not supported by EGF (Walicke and Baird, 1988a). Conversely, EGF-responsive cerebellar neurons did not survive in culture when treated with bFGF (Morrison et al., 1988).

It is important to determine whether or not factors such as bFGF, which are neurotrophic in cultured neurons, also exert similar effects in vivo. One study has demonstrated that bFGF is indeed capable of enhancing the in vivo recovery of brain neurons damaged experimentally. These results showed that exogenously administered bFGF protected some cholinergic neurons in the medial septum and diagonal band of Broca from the lethal effects of axonal transection (Anderson et al., 1988).

Biosynthesis of NGF and EGF

The processes underlying the biosynthetic production of NTFs from transcription to secretion are, like most PGFs not fully understood. The production of NGF and EGF in one tissue, the adult male mouse submaxillary gland, had, because of the relative abundance of material, been studied in somewhat greater detail (Greene and Shooter, 1980). In this tissue, the natural forms of both hormones are associated non-covalently with two glandular kallikreins, with catalytic specificities for bonds contributed by the carboxyl groups of arginine residues, that have been suggested to be involved in precursor processing (Angeletti and Bradshaw, 1971; Taylor et al., 1974). Whether they actually play this role, the elucidation of the molecular basis for the selective interactions that define the complexes provides the opportunity to probe structure/function relationships with respect to both the kallikreins and the hormones.

The precursor structures that yield the mature hormones for both NGF and EGF have been determined from cDNA sequence analyses (Gray et al., 1983; Scott et al., 1983a, b; Ullrich et al., 1983). The NGF precursor can vary in length due to the production of alternate transcripts arising from different splicing events (Edwards et al., 1986). However, the processing events that produce active beta-NGF are the same in all cases. The 118 residue mature form is released from the precursor by carboxyl terminal cleavage to a Lys-Arg site. A carboxyl terminal dipeptide (Arg-Gly) is similarly removed by the hydrolysis of an Arg-Arg bond. The 53 residue EGF molecule arises from a much larger precursor structure (1217 amino acid) by cleavage at single arginine residues. The mature sequence occurs in the middle of the precursor, commencing at residue 977. The active kallikrein sequences of the NGF and EGF complexes (gamma-NGF and EGF-BP, respectively) have also been defined by protein/cDNA sequencing (Thomas et al., 1981; Ullrich et al., 1984; Blaber et al., 1987). They are highly similar in structure sharing identical pre- and prosegments; the active enzymes are

distinguished by 35 differences in 237 positions. The specific association of each kallikrein for its respective growth factor thus resides in a relatively small number of amino acid replacements.

A number of observations suggest that the kallikrein growth factor association is primarily through the carboxyl terminal arginine residue found on the mature form of each growth factor (Isackson et al., 1987). If, as anticipated, this arginine residue occupies the P1 position in the catalytic site of each enzyme, then the preceding two amino acids (threonine and alanine in NGF and leucine and glutamic acid in EGF) would be expected to occupy the P2 and P3 sites as well. Detailed kinetic analyses using synthetic substrates corresponding to the tripeptide sequences in the p-nitroanilide form, suggest that the specificity cannot be limited to these interactions (Blaber et al., 1989). Accordingly, using the cDNA sequences for each kallikrein, constructs were prepared and expressed in E. coli to produce each kallikrein as a fusion product with the ara-B protein of E. coli. Cleavage and isolation allowed the recovery of recombinant EGF-BP and gamma-NGF fully capable of specifically binding beta-NGF and EGF, respectively. These proteins differ from the native molecules in that they are not glycosylated nor fully processed with respect to internal intrachain cleavages. To identify regions of the molecule that could participate in additional binding interactions with the mature growth factors, a series of six chimeric constructs were prepared by exchanging corresponding segments of the kallikrein cDNAs. The pieces that were interchanged were selected on the basis of predicted surface loops, as deduced from the examination of similar proteins whose structures have been determined by X-ray crystallography. Initial characterization of these hybrid molecules suggests a single additional interaction site for EGF on EGF-BP while gamma-NGF may associate in the 7S complex (with alpha- and beta-NGF) through two sites. These findings suggest, that at least in some cases, processing enzymes for growth factors and hormones may be highly specific and could therefore lend themselves to specific regulation for the production of the mature factors in situ.

Mechanistic aspects of FGF and NGF in PC12 cells

Both in vivo and in vitro, a wide spectrum of biochemical events follows the application of NTFs to responsive cells and tissues. A small fraction of these events are direct consequences of binding to receptors, and differentiating the direct from indirect events even when specific enzymatic activities of receptor molecules are known remains a daunting task. In the case of the best characterized NTF, NGF, no specific activity can be attributed directly to the receptor even though the gene for a receptor protein has been cloned and sequenced.

Due to the complexity of cell types in the CNS, biochemical studies of NTF action depend heavily upon cultured cell models. A dominant model is the rat pheochromocytoma line PC12, responsive to several NTFs, and many parallels can be drawn between PC12 cells and CNS neurons (Greene and Tischler, 1982). However, some differences between PC12 cells and CNS neurons should be noted. CNS cells respond to a larger spectrum of factors than PC12 cells; the adhesive interactions which are essential for neurite outgrowth are significantly different in PC12 and CNS cells; and the PC12 line is a transformed cell which certainly responds differently than normal cells in regard to survival. Nonetheless, studies of NTF-induced differentiation of the PC12 line continue to be informative.

Like CNS and PNS neurons, differentiation of PC12 cells is initiated by the binding of NGF to specific plasma membrane receptors. A common feature of these systems is the presence of two classes NGFR, type I (high affinity or slow) and type II (low affinity or fast) (Sutter et al., 1979; Schecter and Bothwell, 1981). Considerable evidence supports the idea that the differentiative response (development of a morphology and biochemistry reminiscent of mature sympathetic neurons) is mediated solely through the type I

NGFR (Sonnenfeld and Ishii, 1982; Stach and Wagner, 1982). Many cell types are known which possess the type II NGFR and do not respond to NGF. All cell types (with the exception noted below) which possess type I NGFR do respond.

The rat (PC12) and human NGF receptor genes have now been cloned (Johnson et al., 1986; Radecke et al., 1987). The receptor is smaller than most other known receptors and is not homologous to any other known receptor protein. Transformation of the receptor gene into fibroblasts does not confer any biological activity; however, transformation of the receptor gene into at least one neuroblastoma cell line results in the acquisition of NGF responsiveness (M. Chao, personal communication). Thus this single gene forms at least part of both type I and type II NGFR species. These observations support the hypothesis that the NGFR is itself unable to generate second messengers but must interact with other cellular machinery, present only in appropriate cells, to generate a response. Several authors have proposed the existence of an accessory protein to account for the difference in the two NGFR types (Yankner and Shooter, 1982; Johnson et al., 1986).

While the immediate post-binding signalling event remains unknown, generation of the differentiative signal appears to depend upon translocation of NGF-receptor complexes to a distinct subcellular compartment. Two lines of evidence support this hypothesis:

(1) *Type I NGFR represents a compartmentalized subpopulation of NGFR*. Several laboratories have shown that the endocytosis of NGF occurs primarily through the type I NGFR (Bernd and Greene, 1984; Hosang and Shooter, 1987). We have proposed a model accounting for the observation of two receptor types based solely upon intracellular sequestration and recycling of NGF and NGFR (Eveleth and Bradshaw, 1988; Fig. 1). Type II receptor, found on both responsive and non-responsive cell types, remains on the cell surface and is not internalized in response to NGF binding. NGF is free to associate and dissociate, limited only by diffusion. Agents which disrupt endocytosis,

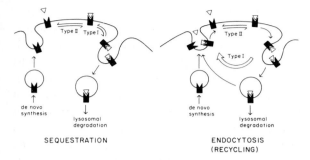

Fig. 1. Models for the cycling of NGF and NGF receptors in PC12 cells. In both the sequestration and the endocytosis models, type II (fast) binding is rapidly reversible binding of NGF to the receptor on the cell surface. Type I (slow) binding involves the reversible sequestration (left) or rapid endocytosis and recycling (right) of both receptor and ligand recruited from the type II pool. Sequestration or endocytosis and thus type I binding are blocked by PAO, while recycling of receptor is inhibited by monensin, resulting in the accumulation of type I binding and depletion of receptor at the cell surface. (Reprinted from Eveleth and Bradshaw, 1988.)

such as phenylarsine oxide and digitonin, cause PC12 cells to exhibit only type II NGF binding. In responsive cells, some of the occupied type II receptor is internalized. NGF is not free to dissociate from the cell while in the internalized compartment and thus this form of the receptor appears to have a much slower dissociation rate and a much higher affinity. Both the NGF and receptor are recycled to the cell surface, where the NGF can dissociate from the cell. Agents which disrupt intracellular vesicle traffic such as monensin and chloroquine disrupt the recycling but not the endocytosis of NGF and result only in type I NGF binding. The novel aspect of this model is not the endocytosis and recycling of receptor but that the NGF is also recycled.

(2) *Cells incapable of receptor compartmentalization are unable to respond to NGF.* Several variants of PC12 cells are known which are incapable of responding to NGF. We have characterized NGF endocytosis in one of these, the PC12nnr5 cell line (D.D. Eveleth and R.A. Bradshaw, manuscript in preparation). These cells express both type I and type II receptors but show no morphological or biochemical response to NGF and also respond poorly or not at all to FGF. The defect is not in the structural machinery required for neurite outgrowth since the cells are capable of extending neurites upon transfection with *v-src* genes (Eveleth et al., 1989). These cells initially sequester bound NGF but are incapable of bringing the bound NGF into lysosomes for degradation.

One of the earliest events following NGF binding to cells is the turnover of membrane lipids, including phosphoinositides. This turnover generates 1,2-diacylglycerol (DAG), inositol phosphates, and inositol glycans (Contreras and Guroff, 1987; Chan et al., 1989). DAG is a stimulator of protein kinase C activity, and some antagonists of this enzyme such as sphingosine and K252a will block the effects of NGF (Hall et al., 1988; Koizumi et al., 1988). However, agonists such as phorbol esters are insufficient to generate the differentiative response and PC12 cells substantially depleted in protein kinase C remain able to respond to NGF (Reinhold and Neet, 1989). PC12 cells produce similar amounts of DAG in response to NGF, FGF and the muscarinic acetylcholine receptor agonist carbachol. However, the amount of phosphoinositide cleaved in response to carbachol is much greater than that hydrolyzed in response to NGF and FGF. Therefore, NGF and FGF must be producing DAG through hydrolysis of a lipid pool comparatively depleted in phosphatidylinositide (Altin and Bradshaw, 1990).

Two types of events may explain this difference between carbachol and the NTFs. Different phospholipases may be involved in the responses to the different agents. Alternatively, the agents may be stimulating similar phospholipases but they in turn may be hydrolyzing different lipid pools. Although the hydrolysis of lipids is thought to be an event closely linked to receptor activation due to the temporal and spatial proximity of the two events, this is not necessarily the case.

The generation of second messengers from an intracellular compartment by NGF-receptor complexes and the possibility of similar mechanisms for other NTFs may be a valuable aspect for responsive neurons. Many differentiated neurons both centrally and peripherally respond to NTFs as survival factors and maintenance factors. Much of this response depends upon influencing the transcriptional machinery in the nucleus while the NTFs are presented to the cell at the nerve terminals some distance away. Transport of NGF-receptor complexes to the cell body by retrograde transport has been demonstrated and may be a convenient way for these cells to transfer the signal between periphery and nucleus (Hendry et al., 1974; Johnson et al., 1987). An interesting corollary of this mechanism is the potential that mature cells might then release (via recycling/exocytosis) intact NGF or NTFs at the cell body to be picked up by adjacent cells, including interneurons, and thus pass a given NTF down or up a chain of neurons in a pathway.

Concluding remarks

The identification of a number of growth factors and hormones, that have well-defined activities outside the nervous system, as neurotrophic agents in both the PNS and CNS is another example of the familiar economy of usage that defines biological systems. It also emphasizes that the superficial differences between trophic and plastic stimulations may be greatly obscured at the mechanistic level. The distinguishing principles will almost certainly occur at the level of gene expression, predetermined by the state of differentiation of the cell. Thus the response of a fibroblast to FGF, that leads to cell division, will not likely be distinguished from the trophic response of a neuron, with the production of neurites, by the signal transduced at the plasma membranes but rather by the genes that are ultimately expressed in response to the stimuli. These conclusions have important ramifications for the events controlling cell proliferation in the CNS and the management of neurodegeneration in pathologies such as Alzheimer's disease.

These conclusions also underscore the important

implication that signal transduction by neurotrophic factors will involve to a very significant degree the same cascade of proto-oncogenes as is used in mitotic responses. When these proteins in cells capable of division undergo structural modification and/or alterations in production, it leads to the transformed phenotype characteristic of tumors and cancer. Since a similar change in a post-mitotic cell would not necessarily be expected to lead to uncontrolled proliferation, its deleterious effect might result rather in cell death (because the stimulus could no longer maintain the viability required by this signal cascade). Neurodegeneration then could be the antithesis of cancer, arising from the same set of lesions but with very different end results. Since cancer is a self-propagating disease, the alteration of a single cell can eventually lead to complete penetration; if the alteration of proto-oncogenes is a significant basis for neurodegeneration, a different mechanism of propagation is required such as might be expected form viral infection, a plausible and often suggested basis for neurodegenerative diseases.

Acknowledgements

This work was supported by U.S.P.H.S. research grants NS 19319 (F.L.) and NS 19664 (R.A.B.), program project grant AG00538 (R.A.B.), and American Cancer Society research grant BC273 (R.A.B.). K.P.C. was supported by a fellowship from the Hereditary Disease Foundation and D.D.E. by a fellowship from the Bank of America – Giannini Foundation. M.B. was a trainee of U.S.P.H.S. grant GM07134.

The authors thank Kisma Stepanich for her expert assistance in preparing the manuscript.

Abbreviations

NGF: nerve growth factor; NTF: neurotrophic factor; CNS: central nervous system; PNS: peripheral nervous system; aFGF: acidic fibroblast growth factor; bFGF: basic fibroblast growth factor; EGF: epidermal growth factor; TGF-alpha: transforming growth factor alpha; IGF-I and -II: insulin-like growth factor I and II; IL-1,2 and 6: interleukin -1,2 and 6; BDNF: brain-derived neurotrophic factor; PDGF: platelet-derived growth factor; IFN alpha, beta and gamma: interferon alpha, beta and gamma; EGF-BP: epidermal growth factor binding protein; NGFR: nerve growth factor receptor; PGF: polypeptide growth factor.

References

Aizenman, Y. and DeVellis, S. (1987) Synergistic action of thyroid hormone, insulin and hydrocortisone on astrocyte differentiation. *Brain Res.,* 414: 301 – 308.

Altin, J.G. and Bradshaw, R.A. (1990) Nerve growth factor and basic fibroblast growth factor primarily stimulate the production of 1,2-diacylglycerol from phospholipids other than phosphoinositides in PC 12 cells. *J. Neurochem.,* 54: 1666 – 1676.

Anderson, K.J., Dam, D., Lee, S. and Cotman, C.W. (1988) Basic fibroblast growth factor prevents death of lesioned cholinergic neurons in vivo. *Nature,* 332: 360 – 361.

Angeletti, R.H. and Bradshaw, R.A. (1971) The amino acid sequence of 2.5S mouse submaxillary gland nerve growth factor. *Proc. Natl. Acad. Sci. U.S.A.,* 68: 2417 – 2420.

Baird, A., Esch, F., Mormede, P., Ueno, N., Ling, N., Bohlen, P., Ying, S.-Y., Wehrenberg, W.B. and Guillemin, R. (1986) Molecular characterization of fibroblast growth factor: distribution and biological activities in various tissues. *Rec. Prog. Horm. Res.,* 42: 143 – 205.

Benveniste, E.N. and Merril, J.E. (1986) Stimulation of oligodendroglial proliferation and maturation by interleukin 2. *Nature,* 321: 610 – 613.

Bernd, P. and Greene, L.A. (1984) Association of ^{125}I nerve growth factor with PC12 pheochromocytoma cells: evidence for internalization via high-affinity receptors only and for long-term regulation by nerve growth factor of both high and low affinity receptors. *J. Biol. Chem.,* 259: 15509 – 15514.

Blaber, M., Isackson, P.J. and Bradshaw, R.A. (1987) A complete cDNA sequence for the major epidermal growth factor binding protein in the male mouse submandibular gland. *Biochemistry,* 26: 6742 – 6749.

Blaber, M., Isackson, P.J., Marsters, J.C., Burnier, J.P. and Bradshaw, R.A. (1989) Substrate specificities of growth factor associated kallikreins of the mouse submandibular gland. *Biochemistry,* 28: 7813 – 7819.

Bradshaw, R.A., Blaber, M., Cavanaugh, K., Eveleth, D.D., Isackson, P.J., Kornblum, H.I., Leslie, F., Morrison, R.S., Schwarz, M. and Sharma, A. (1988) Neurotrophic factors of the central neurons system: synthesis and activities. In: G. Biggio, P.F. Spano, G. Toffano, S.H. Appel and G.L. Gessa (Eds.), *Neuronal Plasticity and Trophic Factors,* Liviana Press – Springer Verlag, Berlin, pp. 9 – 22.

Chan, B.L., Chao, M.V. and Saltiel, A.R. (1989) Nerve growth factor stimulates the hydrolysis of glycosyl-phosphatidylinositol in PC12 cells: a mechanism of protein kinase C regulation. *Proc. Natl. Acad. Sci. U.S.A.,* 86: 1756 – 1760.

Contreras, M.L. and Guroff, G. (1987) Calcium-dependent nerve growth factor-stimulated hydrolysis of phosphoinositides in PC12 cells. *J. Neurochem.,* 48: 1466 – 1472.

Edwards, R.H., Selby, M.J. and Rutter, W.J. (1986) Differential RNA splicing predicts two distinct nerve growth factor precursors. *Nature,* 319: 784 – 787.

Erkman, L., Wuaren, L., Cadelli, D. and Kato, A.C. (1989) Interferon induces astrocyte maturation causing an increase in cholinergic properties of cultured human spinal cord cells. *Dev. Biol.,* 132: 378 – 388.

Esch, F., Baird, A., Ling, N., Ueno, N., Hill, F., Denoroy, L., Klepper, R., Gospodarowicz, D., Bohlen, P. and Guillemin, R. (1985b) Primary structure of bovine pituitary basic fibroblast growth factor (FGF) and comparison with the amino-terminal sequence of bovine brain acidic FGF. *Proc. Natl. Acad. Sci. U.S.A.,* 82: 6507 – 6511.

Esch, F., Ueno, N., Baird, A., Hill, F., Denoroy, L., Ling, N., Gospodarowicz, D. and Guillemin, R. (1985a) Primary structure of bovine brain acidic fibroblast growth factor (FGF). *Biochem. Biophys. Res. Commun.,* 133: 554 – 562.

Eveleth, D.D. and Bradshaw, R.A. (1988) Internalization of cycling of nerve growth factor in PC12 cells: interconversion of type II (fast) and type I (slow) nerve growth factor receptors. *Neuron,* 1: 929 – 936.

Eveleth, D.D., Hanacek, R., Fox, G.M., Fan, H. and Bradshaw, R.A. (1989) *V-src* genes stimulate neurite outgrowth in pheochromocytoma (PC12) variants unresponsive to neurotrophic factors. *J. Neurosci. Res.,* 24: 67 – 71.

Gray, A., Dull, T.J. and Ullrich, A. (1983) Nucleotide sequence of epidermal growth factor cDNA predicts a 128,000-molecular weight protein precursor. *Nature,* 303: 722 – 725.

Greene, L.A. and Shooter, E.M. (1980) The nerve growth factor: biochemistry, synthesis and mechanism of action: *Ann. Rev. Neurosci.,* 3: 353 – 402.

Greene, L.A. and Tischler, A.S. (1982) PC12 pheochromocytoma cultures in neurobiological research. *Adv. Cell. Neurobiol.,* 3: 373 – 414.

Guilian, D. and Lachman, L.B. (1985) Interleukin 1 stimulation of astroglial proliferation after brain injury. *Science,* 228: 497 – 499.

Hall, F.L., Fernyhough, P., Ishii, D.N. and Vulliet, P.R. (1988) Suppression of nerve growth factor-directed neurite outgrowth in PC12 cells by sphingosine, an inhibitor of protein kinase C. *J. Biol. Chem.,* 263: 4460 – 4466.

Hatten, M.E., Lynch, M., Rydel, R.E., Sanchez, J., Joseph-Silverstein, J., Moscatelli, D. and Rifkin, D.B. (1988) In vitro neurite extension by granule neurons is dependent upon astroglial-derived fibroblast growth factor. *Dev. Biol.,* 125: 280 – 289.

Heldin, C.H., Wasteson, A. and Westermark, R. (1977) Partial purification and characterization of platelet factors stimulating the multiplication of normal human glial cells.

Exp. Cell Res., 109: 429–437.

Hendry, I.A., Stoeckel, K., Thoenen, H. and Iversen, L.L. (1974) The retrograde axonal transport of nerve growth factor. *Brain Res.,* 68: 103–121.

Hosang, M. and Shooter, E.M. (1987) The internalization of nerve growth factor by high-affinity receptors on pheochromocytoma PC12 cells. *EMBO J.,* 6: 1197–1202.

Isackson, P.J., Dunbar, J.C. and Bradshaw, R.A. (1987) Role of glandular kallikreins as growth factor processing enzymes: structural and evolutionary considerations. *J. Cell. Biochem.,* 33: 65–75.

Johnson, D., Lanahan, A., Buck, C.R., Sehgal, A., Morgan, C., Mercer, E., Bothwell, M. and Chao, M. (1986) Expression and structure of the human NGF receptor. *Cell,* 47: 545–554.

Johnson, E.M., Taniuchi, M., Clark, H.B., Springer, J.E., Koh, S., Tayrien, M.W. and Loy, R. (1987) Demonstration of the retrograde transport of nerve growth factor receptor in the peripheral and central nervous system. *J. Neurosci.,* 7: 923–929.

Koizumi, S., Contreras, M.L., Matsuda, Y., Hama, T., Lazarovici, P. and Guroff, G. (1988) K-252a: a specific inhibitor of the action of nerve growth factor on PC12 cells. *J. Neurosci.,* 8: 715–721.

Kornblum, H.I., Morrison, R.S., Bradshaw, R.A. and Leslie, F.M. (1986) Effects of epidermal growth factor and basic fibroblast growth factor on postnatal mammalian neurons in culture. *Abstr. Soc. Neurosci. Mtg., Washington, D.C..*

Kornblum, H.I., Raymon, H.K., Morrison, R.S., Cavanaugh, K.P., Bradshaw, R.A. and Leslie, F.M. (1989) Epidermal growth factor and basic fibroblast growth factor affect overlapping populations of neocortical neurons. *Abstr. Soc. Neurosci. Mtg., Phoenix, AZ.*

Levi-Montalcini, R. (1987) The nerve growth factor 35 years later. *Science,* 237: 1154–1162.

Lim, R., Miller, J.F., Hicklin, D.J., Holm, A.C. and Ginsberg, B.H. (1985) Mitogenic activity of glia maturation factor: interaction with insulin and insulin-like growth factor II. *Exp. Cell. Res.,* 159: 335–343.

Lindsay, R.M., Thoenen, M. and Barde, Y.A. (1985) Placode and neural crest-derived sensory neurons are responsive at early developmental stages to brain derived neurotrophic factor. *Dev. Biol.,* 112: 319–328.

McMorris, F.A., Smith, T.M., DeSalvo, S. and Furlanetto, R.W. (1986) Insulin-like growth factor I/somatomedin C: a potent inducer of oligodendrocyte development. *Proc. Natl. Acad. Sci. U.S.A.,* 83: 822–826.

Morrison, R.S. and DeVellis, J. (1981) Growth of purified astrocytes in a chemically defined medium. *Proc. Natl. Acad. Sci. U.S.A.,* 78: 7205–7209.

Morrison, R.S., Sharma, A., DeVellis, J. and Bradshaw, R.A. (1986) Basic fibroblast growth factor supports the survival of cerebral cortical neurons in primary culture. *Proc. Natl. Acad. Sci. U.S.A.,* 83: 7537–7541.

Morrison, R.S., Kornblum, H.I., Leslie, F.M. and Bradshaw, R.A. (1987) Trophic stimulation of cultured neurons from neonatal rat brain by epidermal growth factor. *Science,* 238: 72–75.

Morrison, R.S., Keating, R.F. and Moskal, J.R. (1988) Basic fibroblast growth factor and epidermal growth factor exert differential trophic effects on CNS neurons. *J. Neurosci. Res.,* 21: 71–79.

Needels, D.L. and Cotman, C.W. (1988) Basic fibroblast growth factor (with heparin) increases the survival of rat dentate granule cells in culture. *Abstr. Soc. Neurosci. Mtg., Toronto, Ont.*

Perez-Polo, J.R. and DeVellis, J.R. (Eds.) (1982) Growth and trophic factors. *J. Neurosci. Res.,* 8: 127–574.

Radecke, M.J., Misko, T.P., Hsu, C., Herzenberg, L.A. and Shooter, E.M. (1987) Gene transfer and molecular cloning of the rat nerve growth factor receptor. *Nature,* 325: 593–597.

Recio-Pinto, E. and Ishii, D.N. (1988) Insulin and insulin-like growth factor receptors regulating neurite formation in cultured human neuroblastoma cells. *J. Neurosci. Res.,* 19: 312–320.

Reinhold, D.S. and Neet, K.E. (1989) The lack of a role for protein kinase C in neurite extension and in the induction of ornithine decarboxylase by nerve growth factor in PC12 cells. *J. Biol. Chem.,* 264: 3538–3544.

Rydel, R.E. and Greene, L.A. (1987) Acidic and basic fibroblast growth factors promote stable neurite outgrowth and neuronal differentiation in cultures of PC12 cells. *J. Neurosci.,* 7: 3639–3653.

Satoh, T., Nakamura, S., Taga, T. Matsuda, T., Hirano, T., Kishimoto, T. and Kzairo, Y. (1988) Induction of neuronal differentiation in PC12 cells by B-cell stimulatory factor 2/interleukin 6. *Mol. Cell. Biol.,* 8: 3546–3549.

Schecter, A.L. and Bothwell, M.A. (1981) Nerve growth factor receptors on PC12 cells: evidence for two receptor classes with differing cytoskeletal association. *Cell,* 24: 867–874.

Scott, J., Selby, M., Urdea, M., Quiroga, M., Bell, G.I. and Rutter, W.J. (1983a) Isolation and nucleotide sequence of a cDNA encoding the precursor of mouse nerve growth factor. *Nature,* 302: 538–540.

Scott, J., Urdea, M., Quiroga, M., Sanchez-Pescadoe, R., Fong, N., Selby, M., Rutter, W.J. and Bell, G.I. (1983b) Structure of a mouse submaxillary messenger RNA encoding epidermal growth factor and seven related proteins. *Science,* 221: 236–240.

Simpson, D.L., Morrison, R., DeVellis, J. and Herschman, H.R. (1982) Epidermal growth factor binding and mitogenic activity on purified populations of cells from the central nervous system. *J. Neurosci. Res.,* 8: 453–462.

Sonnenfeld, K.H. and Ishii, D.N. (1982) Nerve growth factor effects and receptors in cultured human neuroblastoma lines. *J. Neurosci. Res.,* 8: 375–391.

Stach, R.W. and Wagner, B.J. (1982) Decrease in the number of lower affinity (type II) nerve growth factor receptors on embryonic sensory neurons does not affect fiber outgrowth. *J. Neurosci. Res.,* 7: 103 – 110.

Sutter, A., Riopelle, R.S., Harris-Warrick, R.M. and Shooter, E.M. (1979) Nerve growth factor receptors: characterization of two distinct classes of binding sites on chick embryo sensory glanglia cells. *J. Biol. Chem.,* 254: 5972 – 5982.

Taylor, J.M., Mitchell, W.M. and Cohen, S. (1974) Characterization of the binding protein for epidermal growth factor. *J. Biol. Chem.,* 249: 2188 – 2194.

Thomas, K.A., Baglan, N.C. and Bradshaw, R.A. (1981) The amino acid sequence of the gamma-subunit of mouse submaxillary gland 7S nerve growth factor. *J. Biol. Chem.,* 256: 9156 – 9166.

Ullrich, A., Gray, A., Berman, C. and Dull, T.J. (1983) Human beta-nerve growth factor gene sequence is highly homologous to that of mouse. *Nature,* 303: 821 – 825.

Ullrich, A., Gray, A., Wood, W., Hayflick, J. and Seeberg, P.H. (1984) Isolation of a cDNA clone coding for the gamma-subunit of mouse nerve growth factor using a high-stringency selection procedure. *DNA,* 3: 387 – 392.

Walicke, P.A. (1988) Basic and acidic fibroblast growth factors have trophic effects on neurons from multiple CNS regions. *J. Neurosci.,* 8: 2618 – 2627.

Walicke, P.A. (1989) Novel neurotrophic factors, receptors, and oncogenes. *Annu. Rev. Neurosci.,* 12: 103 – 126.

Walicke, P.A. and Baird, A. (1988a) Neurotrophic effects of basic and acidic fibroblast growth factors are not mediated through glial cells. *Dev. Brain Res.,* 40: 71 – 79.

Walicke, P.A. and Baird, A. (1988b) Trophic effects of fibroblast growth factor on neural tissue. *Prog. Brain Res.,* 78: 333 – 338.

Walicke, P., Cowan, W.M., Ueno, N., Baird, A. and Guillemin, R. (1986) Fibroblast growth factor promotes survival of dissociated hippocampal neurons and enhances neurite extension. *Proc. Natl. Acad. Sci. U.S.A.,* 83: 3012 – 3016.

Westermark, B. (1976) Density dependent proliferation of human glial cells stimulated by epidermal growth factor. *Biochem. Biophys. Res. Commun.,* 69: 304 – 309.

Yankner, B.A. and Shooter, E.M. (1982) The biology and mechanism of action of nerve growth factor. *Annu. Rev. Biochem.,* 51: 845 – 868.

P. Coleman, G. Higgins and C. Phelps (Eds.)
Progress in Brain Research, Vol. 86
© 1990 Elsevier Science Publishers B.V. (Biomedical Division)

CHAPTER 14

S100β as a neurotrophic factor

Daniel R. Marshak

Cold Spring Harbor Laboratory, Cold Spring Harbor, NY 11724, U.S.A.

Neurite outgrowth

Neurite outgrowth is a process that occurs both in the developing nervous system and in the degenerating brains of Alzheimer disease (AD) patients (Price, 1986; Selkoe, 1989). Ramon y Cajal (1928) first noted the appearance of neuronal regrowth surrounding lesions in degenerating brain and suggested the presence of diffusable neurotrophic factors. The appearance of new neuritic processes surrounding amyloid deposits is characteristic of the later stages of plaque formation in AD autopsy samples (Price, 1986 and this volume). Such observations indicate the presence of neurotrophic substances in the vicinity of AD plaques, and characterization of these factors may provide insight into the mechanism of plaque formation in AD. Understanding the control of neurite outgrowth, particularly in neurons of the central nervous system, may lead to novel therapeutic approaches to degenerative neurological diseases including AD. Patients with Down syndrome (DS) in later life develop a cholinergic neuronal degeneration and dementia similar to AD patients (Epstein, 1986, 1987; Epstein et al., 1987). Because neurite outgrowth is common to both development and AD degeneration, the study of neurotrophic factors may contribute to our understanding of both developmental as well as degenerative neurological diseases.

Several classes of molecules have been shown to be effective neurotrophic agents (Walicke, 1989) including, but not limited to, polypeptides (Barde et al., 1983; Thoenen and Edgar, 1985), gangliosides (Tsuji et al., 1988), neurotransmitters (Lipton et al., 1988a), and extracellular matrix materials (Sanes, 1989). Of these, our research focuses on neurotrophic polypeptides, that comprise a broad family of factors. To aid in the classification of polypeptide neurotrophic factors, it is useful to separate neurite outgrowth into three stages: inititation, propagation, and termination. These stages are intended as a guide for the study of neurite outgrowth, and some polypeptide neurotrophic factors may be important signals in two or more of the stages. Our interest has been the first stage, initiation, and the identification of soluble polypeptide neurotrophic factors that signal the earliest changes in neurons leading to neurite outgrowth.

Initiation

Stage I, the initiation of neurite outgrowth from post-mitotic neurons, includes the changes in gene expression that are required for neurite formation (Masiakowski and Shooter, 1988). For example, the expression of cytoskeletal proteins, such as tubulin and microtubule associate proteins, are increased in neuronal growth (Burgoyne, 1986). Regulation of gene expression could be controlled by transcription factors (Curran et al., 1988) that themselves are sensitive to signal transduction systems stimulated by soluble growth factors (Metz et al., 1988; Walicke, 1989). Such polypeptide molecules may be autocrine factors from the neurons itself or paracrine factors from neighboring neurons or glia. Endocrine factors in the peripheral circulation can be excluded because polypeptides are unlikely to cross the blood-brain barrier (Rubin and Porter, 1989) and because different brain areas appear to initiate neurite outgrowth at different times during development (Rakic, 1988). Candidates for initiation factors are heparin-binding growth factors, such as acidic (Lipton et al., 1988b) and basic (Walicke et al., 1986) fibroblast growth factors (FGF). As discussed in this work, S100β also appears to be an initiation factor for neurite extension.

Propagation

Stage II is the propagation of the neurite in a particular direction or along a path. Propagation may be different for neurites destined to become dendrites rather than axons, but more information on axonal growth is presently available. This stage consists of two related events, the movement of the growth cone at the end of the elongating neurite and the adhesion of the neurite to a surface. These phenomena are related because the pulsatory movement of growth cones requires transient attachment and release of the membrane to the extracellular matrix (Bray and Hollenbeck, 1988). Three major classes of polypeptide neurotrophic factors contribute to stage II: (1) target tissue-derived, soluble polypeptides, such as nerve growth factor (NGF) (Levi-Montalcini and Angeletti, 1968) which bind to receptors on the pre-synaptic neuron, are taken up by the emerging neurite, and transported in a retrograde fashion to the perikaryon (Yankner and Shooter, 1982); (2) extracellular matrix proteins (Sanes, 1989), such as laminin, which provide a favorable surface for neurite outgrowth (Leder et al., 1985); and (3) proteases and protease inhibitors, such as protease nexin I (Guenther et al., 1985; Monard, 1985; Pittman and Patterson, 1987), that contribute to the transient attachment cycle of the growing neurite. Other proteins, such as GAP-43, may play an important role in growth cones of elongating neurites (Skene and Willard, 1981; Basi et al., 1987; Skene, 1989).

Termination

Stage III is the termination phase in which the neurite reaches an appropriate target cell and stops elongating. Cell surface glycoproteins, such as cell adhesion molecules (Edelman, 1985), may contribute to this process. In central nervous system developing neurons, for example, neural cell adhesion molecule is localized to growth cones (Van Den Pol et al., 1986). Subsequent to or concomitant with termination is synaptogenesis that produces a functional connection, the characteristics of which will vary between axon and dendrite as well as among the various neurotransmitters selection. Termination might be reversible, allowing the regeneration of neurites.

Neuronal cell culture

The work of Sensenbrenner and colleagues (Booher and Sensenbrenner, 1972; Sensenbrenner et al., 1978; Pettman et al., 1979) and Kligman (1982) provided the basis for an excellent model of neurite outgrowth in the central nervous system. In the chicken embryo brain, the cells of cerebral cortex of a 7-day embryo are > 95% neuronal, postmitotic, and not fully differentiated (Booher and Sensenbrenner, 1972; Sensenbrenner et al., 1978). These cells can be removed by dissection, separated by trypsinization and gentle trituration, and maintained in serum-free, defined media (Bottenstein and Sato, 1979; Bottenstein et al., 1980) on poly-L-lysine coated polystyrene dishes at low density (5,000 cells/cm^2). Under these conditions, the cells are flat, phase-dark, and have few neurites. They survive well in culture, with > 80% survival over 24 h, but these cells do not proliferate. Upon treatment with neurotrophic factors, the cells elongate neuritic processes, and a quantitative assesment of neurite outgrowth can be made by counting the number of cells with one or more neurites that is at least one cell body in length. Extracts of adult bovine brain have neurotrophic activity, and Kligman (1982) characterized a heat-stable protein fraction of these extracts containing neurotrophic activity. The activity in such preparations is sensitive to trypsin digestion and to reduction and alkylation of sulfhydryls, indicating that protein(s) are required for neurite outgrowth (Kligman and Marshak, 1985). Further fractionation of the heat-stable extracts by anion exchange chromatography and reversed-phase, high-performance liquid chromatography resulted in the identification of a single peak of activity (Kligman and Marshak, 1985). Electrophoretic analysis of the protein showed multiple bands under non-reducing conditions, and a single band upon reduction. Sequence analysis of peptides derived from this protein showed that its primary structure was identical to a known protein, S100β, but reduction and alkylation of the neurite extension factor resulted in complete loss of activity. Thus, neurite extension appeared to be a property of a disulfide form of S100β. These observations provided the foundation for the study of S100β as a neurotrophic factor. This finding was unexpected, since S100β had been recognized for many years (Moore, 1965; Bock, 1978), but its true function was not established. S100β protein is likely to be multifunctional, with both intracellular and extracellular roles. Therefore, before continuing the discussion of the neurotrophic activity of S100β, it is important to review some of the major points in the history of S100β structure and function.

Structure and function of S100β

S100β is a member of family of proteins, the S100 proteins, that is a part of the superfamily of calcium-modulated proteins (Van Eldik et al., 1982). S100 was first identified by Moore (1965) who fractionated bovine brain and liver to define brain-enriched proteins. The name S100 is derived from the original observation that these proteins are soluble in saturated (100%) ammonium sulfate at neutral pH. The S100 proteins are acidic (pH = 4 − 5), small (M_r = 10,000 − 11,000), and bind calcium ions. For many years, S100 was touted as a "nervous system-specific" protein (Bock, 1978), since little or no protein was detected in liver or several other organs. However, during the last ten years this idea has been revised by the discovery of S100 proteins in a variety of tissues including melanocytes of skin (Gaynor et al., 1980; Cocchia et al., 1981), T-lymphocytes (Kanamori et al., 1982), adipocytes (Hidaka et al., 1983; Marshak et al., 1985), pituitary cells (Ishikawa et al., 1983; Girod et al., 1985), chondrocytes (Stefansson et al., 1982), and kidney (Molin et al., 1985). S100 proteins are highly enriched in the nervous system, and the bulk, if not all, of it resides in glia (Bock, 1978; Umekawa et al., 1985). The rat astrocytoma cell line C6 was isolated (Benda et al., 1968) on the basis of the cells' ability to synthesize S100. The C6 glioma cell line remains an important model system for the study of the S100 family of proteins, particularly S100β (Zimmer and Van Eldik, 1987, 1988, 1989).

In recent years several new members of the S100 protein family have been identified and partially characterized. Fig. 1 shows the amino acid sequences of these proteins and their homologies

```
                           *  *    *    *  *                                 *  *  *  *  *  *
S100β         SELEKAVVALIDVFHQYSGREGDKHKLKKSELKELINNELSHFLEEIKEQEVVDKVMETLDSDGDGECDFQEFMAFVAMITTACHEFFEHE

S100α         G    T MET N    AH K      Y S K      LQT    G DAQ DADA       KE EN     V       YVVL  AL V  NN    WENS
S100L         S P  Q LAVMVAT K    Q    F S G M    LHK    PS VG KVDE GLK L GD    ENS QQV     YAV L L  IM ND    QGSPARS
S100G         ARP  E LDVIVST K    K    F N T      LTR    PS LGKRTDEAAFQ    SN    NR N V      YCV LSC AMM N     GCPDKEPRKK
Calcyclin     ACP DQ IGL VAI K          T S K      QK   -TIGSKLQD-AEIARL D    RNK Q VN      YVT LGALALIYN ALKG-
Calpactin LC  PSQMEH METMMFT KFA---    GY T ED RV MEK   FPG L NQ DPLA    I KD  QCR KVG     S FSLI G  I ÑDY -VVHMKQKGKK
Cystic Fib. Ag LT    LNSI  Y K LIK NF AVYRDD  K LET      CPQYIRKKGADVWF-K---E    INT AVN      LIL IKMAWQPTKKAMKKATKSS
Calbindin₉ₖ    -----KSPEELKGI EK AAK    PNQ S E     L LQT FPSL KGPS---TL ELF E    KN      VS E   QVL KKISQ---------
```

Fig. 1. The S-100 family of proteins. The amino acid sequence for bovine S100β is shown on the top row. Potential ligands for coordinating divalent cations (Ca^{2+} and Zn^{2+}) are marked (*) according to Tufty and Kretsinger (1975) and Szebenyi et al. (1982). Below are shown the sequences for the proteins described in the text. Blank spaces represent identities with the S100β sequence, and dashes (−) represent gaps in the sequences introduced for the purposes of alignment (Szebenyi et al., 1982; Glenney et al., 1989).

172

with S100β, aligned according to Szebenyi et al. (1982) and Glenney et al. (1989).

(1) Bovine brain S100α is closely related in structure to S100β (Isobe and Okuyama, 1981). A study by Molin et al. (1985) indicated that immunoreactivity for S100α resides in kidney, raising the possibility that this protein is involved in the regulation of electrolytes.

(2) S100L (Glenney et al., 1989) is a novel S100 protein found in lung, kidney and liver, but not in brain. The localization of S100L appears to be both nuclear and cytosolic (Glenney et al., 1989).

(3) The growth-related protein, here designated S100G, has been identified by several laboratories as: 42A, an NGF inducible gene in PC12 cells (Masiakowski and Shooter, 1988); pEL98, a fibroblast protein (Goto et al., 1988); p9Ka, a cultured myoepithelial cell protein (Barraclough et al., 1987); 18A2 (Jackson-Grusby et al., 1987), a growth related mRNA from mouse fibroblasts; and *mts*-1 (Ebralidze et al., 1989), a gene specifically expressed in metastatic cells.

(4) Calcyclin is a growth regulated gene (Calabretta et al., 1986; Ferrari et al., 1987).

(5) The calpactin light chain (Glenney and Tack, 1985; Gerke and Weber, 1985) is a protein that binds to and regulates the phosphorylation of calpactin (p36), a major tyrosine kinase substrate (Saris et al., 1987; Hagiwara et al., 1988).

(6) The cystic fibrosis antigen (Dorin et al., 1987; Odink et al., 1988) is also a member of this family, indicating that calcium-binding proteins may be involved in this disease.

(7) Calbindin$_{9K}$ is an intestinal protein whose synthesis is induced by vitamin D (Van Eldik et al., 1982). Szebenyi et al. (1982) have analyzed the three-dimensional structure of this protein using X-ray diffraction.

When reading the S100 literature, it is important to remember that "S100 protein" is probably a mixture of S100β (see below) and some or all of these other, related proteins. Activities attributed to S100β must be done with purified, characterized, and homogeneous protein. Special attention should be given to post-translational modification (*N*-α-acetylation) and disulfide bond structure.

Structure

The primary structure of the S100 proteins remained unknown until Isobe et al. (1977) purified two major components of S100 from bovine brain, S100α and S100β, and determined their amino acid sequences (Isobe and Okuyama, 1978, 1981). These proteins consist of 93 and 91 amino acids, respectively (see Fig. 1), and their carboxy-terminal domains comprise a typical "EF-hand" calcium binding loop as described by Tufty and Kretsinger (1975). The amino-terminal portion of each molecule contains a highly basic region, from residues 20–33 of S100β, and a hydrophobic region, from residues 6–17 of S100β. Fig. 2 shows schematically the structural domains of S100β. The primary structure of S100β is highly conserved among mammals with only three amino acid substitutions between the bovine and human proteins (Jensen et al., 1985). Crystals of S100β suitable for diffraction analysis have been reported by Kretsinger et al. (1980), and it will be of interest if the three-dimensional structure of the protein is similar to that of the intestinal calcium-binding protein (Szebenyi et al., 1982). The preliminary crystal analysis indicated that S100β is in a dimeric

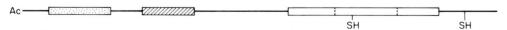

Fig. 2. Structural domains of S100β. The open block with vertical dashed lines represents the E-F hand, calcium ion binding domain (Tufty and Kretsinger, 1975) where the left and right portions are amphipathic α-helices and the central region is the loop containing the ligands for the calcium ion. The stippled region is the hydrophobic domain and the striped region is a cationic domain containing a high proportion of lysinyl, arginyl, and histidinyl residues. The cysteinyl residues are marked SH and the *N*-α-acetylation of the amino terminal serinyl residue is maked Ac. The entire protein is 91 amino acids in length (see Fig. 1) and the cysteinyl residues can form disulfide bonds (see text).

conformation, and Isobe and coworkers have shown that the purified S100 proteins form various sorts of non-covalent dimers (Isobe and Okuyama, 1981). However, all of these experiments are done in vitro, and the active state of any of the S100 proteins in vivo is unproven.

There are two chemical properties of the S100 proteins in general, and of S100β in particular that should be noted: divalent cation binding and reactivity of sulfhydryls. Early studies by Dannies and Levine (1971) revealed that S100 proteins contained sulfhydryl groups whose reactivity is altered by the presence of calcium ions and other divalent cations. Baudier et al. (1983) demonstrated zinc ion as well as calcium ion binding to S100 proteins. Kay and coworkers (Mani et al., 1982, 1983) investigated the changes in physicochemical and optical properties of S100 proteins in various ionic milieus. It is important to note that S100β contains two sulfhydryls (residues 68 and 84), while S100α has only one sulfhydryl (residue 85). The sulfhydryl group at residue 68 in S100β is likely to be significant because it falls between the X and Y coordinating ligands of the calcium binding loop and is likely to be the sulfhydryl regulated by divalent cations (see Fig. 1). S100β is the only known member of the S100 protein family that has a cysteine residue at this position. Thus, activities involving calcium dependent reaction with sulfhydryls is potentially specific to S100β.

Function

The biological activity of S100 proteins has not been established unequivocally. Several types of activities have been reported, most being in vitro biochemical activities. However, it is possible, and in fact likely, that S100β has multiple activities both intracellularly and extracellularly. Our work (Marshak, 1983; Marshak et al., 1981, 1985) and that of Hidaka and co-workers (reviewed in Umekawa et al., 1985) established the calcium-dependent interaction of S100 proteins with phenothiazine and naphthalene sulfonamide drugs. Calcium and zinc ion binding activities have been demonstrated in vitro (Baudier et al., 1986)

and Donato (1988) detailed the mechanism of S100 protein effects on the assembly and disassembly of microtubules in vitro. Baudier and Cole (1988b) have evidence that S100β forms disulfide cross-links to the microtubule associated tau(2) protein. This is significant because tau protein immunoreactivity is associated with neurofibrillary tangles found in Alzheimer disease (Selkoe, 1989). Treatment of C6 cells with anti-microtubular drugs results in a decrease in S100β mRNA (Dunn et al., 1987), suggesting that expression of the mRNA is partially regulated by the level of microtubules. In addition, the phosphorylation of tau protein by protein kinase C may be regulated by S100β (Baudier and Cole, 1988a). Finally, Zimmer and Van Eldik (1986) found that S100 proteins bind to and regulate the enzyme fructose 1,6-bisphosphate aldolase in vitro. All of the aforementioned biochemical activities are interesting but suffer from the lack of demonstration of an effect in vivo or in cells in culture. In many cases, these activities are not selective for S100β over other members of this family of proteins, or this was not tested.

Neurotrophic activity of S100β

The neurotrophic activity of S100β has been demonstrated in cell culture (Kligman and Marshak, 1985; Kligman and Hsieh, 1987; Van Eldik et al., 1988; Winningham-Major et al., 1988), but proof of this function in vivo has not yet been accomplished. Potential models for demonstration of the function are transgenic mice expressing the gene for S100β or expressing a cDNA construct for S100β with alternative promoters. An important role of S100β in vivo has been implicated by Griffin et al. (1989), who have recently shown increased immunoreactivity to S100 antisera in AD and DS brains. The relationships among the neurotrophic activity, the microtubule-associated activities, and the pathology of AD and DS are still unclear. However, the presence of the gene for S100β on human chromosome 21 (Allore et al., 1988) reinforces the notion that the neurotrophic activity of S100β might be involved in the neurological degeneration in AD and DS patients. At present, the information concerning the neurotrophic activity of S100β has two major parts, the expression and secretion of the protein from astrocytes during development and the mechanism of action of S100β as a neurotrophic factor.

Production of S100β by astrocytes

The major site of S100β production in the brain is astrocytes (Bock, 1978). S100β has been shown to be secreted from astrocytes (Suzuki et al., 1987; Zimmer and Van Eldik, 1987) as well as from adipocytes (Suzuki and Kato, 1985) and from novel pituitary cell lines, such as AtT20 (Ishikawa et al., 1983). During the log growth phase, S100β is secreted from C6 cells into the culture media (Zimmer and Van Eldik, 1987), while intracellular accumulation of S100β occurs when the cells are confluent or fully differentiated. Zimmer and Van Eldik (1989) described the localization of S100β to the microtubule organizing region of C6 cells upon differentiation with cAMP, although there is also S100β associated with Golgi. Thus, there appears to be an intracellular form of S100β, presumably associated with the microtubule network and an extracellular, secreted form of S100β. Our working model is that astrocytes synthesize and secrete a disulfide dimer form of S100β, and that this protein acts on neurons to cause neurite outgrowth in a receptor-mediated fashion. Demonstration of a receptor is in progress in several laboratories.

In the developing chicken embryo, the production of S100β correlates with the proliferation of astrocytes in the cerebral cortex and, concomitantly, the elaboration of processes by cortical neurons. We have developed an antiserum from rabbits that reacts with S100β in the monomer, dimer and polymer forms. Using this antiserum, a quantitative radioimmunoassay was performed on extracts of chicken embryo brains at various ages. As shown in Fig. 3, the level of S100β has small increases from days 5 – 10 and then increases linearly from day 10 – 18 of embryogenesis. There appear to be two phases of S100β production: an early

early phase with small changes (days 5 – 10) and a later phase with larger accumulation of protein (days 10 – 18). The cerebral cortical neurons isolated from 7-day embryos show very few glial cells, and astrocyte proliferation in this region occurs between days 7 and 10, during the initial phase of S100β production. This is also correlated in time with extensive neurite outgrowth from cortical neurons. The second phase of S100β accumulation would appear to be associated with confluent, mature astrocytes. Thus, during development of the cerebral cortex, we believe that S100β dimers, the neurite extension factor, are secreted from pro-

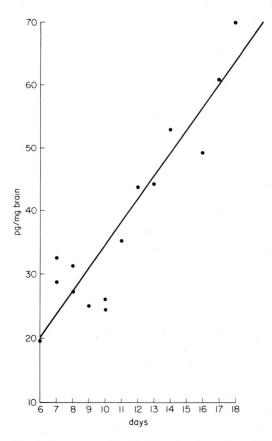

Fig. 3. Immunoreactive S100β in the developing chick brain. Quantitative analysis of S100β was done by radioimmunoassay using antisera specific for S100β. The ordinate shows the amount of immunoreactivity expressed in pg/mg wet weight of brain. The abscissa shows the age, in days, of the chicken embryos after fertilization.

liferating astrocytes and initiate neurite outgrowth from neurons.

Mechanism of action on neurons

Several experiments indicate that the action of S100β as a neurotrophic factor is distinct from that of other agents. First, the cell type specificity of S100β is largely in the central nervous system. Cells of the chick cerebral cortex and optic tectum respond, but dorsal root ganglia and sympathetic ganglia do not respond well to S100β. In culture, Neuro 2a cells can be stimulated by S100β, while PC12 cells cannot. A recent report (Winningham-Major et al., 1988) demonstrates that neonatal rat spinal cord cultures also respond to S100β. Chick cerebral cortical cells, which are sensitive to S100β, are not sensitive to NGF, bFGF, aFGF or EGF under the conditions of our assay (J. Figueiredo and D. Marshak, unpublished observations). Time course analysis of the action of S100β, reported by Winningham-Major et al. (1988), indicates that only 2 h of exposure is sufficient to promote neurite outgrowth, suggesting that S100β is an initiation factor.

The neurotrophic activity for S100β was the first demonstration of an activity that was specific to the oxidized form of S100β and that was demonstrated in a living system (i.e., cell culture). The results in Fig. 4 show that purified neurite extension factor (Kligman and Marshak, 1985; Kligman and Hsieh, 1987) that is predominantly an S100β disulfide dimer, has much higher specific activity than S100β purified by high-performance liquid chromatography (Marshak, 1983), that is predominantly monomer. The related protein, S100α has no neurotrophic activity (Fig. 4). Van Eldik et al. (1988) found that S100β expressed from a synthetic gene cloned in *E. coli* also shows neurotrophic activity, confirming the earlier observation on the native protein. In addition, mutation of the cysteine residues strongly diminishes the activity (Staecker et al., 1988). However, the specific

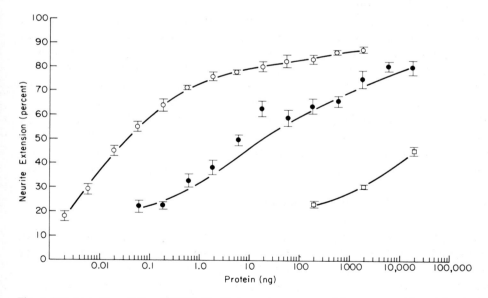

Fig. 4. Neurotrophic activity of S100β. Purified proteins were tested for neurotrophic activity on chick embryo neuronal cultures as described in the text. The ordinate shows the percentage of cells containing a neuritic process at least the length of one cell diameter after 24 h in culture. The abscissa shows the amount of protein in ng, and each assay was 1 ml total volume on 24-well tissue culture plates. The proteins tested are: open circles, S100β dimer, termed neurite extension factor (Kligman and Hsieh, 1987); filled circles, S100β prepared according to Marshak (1983) containing predominantly monomer; and open squares, S100α from bovine brain, prepared according to Marshak (1983). The points shown are the average of quadruplicate assays with standard errors as shown by the bars.

176

activity of the bacterially expressed protein is low, suggesting that a modification found in the mammalian product is lacking or that the protein is partially denatured.

Expression cloning of S100β

The cDNA molecules for S100β have been cloned by at least two groups (Kuwano et al., 1984; Dunn et al., 1987), and a synthetic gene constructed for expression in *E. coli* (Van Eldik et al., 1988). Because of the amino terminal acetylation and the potential for dimerization, we chose to isolate a cDNA clone for S100β from a mammalian expression library. Using synthetic oligonucleotides based on the 5' and 3' ends of the coding region of the clone reported by Kuwano et al. (1984), we selected a cDNA clone from a rat brain cDNA library in the mammalian expression vector pcD2 (Chen and Okayama, 1987). This plasmid contains the SV40 early promoter and is useful for transfection in COS cells. These cells, derived from the monkey cell line CV1, contain high levels of T antigen, allowing replication and expression of the plasmid. Cells were transfected using calcium phosphate precipitation at pH 7.05 for 4 h, followed by glyceral shock for 1 min, and incubation for 48 h. The cells were labeled for 4 h with ^{35}S-methionine, washed, and harvested. The cells were lysed in 50 mM Tris-HCl, 5 mM EDTA, 0.1% (v/v) NP40, and the S100β in the lysate was immunoprecipitated using the methods described by Harlow and Lane (1988). The immunoprecipitated material was subjected to polyacrylamide gel electrophoresis in the presence of sodium dodecyl sulfate and 2-mercaptoethanol, using the buffer system of Laemmli (1970), and subsequently subjected to autoradiography. The results, shown in Fig. 5, demonstrate that cells transfected with 5 μg and 20 μg of plasmid expressed a product that co-migrates with S100β and mock transfected cells show none of this material. Further experiments were performed with transfected, unlabeled cells. The cells were lysed in buffer without detergent, and the extracts were heated to 80°C for 10 min and centrifuged. The resulting

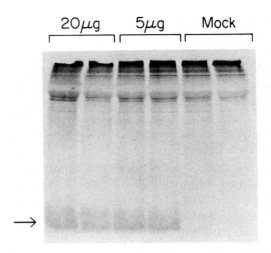

Fig. 5. Immunoprecipitation of S100β expressed in COS I cells. Cells were transfected with 5 μg or 20 μg plasmid (as indicated) or with salmon sperm DNA (mock). The cells were labeled and extracted as described in the text. The extracts were subjected to polyacrylamide gel electrophoresis and autoradiography. The arrow shows the position of migration of S100β.

supernatants were tested for neurotrophic activity and compared with identical extracts from cells that were transfected with non-specific DNA, mock transfected, or untreated (Fig. 6). Transfected cells showed significant neurotrophic activity on the chick embryo cerebral cortical cells, while all three controls were negative. These results demonstrate that expression of S100β cDNA in mammalian cells confers a heat-stable neurotrophic activity that is indistinguishable from S100β.

Summary

S100β is a multifunctional protein that is found in large amounts in astrocytes and a number of other tissues. In the developing nervous system, S100β is secreted from proliferating astrocytes during the time of neurite outgrowth from cortical neurons. The secreted form has neurotrophic activity on primary neurons and neuroblastoma cells. The neurotrophic activity is sensitive to reduction of disulfide bonds, and appears to be a disulfide dimer of S100β. The accumulation of S100β in

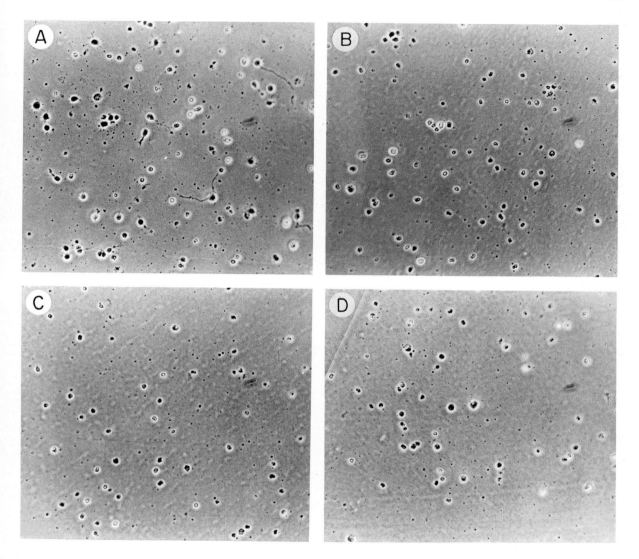

Fig. 6. Neurotrophic activity of transfected cells. COS I cells were transfected with plasmid carrying the S100β cDNA, harvested, and extracted as described in the text. The extracts were heated to 80°C for 10 min and centrifuged to remove precipitate. The resulting supernatants were tested for neurotrophic activity in the chick embryo neuronal culture system as described (Kligman, 1982). Cells were treated with: *A*, plasmid containing S100β cDNA; *B*, salmon sperm DNA; *C*, no DNA; *D*, no DNA and no calcium phosphate precipitation or glycerol shock.

mature glial cells is associated with microtubule network. The transfection and expression of cDNA for S100β in mammalian cells confers neurotrophic activity on extracts of these cells. Based on our observations of a neurotrophic activity for S100β, the occurrence of the gene for S100β on human chromosome 21 (Allore et al., 1988) and the elevated levels of S100β-containing cells in AD and DS brains (Griffin et al., 1989), we suggest that S100β plays a role in the abnormal development of the nervous system in DS and the degeneration of central neurons in AD. It is essential at the present stage to demonstrate the action of S100β in vivo, and to construct animal models, such as transgenic mice, that overexpress S100β. Such models will allow the dissection of the role of S100β in the developing and degenerating central nervous system.

Acknowledgements

This work was supported by the National Science Foundation (NSF Grant BNS8707558), The Esther A. and Joseph Klingenstein Foundation, and The Marie Robertson Fund for Neuroscience.

I thank S. Pesce and R. Tonner for technical assistance; J. Figueiredo, D. Helfman, M. Kessler, and A. Rice for assistance in cloning and transfection experiments; and M. Schmiedeskamp for assistance in characterizing the antisera and performing radioimmunoassays.

References

Allore, R., O'Hanlon, D., Price, R., Neilson, K., Willard, H.F., Cox, D.R., Marks, A. and Dunn, R.J. (1988) Gene encoding the β subunit of S100 protein is on chromosome 21: implications for Down syndrome. *Science, 239*: 1311 – 1313.

Barde, Y.-A., Edgar, D. and Thoenen, H. (1983) New neurotrophic factors. *Annu. Rev. Physiol., 45*: 601 – 612.

Barraclough, R., Savin, J., Dube, S.K. and Rudland, P.S. (1987) Molecular cloning and sequence of the gene for p9Ka, a cultured myoepithelial cell protein with strong homology to S-100, a calcium binding protein. *J. Mol. Biol., 198*: 13 – 20.

Basi, G.S., Jacobson, R.D., Virag, I., Schilling, J. and Skene, J.H.P. (1987) Primary structure and transcriptional regulation of GAP-43, a protein associated with nerve growth. *Cell, 49*: 785 – 791.

Baudier, J. and Cole, R.D. (1988a) Interactions between the microtubule-associated proteins and S100b regulate τ phosphorylation by the Ca^{2+}/calmodulin-dependent protein kinase II. *J. Biol. Chem., 263*: 5876 – 5883.

Baudier, J. and Cole, R.D. (1988b) Reinvestigation of the sulfhydryl reactivity in bovine brain S100b ($\beta\beta$) protein and the microtubule-associated τ proteins. Ca^{2+} stimulates disulfide cross-linking between the S100b β-subunit and the microtubule-associated $\tau(2)$ protein. *Biochemistry, 27*: 2728 – 2736.

Baudier, J., Haglid, K., Haiech, J. and Gerard, D. (1983) Zinc ion binding to human brain calcium binding proteins calmodulin and S100B. *Biochem. Biophys. Res. Commun., 114*: 1138 – 1146.

Baudier, J., Glasser, N. and Gerard, D. (1986) Ions binding to S100 proteins. *J. Biol. Chem., 261*: 8192 – 8203.

Benda, P., Lightbody, J., Sato, G.H., Levine, L. and Sweet, W. (1968) Differentiated rat glial cell strain in tissue culture. *Science, 161*: 370 – 371.

Bock, E. (1978) Nervous system specific proteins. *J. Neurochem., 30*: 7 – 14.

Booher, J. and Sensenbrenner, M. (1972) Growth and cultivation of dissociated neurons and glial cells from embryonic chick, rat and human brain in flask cultures. *Neurobiology, 2*: 97 – 105.

Bottenstein, J.E. and Sato, G.H. (1979) Growth of a rat neuroblastoma cell line in serum-free, supplemented medium. *Proc. Natl. Acad. Sci. U.S.A., 76*: 514 – 517.

Bottenstein, J.E., Skaper, S.D., Varon, S.S. and Sato, G. (1980) Selective survival of neurons from chick embryo sensory ganglionic dissociates utilizing serum-free supplemented medium. *Exp. Cell Res., 125*: 183 – 190.

Bray, D. and Hollenbeck, P.J. (1988) Growth cone motility and guidance. *Annu. Rev. Cell Biol., 4*: 43 – 61.

Burgoyne, R.D. (1986) Microtubule proteins in neuronal differentiation. *Comp. Biochem. Physiol., 83B*: 1 – 8.

Calabretta, B., Battini, R., Kaczmarek, L., De Riel, J.K. and Baserga, R. (1986) Molecular cloning of the cDNA for a growth factor-inducible gene with strong homology to S-100, a calcium-binding protein. *J. Biol. Chem., 261*: 12628 – 12632.

Chen, C. and Okayama, H. (1987) High-efficiency transformation of mammalian cells by plasmid DNA. *Mol. Cell. Biol., 7*: 2745 – 2752.

Cocchia, D., Michetti, F. and Donato, R. (1981) Immunochemical and immunocytochemical localization of S100 antigen in normal human skin. *Nature, 294*: 85 – 87.

Curran, T., Rauscher, F.J., III, Cohen, D.R. and Franza, B.R., Jr. (1988) Beyond the second messenger: oncogenes and transcription factors. *C.S.H. Symp. Quant. Biol., 53*: 769 – 778.

Dannies, P.S. and Levine, L. (1971) The role of sulfhydryl groups in serological properties of bovine brain S-100 protein. *J. Biol. Chem., 246*: 6284 – 6287.

Donato, R. (1988) Calcium-dependent, pH-regulated effects of S-100 proteins on assembly – disassembly of brain microtubules in vitro. *J. Biol. Chem., 263*: 235 – 238.

Dorin, J.R., Novak, M., Hill, R.E., Brock, D.J.H., Secher, D.S. and Van Heyningen, V. (1987) A clue to the basic defect in cystic fibrosis from cloning the CF antigen gene. *Nature, 326*: 614 – 617.

Dunn, R., Landry, C., O'Hanlon, D., Dunn, J., Allore, R., Brown, I. and Marks, A. (1987) Reduction in S100 protein β subunit mRNA in C6 rat glioma cells following treatment with anti-microtubular drugs. *J. Biol. Chem., 262*: 3562 – 3566.

Ebralidze, A., Tulchinsky, E., Grigorian, M., Afanasyeva, A., Senin, V., Revazova, E. and Lukanidin, E. (1989) Isolation and characterization of a gene specifically expressed in different metastatic cells and whose deduced gene product has a high degree of homology to a calcium-binding protein family. *Genes Dev.,* 3: 1086 – 1095.

Edelman, G.M. (1985) Cell adhesion and the molecular processes of morphogenesis. *Ann. Rev. Biochem.,* 54: 135 – 170.

Epstein, C.J. (1986) Trisomy 21 and the nervous system: from cause to cure. In: C.J. Epstein (Ed.), *The Neurobiology of Down Syndrome,* Raven Press, New York, pp. 1 – 15.

Epstein, C.J. (1987) The consequences of altered gene dosage in trisomy 21. In: S.M. Pueschel, C. Tingey, J.E. Rynders, A.C. Crocker and D.M. Crutcher (Eds.), *New Perspectives on Down Syndrome,* Paul H. Brookes, Baltimore, MD, pp. 69 – 80.

Epstein, C.J., Anneren, K.G., Foster, D., Groner, Y., Prusiner, S.B. and Smith, S.A. (1987) Pathogenic relationships between Down's syndrome and Alzheimer's disease: studies with animal models. In: P. Davies and C.E. Finch (Eds.), *Banbury Report 27: Molecular Neuropathology of Aging,* Cold Spring Harbor Laboratory, Cold Spring Harbor, NY, pp. 339 – 352.

Ferrari, S., Calabretta, B., DeRiel, J.K., Battini, R., Ghezzo, F., Lauret, E., Griffin, C., Emanuel, B.S., Gurrieri, F. and Baserga, R. (1987) Structural and functional analysis of a growth regulated gene, the human calcyclin. *J. Biol. Chem.,* 262: 8325 – 8332.

Gaynor, R., Irie, R., Morton, D. and Herschman, H.R. (1980) S100 protein is present in cultured human malignant melanomas. *Nature,* 286: 400 – 401.

Gerke, V. and Weber, K. (1985) The regulatory chain in the p36-kd substrate complex of viral tyrosine-specific protein kinases is related in sequence to the S-100 protein of glial cells. *EMBO J.,* 4: 2917 – 2920.

Girod, C., Trouillas, J. and Dubois, M.P. (1985) Immunocytochemical localization of S-100 protein in stellate cells (folliculo-stellate cells) of the anterior lobe of the normal human pituitary. *Cell Tiss. Res.,* 241: 505 – 511.

Glenney, J.R., Jr. and Tack, B.F. (1985) Amino-terminal sequence of p36 and associated p10: identification of the site of tyrosine phosphorylation and homology with S-100. *Proc. Natl. Acad. Sci. U.S.A.,* 82: 7884 – 7888.

Glenney, J.R., Jr., Kindy, M.S. and Zokas, L. (1989) Isolation of a new member of the S100 protein family: amino acid sequence, tissue and subcellular distribution. *J. Cell Biol.,* 108: 569 – 578.

Goto, K., Endo, H. and Fujiyoshi, T. (1988) Cloning of the sequence expressed abundantly in established cell lines: identification of a cDNA clone homologous to S-100, a calcium binding protein. *J. Biochem.,* 103: 48 – 53.

Griffin, W.S.T., Stanley, L.C., Ling, C., White, L., MacLeod, V., Perrot, L.J., White, C.L., III, and Araoz, C. (1989) Brain interleukin 1 and S100 immunoreactivity are elevated in Down's syndrome and Alzheimer's disease. *Proc. Natl. Acad. Sci. U.S.A.,* in press.

Guenther, J., Hanspeter, N. and Monard, D. (1985) A glia-derived neurite promoting factor with protease inhibitory activity. *EMBO J.,* 4: 1963 – 1966.

Hagiwara, M., Ochiai, M., Owanda, K., Tanaka, T. and Hidaka, H. (1988) Modulation of tyrosine phosphorylation of p36 and other substrates by the S-100 protein. *J. Biol. Chem.,* 263: 6438 – 6441.

Harlow, E. and Lane, D. (1988) *Antibodies, a Laboratory Manual,* Cold Spring Harbor Laboratory, Cold Spring Harbor, NY, pp. 421 – 461.

Hidaka, H., Endo, T., Kawamoto, S., Yamada, E., Umekawa, H., Tanabe, K. and Hara, K. (1983) Purification and characterization of adipose tissue S-100b protein. *J. Biol. Chem.,* 258: 2705 – 2710.

Ishikawa, H., Nogami, H. and Shirasawa, N. (1983) Novel clonal strains from adult rat anterior pituitary producing S-100 protein. *Nature,* 303: 711 – 713.

Isobe, T. and Okuyama, T. (1978) The amino acid sequence of S100 protein (PAPI-b protein) and its relation to the calcium-binding proteins. *Eur. J. Biochem.,* 89: 379 – 388.

Isobe, T. and Okuyama, T. (1981) The amino-acid sequence of the alpha subunit in bovine brain S-100a protein. *Eur. J. Biochem.,* 116: 79 – 86.

Isobe, T., Nakajima, T. and Okuyama, T. (1977) Reinvestigation of the extremely acidic proteins in bovine brain. *Biochim. Biophys. Acta,* 494: 222 – 232.

Jackson-Grusby, L.L., Swiergiel, J. and Linzer, D.I.H. (1987) A growth related mRNA in cultured mouse cells encodes a placental calcium binding protein. *Nucleic Acids Res.,* 15: 6677 – 6690.

Jensen, R., Marshak, D.R., Anderson, C., Lukas, T.J. and Watterson, D.M. (1985) Purification and characterization of human brain S100 protein components: amino acid sequence of human S100β. *J. Neurochem.,* 45: 700 – 705.

Kanamori, M., Endo, T., Shirikawa, S., Sakurai, M. and Hidaka, H. (1982) S-100 antigen in human T-lymphocytes. *Biochem. Biophys. Res. Commun.,* 108 1447 – 1452.

Kligman, D. (1982) Isolation of a protein from bovine brain which promotes neurite extension from chick embryo cerebral cortex neurons in defined medium. *Brain Res.,* 250: 93 – 100.

Kligman, D. and Hsieh, L.-S. (1987) Neurite extension factor induces rapid morphological differentiation of mouse neuroblastoma cells in defined medium. *Dev. Brain Res.,* 33: 296 – 300.

Kligman, D. and Marshak, D.R. (1985) Isolation and characterization of a neurite extension factor from bovine brain. *Proc. Natl. Acad. Sci. U.S.A.,* 82: 7136 – 7139.

Kretsinger, R.H., Rudnick, S.E., Sneden, D.A. and Schatz, V.B. (1980) Calmodulin, S-100 and crayfish sarcoplasmic calcium-binding protein crystals suitable for X-ray diffraction studies. *J. Biol. Chem.,* 255: 8154 – 8156.

Kuwano, R., Usui, H., Maeda, T., Fukui, T., Yamanari, N., Ohtsuka, E., Ikehara, M. and Takahashi, Y. (1984) Molec-

180

ular cloning and complete nucleotide sequence of cDNA to mRNA for S-100 protein of rat brain. *Nucleic Acids Res.,* 12: 7455 – 7465.

Laemmli, U.K. (1970) Cleavage of structural proteins during the assembly of the head of bacteriophage T4. *Nature,* 227: 680 – 681.

Leder, A.D., Fuji, D.K. and Reichardt, L.F. (1985) Purification of a factor that promotes neurite outgrowth: isolation of laminin and associated molecules. *J. Cell Biol.,* 101: 898 – 913.

Levi-Montalcini, R. and Angeletti, P.U. (1986) Nerve growth factor. *Physiol. Rev.,* 48: 534 – 569.

Lipton, S.A., Frosch, M.P., Phillips, M.D., Tauck, D.L. and Aizenman, E. (1988a) Nicotinic antagonists enhance process outgrowth by rat retinal ganglion cells in culture. *Science,* 239: 1293 – 1296.

Lipton, S.A., Wagner, J.A., Madison, R.D. and D'Amore, P.A. (1988b) Acidic fibroblast growth factor enhance regeneration of processes by postnatal mammalian retinal ganglion cells in culture. *Proc. Natl. Acad. Sci. U.S.A.,* 85: 2388 – 2392.

Mani, R.S., Boyes, B.E. and Kay, C.M. (1982) Physicochemical and optical studies on calcium and potassium-induced conformational changes in bovine brain S-100b protein. *Biochemistry,* 21: 2607 – 2612.

Mani, R.S., Shelling, J.G., Sykes, B.D. and Kay, C.M. (1983) Spectral studies of the calcium binding properties of bovine brain S-100b protein. *Biochemistry,* 22: 1734 – 1740.

Marshak, D.R. (1983) *Comparative Biochemistry of Drug-Binding Proteins in the Calmodulin/S100 Family.* Doctoral Dissertation, The Rockefeller University, New York, pp. 37 – 40.

Marshak, D.R., Watterson, D.M. and Van Eldik, L.J. (1981) Calcium-dependent interaction of S100b, troponin C and calmodulin with an immobilized phenothiazine. *Proc. Natl. Acad. Sci. U.S.A.,* 78: 6793 – 6797.

Marshak, D.R., Umekawa, H., Watterson, D.M. and Hidaka, H. (1985) Structural characterization of the calcium binding protein S100 from adipose tissue. *Arch. Biochem. Biophys.,* 240: 777 – 780.

Masiakowski, P. and Shooter, E.M. (1988) Nerve growth factor induces the genes for two proteins related to a family of calcium-binding proteins in PC12 cells. *Proc. Natl. Acad. Sci. U.S.A.,* 85: 1277 – 1281.

Metz, R., Gorham, J., Siegfried, Z., Leonard, D., Gizang-Ginsberg, A., Thompson, M.A., Lawe, D., Kouzarides, T., Vosatka, R., MacGregor, D., Jamal, S., Greenberg, M.E. and Ziff, E.B. (1988) Gene regulation by growth factors. *C.S.H. Symp. Quant. Biol.,* 53: 727 – 738.

Molin, S.-O., Rosengren, L., Baudier, J., Hamberger, A. and Haglid, K. (1985) S-100 alpha-like immunoreactivity in tubules of rat kidney. A clue to the function of a "brain-specific" protein. *J. Histochem. Cytochem.,* 33: 367 – 374.

Monard, D. (1985) Neuronal cell behavior: modulation by pro-

tease inhibitors derived from non-neuronal cells. *Cell Biol. Int. Rep.,* 9: 297 – 305.

Moore, B. (1965) A soluble protein characteristic of the nervous system. *Biochem. Biophys. Res. Commun.,* 19: 739 – 744.

Odink, K., Cerletti, N., Bruggen, J., Clerc, R.G., Tarcsay, L., Zwadlo, G., Schlegel, R. and Sorg, C. (1987) Two calcium-binding proteins in infiltrate macrophages of rheumatoid arthritis. *Nature,* 330: 80 – 82.

Pettman, B., Louis, J.C. and Sensenbrenner, M. (1979) Morphological and biochemical maturation of neurones cultures in the absence of glial cells. *Nature,* 281: 378 – 380.

Pittman, R.N. and Patterson, P.H. (1987) Characterization of an inhibitor of neuronal plasminogen activator released by heart cells. *J. Neurosci.,* 7: 2664 – 2673.

Price, D.L. (1986) New perspectives on Alzheimer's disease. *Annu. Rev. Neurosci.,* 9: 489 – 517.

Rakic, P. (1988) Specification of cerebral cortical areas. *Science,* 241: 170 – 176.

Ramon y Cajal, S. (1928) *Degeneration and Regeneration in the Nervous System* (translated by R.M. May), Oxford Univ. Press, London, pp. 329 – 361.

Rubin, L.L. and Porter, S. (1989) Cell biology of the blood-brain barrier. In: D.R. Marshak and D.T. Liu (Eds.), *Therapeutic Peptides and Proteins: Formulation, Delivery and Targeting,* Cold Spring Harbor Laboratory, Cold Spring Harbor, NY, pp. 81 – 83.

Sanes, J.R. (1989) Extracellular matric molecules that influence neural development. *Annu. Rev. Neurosci.,* 12: 491 – 516.

Saris, C.J.M., Kristensen, T., D'Eustachio, P., Hicks, L.J., Noonan, D.J., Hunter, T. and Tack, B.F. (1987) cDNA sequence and tissue distribution of the mRNA for bovine and murine p11, the S100-related light chain of the protein tyrosine kinase substrate p36 (calpactin I). *J. Biol. Chem.,* 262: 10663 – 10671.

Selkoe, D.J. (1989) Biochemistry of altered brain proteins in Alzheimer's disease. *Annu. Rev. Neurosci.,* 12: 463 – 490.

Sensenbrenner, M., Maderspach, K., Latzkovits, L. and Jaros, G.G. (1978) Neuronal cells from chick embryo cerebral hemispheres cultivated on polylysine-coated surfaces. *Dev. Neurosci.,* 1: 90 – 101.

Skene, J.H.P. (1989) Axonal growth-associated proteins. *Annu. Rev. Neurosci.,* 12: 127 – 156.

Skene, J.H.P. and Willard, M. (1981) Axonally transported proteins associated with axon growth in rabbit central and peripheral nervous system. *J. Cell Biol.,* 89: 96 – 103.

Staecker, J.L., Winningham-Major, F. and Van Eldik, L.J. (1988) Mutation of the cysteines in S100β affects neurotrophic activity. *J. Cell Biol.,* 107: 510a.

Stefansson, K., Wollmann, R.L., Moore, B.W. and Arnason, B.G.W. (1982) S-100 protein in human chondrocytes. *Nature,* 295: 63 – 65.

Suzuki, F. and Kato, K. (1985) Inhibition of adipose S-100 protein release by insulin. *Biochim. Biophys. Acta,* 845: 311 – 316.

Suzuki, F., Kato, K., Kato, T. and Ogasawara, N. (1987) S-100 protein in clonal astroglioma cells is released by adrenocorticotropic hormone and corticotropin-like intermediate-lobe peptide. *J. Neurochem.*, 49: 1557 – 1563.

Szebenyi, D.M.E., Obendorf, S.K. and Moffat, K. (1982) Structure of vitamin D-dependent calcium-binding protein from bovine intestine. *Nature,* 294: 327 – 332.

Thoenen, H. and Edgar, D. (1985) Neurotrophic factors. *Science,* 229: 238 – 242.

Tsuji, S., Yamashita, T., Tanaka, M. and Nagai, Y. (1988) Synthetic sialyl compounds as well as natural gangliosides induce neuritogenesis in a mouse neuroblastoma cell line (Neuro 2a). *J. Neurochem.*, 50: 414 – 423.

Tufty, R.M. and Kretsinger, R.H. (1975) Troponin and parvalbumin calcium binding regions predicted in myosin light chain and T4 lysozyme. *Science,* 187: 167 – 169.

Umekawa, H., Naka, M., Inagaki, M. and Hidaka, H. (1985) Interaction of W-7, a calmodulin antagonist, with another Ca^{2+}-binding protein. In: H. Hidaka and D.J. Hartshorne (Eds.), *Calmodulin Antagonists and Cellular Physiology,* Academic Press, New York, pp. 511 – 524.

Van Den Pol, A.N., di Porzio, U. and Rutishauser, U. (1986) Growth cone localization of neuronal cell adhesion molecule on central nervous system neurons in vitro. *J. Cell Biol.,* 102: 2281 – 2294.

Van Eldik, L.J., Zendegui, J.G., Marshak, D.R. and Watterson, D.M. (1982) Calcium binding proteins and the molecular basis of calcium action. *Int. Rev. Cytol.,* 77: 1 – 61.

Van Eldik, L.J., Staecker, J.L. and Winningham-Major, F.W. (1988) Synthesis and expression of a gene coding for the calcium modulated protein S100β and designed for casette-based, site-directed mutagenesis. *J. Biol. Chem.,* 263: 7830 – 7837.

Walicke, P.A. (1989) Novel neurotrophic factors, receptors, and oncogenes. *Annu. Rev. Neurosci.,* 12: 103 – 126.

Walicke, P., Cowan, W.M., Ueno, N., Baird, A. and Guillemin, R. (1986) Fibroblast growth factor promotes survival of dissociated hippocampal neurons and enhances neurite extension. *Proc. Natl. Acad. Sci. U.S.A.,* 83: 3012 – 3016.

Winningham-Major, F., Whetsell, W.O. and Van Eldik, L.J. (1988) Recombinant neurotrophic factor stimulates neurite outgrowth in nervous system cultures. *J. Cell Biol.,* 107: 729a.

Yankner, B.A. and Shooter, E.M. (1982) The biology and mechanism of action of nerve growth factor. *Annu. Rev. Biochem.,* 51: 845 – 868.

Zimmer, D.B. and Van Eldik, L.J. (1986) Identification of a molecular target for the calcium-modulated protein S100: fructose-1,6-biphosphate aldolase. *J. Biol. Chem.,* 261: 11424 – 11428.

Zimmer, D.B. and Van Eldik, L.J. (1987) Secretion of S-100 from rat C6 glioma cells. *Brain Res.,* 436: 367 – 370.

Zimmer, D.B. and Van Eldik, L.J. (1988) Levels and distribution of the calcium-modulated proteins S100 and calmodulin in rat C6 glioma cells. *J. Neurochem.,* 50: 572 – 579.

Zimmer, D.B. and Van Eldik, L.J. (1989) Analysis of the calcium-modulated proteins, S100 and calmodulin, and their target proteins during C6 glioma cell differentiation. *J. Cell Biol.,* 108: 141 – 151.

P. Coleman, G. Higgins and C. Phelps (Eds.)
Progress in Brain Research, Vol. 86
© 1990 Elsevier Science Publishers B.V. (Biomedical Division)

CHAPTER 15

Growth factor-mediated protection in aging CNS

Karin Werrbach-Perez, George Jackson, Dario Marchetti, Brent Morgan, Larry Thorpe and J. Regino Perez-Polo

Department of Human Biological Chemistry and Genetics, The University of Texas Medical Branch, Galveston, TX 77550-2777, U.S.A.

Introduction

Much of the research that has taken place during the last decade on aging and degenerative diseases of the aged nervous system attempted to define those cellular and molecular parameters that might be labeled as "markers" for the aging process. It was often assumed that age-associated cognitive or physiological deficits reflected metabolic deficiencies. This approach to the study of the aging phenomena is in line with strategies being applied to brain and spinal trauma research and, in the periphery, PNS, to the study of neuronal development. Not surprisingly, it has been difficult to elaborate unitary hypotheses that can withstand close scrutiny. It is true that aging, aging-associated neurological diseases, injury to the CNS and certain aspects of PNS development are characterized by restriction of growth factor availability to neurons and the resulting neuronal cell death of deprived neurons. These events can also lead to glial activation and gliosis with increases in the levels of cytokines, hormones and other growth factors in situ. Some examples of this kind of behavior have been described for the hippocampus, where lesions can lead to sympathetic sprouting into hippocampal areas, and in contused monkey spinal cord, where the introduction of nerve growth factor (NGF) can dramatically increase peripheral sprouting with deleterious effects on functional recovery (Nieto-Sampedro et al.,

1982, 1983, 1984; Eidelberg et al., 1984). More recently, Cotman has suggested that such sprouting in brain may take place in Alzheimer's disease (AD) in response to the neuronal cell death and atrophy that has been reported for aged rodent and human CNS. Thus, the reported neuronal tangles and plaques present in AD may be but a dramatic accumulation of aberrant axonal sprouting (Cotman, this volume). This would suggest that cell injury and death can themselves trigger increased availability of trophic and tropic substances which can then act in a paracrine fashion. Stimulatory effects on other non-neuronal cell targets may bring about a disruption of intercellular communication that results in a secondary wave of damaging events. Perhaps, this is the phenomenon that is expressed as a neurotoxic activity, described as being lesion-induced in the hippocampus (Nieto-Sampedro and Cotman, 1985). Complementary events have been described where relatively low concentrations of toxic substances, such as hydrogen peroxide, can have trophic effects in vitro (Nishimura et al., 1988; Jackson et al., 1990). It has been proposed that there is a xenobiotic response that is responsible for the inductive effects of conditioning lesions in vivo and in vitro (Jackson et al., 1990).

Since neuronotrophic factors have been shown to have cell sparing effects in CNS and PNS following injury (Williams et al., 1986; Windebank and Poduslo, 1986; Kromer, 1987; Montero and

184

Hefti, 1988), it has been proposed that they may play an important role in the three physiological events here discussed: neuronal development, injury and aging. Thus, it would be of interest to understand how neuronotrophic activity abrogates neuronal cell death. Our hypothesis is that neuronal cell death is mediated in part by a shift in neuronal oxidant – antioxidant balance and that at least one neuronotrophic factor, NGF, regulates cell death by stimulating antioxidant systems (Perez-Polo et al., 1986). In particular, we have found that NGF does protect neurons in culture from peroxyl radical generators such as 6-hydroxy-dopamine and hydrogen peroxide, in part, by inducing catalase activity, low levels of which are expressed by neuronal as compared to non-neuronal cell lines (Perez-Polo and Werrbach-Perez, 1985, 1987, 1988). In the rodent brain, we also have preliminary evidence that NGF induces catalase activity. Thus, aging-associated deficits in cholinergic NGF-responsive neurons and the suggested beneficial effects of NGF treatment in CNS may be due to shifts in the oxidant – antioxidant balance as a consequence of changes in NGF activity (Fig. 1).

NGF deficits

What is meant by NGF activity deficits and how can they be measured? Although a list can easily be generated based on the known effects of NGF (See Table I and II), the first obligatory event that is required for NGF action is the binding of the NGF molecule to NGF receptors on cell surfaces, NGFR (Banerjee et al., 1973; Herrup and Shooter, 1973; Frazier et al., 1974). Here we will discuss one approach to the characterization of NGF action in CNS by discussing the properties of the NGF receptor. Also, we will consider the significance of reported deficits in NGF binding to some regions of the CNS of the aged rat with specific emphasis on one outcome of cellular behavior that appears to be under NGF control in vivo and in vitro development, injury and aging: cell death.

Cell death

Cell death during the ontogeny of the nervous system allows for competitive innervation of targets (Hamburger and Oppenheim, 1982; Oppenheim, 1985). At critical stages in development,

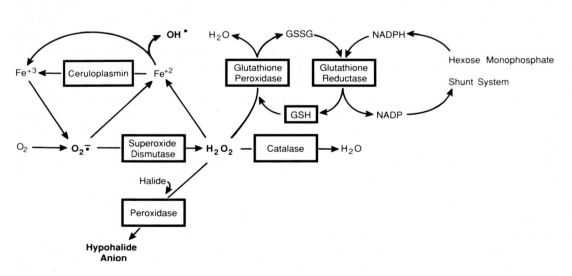

Fig. 1. Some aspects of oxidant – antioxidant balance.

TABLE I

Effects of NGF on PC-12 and SY5Y

1. Development of membrane electrical excitability
2. Increased synthesis, assembly and stabilization of cytoskeletal structures
3. Increased cell adhesion
4. Hypertrophy and increased anabolic activity
5. Diminished DNA synthesis and cellular proliferation
6. Selective induction of antioxidant and energy metabolism
7. Permissive stimulation of neurotransmitter metabolism
8. Altered gene expression

TABLE II

Deficits in NGF action

1. Reduced synthesis, processing, post-translational processing and secretion of NGF
2. Expression and processing of NGF with altered structure
3. Reduced synthesis, processing, post-translational processing and membrane insertion of NGFR
4. Expression and processing of NGFR with altered structure
5. Altered association of low affinity NGFR or conversion to high affinity NGFR by interaction with a receptor-associated protein or altered glycosylation of the NGFR apoprotein
6. Losses of NGFR bearing cells
7. Reduced intracellular transport of NGFR-bound NGF
8. Altered or reduced second messenger systems present for NGF – NGFR action following binding of the NGF

neurons that successfully compete for target-derived trophic factors, such as NGF, are spared cell death (Hamburger and Yip, 1984; Levi-Montalcini, 1987). Withdrawal of NGF by anti-NGF has been shown to have significant and permanent stimulatory effects on axonal sprouting, while reducing survival of sympathetic, sensory and striatal neurons (Yip and Johnson, 1984; Hulsebosch et al., 1987; Levi-Montalcini, 1987; Montero and Hefti, 1988). The relationship among neuronal cell death during development and its counterparts in injury and aging is not known. Cycloheximide, a protein synthesis inhibitor, protects sympathetic neurons from developmental

neuronal death where it may suppress expression of "suicide genes" (Martin et al., 1988). However, there are other alternatives to this explanation. Since neurons have low endogenous levels of antioxidants, the regulation of the intracellular oxidant – antioxidant balance by NGF may be the controlling agent that regulates neuronal death in development, injury and aging. It is a corollary of this hypothesis that aging-associated deficits may be due to reductions in neuronotrophic activity leading to shifts in oxidant – antioxidant balance. Such metabolic shifts could impair the ability of neurons to cope with free-radical induced damage and also diminish energy metabolism directly by acting on the glutathione pathway and thus the glucose phosphate shunt (Fig. 1) and indirectly on mitochondria, where free radical generating systems are normally operating (Agranoff, 1984). One consequence of such a shift is likely to be an increased release of calcium from mitochondrial stores or an increased calcium influx into cells due to membrane peroxidation induced damage that in turn will activate calcium-dependent proteases and will increase crosslinking of cellular proteins and nucleic acids (Davies, 1987; Richter, 1987; Richter and Frei, 1988; Richter et al., 1988). These alternative explanations for cell death in the nervous system are not mutually exclusive, but rather could be coupled. For example, expression of a "suicide gene" could result in increased levels of superoxide dismutase while catalase activity remains at low levels, or increased levels of proteases or of transport of calcium into the cytoplasm from extracellular spaces or the mitochondrial domain. One further complication is that NGF has been shown to have active responses to free radicals (Thorpe et al., 1988, 1989). Similar mechanisms have been proposed to be at work following spinal cord injury and head trauma (Perez-Polo et al., 1983; Perez-Polo and Werrbach-Perez, 1985, 1988).

With advancing age, the functional capacity of the immune system declines dramatically (Fabris, 1982; Lal and Forster, 1988). One set of age-related disorders, such as AD, may result in part from changes in immune function (Rogers and Luber-Narod, 1988). Here, also, it is known that one consequence of aging is increased oxidative stress usually manifested in part by an increase in the amount of peroxidative events (Agranoff, 1984). This perturbation of oxidant – antioxidant balance may damage cell proteins and membranes and affect proper cytokine action (Kay, 1978; Proust et al., 1988). The issue is complicated since, at low concentrations, H_2O_2 has inductive effects on lymphoid cells whereas at high concentrations it has toxic effects. The regulation of free radical scavenging mechanisms is particularly important to neural tissue, because free radicals can accumulate and adversely affect the functions of neurons which are highly specialized and have a limited regenerative capacity and a relatively high requirement for oxygen.

NGF

The protein is highly conserved (Levi-Montalcini, 1987; Perez-Polo, 1987; Whittemore et al., 1988). The highest levels of NGF mRNA and protein are in cortex and hippocampus, terminal axonal regions for basal forebrain cholinergic neurons (Selby et al., 1987; Whittemore and Seiger, 1987). This is where NGF effects on ChAT induction and cell sparing have been best documented (Selby et al., 1987; Whittemore and Seiger, 1987). There is NGF mRNA present in the thalamus/hypothalamus, brain stem, striatum, cerebellum and spinal cord, in that order (Ernfors et al., 1988). In these areas NGF mRNA and protein levels in the periphery and brain have been shown to correlate well with expression of NGF activity during the development of NGF-responsive neurons. Thus, the extent of innervation to hippocampus was found to reflect the levels of NGF expression. The hippocampus, the target tissue, expresses NGF mRNA followed by NGF protein. The NGF protein is secreted and, after binding to NGF receptors (NGFR) at nerve terminals, is transported retrogradely to neuronal soma in basal forebrain, where it accumulates (Whittemore and Seiger,

1987; Ernfors et al., 1988). There is also evidence for the internalization of NGF by glial cells in sensory ganglia, although less is known here about its physiological role (Khan et al., 1987). It should be emphasized that low levels of NGF mRNA have been reported for non-cholinergic regions of brain and spinal cord at early developmental stages in rat, although nothing is known about the function of NGF there (Whittemore and Seiger, 1987).

NGF effects

NGF can directly influence lymphoid cells, acting on mast cell accumulation (Aloe and Levi-Montalcini, 1977; Stead et al., 1987; Aloe, 1988), histamine release (Stead et al., 1987) or as a chemotactic agent for human neutrophils (Gee et al., 1983; Boyle et al., 1985). The synthesis of NGF by macrophages has been suggested (Otten et al., 1987). There are NGF receptors on B-cells and T-cells and NGF has mitogenic properties on lymphocytes and thymocytes (Stead et al., 1987; Fig. 2). Very high levels of NGFR mRNA and NGFR protein have been reported for rat and chick lymphoid organs in vivo and in vitro (Ernfors et al., 1988; Thorpe et al., 1988). Whether NGF is here internalized has not been demonstrated but crosslinking studies that rely on the use of EDAC to crosslink ^{125}I-NGF to the NGFR on rodent splenocytes and thymocytes would suggest that the NGFR molecular species present are not very dif-

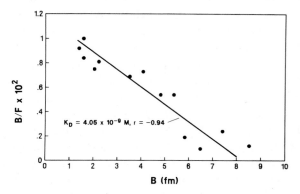

Fig. 2. Scatchard analysis of ^{125}I-NGF binding to human peripheral blood derived lymphocytes.

ferent from those reported for neuronal cells (Shan et al., 1989).

Treatment of sensory and sympathetic ganglia with NGF, at appropriate stages in development, results in a decrease in neuronal cell death, neuronal hypertrophy, increased anabolic activity, neurotransmitter synthesis and exaggerated neurite outgrowth (Johnson et al., 1986; Levi-Montalcini, 1987; Perez-Polo, 1987). Depression of NGF levels in early development, due to injections of anti-NGF, results in irreversible sympathectomy, neuronal cell loss and axonal sprouting in sensory ganglia (Greene and Shooter, 1980; Thoenen et al., 1981; Hulsebosch et al., 1987; Fig. 3). In the CNS, NGF stimulates ChAT in the hippocampus, septum and cortex of rat neonates and adult rats following fimbrial lesions (Hefti et al., 1984) and neurite outgrowth in cultures of dissociated fetal basal forebrain and septal cells (Bostwick et al., 1987; Gahwiler et al., 1987; Whittemore and Seiger, 1987; Hartikka and Hefti, 1988; Hatanaka et al., 1988). The retrograde transport of NGF from innervated tissues to cell bodies has been demonstrated for PNS and CNS neurons (Hendry et al., 1974; Stoekel et al., 1974; Johnson et al., 1987). NGF in spinal cord is also retrogradely transported by central processes to sensory neurons (Johnson et al., 1987; Khan et al., 1987). As a first obligatory step NGF binds to a cell surface receptor (Stach and Perez-Polo, 1987).

AXON NUMBERS IN LISSAUER'S TRACT

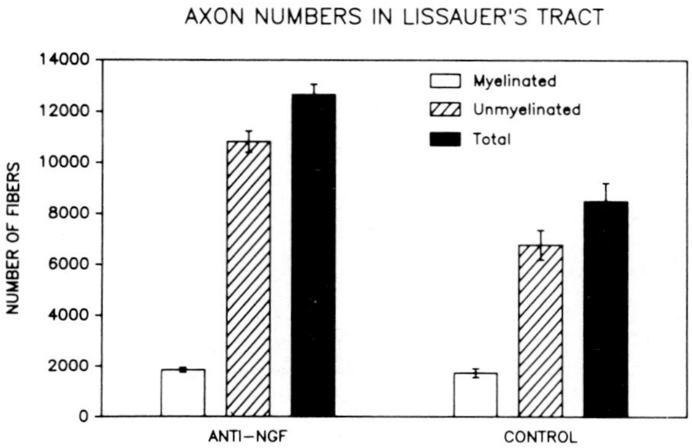

Fig. 3. Effect of anti-NGF on sensory neuron axonal sprouting.

NGF receptors

Studies on NGF receptors are of three different types: binding studies, detection of NGFR protein and detection of NGFR mRNA. Binding studies use ^{125}I-NGF as a ligand for in vitro kinetic and equilibrium studies or as a probe for the localization of NGFR by autoradiography of tissues (Richardson and Riopelle, 1984; Stach and Perez-Polo, 1987). Results obtained from binding studies would suggest that there are two binding activities present in both PNS and CNS neurons. These two binding activities are described as belonging to a type II receptor that is a low-affinity, high-capacity, or quickly dissociating NGF receptor (with reference to the dissociation of NGF from NGFR) with an equilibrium binding constant in the nanomolar range and a dissociation constant of seconds as opposed to a type I receptor that is a high-affinity, low-capacity, or slowly dissociating NGF receptor with an equilibrium binding constant in the picomolar range and a dissociation constant of minutes. Typically, neurons will display several thousand type I NGFR and $25-30$ times that number of the type II NGFR (Greene and Shooter, 1980; Stach and Perez-Polo, 1987; Figs. 4, 5). Non-neuronal cells like Schwann cells, astrocytes and NGF-responsive lymphoid cells typically display only the type II NGFR (Zimmermann and Sutter, 1983; Bernd, 1986; Marchetti et al., 1987). For these cells, NGF action appears to be linked to the regulation of cellular proliferation (Lillien and Claude, 1985; Thorpe et al., 1988, 1989).

NGFR protein has been characterized by affinity crosslinking of ^{125}I-NGF to NGFR followed by immunoprecipitation and SDS-PAGE or SDS-PAGE without immunoprecipitation (see Eveleth and Bradshaw, 1988, for discussion). The iodination of cell surface proteins followed by immunoprecipitation or the iodination of cell surface proteins followed by partial purification and characterization of the receptor has also provided useful structural information on NGFR (Marchetti et al., 1987; Shan et al., 1989). There is evidence for a 93 – 97 kDa NGFR molecule that is associated with the low-affinity type of binding and also for a higher molecular weight species of 158 – 200 kDa that is associated with the high-affinity species (Marchetti et al., 1987; Figs. 6 – 8). There is also evidence for a receptor-associated protein that allows for the conversion of low-affinity binding sites to their high-affinity counterparts for PC12, a rodent phenochromocytoma line, and LAN-1, a human neuroblastoma line

(Hosang and Shooter, 1985; Marchetti et al., 1987; Shan et al., 1989; Fig. 8).

NGFR can be partially isolated after solubilization by lectin chromatography and preparative electrofocusing on a granulated gel, PEGG. One advantage of this technique is that NGF binding can be carried out on samples that are chromatographed by PEGG with sufficient recoveries of NGF binding activities to allow for further analysis by immunoprecipitation and SDS PAGE. When LAN-1 human neuroblastoma cells known to display both type I and type II NGF binding activities are analyzed by labeling cell surface proteins with ^{125}I and assays of this solubilized preparation are carried out with ^{131}I-NGF, one

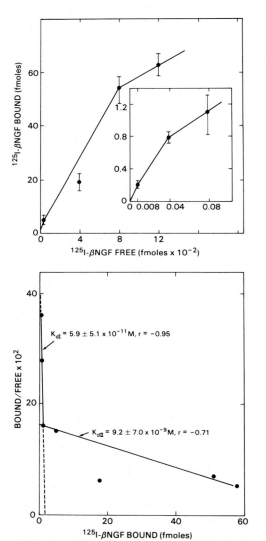

Fig. 4. Equilibrium binding and Scatchard analysis of ^{125}I-NGF to human neuroblastoma cells (LAN-1).

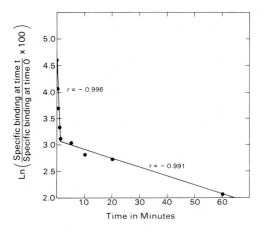

Fig. 5. Dissociation of ^{125}I-NGF from human neuroblastoma cells (LAN-1).

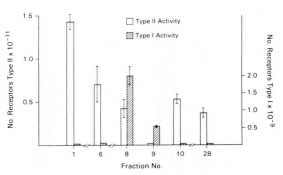

Fig. 6. NGF binding properties of partially purified NGFR from LAN-1. (From Marchetti et al., 1987.)

can isolate the low-affinity NGF binding activity as a 93 kDa protein and the high-affinity NGF binding activity as a 200 kDa protein. Reconstitution experiments carried out using this protocol would suggest that there is a receptor-associated glycoprotein that increases the levels of high-affinity binding activity and high molecular weight NGFR protein while decreasing the level of the low-affinity binding NGFR species and low molecular weight NGFR protein. That is, this receptor associated protein can convert NGFR II to NGFR I (Marchetti and Perez-Polo, 1987). In other experiments, where PC12 NGFR is chromatographed by reverse phase high-performance liquid chromatography, RP-HPLC, it would appear that the NGFR-associated protein may have a molecular weight of 55 − 58 kDa (Shan

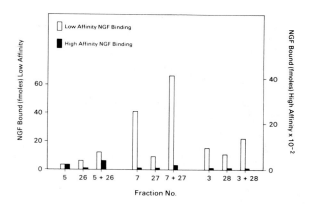

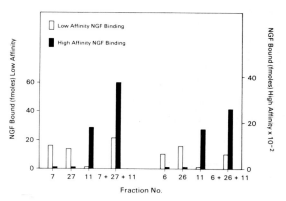

Fig. 8. NGF binding after mixing individual PEGG fractions containing only low-affinity NGF binding type II NGFR (top) or mixing fractions with low-affinity and high-affinity NGF binding activity type I NGFR (bottom). (From Marchetti and Perez-Polo, 1987.)

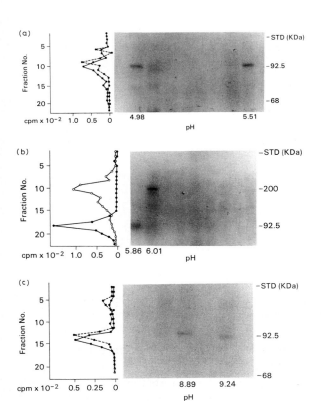

Fig. 7. a − c. SDS-PAGE analysis of partially purified NGFR from LAN-1 immunoprecipitated with NGF and anti-NGF. (From Marchetti et al., 1987.)

et al., 1989). Whether such shifts in specific binding activity can also take place for those non-neuronal cells such as astrocytes and lymphocytes, that display NGFR but respond to NGF mitogenic action is not known (Marchetti et al., 1987). Estimates for the molecular weight of the receptor-associated proteins range from 16 to 60 kDa (Hosang and Shooter, 1985; Shan et al., 1989).

NGFR mRNA has been detected by Northern analysis using two independently derived cDNA probes (Chao et al., 1986; Radeke et al., 1987; Ernfors et al., 1988). NGFR is expressed as a 3.7

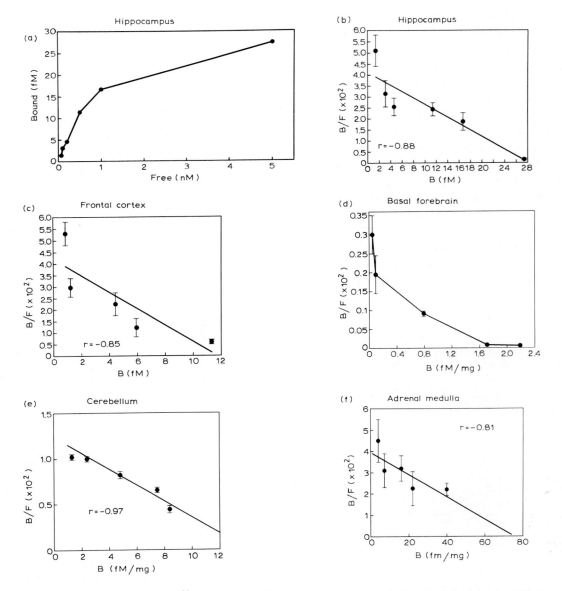

Fig. 9. *a*, Equilibrium binding of ^{125}I-NGF to solubilized rodent hippocampus; *b*, Scatchard analysis of equilibrium binding of ^{125}I-NGF to solubilized rodent hippocampus; *c*, frontal cortex; *d*, basal forebrain area; *e*, cerebellum; *f*, adrenal medulla.

kb mRNA in rodent, primate and human tissues and as a 4.5 kb mRNA in chick tissues (Ernfors et al., 1988). It should be emphasized that this is the predominant species reported but that there is also a minor 1 kb mRNA species present in chick and a 4.2 kb mRNA species that is present in the rodent brain. The significance of these variations is not

fully understood. In the chick the highest levels of NGFR mRNA reported are in cerebellum, brain stem and optic lobe, in that order; whereas in the rodent brain, the highest distribution of NGFR mRNA is in the septal area, including the diagonal band of Broca and nucleus basalis of Meynert (Ernfors et al, 1988). Here also, cerebellum has very high levels of NGFR mRNA. At earlier stages of embryonic development, NGFR mRNA appears to be more ubiquitous through the embryo. It is of interest that for both the chick and the rat the levels of NGFR mRNA and NGF binding remain at relatively high levels during adulthood. Thus, it would appear that NGF binding is present in neuronal tissues where it regulates innervation of targets in early development and the ability of neurons to overcome injury, perhaps by similar mechanisms in adulthood.

NGF mitogenic effects on glial and lymphoid cells may be most relevant following neuronal injury when gliosis and inflammation are highly regulated by several lymphokines, of which NGF may be one. In this instance, NGF may act in a paracrine fashion on neurons after being synthesized by glia and macrophages and in an autocrine fashion on the glia and macrophages themselves. Similar complex paracrine and autocrine effects may also be at play in aging where cholinergic neuronal cell losses may trigger similar reactions in the surrounding astrocytes. Events resulting from neuronal aging will yield free radical generation that may account for deficits in metabolic expression and altered energy and diminished immunogenic response. There are events subsequent to free radical generation that involve permanent changes at the blood-brain barrier and astrocytic activation that cannot be addressed here, although they are important and free radical metabolism may be involved.

It is established that various forms of NGFR mRNA and protein are present throughout the CNS, albeit it is not clear what the function of these are in all cases. Certainly there are reductions in NGF and NGF mRNA in the aged rodent and human CNS in those cholinergic areas that have been demonstrated to be NGF responsive. It has been demonstrated that NGF binding activity in these CNS tissues is not dissimilar from that expressed by PNS NGF responsive neurons or cell lines such as PC12 and several human neuroblastoma (Angelucci et al., 1988; Figs. 9, 10). There are dramatic decreases in overall NGF bind-

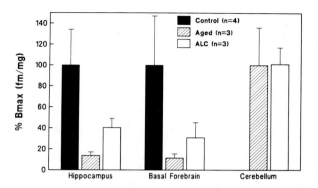

Fig. 10. Relative B_{max} values for NGF binding in 26 month old rats compared to 4 month old rats or acetyl-L-carnitine treated 26 months old rats (ALC). (From Angelucci et al., 1988.)

ing in the aged rodent CNS in those regions shown to have NGF responsive neurons such as the hippocampus, the basal forebrain and the frontal cortex but not the cerebellum (Angelucci et al., 1988). The significance of the manipulation of the level of NGF binding activity in CNS by exogenous NGF and acetyl-L-carnitine, ALC (Angelucci et al., 1988), is being further explored but as of yet, it is premature to speculate as to whether such manipulations will stimulate the development of therapeutic strategies relying on NGF or ALC. It must be emphasized that the spectrum of NGF action in the CNS and the immune system is not known at this time and that the role of CNS structures in response to stress in the aged CNS as it relates to NGF action in adult and aged mammals is totally unknown. It is our speculation that much of what we call aging-associated deficits in the limbic system is a consequence of stress-associated deficits that result from an aging-induced lowering of the threshold for stressful responses to stimuli.

Acknowledgements

This study was supported in part by grants of the NINDS, ONR and the Sigma Tau Company.

It is a pleasure to acknowledge the collaboration of Luciano Angelucci, Carol Beck, Jay Foreman, Claire Hulsebosch, Maria-Teresa Ramacci, Joan

Rhyne, Din E. Shan, Robert Stach and Giulio Taglialatela. Thanks to Donna Masters for manuscript preparation.

References

Agranoff, B.W. (1984) Lipid peroxidation and membrane aging. *Neurobiol. Aging,* 5: 337 – 338.

Aloe, L. (1988) The effect of nerve growth factor and its antibody on mast cells in vivo. *J. Neuroimmunol.,* 18: 1 – 12.

Aloe, L. and Levi-Montalcini, R. (1977) Mast cells increase in tissues of neonatal rats injected with the nerve growth factor. *Brain Res.,* 133: 358 – 366.

Angelucci, L., Ramacci, M.T., Taglialatela, G., Hulsebosch, C., Morgan, B., Werrbach-Perez, K. and Perez-Polo, R. (1988) Nerve growth factor binding in aged rat central nervous system: effects of acetyl-L-carnitine. *J. Neurosci. Res.,* 20: 491 – 496.

Banerjee, S.P., Snyder, S.H., Cuatrecasas, P. and Greene, L.A. (1973) Binding of nerve growth factor in superior cervical ganglia. *Proc. Natl. Acad. Sci. U.S.A.,* 70: 2519 – 2523.

Bernd, P. (1986) Characterization of nerve growth factor binding to cultured neural crest cells: evidence of an early developmental form of the nerve growth factor receptor. *Dev. Biol.,* 115: 415 – 424.

Bostwick, J.R., Appel, S.H. and Perez-Polo, J.R. (1987) Distinct influences of nerve growth factor and central nervous system cholinergic factor on medial septal explants. *Brain Res.,* 422: 92 – 98.

Boyle, M.D.P., Lawman, M.J.P., Gee, A.P. and Young, M. (1985) Nerve growth factor: a chemotactic factor for polymorphonuclear leukocytes in vivo. *J. Immunol.,* 134: 564 – 568.

Chao, M.V., Bothwell, M., Ross, A., Koprowski, H., Lanahan, A., Buck, C. and Sengal, P. (1986) Gene transfer and molecular cloning of the human nerve growth factor receptor. *Science,* 232: 518 – 521.

Davies, K. (1987) Protein damage and degradation by oxygen radicals. *J. Biol. Chem.,* 262: 9895 – 9920.

Eidelberg, E., Hansen, J.T. and Perez-Polo, J.R. (1984) Effects of nerve growth factor on recovery from spinal cord hemisection. *Soc. Neurosci. Abstr.,* 10: 175.

Ernfors, P., Hallbook, F., Ebendal, T., Shooter, E.M., Radeke, M.J., Misko, T.P. and Persson, H. (1988) Developmental and regional expression of beta-nerve growth factor receptor mRNA in the chick and rat. *Neuron,* 1: 983 – 996.

Eveleth, D.D. and Bradshaw, R.A. (1988) Internalization and cycling of nerve growth factor in PC12 cells: interconversion of type II (fast) and type I (slow) nerve growth factor receptors. *Neuron,* 1: 929 – 936.

Fabris, N. (1982) Neuroendocrine-immune network in aging.

Dev. Immunol. Clin. Probl. Aging, 1: 291 – 298.

Frazier, W.A., Boyd, L.F., Szutowicz, A., Pulliam, M.W. and Bradshaw, R.A. (1974) Specific binding sites for ^{125}I-nerve growth factor in peripheral tissues and brain. *Biochem. Biophys. Res. Commun.,* 57 (4): 1096 – 1103.

Gahwiler, B.H., Enz, A. and Hefti, F. (1987) Nerve growth factor promotes development of the rat septo-hippocampal cholinergic projection in vitro. *Neurosci. Lett.,* 75: 6 – 10.

Gee, A.P., Boyle, M.D.P., Munger, K.L., Lawman, M.J.P. and Young, M. (1983) Nerve growth factor: stimulation of polymorphonuclear leukocyte chemotaxis in vitro. *Proc. Natl. Acad. Sci. U.S.A.,* 80: 7215 – 7218.

Greene, L.A. and Shooter, E.M. (1980) The nerve growth factor: biochemistry, synthesis, and mechanism of action. *Annu. Rev. Neurosci.,* 3: 353 – 402.

Hamburger, V. and Oppenheim, R.W. (1982) Cell death. *Neurosci. Commun.,* 1: 39 – 55.

Hamburger, V. and Yip, J.W. (1984) Reduction of experimentally induced neuronal death in spinal ganglia of the chick embryo by nerve growth factor. *J. Neurosci.,* 4: 767 – 774.

Hartikka, J. and Hefti, F. (1988) Development of septal cholinergic neurons in culture: plating density and glial cells modulate effects of NGF on survival, fiber growth, and expression of transmitter-specific enzymes. *J. Neurosci.,* 8: 2967 – 2985.

Hatanaka, H., Nihonmatsu, I. and Tsukui, H., (1988) Nerve growth factor promotes survival of cultured magnocellular cholinergic neurons from nucleus basalis of Meynert in postnatal rats. *Neurosci. Lett.,* 90: 63 – 68.

Hefti, F., Dravid, A. and Hartikka, J. (1984) Chronic intraventricular injections of nerve growth factor elevate hippocampal choline acetyltransferase activity in adult rats with partial septo-hippocampal. *Brain Res.,* 293: 305 – 311.

Hendry, I.A., Stockel, K., Thoenen, H. and Iversen, L.L. (1974) The retrograde axonal transport of nerve growth factor. *Brain Res.,* 68: 103 – 121.

Herrup, K. and Shooter, E.M. (1973) Properties of the beta nerve growth factor receptor of avian dorsal root ganglia. *Proc. Natl. Acad. Sci. U.S.A.,* 70: 3884 – 3888.

Hosang, M. and Shooter, E.M. (1985) Molecular characteristics of nerve growth factor receptors on PC12 cells. *J. Biol. Chem.,* 260: 655 – 662.

Hulsebosch, C., Coggeshall, R. and Perez-Polo, R. (1987) Persistence of anti-nerve growth factor induced sensory axons: possible penetration in mammalian spinal cord. *Brain Res.,* 411: 267 – 274.

Jackson, G.R., Apffel, L., Werrbach-Perez, K. and Perez-Polo, J.R. (1990) Role of nerve growth factor in oxidant – antioxidant balance and neuronal injury. I. Stimulation of hydrogen peroxide resistance. *J. Neurosci.,* in press.

Jackson, G.R., Werrbach-Perez, K. and Perez-Polo, J.R. (1990) Role of nerve growth factor in oxidant – antioxidant balance and neuronal injury. II. A conditioning lesion paradigm. *J. Neurosci.,* in press.

Johnson, E.M., Rich, K. and Kip, H. (1986) The role of nerve growth factor in sensory neurons in vivo. *Trends Neurosci.,* 9: 33–37.

Johnson, E.M., Taniuchi, M., Clark, H.B., Springer, J.E., Koh, S.Y., Tayrien, M.W. and Loy, R. (1987) Demonstration of retrograde transport of nerve growth factor receptor in peripheral nervous system and central nervous system. *J. Neurosci.,* 7: 923–929.

Kay, M.M.B. (1978) Effect of age on T-cell differentiation. *Fed. Proc.,* 37: 1241.

Khan, R., Green, B. and Perez-Polo, J.R. (1987) Effect of injury on nerve growth factor uptake by sensory ganglia. *J. Neurosci. Res.,* 18: 562–567.

Kromer, L.F. (1987) Nerve growth factor treatment after brain injury prevents neuronal death. *Science,* 235: 214–216.

Lal, H. and Forster, M.J. (1988) Autoimmunity and age-associated cognitive decline. *Neurobiol. Aging,* 9: 733–742.

Levi-Montalcini, R. (1983) The nerve growth factor – target cells interaction: a model system for the study of directed axonal growth and regeneration. In: B. Haber, J.R. Perez-Polo, G.A. Hashim and A.M. Giuffrida-Stella (Eds.), *Nervous System Regeneration, Vol 19,* Alan Liss, New York, pp. 3–22.

Levi-Montalcini, R. (1987) The nerve growth factor 35 years later. *Science,* 237: 1154–1162.

Lillien, L. and Claude, P. (1985) Nerve growth factor mitogen for chromaffin cells. *Nature,* 317: 632–634.

Marchetti, D. and Perez-Polo, R. (1987) Nerve growth factor receptor in human neuroblastoma cells. *J. Neurochem.,* 49: 475–486.

Marchetti, D., Stach, R.W., Saneto, R.P., DeVellis, J. and Perez-Polo, J.R. (1987) Binding constants of soluble nerve growth factor receptors in rat oligodendrocytes and astrocytes in culture. *Biochem. Biophys. Res. Commun.,* 147: 422–427.

Martin, D.P., Schmidt, R.E., DiStefano, P.S., Lowry, O.H., Carter, J.G. and Johnson, E.M., Jr. (1988) Inhibitors of protein synthesis and RNA synthesis prevent neuronal death caused by nerve growth factor deprivation. *J. Cell Biol.,* 106: 829–844.

Montero, C.N. and Hefti, F. (1988) Rescue of lesioned septal cholinergic neurons by nerve growth factor: specificity and requirement for chronic treatment. *J. Neurosci.,* 8: 2986–2999.

Nieto-Sampedro, M. and Cotman, C.W. (1985) Growth factor induction and temporal order in central nervous system repair. In: C.W. Cotman (Ed.), *Synaptic Plasticity, Vol. 14,* Guilford Press, New York, pp. 407, 455.

Nieto-Sampedro, M., Lewis, E.R., Cotman, C.W., Manthorpe, M., Barbin, G., Longo, F.M. and Varon, S. (1982) Brain injury causes a time-dependent increase in neuronotrophic activity at the lesion site. *Science,* 217: 860–861.

Nieto-Sampedro, M., Manthorpe, M., Barbin, G., Varon, S. and Cotman, C.W. (1983) Injury-induced neuronotrophic activity in adult rat brain: correlation with survival of delayed implants in the wound cavity. *J. Neurosci.,* 3: 2219–2229.

Nieto-Sampedro, M., Whittemore, S.R., Needels, D.L., Larson, J. and Cotman, C.W. (1984) The survival of brain transplants is enhanced by extracts from injured brain. *Proc. Natl. Acad. Sci. U.S.A.,* 81: 6250–6254.

Nishimura, R.N., Dwyer, B.E., Cole, R. and DeVellis, J. (1988) Induction of the 68/72 Kd heat-shock. Protein during hydrogen peroxide toxicity. In: A. Gorio, R. Perez-Polo, J. DeVellis and B. Haber (Eds.), *Neural Development and Regeneration. Cellular and Molecular Aspects,* Springer-Verlag, Heidelberg, pp. 583–594.

Oppenheim, R.W. (1985) Naturally occurring cell death during neural development. *Trends Neurosci.,* 8: 487–493.

Otten, U., Weskamp, G., Hardung, M. and Meyer, D.K. (1987) NGF synthesis by macrophages. *Soc. Neurosci. Abstr.,* 13: 184.

Perez-Polo, J.R. (1987) *Neuronal Factors,* CRC Press, Boca Raton, FL, 202 pp.

Perez-Polo, J.R. and Werrbach-Perez, K. (1985) Effects of nerve growth factor on the response of neurons to injury. In: J. Eccles and J.R. Dimitrijevic (Eds.), *Recent Achievements in Restorative Neurology: Neuronal Function and Dysfunction, Vol. 30,* Karger, Basel, pp. 321–377.

Perez-Polo, J.R. and Werrbach-Perez, K. (1987) In vitro model of neuronal aging and development in the nervous system. In: A. Vernadakis (Ed.), *Model Systems of Development and Aging of the Nervous System,* Nijhoff, Boston, pp. 433–442.

Perez-Polo, J.R. and Werrbach-Perez, K. (1988) Role of nerve growth factor in neuronal injury and survival. In: A. Gorio, J.R. Perez-Polo, J. DeVellis and B. Haber (Eds.), *Neural Development and Regeneration. Cellular and Molecular Aspects,* Springer-Verlag, Heidelberg, pp. 399–410.

Perez-Polo, J.R., Tiffany-Castiglioni, E. and Werrbach-Perez, K. (1983) Model clonal system for study of neuronal cell injury. In: A.M. Giuffrida, B. Haber, G. Hashim and J.R. Perez-Polo (Eds.), *Nervous System Regeneration,* Alan Liss, New York, pp. 201–220.

Perez-Polo, J.R., Apffel, L. and Werrbach-Perez, K. (1986) Role of central nervous system and peripheral nervous system trophic factors on free radical mediated aging events. *Clin. Neuropharmacol.,* 9: 98–100.

Proust, J.J., Kittur, D.S., Buchholz, M.A. and Nordin, A.A. (1988) Restricted expression of mitogen-induced high-affinity IL-2 receptors in aging mice. *J. Immunol.,* 141: 4209–4216.

Radeke, M.J., Misko, T.P., Hasu, C., Herzenberg, L.A. and Shooter, E.M. (1987) Gene transfer and molecular cloning of rat nerve growth factor receptor. *Nature,* 325: 593–597.

Richardson, P.M. and Riopelle, R.J. (1984) Uptake of nerve

growth factor along peripheral and spinal axons of primary sensory neurons. *J. Neurosci.,* 4: 1683 – 1689.

Richter, C. (1987) Biophysical consequences of lipid peroxidation in membranes. *Chem. Phys. Lipids,* 44: 175 – 189.

Richter, C. and Frei, B. (1988) Ca^{2+} release from mitochondria induced by peroxidants. *Free Radical Biol. Med.,* 4: 365 – 375.

Richter, C., Park, J.W. and Ames, B.N. (1988) Normal oxidative damage to mitochondrial and nuclear DNA is extensive. *Proc. Natl. Acad. Sci. U.S.A.,* 85: 6465 – 6467.

Rogers, J. and Luber-Narod, J. (1988) Immune actions in the nervous system: a brief review with special emphasis on Alzheimer's disease. *Drug Dev. Res.,* 15: 227 – 235.

Selby, M.J., Edwards, R., Sharp, F. and Rutter, W.J. (1987) Mouse nerve growth factor gene: structure and expression. *Mol. Cell. Biol.,* 7: 3057 – 3064.

Shan, D.E., Beck, C., Marchetti, D. and Perez-Polo, J.R. (1989) Characterization of nerve growth factor receptor on PC12 cells using receptor binding assay and high-performance liquid chromatography. *12th ISN Mtg., Algarve, Portugal.*

Stach, W. and Perez-Polo, R. (1987) Binding of nerve growth factor to nerve growth factor receptor. *J. Neurosci. Res.,* 17: 1 – 10.

Stead, R.H., Bienenstock, J. and Stanisz, A.M. (1987) Neuropeptide regulation of mucosal immunity. *Immunol. Rev.,* 100: 333 – 360.

Stoekel, K., Paravicini, U. and Thoenen, H. (1974) Specificity of the retrograde axonal transport of nerve growth factor. *Brain Res.,* 76: 413 – 421.

Thoenen, H., Barde, Y.A., Davies, A.M. and Johnson, J.E. (1981) Neuronotrophic factors and neuronal death. *Ciba Found. Symp.,* 126: 838 – 840.

Thorpe, L.W., Morgan, B., Beck, C., Werrbach-Perez, K. and Perez-Polo, R. (1988) Nerve growth factor and the immune system. In: A. Gorio, R. Perez-Polo, J. DeVellis and B. Haber (Eds.), *Neural Development and Regeneration. Cellular and Molecular Aspects,* Springer-Verlag, Heidelberg, pp. 583 – 594.

Thorpe, L.W., Stach, R.W., Morgan, B. and Perez-Polo, J.R. (1989) In: J.M. Lakoski, J.R. Perez-Polo and D.K. Rassin (Eds.), *Neural Control of Reproductive Function,* Alan Liss, New York, pp. 351 – 369.

Whittemore, S.R. and Seiger, A. (1987) The expression, localization and functional significance of beta-nerve growth factor in the central nervous system. *Br. Res. Rev.,* 12: 439 – 464.

Whittemore, S.R., Persson, H., Ebendal, T., Larkfors, L., Larhammar, D. and Ericsson, A. (1988) Structure and expression of beta-nerve growth factor in rat central nervous system. In: A. Gorio, J.R. Perez-Polo, J. DeVellis and B. Haber (Eds.), *Neural Development and Regeneration. Cellular and Molecular Aspects,* Springer-Verlag, Heidelberg.

Wiiliams, L.R., Varon, S., Peterson, G.M., Wictorin, K., Fischer, W., Bjorklund, A. and Gage, F.H. (1986) Continuous infusion of nerve growth factor prevents basal forebrain neuronal death after fimbria fornix transection. *Proc. Natl. Acad. Sci. U.S.A.,* 83: 9231 – 9235.

Windebank, A. and Poduslo, J.F. (1986) Neuronal growth factors produced by adult peripheral nerve after injury. *Brain Res.,* 385: 197 – 200.

Yip, H. and Johnson, R. (1984) Developing dorsal root ganglia require trophic support from central processes: evidence for a role for retrogradely transported nerve growth factor from central nervous system to peripheral nervous system. *Proc. Natl. Acad. Sci. U.S.A.,* 81: 6245 – 6249.

Zimmerman, A. and Sutter, A. (1983) Beta-nerve growth factor (β-NGF) receptors on glial cells. Cell – cell interaction between neurones and Schwann cells in cultures of chick sensory ganglia. *EMBO J.,* 2: 879 – 885.

P. Coleman, G. Higgins and C. Phelps (Eds.)
Progress in Brain Research, Vol. 86
© 1990 Elsevier Science Publishers B.V. (Biomedical Division)

CHAPTER 16

The brain nicotinic acetylcholine receptor gene family

S. Heinemann, J. Boulter, E. Deneris, J. Conolly, R. Duvoisin, R. Papke and J. Patrick[1]

Molecular Neurobiology Laboratory, The Salk Institute, San Diego, CA 92138, U.S.A.

The history of the cultivation of tobacco suggests that early man appreciated the behavioral effects of nicotine. During the past decade the availability of radiolabeled nicotine with high specific activity has led to the discovery and mapping of nicotine binding sites in the mammalian brain (Clarke et al., 1985, 1986; for review see Martin, 1986; Clarke, 1988). These data suggested that the mammalian brain contains an important nicotinic receptor system. In order to investigate this possibility we decided to use a molecular genetic approach to identify genes that code for nicotinic receptors expressed in the brain. We reasoned that the brain nicotinic receptors should be evolutionarily related to the *Torpedo* electric organ and skeletal muscle nicotinic receptors that we and others had cloned previously (Ballivet et al., 1981, 1982; Claudio et al., 1983; Patrick et al., 1983; Boulter et al., 1985, 1986a). Based upon this assumption we screened genomic and brain cDNA libraries at low stringency using the muscle nicotinic receptor cDNAs as probes. The subject of this paper is the family of brain nicotinic acetylcholine receptors that we have discovered in the past few years through the use of this molecular genetic approach (Boulter et al., 1985, 1986a, b, 1987; Goldman et al., 1986, 1987; Deneris et al., 1988, 1989; Wada et al., 1988).

We have identified seven genes in the rat or mouse genome that code for proteins with homology to the nicotinic acetylcholine receptor. These genes are expressed in the mammalian brain and in some peripheral neurons. We have named these genes alpha2, alpha3, alpha4, alpha5, beta2, beta3, and beta4. In our terminology the genes coding for the muscle nicotinic acetylcholine receptors are called alpha1, beta1, gamma, delta and epsilon. Thus, the nicotinic acetylcholine receptor family is encoded by at least twelve genes in the mammalian genome. A similar set of genes has been identified in chicken (Nef et al., 1988). Recently the GABA and glycine receptors have also been cloned and shown to be structurally related to the nicotinic receptor (Grenningloh et al., 1987; Schofield et al., 1987; Levitan et al., 1988). Thus, the major inhibitory receptors in the nervous system are similar in structure to the nicotinic receptor, an excitatory receptor. This was an unexpected finding and raises the exciting possibility that all ligand gated channels are members of one super-family of related proteins. Thus, it is reasonable to expect that knowledge about one receptor will be useful in understanding the role and function of other ligand gated channel receptors.

The primary structures of the brain nicotinic receptor subunits expressed in the brain have been deduced from the sequences of the cDNA clones (see Fig. 1). Analysis of the hydrophobicity profiles of the brain nicotinic receptor subunits suggests that they fold through the membrane in an identical manner to the *Torpedo* fish nicotinic

---

[1] Present address: Baylor College of Medicine, Houston, TX, U.S.A.

NEURONAL NICOTINIC ACETYLCHOLINE RECEPTOR SUBUNITS

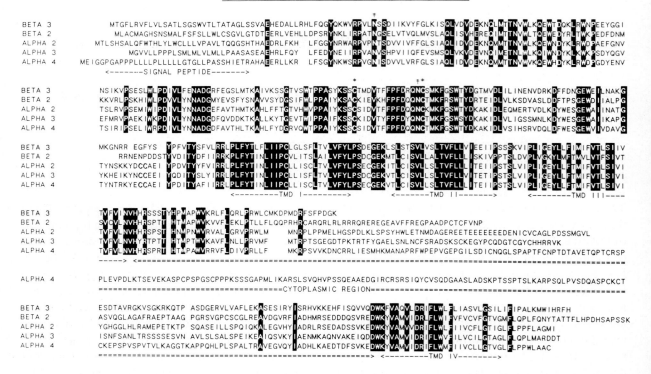

Fig. 1. Amino acid sequence alignment of the beta3 subunit with neuronal nAChR subunits. Aligned with the beta3 subunit are the rat beta2, alpha2, alpha3 and alpha4 – 1 subunits. Indicated in the figure are the positions of the predicted leader peptide, potential *N*-linked glycosylation sites (double crosses), cysteine residues conserved in each member of the neurotransmitter-gated ion-channel subunit superfamily (asterisks), putative transmembrane domains (TMD I – IV) and cytoplasmic domain.

receptor. Each subunit contains four stretches of about 25 amino acids that are very hydrophobic. We have suggested that these hydrophobic stretches are membrane spanning regions. Thus, we have proposed that each subunit spans the membrane four times placing the N-terminal and C-terminal outside the cell (Claudio et al., 1983). This four trans-membrane model places about half the protein bulk outside the cell, consistent with structural studies of the *Torpedo* receptor (Stroud and Finer-Moore, 1985; Karlin et al., 1986; Toyoshima and Unwin, 1988). This model also predicts that a number of potential phosphorylation sites are cytoplasmic and, in one case phosphorylation at one of these sites is known to regulate receptor function (Huganir et al., 1986; Safran et al., 1986). In addition the model predicts that the C-terminal

is outside the cell and this has been recently confirmed by McCrea et al. (1987). The brain alpha subunits all contain adjacent cysteines at homologous positions to the *Torpedo* alpha subunit cysteines 192 and 193, which are known to be near the acetylcholine binding site (Heinemann et al., 1986; Karlin et al., 1986). At present it is not known how many copies of each subunit form a brain nicotinic receptor. However, because of the observed structural homology between the ligand-gated channels, we have proposed that the brain receptors have a pentameric structure, as has been shown to be the case for the *Torpedo* fish nicotinic acetylcholine receptor, and recently, the glycine receptor (Popot and Changeux, 1984; Langosch et al., 1988). The results of the physiological experiments described below indicate that the brain nicotinic receptors are composed of two different gene products, an alpha and a beta subunit. This conclusion is also compatible with the recent biochemical analysis of a nicotine binding site isolated from rat brain (Whiting and Lindstrom, 1987). The availability of cDNA clones coding for the brain nicotinic receptors has made it possible to study their function. Expression studies in *Xenopus* oocytes have shown that the following combinations of subunits form functional nicotinic receptors: alpha2/beta2; alpha3/beta2 and alpha4/beta2 (Figs. 2 and 3; Boulter et al., 1987; Wada et al., 1988). Thus, beta2 is a promiscuous subunit which can combine with three different alpha subunits to form a functional receptor. This is consistent with its wide distribu-

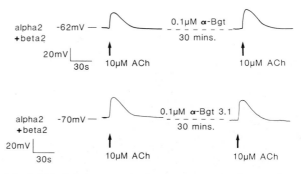

Fig. 3. This figure shows the effect of two different neurotoxins on the activation by acetylcholine of the neuronal nicotinic acetylcholine receptor subtype, alpha2/beta2. The voltage tracing on the left shows the response before application of the toxin and the voltage tracing on the right shows the response following a brief washing and a 30-min incubation in the indicated concentrations of the two toxins.

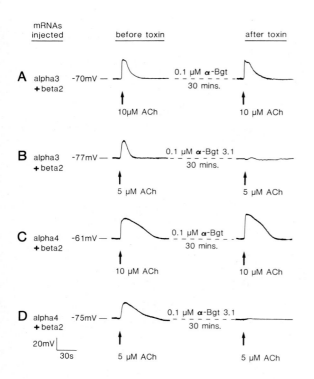

Fig. 2. This figure shows the effect of two different neurotoxins on the activation by acetylcholine of two neuronal nicotinic acetylcholine receptor subtypes, alpha3/beta2 and alpha4/beta 2. The voltage tracing on the left shows the response before application of the toxin and the voltage tracing on the right shows the response following a brief washing and a 30-min incubation in the indicated concentrations of the two toxins.

tion of expression in the brain (Wada et al., 1989; and see below). Each of the three functional combinations of subunits forms a pharmacologically distinct subtype which is activated by acetylcholine and nicotine and is resistant to alpha-bungarotoxin (Figs. 2, 3). Alpha3/beta2 and alpha4/beta2 are blocked by *Bungarus* toxin 3.1, consistent with a ganglionic nicotinic type pharmacology (Fig. 2). However, the alpha2/beta2 receptor is resistant to *Bungarus* toxin 3.1 and is a new receptor subtype with a pharmacology that has not been observed previously (Boulter et al., 1987; Wada et al., 1988; Fig. 3).

In order to determine where these nicotinic receptors are expressed in the brain we have utilized the method of in situ hybridization to visualize the distribution of expression of the mRNA coding for each nicotinic receptor subtype. These experiments demonstrated that each of the three alpha subunit mRNAs has a unique distribution of expression in the brain, consistent with the proposal that they are part of three independent nicotinic receptor systems (Fig. 4). The beta2 transcript is widely distributed throughout the brain consistent with the hypothesis that it is a common subunit used to form at least three different receptor subtypes (Fig. 5). On the other hand the beta3 transcript shows a much more

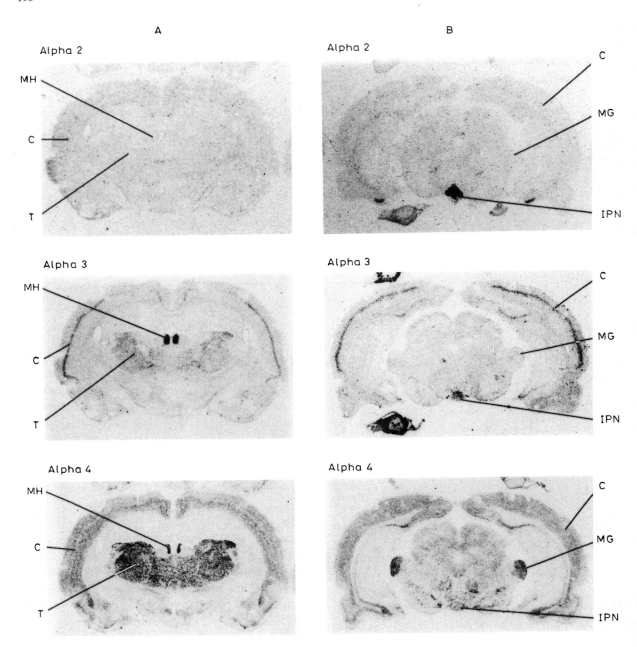

Fig. 4. Comparison of the distribution of alpha2, alpha3 and alpha4 transcripts by in situ hybridization histochemistry. Serial coronal sections through the medial habenula (*A*) and the interpeduncular nucleus (*B*) were hybridized with the probes for alpha2, alpha3 and alpha4. In *B* slides contain sections of the trigeminal ganglion. Abbreviations: C, cortex; IPN, interpeduncular nucleus; MH, medial habenula; MG, medial geniculate nucleus; T, thalamus. Tissue preparation and hybridization were performed with minor modifications. Briefly, paraformaldehyde-fixed rat brain sections. (25μm) were mounted on poly-L-lysine-coated slides, digested with proteinase K (10 μg/ml, 37°C, 30 min), acetylated, and dehydrated. Hybridization with ^{35}S-radiolabeled RNA probe (5 – 10 · 10^6 cpm/ml) was performed at 55°C for 12 – 18 h in a solution containing 50% formamide, 0.3 M NaCl, 10 mM Tris (pH 8.0), 1 mM EDTA, 0.05% tRNA, 10 mM DTT, 1 × Denhardt's solution and 10% dextran sulfate. Because of the high sequence similarities

localized distribution of expression (Fig. 6). In general the distribution of mRNA coding for the nicotinic receptor family parallels the map of nicotine binding (Boulter et al., 1986b, 1987; Goldman et al., 1986, 1987; Deneris et al., 1988, 1989; Wada et al., 1988, 1989).

The finding that these nicotinic receptor genes are expressed widely in the brain indicates that the nicotinic receptor is a major excitatory system. In the past few years physiologists using recently developed sophisticated techniques such as the slice preparation and patch clamp recording methods have found extensive evidence for nicotinic receptor function in the brain. The in situ hybridization results demonstrated that the alpha3, alpha4, beta2 and beta3 genes are expressed at high levels in the medial habenula (Figs. 4 – 6). The presence of functional nicotinic receptors has been confirmed in the medial habenula by intracellular recording techniques (McCormick and Prince, 1987a). Nicotine has also been shown to increase glucose utilization in the medial habenula (London et al., 1988). There is now good evidence for functional nicotinic receptors in many other regions of the brain that have high levels of nicotinic receptor gene expression, including the interpeduncular nucleus, the retina, the lateral and medial geniculate and the neocortex (Brown et al., 1984; Lipton et al., 1987; McCormick and Prince, 1987b; Lipton, 1988; Vidal and Changeux, 1989).

The discovery of a family of genes coding for nicotinic acetylcholine receptors expressed in the brain brings for the first time the full power of molecular biology to the study of this important receptor system. The existence of multiple subtypes and the fact that they are expressed throughout the brain suggests that the nicotinic receptor is a major excitatory system. The anatomical distribution of these receptors can now be studied using specific antibodies to localize the receptor subtypes in the brain. In situ hybridization methods can be used to localize the cell bodies that synthesize the receptor protein. The regulation of receptor gene expression can be studied under various experimental conditions. Understanding the promoters of these receptor genes will provide insight into how the brain builds, regulates and maintains specific neural networks. At present there are little reliable pharmacological data on the properties of the nicotinic acetylcholine receptor in the brain. The receptors can now be expressed in the oocyte system where rigorous pharmacology can be performed without the complications that are inherent in pharmacological studies in the brain. By engineering mammalian cell lines it will be possible to study these receptors in a number of convenient cell systems to ask specific questions about their function. The availability of the primary structure of the brain and muscle receptors makes it possible to build models that relate structure to pharmacology and function. These models can be tested by site specific mutagenesis. At present the only ligand gated channel that can be isolated in milligram amounts is the *Torpedo* nicotinic receptor. Thus, it is the only candidate for structural studies leading to a complete high-resolution three-dimensional structure. Because of the structural homologies between the ligand gated channels it should be possible to apply the results of the structural studies of the *Torpedo* nicotinic receptor to the muscle and brain nicotinic receptors and even to the glycine and GABA receptors.

Interesting mutations can be introduced into the receptors and expressed in transgenic mice and the mutant mice studied in order to gain insight into the function of the nicotinic receptors. The diversity of structure and function in this receptor system can now be studied with the long range goal of

---

in the protein coding regions of the cDNAs, 3′ untranslated sequences were used to make probes. The *Eco*RI/3′ end, *Bal*I/3′ end and *Bgl*I/3′ end fragments derived from C183, PCA48 and α4 – 2 cDNA clones, respectively, were subcloned into the plasmid, pSP65 and used to synthesize antisense RNA probes in vitro. After hybridization sections were treated with RNaseA (20 μg/ml, 37°C, 30 min) and washed in 0.1 × SSC at 55°C. Dehydrated slides were exposed to X-ray films for 3 – 16 days at 4°C. A RNA probe coding the sense strand of C183 clone was used as a control.

(A) Antisense

(B) Sense

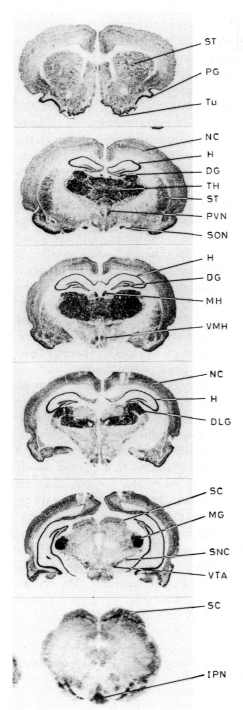

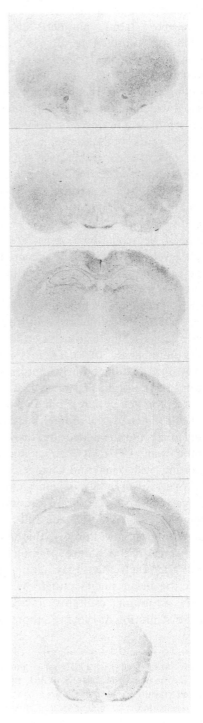

understanding the functional roles that the nicotinic receptors play in the nervous system.

At present little is known about the role of the

nicotinic receptor system in the brain. However, nicotine is one of the most widely consumed and addictive drugs. Many behavioral effects have been observed which include mood changes, effects on learning and memory and weight loss (Wellman et al. 1986; for review, see Clarke, 1988). Under some conditions nicotine is a relaxant and under other conditions nicotine is a stimulant. Many of these effects may be beneficial and this raises the possibility of designing better and more specific nicotinic drugs (Luyten and Heinemann, 1987).

The nicotinic receptor system has been implicated in a number of serious health problems. Nicotine is a widely consumed and addictive drug and is a major factor in the present smoking epidemic. Behavioral studies have linked the nicotinic receptor system to learning and memory which is intriguing given the finding that Alzheimer's patients have a deficiency in memory and cortical nicotinic receptors (Perry et al., 1987). The possibility that one or more of the nicotinic receptor subtypes is depressed in patients with Alzheimer's disease can now be explored. The fact that in Alzheimer's disease both the number of nicotine binding sites is depressed and the fraction of high-affinity and low-affinity sites is altered, suggests that one nicotinic receptor subtype may be specifically impacted by the disease (Whitehouse et al., 1986; Nordberg et al., 1988).

The existence of receptor subtypes and the availability of cDNA clones may make it possible to design new drugs that are subtype-specific and which will prove useful in the battle against the smoking and Alzheimer's epidemics. The known ability of nicotine to effect mood suggests that new nicotinic drugs may also prove useful in the treatment of various mood disorders.

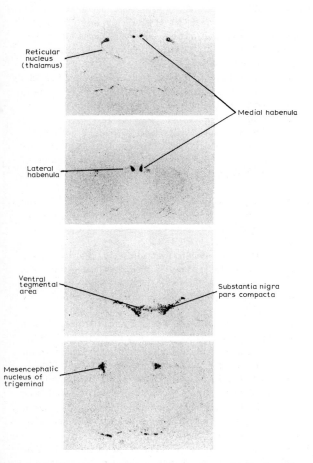

Fig. 6. Localization of beta3 transcripts in the rat forebrain and midbrain. Rat brain sections were probed with [^{35}S]-UTP radiolabeled antisense RNA transcribed in vitro from pESD77. Regions where hybridization signals were detected are indicated. Magnification: × 10.

Fig. 5. In situ hybridization analysis. Rat forebrain and midbrain sections were probed with [^{35}S]-radiolabeled antisense (A) or sense (B) beta2 RNA transcribed in vitro using a plasmid into which a 571bp Pst1/EcoR1 fragment of PCX49 was subcloned. Abbreviations are: DLG, lateral geniculate nucleus (dorsal part); DG, dentate gyrus; H, Ammon's horn (hippocampus); IPN, interpeduncular nucleus; MG, medial geniculate nucleus; MH, medial habenular nucleus; NC, neocortex; PC, piriform cortex; PVN, paraventricular hypothalamic nucleus; SON, supraoptic hypothalamic nucleus; SNC, substantia nigra, pars compacta; SC, superior colliculus; ST, striatum; TH, thalamus; Tu, olfactory tubercle; VTA, ventral tegmental area; VMH, ventromedial hypothalamic nucleus.

Acknowledgements

The work reviewed in this paper was supported by the National Institutes of Health, U.S.A., National Institute of Neurological and Communicative Disorders and Stroke (S.H. and J.P.), and the Muscular Dystrophy Association of America (S.H. and J.P.).

References

Ballivet, M., Patrick, J., Lee, J. and Heinemann, S. (1981) Progress in cloning of the acetycholine receptor cDNAs and genes. *Cold Spring Harbor Symposium on Molecular and Cellular Control of Muscle Development,* Cold Spring Harbor Press, Cold Spring Harbor, NY.

Ballivet, M., Patrick, J., Lee, J. and Heinemann, S. (1982) Molecular cloning of cDNA coding for the gamma subunit of the *Torpedo* acetylcholine receptor. *Proc. Natl. Acad. Sci. U.S.A.,* 79: 4466–4470.

Ballivet, M., Nef, P., Couturier, S., Rungger, D., Bader, C.R., Bertrand, D. and Cooper, E. (1988) Electrophysiology of a chick neuronal nicotinic acetylcholine receptor expressed in *Xenopus* oocytes after cDNA injection. *Neuron,* 1: 847–852.

Boulter, J., Luyten, W., Evans, K., Mason, P., Ballivet, M., Goldman, D., Stengelin, S., Martin, G., Heinemann, S. and Patrick, J. (1985) Isolation of a clone coding for the alpha subunit of a mouse acetylcholine receptor. *J. Neurosci.,* 5: 2545–2552.

Boulter, J., Goldman, D., Evans, K., Martin, G., Mason, P., Stengelin, S., Heinemann, S. and Patrick, J. (1986a) Isolation and sequence of cDNA clones coding for the precursor to the gamma-subunit of mouse muscle acetylcholine receptor. *J. Neurosci. Res.,* 16: 37–49.

Boulter, J., Evans, K., Goldman, D., Martin, G., Treco, D., Heinemann, S. and Patrick J. (1986b) Isolation of a cDNA clone coding for a possible neural nicotinic acetylcholine receptor alpha subunit. *Nature,* 319: 368–374.

Boulter, J., Connolly, J., Deneris, E., Goldman, D., Heinemann, S. and Patrick, J. (1987) Functional expression of two neuronal nicotinic acetylcholine receptors from cDNA clones identifies a gene family. *Proc. Natl. Acad. Sci. U.S.A.,* 84: 7763–7767.

Briggs, C.A. and Cooper, J.R. (1982) Cholinergic modulation of the release of [^{3}H] acetylcholine from synaptosomes of myenteric plexus. *J. Neurochem.,* 38: 501–508.

Brown, D.A., Docherty, R.J. and Halliwell, J.V. (1984) The action of cholinomimetic substances on impulse conduction in the habenulointerpeduncular pathways of the rat in vitro. *J. Physiol. (Lond.),* 353: 101–109.

Clarke, P.B.S. (1988) The central pharmacology of nicotine:

electrophysiological approaches. In: I.P. Stolerman, S. Wonnacott and M.A.H. Russel (Eds.), *Actions and Medical Implications,* Oxford University Press, Oxford, pp. 2–55.

Clarke, P.B.S., Schwartz, R.D., Paul, S.M., Pert, C.B. and Pert, A. (1985) Nicotinic binding in rat brain: autoradiographic comparison of [^{3}H] acetylcholine, [^{3}H] alicotine, and [^{125}I]-alpha-bungarotoxin. *J. Neurosci.,* 5: 1307–1315.

Clarke, P.B.S., Hamill, G.S., Nadi, N.S., Jacobowitz, D.M. and Pert, A. (1986) ^{3}H-nicotine- and ^{125}I-alpha-bungarotoxin-labeled nicotinic receptors in the interpeduncular nucleus of rats. II. Effects of habenular deafferentation. *J. Comp. Neurol.,* 251: 407–413.

Claudio, T., Ballivet, M., Patrick, J. and Heinemann, S. (1983) Nucleotide and deduced amino acid sequences of *Torpedo californica* acetylcholine receptor gamma subunit. *Proc. Natl. Acad. Sci. U.S.A.,* 80: 1111–1115.

Deneris, E.S., Connolly, J., Boulter, J., Wada, E., Wada, K., Swanson, L., Patrick, J. and Heinemann, S. (1988) Primary structure and expression of beta2: a novel subunit of neuronal nicotinic acetylcholine receptors. *Neuron,* 1: 45–54.

Deneris, E., Boulter, J., Swanson, L., Patrick, J. and Heinemann, S. (1989) β_3: a new member of nicotinic acetylcholine receptor gene family is expressed in brain. *J. Biol. Chem.,* 264(11): 6268–6272.

Goldman, D., Simmons, D., Swanson, L.W., Patrick, J. and Heinemann S. (1986) Mapping brain areas expressing RNA homologous to two different acetylcholine receptor alpha-subunit cDNAs. *Proc. Natl. Acad. Sci. U.S.A.,* 83: 4076–4080.

Goldman, D., Deneris, E., Kochhar, A., Patrick, J. and Heinemann, S. (1987) Members of a nicotinic acetylcholine receptor gene family are expressed in different regions of the mammalian central nervous system. *Cell,* 48: 965–973.

Grenningloh, G., Rienitz, A., Schmitt, B., Methfessel, C., Zensen, M., Beyreuther, K., Gundelfinger, E.D. and Betz, H. (1987) The strychnine-binding subunit of the glycine receptor shows homology with nicotinic acetylcholine receptors. *Nature,* 328: 215–220.

Heinemann, S., Asouline, G., Ballivet, M., Boulter, J., Connolly, J., Deneris, E., Evans, K., Evans, S., Forrest, J., Gardner, P., Goldman, D., Kochhar, A., Luyten, W., Mason, P., Treco, D., Wada, K. and Patrick, J. (1986) Molecular biology of the neural and muscle acetylcholine receptors. In: J. Patrick and S. Heinemann (Eds.), *Molecular Neurobiology,* Plenum, New York.

Heinemann, S., Boulter, J., Deneris, E.S., Gardner, P., Connolly, J., Wada, E., Wada, W., Ballivet, M., Swanson, L.W. and Patrick, J. (1988) Brain nicotinic acetylcholine receptors: a gene family. In: *Methods in Protein Sequence Analysis,* Springer-Verlag, Heidelberg, in press.

Heinemann, S., Boulter, J., Deneris, E.S., Gardner, P., Connolly, J., Wada, E., Wada, K., Ballivet, M., Swanson, L.W. and Patrick, J. (1989) The nicotinic acetylcholine receptor gene family. In: *The Neuronal Nicotinic Acetylcholine Receptors,* Springer-Verlag, Heidelberg, in press.

Huganir, R.L., Delcour, A.H., Greengard, P. and Hess, G.P. (1986) Phosphorylation of the nicotinic acetylcholine receptor regulates its rate of desensitization. *Nature,* 321: 774 – 776.

Karlin, A., DiPaola, M., Kao, P.N. and Lobel, P. (1986) Functional sites and transient states of the nicotinic acetylcholine receptor. In: B. Hille and D.M. Fambrough (Eds.), *Proteins of Excitable Membrane,* Wiley, New York.

Langosch, D., Thomas, L. and Betz, H. (1988) Conserved quaternary structure of ligand-gated ion channels: the postsynaptic glycine receptor is a pentamer. *Proc. Natl. Acad. Sci. U.S.A.,* 85: 7394 – 7398.

Levitan, E.S., Schofield, P.R., Burt, D.R., Rhee, L.M., Wisden, W., Kohler, M., Fujita, N., Rodriguez, H.F., Stephenson, A., Darlison, M.G., Barnard, E.A. and Seeburg, P.H. (1988) Structural and functional basis for GABA$_A$ receptor heterogeneity. *Nature,* 335: 76 – 79.

Lipton, S. (1988) Spontaneous release of acetylcholine affects the physiological nicotinic responses of rat retina ganglion cells in culture. *J. Neurosci.,* 8: 3857 – 3868.

Lipton, S., Aizenman, E. and Loring, R. (1987) Neural nicotinic responses in solitary mammalian retinal ganglion cells. *Pflugers Arch.,* 410: 37 – 43.

London, E.D., Connolly, R.J., Szikszay, M., Wamsley, J.K. and Dam, M. (1988) Effects of nicotine on local cerebral glucose utilization in the rat. *J. Neurosci.,* 8: 3920 – 3928.

Luyten, H.W.M.L. and Heinemann, S.F. (1987) Molecular cloning of the nicotinic acetylcholine receptor: new opportunities in drug design? *Rep. Med. Chem.,* 22: 281 – 291.

Martin, B.R. (1986) Nicotine receptors in the central nervous system. In: *The Receptors, Vol. III,* Academic Press, Orlando, FL, pp. 393 – 415.

McCormick, D.A. and Prince, D. (1987a) Acetylcholine causes rapid nicotinic excitation in the medial habenular nucleus of guinea pig in vivo. *J. Neurosci.,* 7(3): 742 – 752.

McCormick, D.A. and Prince, D. (1987b) Actions of acetylcholine in the guinea-pig and cat medial and lateral geniculate nuclei in vitro. *J. Physiol. (Lond.),* 392: 147 – 165.

McCrea, P.D., Popot, J. and Engelman, D.M. (1987) Transmembrane topography of the nicotinic acetylcholine receptor δ- subunit. *EMBO J.,* 6: 3619 – 3626.

Nef, P., Oneyser, C., Alliod, C., Couturier, S. and Ballivet, M. (1988) Genes expressed in the brain define three distinct neuronal nicotinic acetylcholine receptors. *EMBO J.,* 7: 595 – 601.

Nordberg, S.M., Adem, A., Hardy, J. and Winblad, B. (1988) Change in nicotinic receptor subtypes in temporal cortex of Alzheimer brains. *Neurosci. Lett.,* 86: 317 – 321.

Patrick, J., Ballivet, M., Boas, L., Caludio, T., Forrest, J., Ingraham, H., Mason, P., Stengelin, S., Ueno, S. and Heinemann, S. (1983) Molecular cloning of the acetylcholine receptor. *Cold Spring Harbor Symposia on Quantitative Biology, Vol. XLVIII,* Cold Spring Harbor, NY, pp. 71 – 78.

Perry, E.K., Perry, R.H., Smith, C.J., Dick, D.J., Candy, J.M., Edwardson, J.A., Fairbairn, A. and Blessed, G. (1987) Nicotinic receptor abnormalities in Alzheimer's and Parkinson's disease. *J. Neurol. Neurosurg. Psychiatry,* 50: 806 – 809.

Popot, J.L. and Changeux, J.-P. (1984) The nicotinic receptor of acetylcholine: structure of an oligomeric integral membrane protein. *Physiol. Rev.,* 64: 1162 – 1239.

Safran, A., Neumann, D. and Fuchs, S. (1986) Analysis of acetylcholine receptor phosphorylation sites using antibodies to synthetic peptides and monoclonal antibodies. *EMBO J.,* 5: 3175 – 3178.

Schofield, P.R., Darlison, M.G., Fujita, N., Burt, D.R., Stephenson, F.A., Rodriguez, H., Rhee, L.M., Ramachandran, J., Reale, V., Glencorse, T.A., Seeburg, P.H. and Barnard, E.A. (1987) Sequence and functional expression of the GABA$_A$ receptor shows a ligand-gated receptor superfamily. *Nature,* 328: 221 – 227.

Stroud, R.M. and Finer-Moore, J. (1985) Acetylcholine receptor structure, function and evolution. *Annu. Rev. Cell Biol.,* 1: 369 – 401.

Toyoshima, C. and Unwin, N. (1988) Ion channel of acetylcholine receptor reconstructed from images of postsynaptic membranes. *Nature,* 336: 247 – 250.

Vidal, C. and Changeux, J. (1989) Pharmacological profile of nicotinic acetylcholine receptors in the rat prefrontal cortex: an electrophysiological study in a slice preparation. *Neuroscience,* 29: 261 – 270.

Wada, E., Wada, K., Boulter, J., Deneris, E., Heinemann, S., Patrick, J. and Swanson, L.W. (1989) The distribution of alpha2, alpha3, alpha4, and beta2 neuronal nicotinic receptor subunit mRNAs in the central nervous system. A hybridization histochemical study in the rat. *J. Comp. Neurol.,* in press.

Wada, W., Ballivet, M., Boulter, J., Connolly, J., Wada, E., Deneris, E.S., Swanson, L.W., Heineman, S. and Patrick, J. (1988) Functional expression of a new pharmacological subtype of brain nicotinic acetylcholine receptor. *Science,* 240: 330 – 334.

Wellman, P.J., Marmon, M.M., Reich, S. and Ruddle, J. (1986) Effects of nicotine on body weight, food intake and brown adipose tissue thermogenesis. *Pharmacol. Biochem. Behav.,* 24: 1605 – 1609.

Whitehouse, P., Martino, A., Antuono, P., Lowenstein, P., Coyle, J., Price, D. and Kellar, K. (1986) Nicotinic acetylcholine binding sites in Alzheimer's disease. *Brain Res.,* 371: 146 – 151.

Whiting, P. and Lindstrom, J. (1987) Purification and characterization of a nicotinic acetylcholine receptor from rat brain. *Proc. Natl. Acad. Sci. U.S.A.,* 84: 595 – 599.

P. Coleman, G. Higgins and C. Phelps (Eds.)
Progress in Brain Research, Vol. 86
© 1990 Elsevier Science Publishers B.V. (Biomedical Division)

CHAPTER 17

Gene therapy in the CNS: intracerebral grafting of genetically modified cells

Fred H. Gage[1], Michael B. Rosenberg[2], Mark H. Tuszynski[1], Kazunari Yoshida[1], David M. Armstrong[1], Robert C. Hayes[1] and Theodore Friedmann[2]

Departments of [1]Neurosciences and [2]Pediatrics, University of California at San Diego, La Jolla, CA 92093, U.S.A.

Grafting cells to the CNS has been suggested and applied as a potential approach to CNS therapy through the selective replacement of cells lost as a result of disease or damage. Independently, studies aimed at direct genetic therapy in model systems have recently begun to suggest conceptually new approaches to the treatment of several kinds of human genetic disease, especially those caused by single gene enzyme deficiencies. We suggest that a combination of these two approaches, namely the graftment into the CNS of genetically modified cells, may provide a new approach toward the restoration of some functions in the damaged or diseased CNS. We present evidence for the feasibility of this approach, including a description of some current techniques for mammalian cell gene transfer and CNS grafting, and several possible approaches to clinical applications. Specifically, we report that fibroblasts, genetically modified to secrete NGF by infection with a retroviral vector and implanted into the brains of rats with a surgical lesion of the fimbria-fornix, prevented the degeneration of cholinergic neurons that would die without treatment.

Introduction

During the past decade techniques aimed at a conceptually new view of disease therapy based on the direct correction of a genetic deficit have begun to be developed. The extension of this approach to whole animals, that is, the correction of a disease phenotype in vivo through the use of the functional genes as a pharmacological agent, has come to be called gene therapy (Friedmann, 1983). Such a therapy is based on the assumption that the correction of a disease phenotype can be accomplished either by modification of the expression of a resident mutant gene or by the introduction of new genetic information into defective cells or organs in vivo.

At present, techniques for the ideal type of gene therapy, that is through site-specific gene sequence correction or replacement, are just beginning to be conceived, but are not well developed. Therefore, most current models of gene therapy are really genetic augmentation rather than replacement models, and rely on the development of efficient gene transfer systems to introduce functional wild-type genetic information into genetically defective cells in vitro and in vivo.

We have recently proposed that a combination of gene transfer into cultured cells followed by intracerebral grafting of the genetically modified cells may constitute an effective approach to some disorders of CNS function (Gage et al., 1987; Fig. 1). This approach relies on the development of methods to introduce the foreign genes (transgenes) into appropriate neuronal and other target cells efficiently and functionally in vitro, as well as on the long-term survival of these cells and continued stable gene expression following intracerebral grafting. The conceptual and methodological development of these general objectives depends on the solutions to a variety of questions and problems including:

(1) What is the susceptibility of the variety of

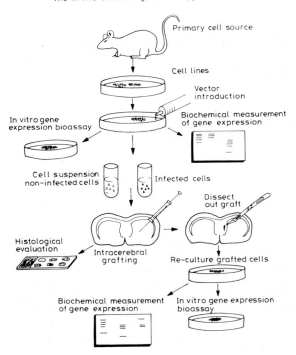

The in vivo selective gene therapy

Primary cell source

Cell lines

Vector introduction

In vitro gene expression bioassay

Biochemical measurement of gene expression

Cell suspension non-infected cells

Infected cells

Dissect out graft

Histological evaluation

Intracerebral grafting

Re-culture grafted cells

Biochemical measurement of gene expression

In vitro gene expression bioassay

Fig. 1. Grafting of genetically modified cells to the CNS. Established cell lines or primary cell cultures are infected in vitro with retroviral vectors containing "reporter" genes encoding proteins whose activity can be easily assayed and/or selected for. The cells are then grown in selective media so that only infected cells survive. Expression of the genes in the recipient cells in vitro is characterized. The cells are injected intracerebrally, and uninfected control cells are injected contralaterally. Subsequently, the brains are examined histologically to evaluate cell survival. Alternatively, the grafted regions are dissected and expression of the reporter genes in vivo is measured. In addition, portions of the graft can be recultured and the continued presence and expression of the transgenes can be determined.

appropriate target CNS cells to the introduction of transgenes? What vectors are most suitable?

(2) Does the introduction of foreign sequences cause metabolic or genetic damage to recipient cells, or to the organism as a whole?

(3) Are the transgenes structurally and functionally stable? Are they efficiently expressed?

(4) What is the immunological response of the animal to the presence in the brain of genetically modified autologous or heterologous cells, or to the expressed gene product?

(5) Does a foreign gene product provide a needed and physiologically useful new function that can lead to correction of a particular disease phenotype?

We have addressed some of these questions and present data to test the potential applications of this approach (Gage et al., 1987). We have identified some of the technical and conceptual problems inherent in the techniques, and have suggested some of the human disease models for which this approach may be applicable and the issues that must be addressed before this approach can be considered for clinical use. We have also presented data based on the use of several prototype marker vectors expressing: (1) the human hypoxanthine-guanine phosphoribosyltransferase (HPRT) cDNA; (2) the transposon Tn5 neomycin-resistance gene (neoR); and (3) the firefly luciferase cDNA. These reporter genes were chosen for their availability and the availability of sensitive assays to measure the gene products.

Choice of vector

While several procedures exist for inserting DNA into cells (see Table I), murine retroviral vectors offer at present the most efficient, useful, and best characterized means of introducing and expressing foreign genes in mammalian cells. Briefly, these vectors have very broad host and cell type ranges, integrate by reasonably well understood mechanisms into random sites in the host genome, ex-

TABLE I

Methods of gene insertion

(A)	Microinject DNA in nucleus
(B)	(Electric field) electroporation
(C)	Calcium phosphate transfection
(D)	Liposomal transfection (lipofection)
(E)	Retroviral infection
(F)	Viral infection

press genes stably and efficiently, and under most conditions do not kill or obviously damage their host cells. Because retroviral vectors integrate at predominantly random sites in the cellular genome, insertional mutagenesis is a theoretical, and in fact a well documented, occasional consequence of viral infection (Hayward et al., 1981; Lohler et al., 1984), and can occur either by interruption of an essential cellular gene or by insertion of regulatory sequences such as promoters and enhancers near cellular genes with resulting inappropriate regulation of expression of such genes.

The methods of preparation of retroviral vectors have been reviewed extensively elsewhere (Mann et al., 1983; Anderson, 1984; Miller et al., 1985; Constantini et al., 1986; Gilboa et al., 1986; Mason et al., 1986; Readhead et al., 1987) and are now in common use in many laboratories. In principle, the aim is to design a vector in which the transgene is brought under the control of either the viral long terminal repeat (LTR) promoter-enhancer signals, or of a powerful internal promoter, and further, in which retained signals within the retroviral LTR can still bring about efficient integration of the vector into the host cell genome. To prepare transmissible virus, recombinant DNA molecules of such defective vectors are transfected into "producer" cell lines that contain a provirus expressing all of the retroviral functions required for packaging of viral transcripts into transmissible virus particles, but lacking the crucial packaging signal. Because of this deletion, transcripts from the helper cannot be packaged into viral particles. However, an integrated defective vector introduced into the same cell by means of calcium-phosphate-mediated transfection produces transcripts that can be packaged in trans since they do contain the packaging sequence. Ideally, the result is the production of infectious particles carrying the transgene completely free of replication-competent wild-type helper virus. In most models of gene therapy, the production of helper virus is probably undesirable since it may lead to spreading infection and possibly proliferative disease in lymphoid or other tissue in the host animal. An exam-

ple of the prototype retrovirus and the reconstructed retroviral vector is shown in Fig. 2.

Choice of donor cells

The choice of donor cells for implantation depends heavily on the nature of the expressed gene, characteristics of the vector, and the desired phenotypic result. Because retroviral vectors are thought to require cell division and DNA synthesis for efficient infection, integration and gene expression (Varmus and Swanstrom, 1982; Gage and Bjorklund, 1986) our present model may be restricted to actively growing cells such as primary fibroblast cultures or established cell lines, replicating embryonic neuronal cells or replicating adult neuronal cells in selected areas such as the olfactory mucosa and possibly developing or reactive glia. The eventual use of other viral vectors, or of methods to induce a state of susceptibility in stationary, non-replicating target cells may make many other cell types suitable targets for viral transduction. For instance, we have recently developed methods that have permitted the successful retroviral vector infection of primary cultures of adult rat hepatocytes, ordinarily refrac-

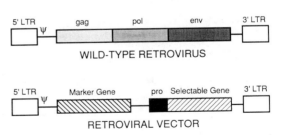

Fig. 2. Structure of integrated vectors. LTR, long terminal repeat. Helper functions required for the production of transmissible virus particles include the GAG and ENV genes which encode the capsid proteins as well as the reverse transcriptase (POL). The wild type virus also contains the packaging (psi) sequence essential for the encapsidation of RNA transcripts of the provirus into the mature virus particles. The prototype transmissible retrovirus is prepared by constructing a plasmid in which the GAG, POL and ENV genes have been replaced by the reporter gene (marker gene), and selector gene which is controlled by an internal promoter separate from the intact retroviral LTR which controls the marker gene.

tory to infection with such vectors, and similar methods may be helpful for a number of other cells (Wolff et al., 1987). The development of other kinds of vectors derived from herpes, vaccinia, or other viruses, as well as the use of efficient, non-viral methods for introducing DNA into donor cells such as the recently developed electroporation technique (Toneguzzo et al., 1986), may allow successful gene transfer into many other cells presently not susceptible to retroviral vector infection.

One can envision several mechanisms by which one can introduce a new function into target cells in a phenotypically useful way (see Fig. 3). The most direct approach, which would bypass the need for cellular grafting entirely, would be the introduction of a transgene directly into the cells in which that function is aberrant as a consequence of a genetic defect; e.g., neuronal cells in the case of Tay Sachs disease, possibly Lesch-Nyhan disease,

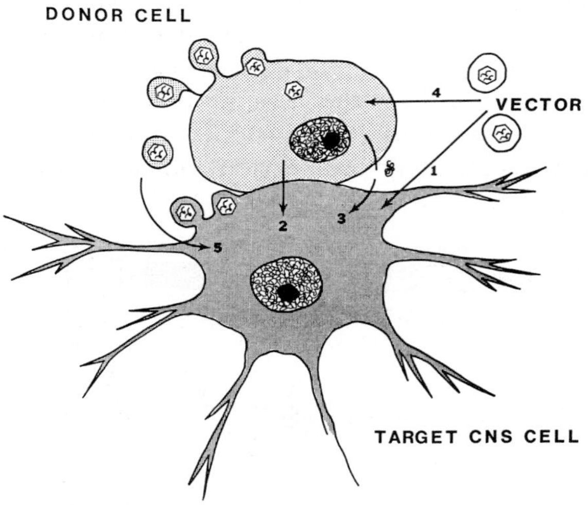

and probably Parkinson's disease. Alternatively, one could express a new function in such defective target cells by introducing a genetically modified donor cell that could establish tight junction or other contacts with the target cell. Some such contacts are known to permit the efficient diffusion of metabolically important small molecules from one cell to another, leading to phenotypic changes in the recipient cell (Loewenstein, 1979). This process has been called "metabolic cooperation" and is known to occur between fibroblasts and glial cells (Gruber et al., 1985), although it has not yet been demonstrated conclusively in neurons. Still other donor cells could express and secrete a diffusible gene product that can be taken up and used by nearby defective target cells. The donor cells may be genetically modified in vitro or, alternatively they may be directly infected in vivo. Finally, an introduced donor cell infected with not only replication-defective vector but also replication-competent helper virus, could produce locally high titers of progeny virus that might in turn infect nearby target cells to provide a functional new transgene.

Marker genes

Initial studies have provided support for the concept that a combination of gene transfer and neural grafting can be used as a new approach toward the restoration of some functions in the damaged or diseased brain (Gage et al. 1987). An essential requirement for the development of this approach is the availability of a reporter gene which can be easily and accurately detected by histochemical and/or biochemical methods.

Retrovirus-mediated transfer of the *Escherichia coli* (*E. coli*) β-galactosidase gene (*lacZ*), combined with histochemical staining for β-galactosidase activity (Sanes et al., 1986; Price et al., 1987; Turner et al., 1987), has recently been used to mark cell lineages in the CNS. These studies are based on the assumption that exogenous *E. coli* β-galactosidase can be distinguished from the endogenous lysosomal β-galactosidase that is widely distributed

DONOR CELL

VECTOR

TARGET CNS CELL

Fig. 3. Introduction of new function into target cells. In the most straightforward approach, transgenes would be introduced into the target cells directly (1). Alternatively, donor cells may be used to introduce the new function into the target cells through tight junctions (2), or through secretion and uptake of the gene products (3). The donor cells may express the new function naturally or may be genetically modified to express the function (4), either in vitro or in vivo. Finally, donor cells genetically engineered to produce transmissible retrovirus (see Fig. 1) could be used to produce virus that can, in turn, infect target cells (5).

in mammalian cells (Furth and Robinson, 1965; Dannenberg and Suga, 1981; Mann et al., 1983), taking advantage of the widely different pH optima for the two enzymes. The pH optimum for *E. coli* β-galactosidase is approximately 7.3 and that or rat brain is approximately 3.5.

Based on these important features, we chose *lacZ* as a reporter gene for the grafting of retrovirus-infected cultured cells to the rat brain. We have observed *E. coli* β-galactosidase-positive fibroblasts, stained at pH 7.5, in the brains of rats several weeks after grafting. However, some β-galactosidase-positive cells were also observed in control grafts of cells which had not been infected with the *lacZ* gene. Subsequent studies revealed that this "false" staining was due to endogenous lysosomal activity associated with macrophage infiltration induced by the damage associated with grafting. By using an antibody specific for *E. coli* β-galactosidase we have been able to distinguish between the *E. coli* enzyme and the endogenous mammalian β-galactosidase. We conclude here that *lacZ* is a useful reporter gene for intracerebral grafting studies if appropriate caution is taken for false positives. Our next objective was to test this approach with a gene which we could use to evaluate the consequences of the therapeutic intervention.

The functional gene product (NGF)

NGF is currently the best characterized neurotrophic factor (NTF) (Cohen and Levi-Montalcini, 1957; Greene and Shooter, 1980; Thoenen and Barde, 1980; Barde et al., 1983; Ullrich et al., 1983; Berg, 1984). NGF supports the survival and axonal growth in vitro and in vivo of sensory and sympathetic neurons from the peripheral nervous system (PNS) (Gundersen and Barrett, 1980; Campenot, 1982). Furthermore, NGF can attract and guide regenerating axons, whether provided to the neuron in a soluble or immobilized form (Gundersen and Barrett, 1980; Levi-Montalcini, 1982), and may stimulate the growth rate even of axons whose neurons do not require NGF for survival (Collins and Dawson, 1983). A number of studies have shown that NGF occurs in, and is produced by, the central nervous system (CNS). For example, mammalian CNS tissues have been shown to contain NGF messenger RNA by in situ hybridization (Korshing et al., 1985; Sheldon and Reichardt, 1986), NGF antigen by immunohistochemical and radioimmune assays (Greene and Shooter, 1980; Ayer LeLievre et al., 1983), NGF receptors by autoradiography (Richardson et al., 1986) and NGF by biological assays (Scott et al., 1981; Manthorpe et al., 1983; Nieto-Sampedro et al., 1983; Collins and Crutcher, 1985). The greatest NGF levels in CNS tissues appear within the target areas of the cholinoceptive basal forebrain systems (Scott et al., 1981), and NGF administered into rat brain raises choline acetyltransferase (ChAT) levels in the hippocampus and striatum (Hefti et al., 1984; Mobley et al., 1985). Radiolabeled NGF injected into target regions is taken up and retrogradely accumulated by the cholinergic neurons innervating them, such as the septal/diagonal band neurons for the hippocampus and nucleus basalis neurons for the neocortex (Schwab et al., 1979; Gnahn et al., 1983; Seiler and Schwab, 1984). NGF is also produced by purified cultures of cerebral astroglial cells (Rudge et al., 1985) and accumulates in fluids surrounding rat brain lesions (Manthorpe et al., 1983; Nieto-Sampedro et al., 1983; Assouline et al., 1985). More recently NGF has been shown to increase ChAT activity in CNS neuronal cultures (Honegger and Lenoir, 1982; Hefti et al., 1985; Martinez et al., 1985; Mobley et al., 1985).

The concept that neuronal survival in vivo may depend on the continued presence of an adequate supply of NTFs in general, and NGF in particular, is supported by the existence of such phenomena as: (1) "developmental neuronal death," in which the excessive number of neurons produced during development is decreased to accommodate the limited target cell number (Landmeser and Pilar, 1978; Cunningham, 1982; Hamburger and Oppenheim, 1982; Cowan et al., 1984; Fawcett et al., 1984); (2) "retrograde neuronal degeneration," in which axotomized neurons cut off from their innervation target and surrounding glial cells undergo degeneration or even death (Grafstein, 1977; Feringa et al., 1983; Pearson et al., 1983; Grady et al., 1984); and (3) "pathological neuronal death," in which specific populations of neurons degenerate and die (Terry and Davies, 1980; Appel, 1981; Bartus et al., 1982; Bondareff et al., 1982; Whitehouse et al., 1982). One explanation commonly put forth for such neuronal death-inducing situations is that neurons normally depend for their continued health upon NTFs supplied by their target and associated glial cells, and that disruption in this trophic supply causes their death.

Model system: "retrograde neuronal degeneration"

The cholinergic projection from the adult rat septum and diagonal band to the ipsilateral hippocampus has been a useful model for examining CNS plasticity (Chun and Patterson, 1977; Gnahn et al., 1983; Amaral and Kurz, 1985; Armstrong et al., 1987; Springer et al., 1987). Neurons of the medial septum and the vertical limb of the diagonal band project dorsally to the hippocampus mainly through the fimbria-fornix (Lewis et al., 1967; Armstrong et al., 1983; Gage et al., 1983). About 50% of the septal/diagonal band neurons sending fibers through the fimbria-fornix are cholinergic (Amaral and Kurz, 1985; Wainer et al., 1985) and provide the hippocampus with about 90% of its total cholinergic innervation (Storm-Mathisen, 1974). The cholinergic neurons, axons and terminals can be visualized by acetylcholinesterase (AChE) (Butcher, 1983; Hedreen et al., 1985) and ChAT immunocytochemical analysis (Armstrong et al., 1983; Wainer et al., 1985), and the terminal fields within the hippocampal formation can be quantified biochemically by measuring extracted ChAT activity (Fonnum, 1969, 1984).

Complete transection of the fimbria-fornix pathway in adult rats results in a rapid and consistent retrograde degeneration and death of many of the septum/diagonal band neurons (including the cholinergic neurons) that originally contributed axons through this pathway (Cunningham, 1982; Grady et al., 1984; Kromer and Cornbrooks, 1984; Wainer et al., 1985; Hefti, 1986). One explanation for this axotomy-induced cell death is that the septal neurons become deprived of a critical supply of NTF provided possibly by the post-synaptic neurons or glial cells in the axonal and/or synaptic vicinity within the hippocampal innervation territory (Gnahn et al., 1983; Nieto-Sampedro et al., 1983; Heacock et al., 1984; Collins and Crutcher, 1985; Gage and Bjorklund, 1986). That this hippocampal NTF might be NGF or NGF-like is supported by the previously listed studies from several laboratories reporting an NGF presence within the septo-hippocampal system.

These studies raise the question whether exogenous administration of NGF to axotomized septal neurons might rescue them from the ensuing retrograde degeneration and death and thus allow them to regenerate their already cut axons, or even grow new ones, back to the hippocampal formation. Recently Hefti (1986) and Williams et al. (1986) have independently reported that the intraventricular administration of purified NGF into adult rats from the time of fimbria-fornix transection onward prevents the death of most of the axotomized cholinergic septum/diagonal band neurons. Furthermore, it appears that, as a result of the transection even non-cholinergic septal neurons (Panula et al., 1984) are destined to die (Gage et al., 1986) and may be saved by NGF administration (Williams et al., 1986). NGF administration also seems to prevent the degeneration of the cut septal cholinergic axons and/or stimulate their regrowth, since a large number of AChE-positive fibers appear to form a neuroma-like structure proximal to the transection site (Gage et al., 1986).

Using the above described model system we have tested the possible functional effects of genetically modified cells grafted to the brain. Specifically, we demonstrated that cultured rat fibroblasts, genetically modified to produce and secrete NGF, and then grafted to the cavity formed in creating a fimbria-fornix lesion, prevented retrograde cholinergic degeneration and induced axonal sprouting, thereby demonstrating a functional response (Rosenberg et al., 1988).

A prototypical retroviral vector was constructed that contains NGF cDNA corresponding to the shorter transcript that predominates in mouse tissue receiving sympathetic innervation (Edwards et al., 1986; Fig. 4). This transcript is believed to encode the precursor to NGF that is constitutively secreted. The vector also includes a dominant selectable marker, the transposon Tn5 neomycin-resistance gene. Transmissible retrovirus was generated and used to infect the established rat fibroblast cell line 208F. Individual neomycin-resistant colonies, selected in medium containing the neomycin analog G418, were expanded and tested for NGF production and secretion using a two-site enzyme immunoassay (Korsching and Thoenen, 1983). The clone producing the greatest levels of NGF had 1.7 ng NGF/mg total cellular protein and secreted NGF into the medium at a rate of 50 pg/h/10^5 cells. The NGF secreted by this clone was biologically active, as determined by its ability to induce neurite outgrowth from PC12 rat pheochromocytoma cells. Uninfected 208F cells, in contrast, did not produce detectable levels of NGF in either assay.

Fimbria-fornix (FF) lesions were made in 16 rats; 8 rats received grafts of infected cells while the remaining eight received uninfected control cells. After 2 weeks, all animals were sacrificed and

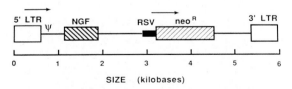

Fig. 4. NGF retroviral vector. Constructed from the Moloney murine leukemia virus, containing the 777-bp HgaI-Pst I fragment of the NGF cDNA under the control of the viral 5′ LTR. The vector also includes the dominant selector marker encoding the neomycin-resistance function of transposon Tn5 under the control of an internal Rous sarcoma virus promoter.

processed for immunohistochemistry. Staining for fibronectin, a fibroblast-specific marker, revealed robust graft survival, which was comparable in both the NGF-secreting cells and the control cells. Sections stained for choline acetyltransferase (ChAT) to evaluate the survival of cholinergic cell bodies indicated a greater number of remaining neurons on the lesioned side of the medial septum in animals that had received grafts of infected cells than in animals that had received control grafts. Neuronal survival was quantitated and, when expressed as a percentage of the remaining cholinergic cells in the septum ipsilateral to the lesion relative to the intact contralateral septum, was shown to be 92% in animals grafted with NGF-secreting cells, but only 49% in animals grafted with control cells (Rosenberg et al., 1988). The latter results from the control group are comparable to our previous observations in lesioned animals that had received no grafts (Williams et al., 1986).

The 208F fibroblasts used in the above described study were chosen because they were immortalized, and were deficient in the HPRT gene, a feature that is useful as an in vitro model of Lesch-Nyhan disease. However, upon careful examination we found that these cells do not survive as well in vivo as the parental line, Rat1, and thus the NGF retroviral vector was used to infect the established rat fibroblast cell line Rat1 cells. As before, individual neomycin-resistant colonies, selected in medium containing the neomycin analog G418, were expanded and tested for NGF production and secretion by two-site enzyme immunoassay. This time the highest producing clone, Rat1-N.8-8, contained 66 pg NGF/10^5 cells and secreted NGF into the medium at a rate of 77 pg/h/10^5 cells. The secreted NGF was biologically active, as determined by its ability to induce neurite outgrowth from PC12 rat pheochromocytoma cells. Uninfected Rat1 cells, in contrast, did not produce detectable levels of NGF.

Again unilateral aspirative cavities were made through the cingulate cortex of Sprague-Dawley rats, completely transecting the fimbria-fornix. Retrovirus-infected (NGF-secreting) and control uninfected fibroblasts were suspended in PBS at $8 \cdot 10^4$ cells/μl, and 4 μl aliquots were injected free-hand into the lesion cavity and lateral ventricle ipsilateral to the cavity. In this experiment, animals were sacrificed after 2 or 8 weeks and processed for immunohistochemistry and for in situ hybridization of mRNA for NGF. Staining for fibronectin, a fibroblast-specific marker, revealed robust graft survival that was comparable in both infected and control groups. Staining for choline acetyltransferase, to evaluate the survival of cholinergic neurons, indicated a significantly greater number of remaining neurons on the lesioned side of the medial septum in animals that had received grafts on infected cells than in animals that had received uninfected control grafts (see Fig. 5A, B). We have further examined these animals for their immunoreactivity to NGR receptor (IGg 192). With this antibody we observed that in the animals with control grafts there was a dramatic decrease in the number and intensity of cell staining in the medial septal area ispilateral to

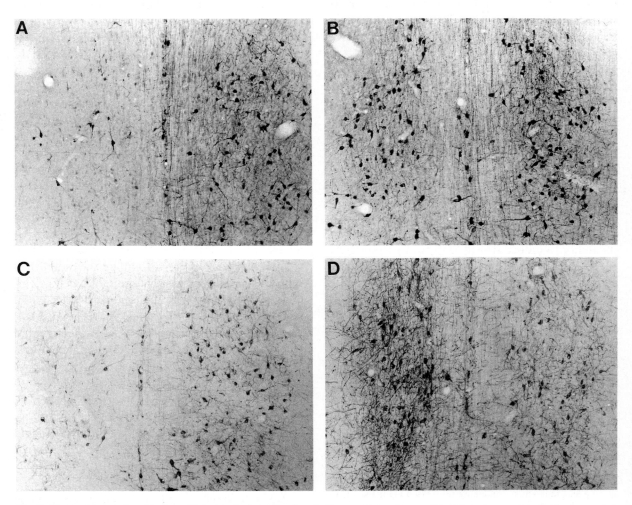

Fig. 5. Photomicrographs of immunohistochemical staining for choline acetyltransferease (ChAT) and nerve growth factor receptor (NGFR). *A, B.* Coronal section through medial septum of tissue stained for ChAT. *C, D.* Coronal section through medial septum of tissue stained for NGFR. *A, C.* Animal with graft of retrovirus-infected cells. *B, D.* Animal with graft of control cells. Lesions were placed on the left side. Magnification: × 220.

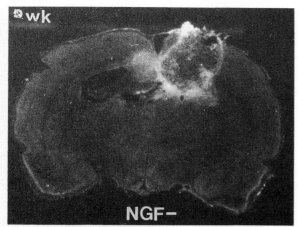

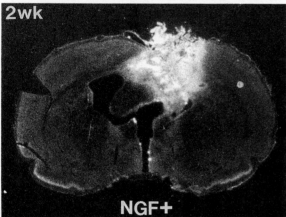

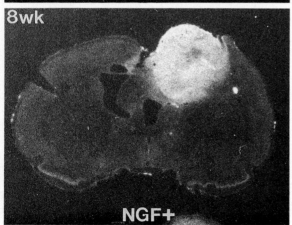

Fig. 6. Photomicrographs of sections prepared for in situ hybridization for NGF mRNA. They are coronal sections taken through the middle of the grafts in the fimbria-fornix cavity.

the fimbria fornix lesion. In stark contrast, the immunoreactivity for this same antibody was intense in the ipsilateral septum for those animals that received grafts of NGF secreting fibroblasts (see Fig. 5C, D). Staining for parvalbumin, to evaluate the survival of GABAergic neurons, which also degenerate following transection of the fimbria-fornix by 8 weeks (Peterson et al., 1987), indicated no increased survival in response to NGF-secreting fibroblasts, indicating the specificity of these grafts for cholinergic neurons. It is interesting to note that uninfected control grafts resulted in 50% survival of cholinergic neurons, whereas previous studies have shown 10 – 50% survival in untreated control animals (Hefti, 1986; Williams et al., 1986). This suggests the possibility that the fibroblasts produce other as yet unknown factors that can affect cholinergic survival. Alternatively, this could reflect the variablity in the location of the lesion with respect to the cholinergic cell bodies. In our previous study with 208F fibroblasts as well as the study described here, we observed that the animals that received NGF-secreting fibroblasts showed an increase in acetylcholine-sterase-positive fiber and cell staining, with a robust sprouting response in the dorsal lateral quadrant of the septum, and the most intense staining abutting the cavity containing the graft. We had previously observed this sprouting in response to chronic NGF infusion (Gage et al., 1988), but not to the extent seen in the 208F study, even though the fibroblasts secrete NGF at a rate significantly lower than administered in the infusion studies. This observation may reflect the fact that the biological activity of the NGF in the pump decreases with time, while the NGF constantly being synthesized in the cells remains more or less constant. Still other alternatives are conceivable.

Recently we have examined the grafts for their ability to express detectable levels of NGF mRNA in parallel sections of brains which had been taken for histochemical evaluation. Individual sections were processed for in situ hybridization. At 2 weeks following implantation, retroviral-infected fibroblast grafts expressed high levels of NGF mRNA in the graft relative to the endogenous levels in the brain, though message was detected in the expected areas of the hippocampus and cortex. Non-infected grafts showed much less specific hybridization. There was, however, clear hybridization around the edges of the cavity in which the grafts were implanted. This may be attributed to the increased expression of NGF mRNA in the reactive astrocytes around the wound, but at present we do not know this be true. In 3 animals with NGF-producing grafts processed for in situ hybridization at 8 weeks there was continued, though slightly decreased expression of NGF mRNA in the graft, compared to those processed at 2 weeks following grafting (see Fig. 6).

Discussion

Our studies have demonstrated that genetically modified fibroblasts can survive intracerebral grafting and continue to express transgenes for at least 2 months. Furthermore, the grafts continue to produce and secrete sufficient NGF to have a biological effect during this period. There are several prerequisites for a neurological disease to be a candidate for this approach:

(1) The pathogenesis of the disease must be sufficiently well understood to allow identification of the relevant lacking function.

(2) The relevant gene must be available as a well-characterized cDNA clone.

(3) The affected region of the CNS must be known and sufficiently localized to permit implantation into the appropriate area(s).

(4) Restoration of normal function must not, at present, require synaptic contact with target cells. Instead, the donor cells must produce a factor that has a mechanism for release by the cells and uptake by neurons. In the example of NGF, these conditions are satisfied because the NGF precursor protein includes a signal sequence for secretion, and the secreted NGF binds to receptors on the target cholinergic neurons. In other systems the gene product may require active transport into storage vesicles or simply diffuse through the cell membrane. Alternatively, the donor cells can act as a toxin "sink" by expressing an enzyme that metabolizes a neurotoxin. This, of course, requires that the neurotoxin has a mechanism for leaving the neuron and entering the donor cell.

(5) Ideally, an animal model should be available.

We conclude that the intracerebral grafting of genetically modified cells could eventually provide a means for CNS therapy. Together with traditional neuronal grafting and the upcoming vectors for direct genetic modification of neurons in vivo, this approach should permit the treatment of numerous CNS disorders that cannot be treated by standard drug therapies.

Acknowledgements

The research presented in this manuscript was supported by NIA AG-0688, HD20034 and HD00669, the Pew Foundation, The Margaret and Herbert Hoover Foundation, Office of Naval Research, and the State of California DHHS. MBR is the recipient of NRSA postdoctoral fellowship GM11013.

We thank Sheryl Christenson for typing and editing the manuscript.

References

Amaral, D.G. and Kurz, J. (1985) An analysis of the origins of the cholinergic and noncholinergic septal projections to the hippocampal formation of the rat. *J. Comp. Neurol.*, 240: 37 – 59.

Anderson, W.F. (1984) Prospects for human gene therapy. *Science*, 226: 401 – 409.

Appel, S.H. (1981) A unifying hypothesis for the cause of amyotrophic lateral sclerosis, parkinsonism, and Alzheimer disease. *Ann. Neurol.*, 10: 499 – 505.

Armstrong, D.M., Saper, C.B., Levey, A.I., Wainer, B.H. and Terry, R.D. (1983) Distribution of cholinergic neurons in rat brain: demonstrated by the immunocytochemical localization of choline acetyltransferase. *J. Comp. Neurol.*, 216: 53 – 68.

Armstrong, D.M., Terry, R.D., Deteresa, R.M., Bruce, G., Hersh, L.B. and Gage, F.H. (1987) Response of septal cholinergic neurons to axotomy. *J. Comp. Neurol.,* 264: 421 – 436.

Assouline, J., Bosch, E.P., Lim, R., Jenson, R. and Pantazis, N.J. (1985) Detection of a neurite promoting factor with some similarity to nerve growth factor in conditioned media from rat primary Schwann cells and astroglia. *Soc. Neurosci. Abstr.,* 11: 933.

Ayer LeLievre, C.S., Ebendal, T., Olsen, L. and Seiger, A. (1983) Localization of NGF-like immunoreactivity in rat neurons tissue. *Med. Biol.,* 61: 296 – 304.

Barde, Y.A., Edgar, D. and Thoenen, H. (1983) New neurotrophic factors. *Annu. Rev. Physiol.,* 45: 601 – 612.

Bartus, R.T., Dean, R.L., Beer, B. and Lippa, A.S. (1982) The cholinergic hypothesis of geriatric memory dysfunction. *Science,* 217: 408 – 417.

Berg, D.K. (1984) New neuronal growth factors. *Annu. Rev. Neurosci.,* 7: 149 – 170.

Bondareff, W., Mountjoy, C.Q. and Roth, M. (1982) Loss of neurons of origin of the adrenergic projection to cerebral cortex (nucleus locus ceruleus) in senile dementia. *Neurology,* 32: 164 – 168.

Butcher, L.L. (1983) Acetylcholinesterase histochemistry. In: *Handbook of Chemical Neuroanatomy,* Elsevier, Amsterdam, pp. 1 – 49.

Campenot, R.B. (1982) Development of sympathetic neurons in compartmentalized cultures. I. Local control of neurite growth by nerve growth factor. *Dev. Biol.,* 93: 1 – 12.

Chun, L.L.Y. and Patterson, P.H. (1977) Role of nerve growth factor in the development of rat sympathetic neurons in vitro. II. Developmental study. *J. Cell Biol.,* 75: 705 – 711.

Cohen, S. and Levi-Montalcini, R. (1957) Purification and properties of a nerve growth-promoting factor isolated from mouse sarcoma. *Cancer Res.,* 17: 15 – 20.

Collins, F. and Crutcher, K.A. (1985) Neurotrophic activity in the adult rat hippocampal formation: regional distribution and increase after septal lesion. *J. Neurosci.,* 5: 2809 – 2814.

Collins, F. and Dawson, A. (1983) An effect of nerve growth factor on parasympathetic neurite outgrowth. *Proc. Natl. Acad. Sci. U.S.A.,* 80: 2091 – 2094.

Constantini, F., Chada, K. and Magram, K. (1986) Correction of murine β-thalassemia by gene transfer into the germ line. *Science,* 233: 1192 – 1194.

Cowan, W.M., Fawcett, J.W., O'Leary, D.D. and Stanfield, B.B. (1984) Regressive events in neurogenesis. *Science,* 225: 1258 – 1265.

Cunningham, T.J. (1982) Naturally occuring neuron death and its regulation by developing neural pathways. *Int. Rev. Cytol.,* 74: 163 – 186.

Dannenberg, A.M. and Suga, M. (1981) Histochemical stains for macrophages. In: S.D.O. Adams, P.J. Edelson and M.S. Koren (Eds.), *Methods for Studying Mononuclear Phagocytes,* Academic Press, New York, pp. 375 – 396.

Edwards, R.H., Selby, M.J. and Rutter, W.J. (1986) Differential RNA splicing predicts two distinct nerve growth factor precursors. *Nature,* 319: 784 – 787.

Fawcett, J.W., O'Leary, D.D.M. and Cowan, W.M. (1984) Activity and the control of ganglian cell death in the rat retina. *Proc. Natl. Acad. Sci. U.S.A.,* 81: 5589 – 5593.

Feringa, E.R., Vahlsing, H.L. and Smith, B.E. (1983) Retrograde transport in spinal cord neurons after spinal transection. *Neurology,* 33: 478 – 482.

Fonnum, F. (1969) Radiochemical micro assays for the determination of choline acetyltransferase and acetylcholinesterase activities. *J. Biochem.,* 115: 465 – 472.

Fonnum, F. (1984) Topographical and subcellular localization of choline acetyltransferase in the rat hippocampal region. *J. Neurochem.,* 24: 407 – 409.

Friedmann, T. (1983) *Gene Therapy – Fact and Fiction in Biology's New Approaches to Disease,* Cold Spring Harbor Laboratory, Cold Spring Harbor, NY.

Furth, A.J. and Robinson, D. (1965) Specificity and multiple forms of β-galactosidase in the rat. *J. Biochem.,* 97: 59 – 66.

Gage, F.H. and Bjorklund, A. (1986a) Neural grafting in the aged brain. *Annu. Rev. Physiol.,* 48: 447 – 459.

Gage, F.H. and Bjorklund, A. (1986b) Enhanced graft survival in the hippocampus following selective denervation. *Neuroscience,* 17: 89 – 98.

Gage, F.H., Bjorklund, A., Stenevi, U. and Dunnett, S.B. (1983) Functional correlates of compensatory collateral sprouting by aminergic and cholinergic afferents in the hippocampal formation. *Brain Res.,* 268: 39 – 47.

Gage, F.H., Wictorin, K., Fisher, W., Williams, L.R., Varon, S. and Bjorklund, A. (1986) Life and death of cholinergic neurons: in the septal and diagonal band region following complete fimbria-fornix transection. *Neuroscience,* 19: 241 – 255.

Gage, F.H., Wolff, J.A., Rosenberg, M.B., Xu, L., Yee, J.E., Shults, C. and Friedmann, T. (1987) Grafting genetically modified cells to the brain: possibilities for the future. *Neuroscience,* 23: 795 – 807.

Gage, F.H., Armstrong, D.M., Williams, L.R. and Varon, S. (1988) Morphologic response of axotomized septal neurons to nerve growth factor. *J. Comp. Neurol.,* 269: 147 – 155.

Gilboa, E., Eglitis, M.A., Kantoff, P.W. and Anderson, W.F. (1986) Transfer and expression of cloned genes using retroviral vectors. *Biotechniques,* 4: 504 – 512.

Gnahn, H., Hefti, F., Heumann, R., Schwab, M.E. and Thoenen, H. (1983) NGF-mediated increase in choline acetyltransferase (ChAT) in the neonatal rat forebrain; evidence for physiological role of NGF in the brain? *Dev. Brain Res.,* 9: 45 – 52.

Grady, S., Reeves, T. and Steward, O. (1984) Time course of retrograde degeneration of the cells of origin of the septohippocampal pathway after fimbria-fornix transections. *Soc. Neurosci. Abstr.,* 10: 463.

Grafstein, B. (1977) Axonal transport and transneuronal transport in mouse visual system following injection of tritiated fucose into the eye. *Exp. Neurol.,* 48: 32 – 51.

Greene, L. and Shooter, E.M. (1980) The nerve growth factor: biochemistry, synthesis, and mechanism of action. *Annu. Rev. Neurosci.,* 3: 353–402.

Gruber, H.E., Koenker, R., Kuchtman, L.A., Willis, R.C. and Seegmiller, J.E. (1985) Glial cells metabolically cooperate: a potential requirement for gene replacement therapy. *Proc. Natl. Acad. Sci. U.S.A.,* 82: 6662–6666.

Gundersen, R.W. and Barrett, J.N. (1980) Characterization of the turning response of dorsal root neurites toward nerve growth factor. *J. Cell Biol.,* 87: 546–554.

Hamburger, V. and Oppenheim, R.W. (1982) Naturally occurring neuronal death in vertebrates. *Neurosci. Comm.,* 1: 55–68.

Hayward, W.S., Neel, B.G. and Astrin, S.M. (1981) Activation of cellular *onc* gene by promoter insertion in ALZ-induced lymphoid lukosis. *Nature,* 290: 475.

Heacock, A.M., Schonfeld, A.P. and Katzman, R. (1984) Relationship of hippocampal trophic activity to cholinergic nerve sprouting. *Soc. Neurosci. Abstr.,* 10: 1052.

Hedreen, J.C., Bacon, J.C. and Price, D.L. (1985) A modified histochemical method to visualize acetylcholinesterase-containing axons. *J. Histochem. Cytochem.,* 33: 134–140.

Hefti, F. (1986) Nerve growth factor (NGF) promotes survival of septal cholinergic neurons after fimbrial transection. *J. Neurosci.,* 6: 2155–2162.

Hefti, F., Dravid, A. and Hartikka, J.J. (1984) Chronic intraventricular injections of nerve growth factor elevate hippocampal choline acetyltransferase activity in adult rats with partial septohippocampal lesions. *Brain Res.,* 293: 305–311.

Hefti, F., Hartikka, J.J., Eckenstein, F., Gnahn, H., Heumann, R. and Schwab, M. (1985) Nerve growth factor increases choline acetyltransferase but not survival or fiber outgrowth of cultured fetal septal cholinergic neurons. *Neuroscience,* 14: 55–68.

Honegger, P. and Lenoir, D. (1982) Nerve growth factor (NGF) stimulation of cholinergic telencephalic neurons in aggregating cell cultures. *Dev. Brain. Res.,* 3: 229–238.

Korsching, S. and Thoenen, H. (1983) Nerve growth factor in sympathetic ganglia and corresponding target organs of the rat: correlation with density of sympathetic innervation. *Proc. Natl. Acad. Sci. U.S.A.,* 80: 3513–3516.

Korsching, S., Auburger, G., Heumann, R., Scott, J. and Thoenen, H. (1985) Levels of nerve growth factor and its mRNA in the central nervous system of the rat correlate with cholinergic innervation. *EMBO J.,* 4: 1389–1393.

Kromer, L.R. and Cornbrooks, C. (1984) Laminin and a Schwann cell surface antigen present within transplants of cultured CNS cells colocalize with CNS axons regenerating in vivo. *Soc. Neurosci. Abstr.,* 10: 1084.

Landmeser, L. and Pilar, G. (1978) Interactions between neurons and their targets during in vivo synaptogenesis. *Fed. Proc.,* 37: 2016–2021.

Levi-Montalcini, R. (1982) Developmental neurobiology and the natural history of nerve growth factor. *Annu. Rev.*

Neurosci., 5: 341–361.

Lewis, P.R., Shute, C.C.D. and Silver, A. (1967) Confirmation from cholineacetylase of a massive cholinergic innervation to the rat hippocampus. *J. Physiol. (Lond.),* 191: 215–224.

Loewenstein, W.R. (1979) Junctional intercellular communication and the control of cell growth. *Biochim. Biophys. Acta,* 560: 1–66.

Lohler, J., Timpl, R. and Jaenisch, R. (1984) Embryonic lethal mutation in mouse collagen: gene causes rupture of blood vessels and is associated with erythropoietic and mesenchymal cell death. *Cell,* 38: 597–607.

Mann, R., Mulligan, R. and Baltimore, D. (1983) Construction of a retrovirus packaging mutant and its use to produce helper-free defective retrovirus. *Cell,* 33: 153–159.

Manthorpe, M., Nieto-Sampedro, M., Skaper, S.D., Barbin, G., Longo, F.M., Lewis, E.R., Cotman, C.W. and Varon, S. (1983) Neurotrophic activity in brain wounds of the developing rat. *Brain Res.,* 267: 47–56.

Martinez, H.J., Dreyfus, C.F., Jonakait, G.M. and Black, I.B. (1985) Nerve growth factor promotes cholinergic development in brain striatal cultures. *Proc. Natl. Acad. Sci. U.S.A.,* 82: 7777–7781.

Mason, A.J., Pitts, S.L., Nikolics, K., Szonyi, E., Wilcox, J.N., Seeburg, P.H. and Steward, T.A. (1986) The hypogonadal mouse: reproductive functions restored by gene therapy. *Science,* 234: 1372–1378.

Miller, A.D., Law, M.-F. and Verma, I. (1985) Generation of helper free amphotropic retroviruses that transduce a dominant-acting, methotrexate-resistant dihydrofolate reductase gene. *Mol. Cell. Biol.,* 5: 431–437.

Mobley, W.C., Rutkowski, J.L., Tennekoon, G.I., Buchanan, K. and Johnston, M.W. (1985) Choline acetyltransferase activity in striatum of neonatal rats increased by nerve growth factor. *Science,* 229: 284–287.

Nieto-Sampedro, M., Manthorpe, M., Barbin, G., Varon, S. and Cotman, C.W. (1983) Injury-induced neuronotrophic activity in adult rat brain: correlation with survival delayed implants in the wound cavity. *J. Neurosci.,* 3: 2219–2229.

Panula, P., Revuelta, A.V., Cheney, D.L., Wu, J-Y. and Costa, E. (1984) An immunohistochemical study in the location of GABAergic neurons in rat septum. *J. Comp. Neurol.,* 222: 69–80.

Pearson, R.C.A., Gatter, K.C. and Powell, T.P.S. (1983) Retrograde cell degeneration in the basal nucleus of monkey and man. *Brain Res.,* 261: 321–326.

Peterson, G.M., Williams, L.R., Varon, S. and Gage, F.H. (1987) Loss of GABAergic neurons in the medial septum after fimbria-fornix transection. *Neurosci. Lett.,* 76: 140–144.

Price, J., Turner, D. and Cepko, C. (1987) Lineage analysis in the vertebrate nervous system by retrovirus-mediated gene transfer. *Proc. Natl. Acad. Sci. U.S.A.,* 84: 156–160.

Readhead, C., Popko, B., Takashashi, K., Schine, H.D., Saavedra, R.A., Sidman, R.L. and Hood, L. (1987) Expression of a myelin basic protein gene in transgenic shiverer mice: correction of the dysmyelinating phenotype. *Cell*, 48: 703 – 712.

Richardson, P.M., Verge Isse, V.M.K. and Riopelle, R.J. (1986) Distribution of neuronal receptors for nerve growth factor in the rat. *J. Neurosci.*, 6: 2312 – 2321.

Rosenberg, M.B., Friedman, T., Robertson, R.C., Tuszynski, M., Wolff, J.A., Breakefield, X.O. and Gage, F.H. (1988) Grafting genetically modified cells to the damaged brain: restorative effects of NGF expression. *Science*, 242: 1575 – 1578.

Rudge, J.R., Manthorpe, M. and Varon, S. (1985) The output of neuronotrophic and neurite-promoting agents from rat brain astroglial cells: a micro-culture method for screening potential regulatory molecules. *Dev. Brain Res.*, 19: 161 – 172.

Sanes, J.R., Rubenstein, J.L.R. and Nicolas, J.F. (1986) Use of a recombinant retrovirus to study post-implantation cell lineage in mouse embryos. *EMBO J.*, 5: 3133 – 3142.

Schwab, M.E., Otten, U., Agid, Y. and Thoenen, H. (1979) Nerve growth factor (NGF) in the rat CNS: absence of specific retrograde axonal transport and tyrosine hydroxylase induction in locus coeruleus and substantia nigra. *Brain Res.*, 168: 473 – 483.

Scott, S.M., Tarris, R., Eveleth, D., Mansfield, H., Weichsel, M.E. and Fisher, D.A. (1981) Bioassay detection of mouse nerve growth factor (mNGF) in the brain of adult mice. *J. Neurosci. Res.*, 6: 653 – 658.

Seiler, M. and Schwab, M.E. (1984) Specific retrograde transport of nerve growth factor (NGF) from cortex to nucleus basalis in the rat. *Brain Res.*, 300: 33 – 39.

Sheldon, D.L. and Reichardt, L.F. (1986) Studies on the expression of the beta-nerve growth factor (NGF) gene in the central nervous system; level and regional distribution of NGF mRNA suggest that NGF functions as a trophic factor for several distinct populations of neurons. *Proc. Natl. Acad. Sci. U.S.A.*, 83: 2714 – 2718.

Springer, J.E., Tairien, M.W. and Loy, R. (1987) Regional analysis of age-related changes in the cholinergic system of the hippocampal formation and basal forebrain of the rat. *Brain Res.*, 407: 180 – 184.

Storm-Mathisen, J. (1974) Choline acetyltransferase and acetylcholinesterase in fascia dentata following lesions of the entorhinal afferent. *Brain Res.*, 80: 119 – 181.

Terry, R.D. and Davies, P. (1980) Dementia of the Alzheimer type. *Annu. Rev. Neurosci.*, 3: 77 – 95.

Thoenen, H. and Barde, Y.A. (1980) Physiology of nerve growth factor. *Physiol. Rev.*, 60: 1284 – 1335.

Toneguzzo, F., Hayday, A.C. and Keating, A. (1986) Electric field-mediated DNA transfer: transient and stable gene expression in human and mouse lymphoid cells. *Mol. Cell. Biol.*, 6: 703 – 706.

Turner, D.L. and Cepko, C.L. (1987) A common progenitor for neurons and glia persists in rat retina late in development. *Nature*, 328: 131 – 136.

Ullrich, R., Gray, A., Berman, C. and Dull, T.J. (1983) Human beta-nerve growth factor gene sequence highly homologous to that of mouse. *Nature*, 303: 821 – 825.

Varmus, H. and Swanstrom, R. (1982) Replication of retroviruses. In: R. Weiss, N. Reich, H. Warmus and J. Coffin (Eds.), *RNA Tumor Viruses*, Cold Spring Harbor Laboratory, Cold Spring Harbor, NY, pp. 369 – 512.

Wainer, B.H., Levey, A.I., Rye, D.B., Mesulam, M. and Mufson, E.J. (1985) Cholinergic and non-cholinergic septohippocampal pathways. *Neurosci. Lett.*, 54: 45 – 52.

Whitehouse, P.J., Price, D.I., Struble, R.G., Clark, A.W., Coyle, J.T. and Delong, M.R. (1982) Alzheimer's disease and senile dementia: loss of neurons in the basal forebrain. *Science*, 215: 1237 – 1239.

Williams, L.R., Varon, S., Peterson, G.M., Wictorin, K., Fisher, W., Bjorklund, A. and Gage, F.H. (1986) Continuous infusion of nerve growth factor prevents basal forebrain neuronal death after fimbria-fornix transection. *Proc. Natl. Acad. Sci. U.S.A.*, 83: 9231 – 9235.

Wolff, J.A., Yee, J.K., Skelly, H.F., Moores, J.C., Respess, J.G., Friedmann, T. and Leffert, H. (1987) Expression of retrovirally transduced genes in primary cultures of adult rat hepatocytes. *Proc. Natl. Acad. Sci. U.S.A.*, 84: 3344 – 3348.

SECTION V

Intracellular Molecular Mechanisms

P. Coleman, G. Higgins and C. Phelps (Eds.)
Progress in Brain Research, Vol. 86
© 1990 Elsevier Science Publishers B.V. (Biomedical Division)

CHAPTER 18

Receptors, phosphoinositol hydrolysis and plasticity of nerve cells

Norbert J. Pontzer, L. Judson Chandler, Bruce R. Stevens and Fulton T. Crews

Department of Pharmacology and Therapeutics, College of Medicine, J.H.M. Health Center, Gainesville, FL 32610, U.S.A.

Introduction

Neuronal plasticity is thought to occur through synaptic reorganization, morphological changes in synaptic and dendritic structure, and by changes in synaptic sensitivity, such as long term potentiation (LTP). Excitatory neurotransmission is involved in all of these forms of plasticity. Increases in cytosolic calcium levels (Lynch et al., 1983; Malenka et al., 1988) and/or protein kinase activation (Malenka et al., 1986a; Malinow et al., 1988) are likely to mediate adaptive changes in response to high levels of excitation. We have studied cholinergic and glutaminergic excitatory transmission. Both cholinergic-muscarinic and glutaminergic-quisqualate receptor stimulation cause excitation and increased firing rates, which at high concentrations lead to a complete loss of cell firing, e.g., desensitization (Fig. 1). This desensitization may by secondary to a depolarization block.

Neuronal depolarization increases cytosolic calcium through activation of voltage-dependent calcium channels. Increases in cytosolic calcium stimulate the activity of phospholipase C (Gonzales and Crews, 1988; Homma et al., 1988), which further increases calcium levels through $Ins(1,4,5)$ P_3 mediated intracellular calcium release. Furthermore, potassium depolarization tremendously potentiates receptor-stimulated phosphoinositide hydrolysis which in turn causes greater excitation and depolarization (Baird and Nahorski, 1986;

Eva and Costa, 1986). This feed-forward loop could lead to high levels of the second messengers calcium, IP_3, IP_4 and diacylglycerol (DAG), synergistically increase excitability, and perhaps produce the prolonged changes in neurotransmission associated with plasticity. Depolarization induced PI hydrolysis and increases in cytosolic calcium may thus modulate many of the processes associated with long-term neuronal adaptation.

Excitatory responses in hippocampus

Neuronal plasticity has been extensively studied in the hippocampus due to its well defined cytoarchitecture and pivotal role in memory. Muscarinic cholinergic receptors in the hippocampus are associated with memory function. Antimuscarinic drugs, well known for their amnesic effects, support the cholinergic hypothesis of memory (Bartus et al., 1982). Muscarinic receptors in the hippocampus inhibit a number of potassium currents which lead to neuronal excitation. Inhibition of the calcium-dependent potassium current IK_{ca} and a small "leak" current lead to increased cell firing. In addition, intense stimulation of muscarinic receptors inhibits IK_m, which may lead to depolarization block (Madison et al., 1987). Inhibition of potassium currents would delay repolarization and block accommodation, leading to prolonged depolarization. These current changes summate to modify hippocampal pyramidal cell

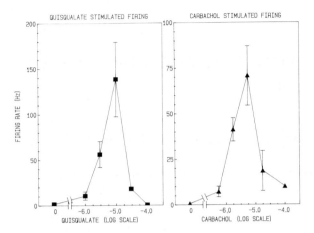

Fig. 1. The extracellular firing rate response to increasing concentrations of the glutaminergic agonist quisqualate (left) and the muscarinic agonist carbachol (right). Hippocampal slices from mature male Sprague-Dawley rats were chopped (375 – 400 μm) and placed in an interface type recording chamber in which buffer containing the various concentrations of drug could be introduced. Firing rate was obtained with 2 – 5 MΩ pipettes and all spikes above noise level were discriminated into 1 or 10 sec bins. The rate of firing was measured 20 – 30 min after exposure when responses had stabilized. Values for carbachol are the average ± S.E.M. compiled from 7 separate experiments. Values for quisqualate are the average ± S.E.M. compiled from 3 separate experiments.

membrane potential and firing rate. Carbachol, a cholinergic agonist which mimics acetylcholine, has a biphasic firing rate concentration – response curve in the hippocampus. Low concentrations increase cell firing while higher concentrations actually decrease cell firing, i.e., desensitize cell firing (Fig. 1). The decreased cell firing may be due to depolarization block, which would be associated with prolonged increases in intracellular calcium due to the opening of voltage-dependent calcium channels. The biphasic excitatory dose – response curve of carbachol appears to be due to excitation of two subtypes of muscarinic receptor, e.g., $M_1 - m_1$ and m_3 (Pontzer and Crews, 1990). The m_3 receptor subtype which appears to be the higher affinity receptor, is linked to inhibition of IK_{ca} and mediates increased cell firing. The $M_1 - m_1$ receptor subtypes appear to have a lower

affinity and inhibit IK_m. Inhibition of both IK_{ca} and IK_m currents could result in prolonged depolarization.

Glutamate receptors are excitatory and have been suggested to be involved in neuronal plasticity. Many studies dealing with LTP and other forms of plasticity have focused on the large calcium currents associated with NMDA receptor activation as a major factor in modifying synaptic transmission (Baudry and Lynch, 1980; Eccles, 1983; Jahr and Stevens, 1987). These currents are blocked by physiological levels of magnesium when the membrane is in the resting state, e.g., polarized. It has thus been hypothesized that there must be simultaneous activation of other receptors that depolarize the membrane in order to allow NMDA-gated calcium flux to occur. Our evidence that both quisqualate and carbachol stimulate neuronal excitation and produce a possible depolarization block (Fig. 1) may allow them to fulfill this function. Muscarinic and/or non-NMDA glutaminergic receptor activation may thus be important in LTP and memory. The membrane depolarization they produce could both increase intracellular calcium and remove the magnesium block of NMDA-gated calcium channels.

Interaction of PI hydrolysis and neuronal plasticity

Phosphoinositide hydrolysis and intracellular calcium both stimulate and enhance neuronal excitability. A variety of excitatory transmitters act on receptors linked through a guanine nucleotide protein (G-protein) to activate phospholipase C (PLC) and produce the second messengers $Ins(1,4,5)P_3$ and DAG. DAG is thought to activate protein kinase C (PKC). $Ins(1,4,5)P_3$ which is thought to release calcium from intracellular stores, can be phosphorylated by $Ins(1,4,5)P_3$ 3-kinase to form $Ins(1,3,4,5)P_4$. Studies have suggested that $Ins(1,3,4,5)P_4$ may also possess second messenger functions by gating a membrane calcium conductance.

PKC activation by DAG may play a crucial role

in LTP. Phorbol esters have been shown to induce a form of LTP (Malenka et al., 1986a), whereas non-specific block of PKC prevents the expression of LTP (Brown et al., 1989). Furthermore, protein substrates of PKC undergo increased phophorylation during LTP and during certain memory-intensive behavioral paradigms (Bank et al., 1988). Activation of PKC has also been found to block IK_{ca}, which may tend to increase voltage-dependent calcium flux by decreasing the afterhyperpolarization (Barbaran et al., 1985; Malenka et al., 1986b). The calcium sensitivity of PKC may thus lead to another positive feed-forward loop.

In addition to receptor-G protein activation of PLC, depolarization can directly activate PLC. Depolarization-dependent stimulation of PI hy-

drolysis is completely dependent upon presence of extracellular calcium (Fig. 2). At least two phosphoinositide-specific phospholipase C enzymes are present in brain (Gonzales and Crews, 1988; Homma et al., 1988). Although all known phosphoinositide-specific phospholipase C's are sensitive to Ca, agonist receptor-G protein interactions are likely to activate some phospholipase C at resting intracellular Ca^{2+} levels. In addition, increases in intracellular calcium may directly activate additional phospholipase C isozymes (Fig. 3), as well as enhancing the transmitter-activated phospholipase C.

Combination of a slightly depolarizing potassium concentration and muscarinic-cholinergic receptor activation, has been reported to synergistically increase phosphoinositide hydrolysis several fold (Baird and Nahorski, 1986; Eva and Costa, 1986), possibly due to increased intracellular calcium. NMDA-gated calcium flux might be expected to both directly stimulate phosphoinositide hydrolysis, and augment PI hydrolysis due to glutaminergic and/or muscarinic receptor activation. Although the mechanisms involved in heterosynaptic control of calcium and phosphoinositide-

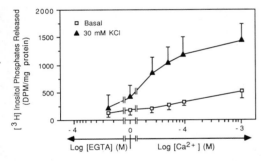

Fig. 2. The effects of increasing extracellular calcium on basal and potassium-stimulated phosphoinositide hydrolysis in rat cerebral cortical synaptoneurosomes over a 60-min time period. Synaptoneurosomes were prepared as described by Hollingsworth et al. (1985). [^{3}H]inositol was incorporated into phospholipids by incubating 5 ml of the synaptoneurosomal suspension with 90 μCi of [^{3}H]inositol for 90 min. The accumulation of [^{3}H]inositol phosphates was assayed by Dowex-1 chromatography. The addition of calcium to the incubation medium caused a concentration-dependent increase in the basal accumulation of [^{3}H]inositol phosphates. Potassium stimulated phosphoinositide hydrolysis was potentiated by extracellular calcium with a steep increase up to 0.1 mM extracellular calcium. No further increase in depolarization-dependent phosphoinositide hydrolysis (potassium-stimulated minus basal) occurred when extracellular calcium was increased to 1.0 mM. The addition of 25 μM EGTA reduced potassium-stimulated phosphoinositide hydrolysis to basal levels. These results demonstrate that both depolarization-dependent and basal phosphoinositide hydrolysis in brain are dependent upon, and sensitive to, extracellular calcium.

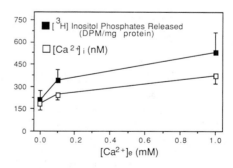

Fig. 3. Shows a comparison of the resting intracellular calcium concentration [Ca^{2+}]$_i$ to the basal accumulation of [^{3}H]inositol phosphates in rat synaptoneurosomes. The [Ca^{2+}]$_i$ was determined in fura-2 loaded synaptoneurosomes by the method of Komulainen and Bondy (1987). In buffer containing no added calcium, the resting [Ca^{2+}]$_i$ was 181 nM. Increasing extracellular calcium to 0.1 mM and 1.0 mM, increased the [Ca^{2+}]$_i$ to 242 nM and 369 nM, respectively. Comparison of [Ca^{2+}]$_i$ levels with [^{3}H]inositol phosphate accumulation, reveals that changes in phosphoinositide hydrolysis follow changes in intracellular calcium.

linked second messengers remain to be worked out, it is likely that the synergistic interactions between receptors causing depolarization and direct G-protein of PLC may be needed to produce the pronounced excitation that triggers long-term plasticity in the CNS (Fig. 4).

Summary

Excitatory amino acid neurotransmission has been shown to be necessary but may not be sufficient, for the production of LTP and other prolonged changes in synaptic transmission. Excitatory

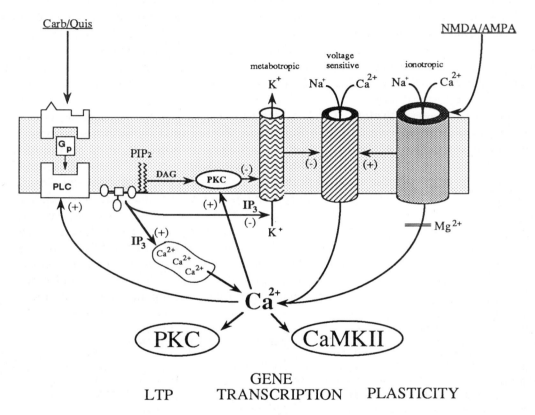

Fig. 4. Schematic illustration of the interactions between the various receptors, second messengers and ion channels which are involved in the induction of LTP and other plastic changes in nervous tissue. Although activation of NMDA receptors is necessary for the establishment of LTP in most systems, it is not sufficient because at resting membrane potential Mg^{2+} blocks NMDA-gated calcium flux. Simultaneous activation of NMDA receptors and receptors mediating depolarization through second messengers (metabotropic) or direct action on ion channels (ionotropic) is thus required for the production of LTP. This depolarization could be accomplished either through closure of potassium channels or the opening of sodium/calcium channels. Stimulation of phospholipase C (PLC) by carbachol (Carb) acting on muscarinic receptors or of quisqualate (Quis) acting on glutaminergic receptors produces the second messengers inositol (1,4,5) trisphosphate (IP_3) and diacylglycerol (DAG). DAG and IP_3 close two separate metabotropic potassium channels. AMPA produces depolarization by acting on non-NMDA glutaminergic receptors to open ionotropic cation (mostly Na^+) channels. Metabotropic and ionotropic mediated depolarization leads to activation of voltage-sensitive sodium channels and further depolarization which removes the Mg^{2+} block from NMDA-gated high-conductance calcium channels. Both membrane depolarization induced calcium flux through voltage-sensitive channels and IP_3 mediated calcium mobilization increase $[Ca^{2+}]_i$ which then acts in a synergistic manner to further increase the activity of PLC and DAG. The high levels of $[Ca^{2+}]_i$ and DAG which are acquired by the feed-forward augmentation in these interacting systems would lead to activation of protein kinase C (PKC) and calcium calmodulin type II kinase (CaMKII) which may in turn cause long-term changes in synaptic strength.

neurotransmission may produce depolarization-induced increases in intracellular calcium that cause PI hydrolysis and synergistically potentiate receptor-G protein induced PI hydrolysis. This synergistic potentiation of phosphoinositide hydrolysis, and increased $[Ca]_i$ due to positive cross stimulation, may lead to depolarization block, a persistent increase in protein kinase activation, altered morphology, oncogene activity and other plasticity changes important in memory.

Acknowledgements

This work was supported by grant AG06660 from NIA and DK38715 from NIH.

References

Baird, J.G. and Nahorski, S.R. (1986) Potassium depolarization markedly enhances muscarinic receptor stimulated inositol tetrakisphosphate accumulation in rat cerebral cortical slices. *Biochem. Biophys. Res. Comm.,* 141: 1130 – 1137.

Bank, B., DeWeer, A., Kuzirian, A.M., Rasmussen, H. and Alkon, D.L. (1988) Classical conditioning induces long-term translocation of protein kinase C in rabbit hippocampal CA1 cells. *Proc. Natl. Acad. Sci. U.S.A.,* 85: 1988 – 1992.

Barbaran, J.M., Snyder, S.H. and Alger, B.E. (1985) Protein kinase C regulates ionic conductance in hippocampal pyramidal neurons: electrophysiological effects of phorbol esters. *Proc. Natl. Acad. Sci. U.S.A.,* 82: 2538 – 2542.

Bartus, R.T., Dean, R.L., Beer, B. and Lippa, A.S. (1982) The cholinergic hypothesis of geriatric memory dysfunction. *Science,* 217: 408 – 414.

Baudry, M. and Lynch, G. (1980) Regulation of hippocampal glutamate receptors: evidence for the involvement of calcium-activated protease. *Proc. Natl. Acad. Sci. U.S.A.,* 77: 2298 – 2302.

Brown, T.H., Chapman, P.F., Kairiss, E.W. and Keenan, C.L. (1989) Long-term synaptic potentiation. *Science,* 242: 724 – 728.

Eccles, J.C. (1983) Calcium in long-term potentiation as a model for memory. *Neuroscience,* 10: 1071 – 1081.

Eva, C. and Costa, E. (1986) Potassium ion facilitation of phosphoinositide turnover activation by muscarinic receptor agonists in rat brain. *J. Neurochem.,* 46: 1429 – 1435.

Gonzales, R.A. and Crews, F.T. (1988) Differential regulation of phosphoinositide phosphodiesterase activity in brain membranes by guanine nucleotides and calcium. *J. Neurochem.,* 50: 1522 – 1528.

Hollingsworth, E.B., McNeal, E.T., Burton, J.L., Williams, R.J., Daly, J.W. and Creveling, C.R. (1985) Biochemical characterization of a filtered synaptoneurosome preparation from guinea pig cerebral cortex: syslic adenosine 3′: monophosphate generating systems, receptors and enzymes. *J. Neurosci.,* 5: 2240 – 2253.

Homma, Y., Imaki, J., Osamu, N. and Takenawa, Y. (1988) Isolation and characterization of two different forms of inositol phospholipid-specific phospholipase C from rat brain. *J. Biol. Chem.,* 263: 6592 – 6598.

Jahr, C.E. and Stevens, C.F. (1987) Glutamate activates multiple single channel conductances in hippocampal neurons. *Science,* 325: 522 – 525.

Komulainen, J. and Bondy, S.C. (1987) Modulation of levels of free calcium within synaptosomes by organochlorine insecticides. *Pharmacol. Exp. Ther.,* 241: 575 – 581.

Lynch, G., Larson, J., Kelso, S., Barrionuevo, G. and Schottler, F. (1983) Intracellular injections of EGTA block induction of long-term potentiation. *Nature,* 305: 719 – 721.

Madison, D.V., Lancaster, B. and Nicoll, R.A. (1987) Voltage-clamp analysis of cholinergic action in the hippocampus. *J. Neurosci.,* 7: 733 – 741.

Malenka, R.C., Madison, D.V. and Nicoll, R.A. (1986a) Potentiation of synaptic transmission in the hippocampus by phorbol esters. *Nature,* 321: 175 – 177.

Malenka, R.C., Madison, R., Andrade, R. and Nicoll, R.A. (1986b) Phorbol esters mimic some cholinergic actions in hippocampal pyramidal neurons. *J. Neurosci.,* 6: 475 – 480.

Malenka, R.C., Kauer, J.A., Zucker, R.S. and Nicoll, R.A. (1988) Post-synaptic calcium is sufficient for potentiation of hippocampal synaptic transmission. *Science,* 242: 81 – 84.

Malinow, R., Madison, D.V. and Tsein, R.W. (1988) Persistent protein kinase activity underlying long-term potentiation. *Nature,* 335: 820 – 824.

Pontzer, N.J. and Crews, F.T. (1990) Desensitization of muscarinic stimulated hippocampal cell firing is related to phosphoinositide hydrolysis and inhibited by lithium. *J. Pharmacol. Exp. Ther.,* 253: 921 – 929.

P. Coleman, G. Higgins and C. Phelps (Eds.)
Progress in Brain Research, Vol. 86
© 1990 Elsevier Science Publishers B.V. (Biomedical Division)

CHAPTER 19

Nerve growth factor induces gene expression of the prion protein and β-amyloid protein precursor in the developing hamster central nervous system

Michael P. McKinley[1], Frank M. Longo[1,3], Janice S. Valletta[1], Fonda Rahbar[1], Rachael L. Neve[5], Stanley B. Prusiner[1,4] and William C. Mobley[1,2,3,*]

Departments of [1]Neurology, [2]Pediatrics, [3]the Neuroscience Program, and [4]Biochemistry and Biophysics, University of California, San Francisco, CA 94143; and the [5] Department of Pediatrics, Children's Hospital, Boston, MA 02115, U.S.A.

Introduction

To understand how information is encoded in the nervous system, and to determine how this process may be perturbed in the diseased or aging brain, it is important to examine the molecular basis by which neuronal viability is established and maintained. Neurotrophic factors are likely to be involved. They are soluble polypeptides which appear to play an important role in enhancing the survival of neurons, in regulating their differentiation, in enhancing neuritic sprouting in target regions, and in inducing expression of genes whose products subserve neuronal form and function (Levi-Montalcini, 1987; Thoenen et al., 1987; Walicke, 1989). To pursue studies of neurotrophic factor actions it is useful to focus on a specific factor and on a defined population of responsive neurons.

Nerve growth factor (NGF) is essential for the survival of developing sensory and sympathetic neurons; studies of NGF have provided a view of the significance and scope of neurotrophic factor

activities in the peripheral nervous system (Levi-Montalcini, 1987). Recently, a number of observations have suggested that NGF acts as a trophic factor for cholinergic neurons of the basal forebrain and, possibly, for those in caudate-putamen (Johnston et al., 1987; Thoenen et al., 1987; Whittemore and Seiger, 1987). To investigate the mechanism of NGF actions on these neurons we have initiated studies of its effects on neuronal gene expression. As candidates for study we sought genes which were expressed predominantly in neurons and developmentally regulated. Our choice was guided further by an interest in genes whose expression may be relevant to neuronal dysfunction in the aging or diseased nervous system. To this end we examined expression of two genes whose proteins are found in certain central nervous system amyloid deposits in specific neurodegenerative disorders.

Scrapie in laboratory rodents is an experimental neurodegenerative disorder, which provides an excellent model for Creutzfeldt-Jakob disease (CJD), kuru, and Gerstmann-Straussler syndrome (Gajdusek, 1977; Prusiner, 1987). Prolonged incubation periods precede clinical illness in each of these disorders. The amyloid protein isolated from scrapie-infected hamster brains is a protease-

* Reprint requests should be adressed to William C. Mobley, Dept. of Neurology, M-794, University of California, School of Medicine, San Francisco, CA 94143 – 0114, U.S.A.

resistant protein of 27 – 30 kDa, designated prion protein (PrP) 27-30. Limited proteolysis generates PrP 27-30 from a protein of 33 – 35 kDa, the scrapie PrP isoform (PrP^{Sc}). Immunohistochemical studies have shown that amyloid plaques in scrapie brains contain intensely staining PrP molecules (Prusiner, 1987). A protease-resistant form of PrP is also found in fractions purified from the brains of CJD patients and antibodies to hamster PrP 27-30 stain amyloid plaques in cases of CJD, kuru, and Gerstmann-Straussler syndrome (Prusiner, 1987; Roberts et al., 1988). PrP^{Sc} appears to differ from its cellular isoform (PrP^C) through posttranslational modification (Basler et al., 1986). The function of PrP^C is unknown, but the protein is membrane bound (Meyer et al., 1986; Stahl et al., 1987) and in the central nervous system is expressed primarily in neurons (Kretzschmar et al., 1986).

The β-protein (4 – 5 kDa) is found in both cerebrovascular and neuritic plaque amyloid in AD; it is derived from a larger precursor (77 kDa) encoded by a gene on human chromosome 21 (Glenner and Wong, 1984; Masters et al., 1985; Goldgaber et al., 1987; Kang et al., 1987; Tanzi et al., 1987). The structure of the β-protein precursor (β-PP) suggests that it is a glycosylated membrane protein (Kang et al., 1987), and there is evidence for this in vivo and in vitro (Dyrks et al., 1988; Shivers et al., 1988). In situ hybridization studies indicate that expression of the β-PP gene within the brain is principally, if not exclusively, within neurons (Bahmanyar et al., 1987; Goedert, 1987). The role, if any, of the β protein in the causation or pathogenesis of AD is unknown. It is clear, however, that β-PP gene expression is not limited to neurons which are selectively vulnerable in AD (Goedert, 1987).

Recent observations have intensified interest in the regulation of the PrP and β-PP genes. The PrP gene in mice (*Prn-p*) is tightly linked to a gene (*Prn-i*) that controls the length of the scrapie incubation period (i.e., the period from inoculation with scrapie prions to the onset of clinical disease) (Carlson et al., 1986). In humans, a mutant allele

of the PrP gene is linked to the development of the ataxic form of the Gerstmann-Straussler syndrome (Hsiao et al., 1989). β-PP is encoded by at least three mRNA species, which may be differentially expressed in the brains of AD patients (Kitaguchi et al., 1988; Ponte et al., 1988; Tanzi et al., 1988). Interestingly, both the PrP gene and the β-PP gene have been found to be regulated during development (McKinley et al., 1987; Tanzi et al., 1987). To investigate the regulation of amyloid gene expression, we examined the pattern of ontogenesis of mRNA levels for these genes in several hamster brain regions during development; distinct regional variations were found. The kinetics of PrP and β-PP gene expression in the basal forebrain were coincident with that of choline acetyltransferase (ChAT) activity, a marker for differentiated cholinergic neurons. Coincident with its enhancement of cholinergic neurochemical differentiation, NGF administration induced regionally specific increases in central nervous system amyloid protein gene expression. Extending these observations, it was determined that the length of the scrapie incubation period is a function of the developmental age at time of inoculation and that NGF injection significantly influences its duration in neonates.

Methods

Dissection of tissues

The birth of Syrian golden hamster litters was recorded as day 0. Dissections were performed as described (Johnston et al., 1987). Subiculum was included with hippocampus. Caudal midbrain plus pons constituted the brain stem. For prenatal determinations, a timed-pregnancy animal was anesthetized with sodium pentobarbital (nembutal) (15 mg, intraperitoneally) and individual embryos were removed and dissected. Whole forebrain was taken in place of frontolateral neocortex in prenatal animals.

Preparation and injection of NGF

NGF was prepared by ion-exchange chromatography as described (Mobley et al., 1986). For injection, lyophilized NGF was redissolved in one part of 0.05% acetic acid followed by 4 parts of phosphate-buffered saline to achieve a final concentration of 3 μg/μl. In experiments in which multiple injections were given, NGF (30μg) was administered intraventricularly (ICV) (Mobley et al., 1985) on postnatal days (PD) 3, 5 and 7, and sacrifice was on PD 9. Vehicle-injected animals served as controls. In gene expression experiments in which a single injection was given, NGF (30 μg) was administered ICV on PD 7 and animals were sacrificed on PD 9. For scrapie incubation period experiments NGF (30μg) was administered ICV in the schedule described in the test. Controls included animals treated with NGF (30μg) denatured by reduction and carbamoylmethylation (Morris et al., 1971) or injection vehicle alone.

NGF studies in vitro

PC12 cells (SPC12; see Schubert et al., 1977) were grown in Dulbeccos modified Eagle's medium (with 3.7 g/l NaHCO, 4.5 g/l glucose; 0.584 g/l L-glutamine) containing 10% fetal bovine serum, 5% heat-inactivated horse serum, 1 $\times$ Pen-Strep and an additional 2 mM glutamine. Cells were fed every other day and the doubling time was 7 days. For NGF treatment cells were plated at a density of 2 $\cdot$ 10^6 per 100 mm dish in the same medium but containing only 2% fetal bovine and 1% heat-inactivated horse serum. NGF, to achieve final concentration of 50 ng/ml, or an equivalent volume (10 μl) of vehicle (0.2% acetic acid) was added to a total volume of 30 ml. At the conclusion of treatment, cells were harvested by centrifugation and briefly washed in phosphate-buffered saline. The cell pellet was immediately taken for RNA preparation.

Purification and analysis of RNA

Total RNA was isolated and prepared as described (Chirgwin et al., 1979; Feramisco et al., 1982; Cathala et al., 1983). Probes for PrP (Oesch et al., 1985) and β-PP mRNA (FB68L) (Tanzi et al., 1987) were prepared according to Oesch et al. (1985). RNA was characterized by slot blot and Northern blot analysis as described (Mobley et al., 1988).

PrP mRNAs were compared to a standard curve for PrP cDNA. The cDNA was ethanol-precipitated and pellets were dried prior to resuspension in 400 μl of TE buffer (10 mM Tris $\cdot$ HCl, pH 7.4; 1 mM EDTA). Serial 1 : 10 dilutions were prepared and the autoradiographic signal for each DNA concentration was determined (Oesch et al., 1985). The poly (A)$^+$ RNA content of RNA samples was estimated by hybridizing radiolabeled polythymidylic acid (poly (dT)) to slot blots of total RNA as described (Mobley et al., 1988).

Measurements of PrP and ChAT

Pooled septal tissues weighing 20 – 30 mg were disrupted by trituration through a Pasteur pipette in 2 ml of ice-cold 50 mM Tris $\cdot$ HCL buffer (pH 7.5) containing 50 mM NaCl, 10 mM EDTA, 0.15% Nonidet P-40, and 0.15% sodium deoxycholate. Extraction was performed on ice for 5 min; cell debris was pelleted 5 min at 1500 $\times$ g and supernatant proteins were precipitated in 80% methanol at $-20°$C for 24 h. Proteins pelleted by centrifugation for 20 min at 2300 $\times$ g were redissolved in 200 μl of 10 mM Tris·HCl buffer (pH 7.5) containing 0.1 mM EDTA. Electrophoresis was performed in 12% polyacrylamide gels according to the method of Laemmli (1976). Proteins were electroblotted to nitrocellulose filter paper (Towbin et al., 1979). The filter was blocked with 5% non-fat dry milk in phosphate-buffered saline, incubated at room temperature with PrP monoclonal antibody 13A5 (Barry and Prusiner, 1986), and staining was developed with the Protoblot alkaline phosphatase system (Promega). Nitrocellulose filters were densitometrically scanned to determine the amount of PrP^C. ChAT activity was determined as described (Mobley et al., 1985).

Measuring the scrapie incubation period

A hamster-adapted isolate of the scrapie agent was passaged and prepared as previously described

(DeArmond et al., 1987). Propagation of prions was performed in Syrian golden hamsters (LVG/LAK) inoculated intracranially (IC) with ~ 10^7 ID_{50} units of scrapie agent and sacrificed 70 days later.

Weanling hamsters were inoculated IC with 50 μl of a 10^{-1} dilution of scrapie brain homogenate. Timed pregnant, random-bred LVG/LAK females were purchased from Charles River Laboratories. The timed pregnant females delivered their pups between midnight and 0800. This was considered PD 0. All inoculations were performed between 0800 and 0900 on the days specified. Pups were briefly separated from their mother and inoculated IC with 20μl of scrapie prions. The IC inoculations were given in the left parietal region with a 26-gauge needle inserted to a depth of approximately 1 – 2 mm. Following inoculation, the needle was held in place for 5 sec; this procedure diminished backstreaming of inocula out of the needle entry point. All pups within a single litter were inoculated with a portion of the same sample. Bioassays for scrapie infectivity were performed by incubation time measurements; these were made as previously described (Prusiner et al., 1982).

Results

PrP gene expression is developmentally regulated

To investigate the regulation of PrP gene expression, PrP mRNA was measured in several regions of the hamster brain during pre- and postnatal development. In each region PrP mRNA increased dramatically in the postnatal period. PrP mRNA levels varied regionally during ontogenesis (Fig. 1). Three developmental patterns for PrP gene expression were found: (i) early expression, observed in brain stem and neocortex; (ii) intermediate expression, seen in hippocampus, thalamus and caudate-putamen; and (iii) delayed expression, found in septum (basal forebrain). Low levels of PrP mRNA were detected in the brain stem in the immediate prenatal period but increased rapidly to levels near those found in adults during the first postnatal week (Fig. 1A). PrP gene expression in

neocortex was similar to the brain stem in its developmental pattern except that greater than adult levels were seen during the second postnatal week. In contrast, there was little or no measurable PrP mRNA in hippocampus, caudate-putamen or thalamus through PD 3 (Fig. 1B, C). By 6 days, PrP mRNA had increased. At this time, PrP mRNA was 40% of adult levels in hippocampus, 97% in thalamus and 124% in caudate-putamen.

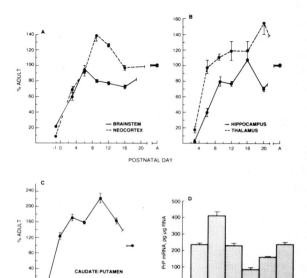

Fig. 1. PrP gene expression in several hamster brain regions during development and in the adult. Tissues were dissected and processed as described. For the prenatal measurement (at PD – 1) the tissues of 4 animals were pooled for examination of forebrain (the result is given in *A* as neocortex), and 7 animals were pooled for brain stem. For each postnatal sample, RNA was prepared from pooled brain regions of entire hamster litters or from 3 to 5 adults. Three separate samples of RNA were examined at each postnatal age for caudate-putamen and hippocampus; two samples were examined for brain stem, neocortex, and thalamus. Values are means ± S.E.M., as percentage of the adult level. In *D* is given the level of PrP mRNA in each of several adult brain regions. Individual samples (n = 2 for each) were compared to a standard curve prepared by blotting PrP cDNA . Values are means ± S.E.M. and are given as pg equivalents of the cDNA insert per μg of total RNA. (Taken from Mobley et al., 1988.)

PrP mRNA increased to adult or greater than adult levels in all three regions over the next 2 weeks. In caudate-putamen, 220% of the adult level was found at PD 16. Individual brain regions also differed in the amount of PrP mRNA found in adult animals (Fig. 1D). Randomly selected postnatal RNA samples were also analyzed by Northern blots; in all instances, the hybridizing species was 2.1 kb (data not shown).

Septum exhibited delayed PrP gene expression (Fig. 2); PrP mRNA was first detected at 9 days of age, at which time it was 17% of the adult level. PrP mRNA levels increased to 60–70% of adult values by 12 days of age and reached maximal values by PD 16. The delayed appearance of PrP mRNA in septum exhibited a pattern reminiscent of the time course followed by septohippocampal cholinergic markers in the rat (Large et al., 1986; Shelton et al., 1989). To determine whether

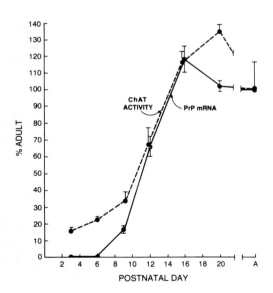

Fig. 2. Comparison of the developmental profiles for ChAT acticity and PrP mRNA in septum. ChAT activity was determined at several postnatal ages and plotted as percentage of the adult value (50.1 ± 8.5 nmol of acetylcholine formed per h/mg protein). Septal PrP mRNA was measured as indicated; three separate samples, each representing pooled septal tissues of an entire litter, were examined at each postnatal age. Values are means ± S.E.M. given as percentage of adult. (Taken from Mobley et al., 1988.)

cholinergic markers followed the same pattern in the hamster, we measured the activity of ChAT. ChAT specific activity in septum was < 20% of adult levels at PD 3 and remained low through 9 days of age, increasing to adult levels over the ensuing week (Fig. 2). From PD 9 – 16, the developmental increase in ChAT activity in the septum was virtually coincident with that for PrP mRNA. Thus, increasing PrP gene expression in the developing hamster septum was temporally coincident with neurochemical differentiation of cholinergic neurons.

NGF induces PrP gene expression

The coincident increases in ChAT activity and PrP mRNA raised the possibility that ChAT and PrP are under coordinate control in developing septal cholinergic neurons. One approach for exploring the regulation of PrP gene expression was suggested by earlier studies with NGF. In rat brain, NGF injections selectively increased septal ChAT activity but had no effect on the neurotransmitter enzyme markers glutamic acid decarboxylase and tyrosine hydroxylase (Mobley et al., 1985, 1986). Moreover, NGF receptors in the rat septum are localized to neuronal cell bodies, which closely resemble cholinergic neurons in their size and distribution (Mesulam et al., 1983; Richardson et al., 1986; Raivich and Kreutzberg, 1987). To determine whether or not NGF influences the expression of PrP mRNA, NGF (30 μg) was administered ICV to neonatal hamsters on PD 3, 5 and 7, and the animals were sacrificed on PD 9. Control littermates received injection vehicle alone. Septal PrP mRNA was increased by NGF about 10-fold relative to controls and exceeded the levels found in adults (Fig. 3A). In NGF-treated animals, ChAT activity was increased almost 2-fold, indicating that hamster basal forebrain cholinergic neurons responded to NGF injection. In uninjected animals, ChAT activity at PD 9 was 34% of adult levels and PrP mRNA was 17% of adult levels (Fig. 2). Similar values were found in vehicle-injected animals.

The NGF-mediated stimulation of ChAT activi-

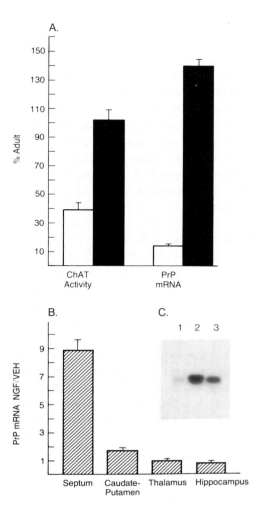

Fig. 3. NGF effects on PrP gene expression. *A*. NGF injection increased septal ChAT activity and PrP mRNA. NGF (30 µg) was injected ICV on PD 3, 5 and 7, and ChAT activity and PrP mRNA were determined at PD 9 (solid bars). Vehicle-injected animals served as controls (open bars). Values are means ± S.E.M. as percentage of adult. ChAT activity increase: control, 18.0 ± 2.8, n = 3; NGF, 51.2 ± 3.7, n = 2; *P* < 0.01, Student's *t*-test. PrP mRNA levels were measured in NGF-treated and control animals on three separate occasions (pooled tissues of 3 – 8 animals in each treatment group on each occasion; *P* < 0.001, Student's *t*-test). *B*. NGF effects were regionally specific. NGF (30 µg) was given on PD 7 and animals were sacrificed on PD 9. Vehicle-injected animals served as controls. Values are the ratio of densitometric scores for PrP mRNA in NGF and vehicle-treated animals (VEH). Results are listed as means ± S.E.M. for two separate determinations (using the pooled tissues of 3 – 8 animals in each treatment group

ty in the septum of rat neonates was first evident 48 h after a single intraventricular injection and persisted for the next several days (Johnston et al., 1987). To determine whether or not an effect of NGF on PrP mRNA would be demonstrable over this time course, NGF (30 µg) was given as a single injection to neonatal hamsters at PD 7 and animals were sacrificed 48 h later, on PD 9. PrP mRNA levels were nearly 9-fold those in control animals (Fig. 3*B*). Septal ChAT activity was increased 100% relative to vehicle-injected animals (mean ± S.E.M.; vehicle injected = 22.3 ± 1.3 nmol of acetylcholine formed per h/mg protein (n = 4); NGF = 44.0 ± 5.0 (n = 4); *P* < 0.005, Student's *t*-test). Northern blot analysis showed that the PrP mRNA induced by NGF treatment migrated identically to that found in vehicle-injected animals and adults (Fig. 3*C*). NGF stimulation required the native form of the molecule since injection of NGF denatured by reduction and carbamoylmethylation failed to produce an increase either in ChAT activity (22.35 ± 1.8 (n = 2)) or in PrP mRNA levels (PrP mRNA in animals receiving denatured NGF was 63.9% ± 20% (S.E.M.) (*n* = 2) of that in vehicle-treated subjects).

The increase in PrP mRNA induced by NGF treatment was confined to specific brain regions. Of note, the caudate-putamen in the rat contains NGF-responsive cholinergic neurons that are distinct from those found in basal forebrain (Mobley et al., 1985). A single NGF injection in

on each occasion). Ratios for septum and caudate-putamen were significantly greater than for thalamus (0.96 ± 0.05; *P* < 0.05, Student's *t*-test). Relative to untreated animals, vehicle injection was associated with a small increase in PrP mRNA levels in the septum and caudate-putamen; it was 6% of the NGF-induced increase in septum and 36% in caudate-putamen. *C*. Northern blot analysis of PrP mRNA in the septum of NGF-treated and control animals. The RNA samples were those prepared for *A*. Lanes: *1*, 5 µg of septal RNA from animals injected with vehicle on PD 3, 5 and 7 and sacrificed on PD 9; *2*, 5 µg of septal RNA from animals injected with NGF (30 µg) via the same schedule; *3*, 5 µg of RNA from adult septum. The hybridizing species was 2.1 kb. (Taken from Mobley et al., 1988.)

neonatal hamsters increased PrP mRNA in caudate-putamen by 70% relative to vehicle-injected animals (Fig. 3B). ChAT activity was increased ~65% (vehicle = 56.1 ± 4.5 (n = 3); NGF = 92.4 ± 6.3 (n = 3); $P < 0.01$, Student's t-test). In contrast to the responses in septum and caudate-putamen, NGF did not alter PrP mRNA levels in thalamus or hippocampus (Fig. 3B). Further documenting the selectivity of NGF actions, NGF injection did not produce an increase in the poly $(A)^+$ RNA content of RNA samples from responsive tissues. The extent of hybridization of radiolabeled poly(dT) to samples of total RNA from NGF- and vehicle-treated septum was nearly identical (mean ± S.E.M. for absorbance source (peak area) for NGF = 87% ± 19% (n = 3) of that for vehicle).

We also measured the translation product of PrP mRNA after NGF injection. As determined by Western blot, PrP^C was increased 2.3-fold in the septum 48 h after a single NGF ($30\mu g$) injection on PD 7 (mean ± S.E.M. for absorbance source (peak area) per mg of tissue wet weight: vehicle-injected = 29.8 ± 2.4, n = 3; NGF = 100.9 ± 16.7, n = 3; $P < 0.05$, Student's t-test). The magnitude of the NGF-induced increase in PrP^C was similar to that observed for ChAT (Fig. 3A).

NGF prolongs the scrapie incubation period in neonatal hamsters

A large body of data argues that PrP gene expression is necessary for scrapie (Prusiner, 1987). Therefore, the transient low expression of PrP^C found during early postnatal life may be expected to influence the development of clinical disease. We predicted that inoculation in neonates would lead to a prolonged incubation interval. Instead, the scrapie incubation period was found to be shorter in neonatal hamsters than in weanling hamsters. When neonates were inoculated with scrapie at PD 0, clinical symptoms occurred 16 days earlier than for animals inoculated as weanlings (68.0 ± 1.15 days vs. 84.0 ± 1.58 days). In addition, death of inoculated neonates occurred at 74 days, approximately 26 days earlier than for inoculated weanlings (Table I). To confirm and extend these observations, individual litters of animals were inoculated IC at PD 0, 2, 4, 6, 8, 10, 12 or 14 and the incubation periods recorded. The interval from inoculation to either illness or death

TABLE I

Nerve growth factor prolongs the intervals from prion inoculation to illness and to death in neonatal hamsters*

Age at inoculation[1] with prions	Age at injection of[1]		Incubation times			
	NGF	VEH	Illness		Death	
			(day ± S.E.M.)	P-value[2]	(day ± S.E.M.)	P-value[2]
30	−[3]	−	84.0 ± 1.58		99.7 ± 1.43	
2	−	−	69.0 ± 0.57	< 0.001	82.5 ± 1.71	< 0.001
2	−	0	70.5 ± 0.50	< 0.001	82.5 ± 1.26	< 0.001
2	0	−	76.5 ± 1.50[4]	< 0.001	89.5 ± 0.95	< 0.002

* Number of animals (n) in each experimental sample is 8.
[1] Amount of inoculum, method of inoculation, and preparation of NGF and vehicle are described in the Methods section.
[2] Incubation times of neonatal hamsters are compared to those of weanling hamsters 30 days of age.
[3] (−) represents no treatment.
[4] Incubation times of NGF-injected animals were significantly prolonged compared to neonatal hamsters receiving no NGF or vehicle on day 0. Comparing times from inoculation to illness (69.0 ± 0.57 vs 76.5 ± 1.50) $P < 0.001$ and to death (82.5 ± 1.71 vs 89.5 ± 0.95) $P < 0.05$.

was developmentally dependent upon age at inoculation (Fig. 4). There was an excellent correlation in the postnatal age at inoculation with the age at death; the correlation coefficient was $r = 0.86$. The correlation coefficient for the interval to clinical illness was 0.60.

The induction of PrP gene expression with NGF suggested a means to modify experimentally the incubation intervals. Therefore, NGF (30 μg) was given ICV on PD 0, 48 h before scrapie inoculation on PD 2. In a series of 3 experiments involving 8 hamster pups, a partial but significant reversal of the acceleration of scrapie was found (Table I). NGF increased the time to illness by 6 days and the time to death by 7 days. For each of these measures NGF produced an increase equal to $40-50\%$ of the difference which distinguished neonates and weanlings. Protocols in which NGF was given at the same time as scrapie inoculation or 2 days after inoculation failed to alter significantly the incubation periods (data not shown).

NGF modulates developmental regulation of β-PP gene expression

β-PP mRNA was found in all brain regions sampled. The patterns for the ontogenesis of β-PP mRNA levels in the septum and thalamus were similar to those seen for PrP mRNA (Fig. 5A). β-

PP mRNA was first detected in septum at PD 9 when it was 12% of the adult level and increased to a maximum between PD 12 and PD 16.

Three NGF injections increased β-PP mRNA levels in septum by > 10-fold relative to vehicle-treated animals (Fig. 5B). Even a single NGF injection on PD 7 induced approximately a 3-fold increase in β-PP mRNA (Fig. 5C). The β-PP mRNA induced by NGF migrated identically to that found in vehicle-injected and adult animals at 3.2 kb. Alternative forms of β-PP mRNA have been detected that differ in the inclusion, or lack thereof, of a segment encoding an apparent protease inhibitor domain (Kitaguchi et al., 1988; Ponte et al., 1988; Tanzi et al., 1988). The probe used for this study, FB68L, will hybridize to all these transcripts but will not distinguish them on Northern blots. Like the studies on PrP mRNA, the effect of NGF was regionally selective in that NGF did not alter β-PP mRNA in the thalamus (Fig. 5B, C).

Extending our studies in vitro we asked whether β-PP mRNA levels would be increased in PC12 cells, a pheochromocytoma cell line which responds to NGF by demonstrating a number of neuronal properties (Greene and Tischler, 1976). Incubated with NGF for 24 h, β-PP mRNA levels were increased approximately 2-fold (mean (peak area) $\pm$ S.E.M. as fold-increase over control $= 2.31 \pm 0.31$). The NGF-induced transcript migrated identically to that in control cultures.

Discussion

The studies reported herein demonstrate that both the PrP and β-PP genes are highly regulated in the hamster central nervous system. We show that: (i) expression of both genes increases during the early postnatal period; (ii) the pattern for mRNA ontogenesis varies regionally; (iii) regional differences in gene expression persist into adulthood; and (iv) the expression of these genes in the basal forebrain septum is stimulated by NGF.

The delay in PrP and β-PP gene expression during development of the basal forebrain may be a

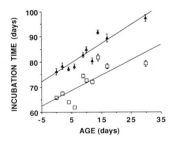

Fig. 4. Reduction in scrapie incubation times and death times in neonatally inoculated hamsters. Neonatal hamster pups were inoculated with $\sim 10^7$ ID$_{50}$ units of prions on the postnatal day indicated on the abscissa. The number of days to illness ($\square$) or death ($\blacktriangle$) is shown on the ordinate. Bars represent S.E.M. for each determination. Note: inoculation of neonates with prions at a 10-fold greater concentration did not further shorten the incubation intervals. (Taken from McKinley et al., 1989.)

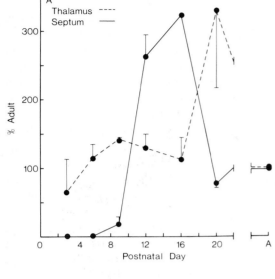

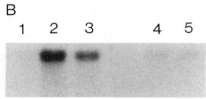

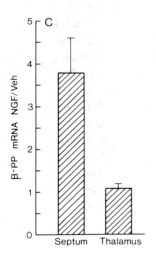

Fig. 5. β-PP gene expression during development. *A*. Ontogenesis of β-PP mRNA in septum and thalamus. Tissues were dissected and processed as described. Each postnatal sample consisted of the RNA from an entire hamster litter or from 3 to 5 adults. Two samples were examined at each postnatal age. Values are means ± S.E.M., as percentage of the adult level.

consequence of neuronal differentiation. In the rat, a mature pattern for the organization of cholinergic fibers is not seen until the second postnatal week (Milner et al., 1983), at which time there is a prominent increase in basal forebrain ChAT activity (Large et al., 1986). The abrupt increase in mRNA for both amyloid genes coincided with ChAT expression in hamster basal forebrain. These observations suggest that, like ChAT, the products of the PrP and β-PP genes are first required at the time neurons begin to establish mature patterns of innervation. The exact role played by PrP^C and β-PP in developing neurons is uncertain, but their localization on neuronal surface membranes suggests that they may mediate cell – cell contacts (Stahl et al., 1987) or perhaps act as membrane receptors (Schubert et al., 1977; Kang et al., 1987).

NGF is a neurotrophic factor (Levi-Montalcini, 1987). It acts, in part, by altering the abundance of proteins involved in neuronal differentiation (Tiercy and Shooter, 1986; Leonard et al., 1988; Masiakowski and Shooter, 1988). Recent studies suggest that NGF acts as a neurotrophic factor for cholinergic neurons in the basal forebrain and, possibly, for those in caudate-putamen (Whittemore and Seiger, 1987). Our results are consis-

B. NGF treatment induced an increase in β-PP mRNA. Northern blot analysis of RNA from hamster pups injected ICV with NGF (30 μg) or vehicle on PD 3, 5 and 7 sacrificed on PD 9. Lanes: *1*, 5 μg of septal RNA from vehicle-treated animals; *2*, 5 μg of septal RNA from NGF-treated animals; *3*, 5 μg of RNA from adult septums; *4*, 0.5 μg of thalamic RNA from vehicle-injected animals; *5*, 0.5 μg of thalamic RNA from NGF-injected animals. The hybridizing species migrated at ~3.2 kb. Note that only a very faint signal is seen in lane *1*. *C*. The NGF-induced increase was regionally specific. NGF (30 μg) was given on PD 7 and animals were sacrificed on PD 9. Vehicle-injected animals were controls. Values are the ratio of densitometric scores for β-PP mRNA in NGF and vehicle-treated animals. Results are means ± S.E.M. for two separate determinations (using the pooled tissues of 3 – 8 animals in each treatment group on each occasion; $P < 0.05$, Student's t-test, one-tailed). β-PP mRNA levels in septum of vehicle-injected animals were comparable to those of untreated animals. Veh, vehicle. (Taken from Mobley et al., 1988.)

tent with this assertion. NGF-induced increases in PrP and β-PP mRNA coincided in time with its stimulation of ChAT activity in these regions. These data suggest that NGF increases the level of mRNA for PrP and β-PP in cholinergic neurons; however, in situ hybridization studies will be required to define more precisely the locus of NGF actions.

The cholinergic neurons of the basal forebrain project prominently to the hippocampus and neocortex (Mesulam et al., 1983). The expression of ChAT activity in developing rat basal forebrain neurons coincides temporally with the expression of NGF in these target regions (Large et al., 1986; Auburger et al., 1987). The coincident increases for ChAT activity and PrP and β-PP mRNA levels in the developing basal forebrain and the response of PrP and β-PP mRNA levels to NGF injection raise the possibility that NGF regulates the expression of these genes in developing basal forebrain neurons. How NGF exerts its effects on the mRNA levels for PrP and β-PP is unknown; actions at the level of transcription, RNA processing or mRNA stability are all possible. In view of recent studies which show that increased mRNA levels for PrP in developing rat brain are correlated with an increased rate of transcription, it is possible that NGF induces activation of this gene (Lieberburg, 1987). Since the PrP and β-PP genes are located on separate chromosomes in humans and mice, it is unlikely that they are syntenic in the hamster. Thus, if NGF induces transcriptional activation of both genes, it probably does so through some *trans* mechanism. Success in inducing increased PrP and β-PP mRNA levels in PC12 cells with NGF will provide a cell culture system for examining further NGF actions. Recent studies on the PrP and β-PP genes have pointed to potential transcriptional regulatory elements common to both (Basler et al., 1986; Salbaum et al., 1988). Studies in vivo and in vitro may help to discern which regulatory elements are used to induce transcription and whether NGF acts to increase mRNA levels via the same or a different mechanism for these two genes.

The role of amyloid gene expression in the pathogenesis of neurodegenerative disorders is an active area for investigation. In the case of the prion diseases, there is persuasive evidence that PrP^{Sc} has a central role (Prusiner, 1987; Hsiao et al., 1989; Westaway et al., 1989). It was of note that development influenced the incubation period. Though the etiology of this finding is unknown, the pathogenetic role played by PrP^{Sc} invites attention to the developmental regulation of PrP mRNA which occurs over the same time course. These data raise the possibility that the abundance of the PrP mRNA translation product may influence disease progression. This could occur through an effect on the amount of PrP^{Sc} which gains access to neurons, the rate at which PrP^{Sc} accumulates, or the extent of its influence on normal cellular processes. The hypothesis that the endogenous level of PrP^{C} at the time of inoculation modulates the initiation of scrapie infection is supported by studies with NGF. The NGF treatment-induced increase in the incubation period is consistent with an effect of NGF on the level of PrP gene expression. A caveat to this interpretation is that NGF effects are likely to have been registered on a number of aspects of neuronal differentiation. In addition, NGF actions are regionally specific and would not be recorded in all neurons. Nevertheless, the pivotal role of PrP^{Sc} in the pathogenesis of scrapie and the marked involvement of the basal forebrain (DeArmond et al., 1987) suggest that NGF may influence scrapie pathogenesis by increasing PrP^{C} levels. The acceleration of scrapie in newborn hamsters, and the ability to modulate PrP gene expression with NGF, has provided important insights into the molecular basis of this neurodegenerative disorder.

Acknowledgements

The authors acknowledge helpful discussions with Drs. David Holtzman, Stephen DeArmond, and David Westaway. This work was supported by National Institutes of Health grants (NS01015, NS24054, NS14069, AG02132); the Senator Jacob Javits Center of Excellence in Neuroscience

(NS22786) (S.B.P.); the March of Dimes Birth Defects Foundation (W.C.M.); the California State Department of Health Services (87-92057) (M.P.M.); and by gifts from Sherman Fairchild Foundation, RJR-Nabisco Inc. and the Transamerica Foundation.

References

Auburger, G., Heumann, R., Hellweg, R., Korsching, S. and Thoenen, H. (1987) Developmental changes of nerve growth factor and its mRNA in rat hippocampus: comparison with choline acetyltransferase. *Dev. Biol.,* 120: 322 – 328.

Bahmanyar, S., Higgins, G., Goldgaber, D., Leuri, D.A., Morrison, J.H., Wilson, M.C., Shankar, S.K. and Gajdusek, D.C. (1987) Localization of amyloid β protein messenger RNA in brains from patients with Alzheimer's disease. *Science,* 237: 77 – 80.

Barry, R.A. and Prusiner, S.B. (1986) Monoclonal antibodies to the cellular and scrapie prion proteins. *J. Infect. Dis.,* 154: 518 – 521.

Basler, K., Oesch, B., Scott, M., Westaway, D., Walchli, M., Groth, D.F., McKinley, M.P., Prusiner, S.B. and Weissman, C. (1986) Scrapie and cellular PrP isoforms are encoded by the same chromosomal gene. *Cell,* 46: 417 – 428.

Carlson, G.A., Kingsbury, D.T., Goodman, P., Coleman, S., Marshall, S.T., DeArmond, S.J., Westaway, D. and Prusiner, S.B. (1986) Prion protein and scrapie incubation time genes are linked. *Cell,* 46: 503 – 511.

Cathala, G., Savouret, J.F., Mendez, B., West, B.L., Karin, M., Martial, J.A. and Baxter, J.D. (1983) A method for isolation of intact, translationally active ribonucleic acid. *DNA,* 2: 329 – 335.

Chirgwin, J.M., Przybyla, A.E., MacDonald, R.J. and Rutter, W.J. (1979) Isolation of biologically active ribonucleic acid from sources enriched in ribonuclease. *Biochemistry,* 18: 5294 – 5299.

DeArmond, S.J., Mobley, W.C., DeMott, D.L., Barry, R.A., Beckstead, J.H. and Prusiner, S.B. (1987) Changes in the localization of brain prion proteins during scrapie infection. *Neurology,* 37: 1271 – 1280.

Dyrks, T., Weidemann, A., Multhaup, G., Salbaum, J.M., Lemaire, H-G., Kang, J., Muller-Hill, B., Masters, C.L. and Beyreuther, K. (1988) Identification, transmembrane orientation and biogenesis of the amyloid A4 precursor of Alzheimer's disease. *EMBO J.,* 7: 949 – 957.

Feramisco, J.R., Smart, J.E., Burridge, K., Helfman, D.M. and Thomas, G.P. (1982) Coexistence of vinculin and a vinculin-like protein of higher molecular weight in smooth muscle. *J. Biol. Chem.,* 257: 11024 – 11031.

Gajdusek, D.C. (1977) Unconventional viruses and the origin and disappearance of kuru. *Science,* 197: 943 – 960.

Glenner, G.G. and Wong, C.W. (1984) Alzheimer's disease and Down's syndrome: sharing of a unique cerebrovascular amyloid fibril protein. *Biochem. Biophys. Res. Comm.,* 122: 1131 – 1135.

Goedert, M. (1987) Neuronal localization of amyloid beta protein precursor mRNA in normal brain and in Alzheimer's disease. *EMBO J.,* 6: 3627 – 3632.

Goldgaber, D., Lerman, M.I., McBride, O.W., Saffioti, U. and Gajdusek, D.C. (1987) Characterization and chromosomal localization of a cDNA encoding brain amyloid of Alzheimer's disease. *Science,* 235: 877 – 880.

Greene, L.A. and Tischler, A.S. (1976) Establishment of a noradrenergic clonal line of rat adrenal pheochromocytoma cells which respond to nerve growth factor. *Proc. Natl. Acad. Sci. U.S.A.,* 73: 2424 – 2428.

Hsaio, K., Baker, H.F., Crow, T.J., Poulter, M., Owen, F., Terwilliger, J.D., Westaway, D., Ott, J. and Prusiner, S.B. (1989) Linkage of a prion protein misseuse variant to Gerstmann-Straussler syndrome. *Nature,* 338: 342 – 345.

Johnston, M.V., Rutkowski, J.L., Wainer, B.H., Long, J.B. and Mobley, W.C. (1987) NGF effects on developing forebrain cholinergic neurons are regionally specific. *Neurochem. Res.,* 12: 985 – 994.

Kang, J., Lemaire, H.-G., Unterbeck, A., Salbaum, J.M., Masters, C.L., Grzeschik, K.-H., Multhaup, G., Beyreuther, K. and Muller-Hill, B. (1987) The precursor of Alzheimer's disease amyloid A4 protein resembles a cell-surface receptor. *Nature,* 325: 733 – 736.

Kitaguchi, N., Takahaski, Y., Tokushima, Y., Shiojiri, S. and Ito, H. (1988) Novel precursor of Alzheimer's disease amyloid protein shows protease inhibitory activity. *Nature,* 331: 530 – 532.

Kretschmar, H.A., Prusiner, S.B., Stowring, L.E. and DeArmond, S.J. (1986) Scrapie prion proteins are synthesized in neurons. *Am. J. Pathol.,* 122: 1 – 5.

Laemmli, U.K. (1970) Cleavage of structured proteins during the assembly of the head of bacteriophage T-4. *Nature,* 227: 680 – 685.

Large, T.H., Bodary, S.C., Clegg, D.O., Weskamp, G., Otten, U. and Reichardt, L.F. (1986) Nerve growth factor gene expression in the developing rat brain. *Science,* 234: 352 – 355.

Leonard, D.B.G., Gorham, J.D., Cole, P., Greene, L.A. and Zipf, E.B. (1988) A nerve growth factor-regulated messenger RNA encodes a new intermediate filament protein. *J. Cell Biol.,* 106: 181 – 193.

Levi-Montalcini, R. (1987) The nerve growth factor 35 years later. *Science,* 237: 1154 – 1162.

Lieberburg, I. (1987) Developmental expression and regional distribution of the scrapie-associated protein mRNA in the rat central nervous system. *Brain Res.,* 417: 363 – 366.

Masiakowski, P. and Shooter, E.M. (1988) Nerve growth factor induces the genes for two proteins related to a family of calcium-finding proteins in PC12 cells. *Proc. Natl. Acad. Sci. U.S.A.,* 85: 1277 – 1281.

Masters, C.L., Simms, G., Weinman, N.A., Multhaup, G., Beyreuther, K. and McDonald, B.L. (1985) Amyloid plaque core protein in Alzheimer's disease and Down's syndrome. *Proc. Natl. Acad. Sci. U.S.A.,* 82: 4245–4249.

McKinley, M.P., Hay, B., Lingappa, V.R., Lieberburg, I. and Prusiner, S.B. (1987) Developmental expression of prion protein gene in brain. *Dev. Biol.,* 121: 105–110.

McKinley, M.P., DeArmond, S.J., Torchia, M., Mobley, W.C. and Prusiner, S.B. (1989) Acceleration of scrapie in neonatal Syrian hamsters. *Neurology,* in press.

Mesulam, M.-M., Mufson, E.J., Wainer B.H. and Levey, A.I. (1983) Central cholinergic pathways in the rat: an overview based on an alternative nomenclature (Ch1–Ch6). *Neuroscience,* 10: 1185–1201.

Meyer, R.K., McKinley, M.P., Bowman, K.A., Barry, R.A. and Prusiner, S.B. (1986) Separation and properties of cellular and scrapie prion proteins. *Proc. Natl. Acad. Sci. U.S.A.,* 83: 2310–2314.

Milner, T.A., Loy, R. and Amaral, D.G. (1983) An anatomical study of the development of the septo-hippocampal projection in the rat. *Dev. Brain. Res.,* 8: 343–371.

Mobley, W.C., Rutkowski, J.L., Tennekoon, G.I., Buchanan, K. and Johnston, M.V. (1985) Choline acetyltransferase activity in striatum of neonatal rats increased by nerve growth factor. *Science,* 229: 284–287.

Mobley, W.C., Rutkowski, J.L., Tennekoon, G.I., Gemski, J., Buchanan, K. and Johnston, M.V. (1986) Nerve growth factor increases choline acetyltransferase activity in developing basal forebrain neurons. *Mol. Brain Res.,* 1: 53–62.

Mobley, W.C., Neve, R.L., Prusiner, S.B. and McKinley, M.P. (1988) Nerve growth factor increases mRNA levels for the prion protein and the β-amyloid protein precursor in developing hamster brain. *Proc. Natl. Acad. Sci. U.S.A.,* 85: 9811–9815.

Morris, S.J., Louis, C.F. and Shooter, E.M. (1971) *Neurobiology,* 1: 64–67.

Oesch, B., Westaway, D., Walchli, M., McKinley, M.P., Kent, S.B.H., Aebersold, R., Barry, R.A., Tempst, P., Teplow, D.B., Hood, L.E., Prusiner, S.B. and Weissmann, C. (1985) A cellular gene encodes scrapie PrP 27–30 protein. *Cell,* 40: 735–746.

Ponte, P., Gonzalez-DeWhitt, P., Schilling, J., Miller, J., Hsu, D., Greenberg, B., Davis, K., Wallace, W., Lieberburg, I., Fuller, F. and Cordell, B. (1988) A new A4 amyloid mRNA contains a domain homologous to serine proteinase inhibitors. *Nature,* 331: 525–527.

Prusiner, S.B. (1987) Prions and neurodegenerative diseases. *N. Engl. J. Med.,* 317: 1571–1581.

Prusiner, S.B., Cochran, S.P., Groth, D.F., Downey, D.E., Bowman, K.A. and Martinez, H.M. (1982) Measurement of the scrapie agent using an incubation time interval assay. *Ann. Neurol.,* 11: 353–358.

Raivich, G. and Kreutzberg, G.W. (1987) The localization and distribution of high affinity β NGF binding sites in the central nervous system of the adult rat. A light microscopic autoradiographic study using [^{125}I]β-NGF. *Neuroscience,* 20: 23–36.

Richardson, P.M., Verge Issa, V.M.K. and Riopelle, R.J. (1986) Distribution of neuronal receptors for nerve growth factor in the rat. *J. Neurosci.,* 6: 2312–2321.

Roberts, G.W., Lofthouse, R., Allsop, D., Landon, M., Kidd, M., Prusiner, S.B. and Crow, T.J. (1988) CNS amyloid proteins in neurodegenerative diseases. *Neurology,* 38: 1534–1540.

Salbaum, J.M., Weidemann, A., Lemaire, H-G., Masters, C.L. and Beyreuther, K. (1988) The promoter of Alzheimer's disease amyloid A4 precursor gene. *EMBO J.,* 7: 2807–2813.

Schubert, D., Heinemann, S. and Kidokoro, Y. (1977) Cholinergic metabolism and synapse formation by a rat nerve cell line. *Proc. Natl. Acad. Sci. U.S.A.,* 74: 2579–2583.

Shelton, D.L., Nadler, J.V. and Cotman, C.W. (1979) Development of high-affinity choline uptake and associated acetylcholine synthesis in the rat fascia dentata. *Brain Res.,* 163: 263–275.

Shivers, B., Hilbich, C., Multhaup, G., Salbaum, M., Beyreuther, K. and Seeburg, P. (1988) Alzheimer's disease amyloidogenic glycoprotein: expression pattern in rat brain suggests a role in cell contact. *EMBO J.,* 7: 1365–1370.

Stahl, N., Borchelt, D.R., Hsaio, K. and Prusiner, S.B. (1987) Scrapie prion protein contains a phosphatidylinositol glycolipid. *Cell,* 51: 229–240.

Tanzi, R., Gusella, J.F., Watkins, P.C., Bruns, G.A.P., St. George-Hyslop, P., Van Keuren, M.L., Patterson, D., Pagan, S., Kurnit, D.M. and Neve, R.L. (1987) Amyloid β protein gene: cDNA, mRNA distribution, and genetic linkage near the Alzheimer locus. *Science,* 235: 880–884.

Tanzi, R., McClatchey, A.I., Lamperti, E.D., Villa-Komaroff, L., Gusella, J.F. and Neve, R.L. (1988) Protease inhibitor domain encoded by an amyloid protein precursor mRNA associated with Alzheimer's disease. *Nature,* 331: 528–530.

Thoenen, H., Bandtlow, C. and Heumann, R. (1987) The physiological function of nerve growth factor in the central nervous system: comparison with the periphery. *Rev. Physiol. Biochem. Pharmacol.,* 109: 146–178.

Tiercy, J.-M. and Shooter, E.M. (1986) Early changes in the synthesis of nuclear and cytoplasmic proteins are induced by nerve growth factor in differentiating rat PC12 cells. *J. Cell Biol.,* 103: 2367–2378.

Towbin, H., Staehelin, T. and Gordon, J. (1979) Electrophoretic transfer of proteins from polyacrylamide gels to nitrocellulose sheets: procedure and some applications. *Proc. Natl. Acad. Sci. U.S.A.,* 76: 4350–4354.

Walicke, P.A. (1989) Novel neurotrophic factors, receptors, and oncogenes. *Annu. Rev. Neurosci.,* 12: 103–126.

Westaway, D., Carlson, G.A. and Prusiner, S.B. (1989) Unravelling prion diseases through molecular genetics. *Trends Neurosci.,* 12: 221–227.

Whittemore, S.R. and Seiger, A. (1987) The expression, localization and functional significance of β-nerve growth factor in the central nervous system. *Brain Res. Rev.,* 12: 439–464.

P. Coleman, G. Higgins and C. Phelps (Eds.)
Progress in Brain Research, Vol. 86
© 1990 Elsevier Science Publishers B.V. (Biomedical Division)

CHAPTER 20

Trophic regulation of basal forebrain gene expression in aging and Alzheimer's disease

Gerald A. Higgins[1,5], Sookyong Koh[1], Rachael L. Neve[2], Elliot J. Mufson[3], Karen S. Chen[4] and Fred H. Gage[4]

[1] *Department of Neurobiology and Anatomy, University of Rochester Medical Center, Rochester, NY 14642;* [2] *Department of Psychobiology, University of California at Irvine, Irvine, CA 92127;* [3] *Christopher Center for Parkinson's Research, Institute for Biogerontology Research, Sun City, AZ 85351;* [4] *Department of Neurosciences, University of California at San Diego, La Jolla, CA 92093; and* [5] *National Institute on Aging, Baltimore, MD 21224, U.S.A.*

Introduction

Alzheimer's disease (AD) is a devastating neurological disorder which affects a large proportion of the aged U.S. population. The etiology of the disease is unknown, but the neuropathological sequelae include the deposition of amyloid in neuritic plaques and blood vessels, intracellular neurofibrillary tangles, as well as neuronal death and atrophy with a variable distribution within specific cortical, limbic and subcortical regions of the CNS. Degeneration of the "ascending" basal forebrain cholinergic projection system to cortex appears to be characteristic of the disease (Bartus et al., 1982; Whitehouse et al., 1982; Coyle et al., 1983). Deficits in this cholinergic pathway are clearly associated with cognitive impairments in the disease, and in animal models which exhibit similar behavioral impairments (Henke and Lang, 1983; Smith, 1988). Although cholinergic dysfunction cannot account for all of the neuropathological changes that occur in AD, numerous studies have documented extensive neuronal atrophy and loss within the nucleus basalis of Meynert (Ch4 cell group) in the disease (for review, see Vogels et al., 1990).

An individual neuron's vulnerability to the pathological consequences of AD may, in part, be determined by its ability to initiate appropriate "regenerative" or "trophic" programs of gene expression during periods of cellular stress. Stressors may include decreased trophic factor support, metabolic and oxidative stress, glucocorticoid or excitotoxin-mediated damage, loss of target or neighboring neurons, or pathological phenomena specific for the disease. The examination of changes in the expression of specific genes can be documented both within the context of disease-related neuronal deterioration, and within model systems which exhibit the capacity to initiate protective or growth-related responses.

The specific neuronal system which is the focus of this chapter is the nerve growth factor (NGF)-responsive pathway which originates in the cholinergic basal forebrain and terminates in the neocortex and hippocampal formation. NGF is the most well-characterized member of a supergene family of growth factors which have been found in the CNS (Hohn et al., 1990; Maisonpierre et al., 1990). It has been proposed that neurodegenerative changes which occur in the cholinergic basal forebrain in AD may be attributed to deficits in the NGF responsiveness of basal forebrain neurons (Hefti and Weiner, 1986). The basal forebrain cholinergic cell groups appear to depend upon NGF released from cortical target regions during development and periods of stress in the adult CNS, and they contain specific receptors for NGF which have been localized to neurons of the medial septum (Ch1 cell group), nucleus of the diagonal band (Ch2, 3) and nucleus basalis of Meynert (Ch4) in the rodent (Springer et al., 1987; Koh et al., 1989), monkey (Kordower et al., 1988), and human (Higgins and Mufson, 1989; Mufson et al., 1989a). Although reduced levels of cholinergic biosynthetic enzymes such as choline acetyltransferase (ChAT) have been observed in the basal forebrain and in the cortical target regions of basal forebrain neurons in AD, previous studies which have examined NGF and receptor (NGF-R) mRNA levels have not detected changes in the expression of these genes in AD (Goedert et al., 1986, 1989). In contrast to these negative results, recent immunohistochemical studies (Hefti and Mash, 1989; Mufson et al., 1989b) have identified decreased NGF-R immunostaining within basal forebrain magnocellular cholinergic neurons in AD tissue as compared to age-matched controls.

To determine the extent to which deficits in the NGF-responsiveness in the basal forebrain may contribute to neuronal atrophy and amyloid pathology in aging and AD, we have conducted parallel studies in the rodent and human basal forebrain to examine several genes whose expression appears to be regulated by NGF. Specific mRNA species which were examined in these studies include the NGF-R, whose abundance reflects the growth factor sensitivity of basal forebrain neurons (Higgins et al., 1989), and ChAT, a biosynthetic enzyme involved in acetylcholine synthesis. In addition, recent data suggest that expression of the amyloid precursor protein (APP) gene, which encodes the $\beta/A4$ protein found in neuritic plaques and the cerebrovasculature in AD (see Neve et al., this volume), may be differentially regulated by NGF (Wion et al., 1988; Schubert et al., 1989; McKinley et al., this volume). We have used in situ hybridization and other RNA analysis methods to address

the following experimental questions: (1) Is NGF-receptor gene expression altered in AD?; (2) Can NGF infusion into the adult rat brain induce a restorative "trophic" program of gene expression in mature basal forebrain neurons?; and (3) Is the expression of the APP gene altered in NGF-responsive basal forebrain neurons during aging and in AD, providing a possible link between neuronal atrophy and amyloid deposition?

NGF-receptor mRNA levels are specifically decreased in the nucleus basalis (Ch4 cell group) in Alzheimer's disease

It has been proposed that magnocellular cholinergic neurons (Ch1 – Ch4; Mesulam et al., 1983) which project to the neocortex and hippocampal formation, are preferentially affected early in the course of AD (Bartus et al., 1982; Coyle et al., 1983). These same neurons express the NGF-R (Hefti and Mash, 1989; Kordower et al., 1989; Mufson et al., 1989a), presumably as part of a growth factor-dependent relationship with NGF released from cortical structures (Hefti, 1983; Gage et al., 1989b). Pronounced degenerative changes in the nucleus basalis are a characteristic feature of AD (Vogels et al., 1989). However, cortical levels of NGF mRNA have been reported not to be altered in the disease (Goedert et al., 1986), and a recent study using RNA blotting detected no differences in NGF-R mRNA levels in the basal forebrain of AD cases versus normal aged controls (Goedert et al., 1989). In order to resolve these apparently contradictory findings, we have used in situ hybridization and Northern blotting to document and quantify cellular changes in NGF-R mRNA expression in the basal forebrain in AD.

Our recent work shows that NGF-R mRNA hybridization is decreased in the nucleus basalis in AD (Higgins and Mufson, 1989), supporting the observation that decreased NGF-responsiveness may be a primary feature of the disease. Brain tissue was obtained from 6 normal aged individuals and 6 patients with AD. In situ hybridization was performed on formaldehyde-

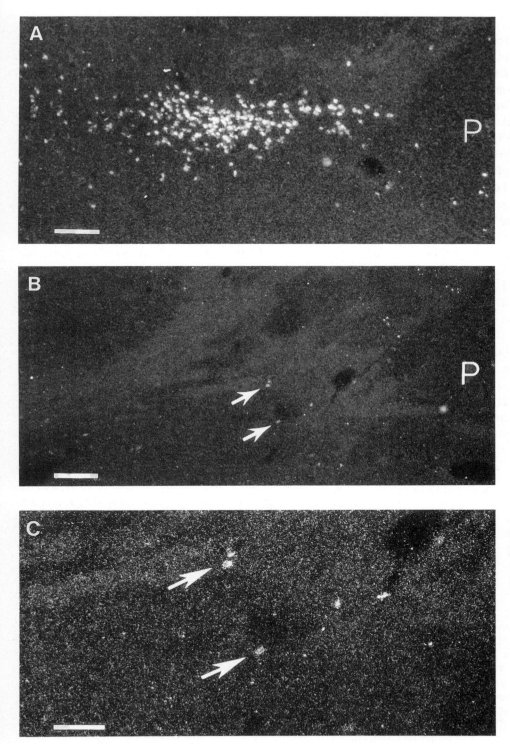

Fig. 1. Example of decreased NGF-R mRNA-positive neuronal hybridization within the posterior subdivision of the nucleus basalis (Ch4p) in AD. *A*. Normal aged individual. *B, C*. Patient with AD. *A* and *B* are low magnification darkfield photomicrographs, and *C* is a higher magnification photograph of *B*. Notice that in this AD case, only a few hybridization profiles are present within Ch4p (arrows). Magnification bars: *A, B* = 500 μM; *C* = 250 μM. (Adapted, with permission, from Higgins and Mufson, 1989.)

fixed coronal tissue sections using an ^{35}S-labeled RNA probe generated from a full-length human NGF-R cDNA clone (Johnson et al., 1986). In situ hybridization shows that the normal distribution of NGF-R mRNA-positive neurons within the basal forebrain is similar to that reported in immunocytochemical studies (Hefti and Mash, 1989; Kordower et al., 1989; Mufson et al., 1989a). Thus NGF-R mRNA hybridization could be observed within components of the medial septum, diagonal band and nucleus basalis, corresponding to the Ch1 – Ch4 cholinergic cell groups.

In comparisons of normal aged versus AD individuals, we observed robust decreases in the number of NGF-R mRNA-positive cells within the basal forebrain, effects which were specific for neurons of the nucleus basalis magnocellularis (Ch4 cell group). The loss of NGF-R mRNA-positive neurons was especially pronounced in the posterior division of the nucleus basalis (Ch4p) in all of the AD cases (Fig. 1). Quantitative studies showed decreases in NGF-R mRNA-positive cell number within all subdivisions of the nucleus basalis (Ch4, Fig. 2), with decreases of approximately 45% in the anterior division (Ch4a), 50%

in the intermediate division (Ch4iv and Ch4id), and over 90% in the posterior division (Ch4p). In contrast, no significant difference in the number of NGF-R mRNA-positive neurons was observed in the medial septum (Ch1) and vertical limb of the nucleus of the diagonal band (Ch2) between normal aged and AD individuals (Fig. 2).

In addition to using in situ hybridization to quantify changes in the number of NGF-R mRNA-containing basal forebrain neurons in AD, we also measured changes in gross NGF-R mRNA levels in the nucleus basalis by use of Northern analysis. For these studies, we examined 2 different AD cases which represented extreme examples in the range of AD cases for NGF-R mRNA-positive cell number. Northern blotting analysis confirmed the finding that NGF-R mRNA levels were reduced in the nucleus basalis-containing samples of basal forebrain tissue in the 2 AD patients relative to the 2 normal aged controls, and the relative magnitude of the NGF-R hybridization signal on the RNA blot was comparable to NGF-R mRNA-positive cell number per case (Fig. 3; Higgins and Mufson, 1989). Thus, both in situ hybridization and Northern blotting showed that NGF-R gene expression is decreased in the nucleus basalis in AD compared with age matched controls.

These results support the hypothesis that loss of NGF-R gene expression in the nucleus basalis (Ch4) is associated with the neurodegenerative process of AD. Whether decreases in NGF-R gene expression in the basal forebrain precede degenerative changes in cortical regions in AD cannot be determined from these findings. However, the loss of NGF-responsiveness in these cases may result from a lack of retrograde NGF support due to cortical atrophy, and not a primary defect within the basal forebrain itself. In contrast with these results in the nucleus basalis, we have not observed significant differences between normal aged and AD patients in the number of NGF-R mRNA-positive neurons within the medial septum and the nucleus of the vertical limb of the diagonal band (Ch1, Ch2). The absence of diminished NGF-R message levels in Ch1 and Ch2 in AD is surpris-

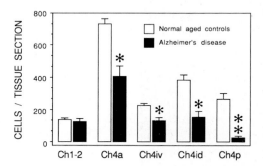

Fig. 2. Decreased numbers of NGF-R mRNA-positive cells within the Ch cholinergic cell groups in AD. Graph shows numbers of cells per tissue section within the various cell groups expressed as mean ± S.E.M. from normal aged individuals (open bars) and AD patients (closed bars). Counts of grain clusters were determined from 2 sections per level from each individual (n = 6 cases each for normal aged (NA) controls and for AD patients). *$P \leq 0.005$, ** $P \leq 0.0005$, as determined by Student's t-test. (Adapted, with permission, from Higgins and Mufson, 1989.)

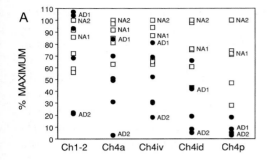

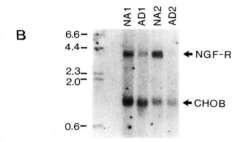

Fig. 3. Correlation between loss of NGF-R mRNA positive neurons, determined by in situ hybridization, and decreased levels of NGF-R message as determined by Northern blotting. Tissue samples from the contralateral sides of the same brains of age-matched normal aged individuals (NA1, NA2) and AD cases (AD1, AD2) were processed for (A) in situ hybridization and (B) Northern analysis. (Adapted, with permission, from Higgins and Mufson, 1989.) A. Scattergram plot showing the distribution of all normal aged controls (□) and AD cases (●) within the Ch cell groups. The average number (determined from 2 tissue sections) of cells for each case is plotted as a percentage of cells in case NA2, which contained the maximum number of cells per cell group of the control cases. Specific AD cases, such as AD1, showed considerable overlap with the distribution of normal aged cases, and other AD cases, such as AD2, showed very little overlap. However, large differences between controls and all of the AD cases occurred in Ch4p. Note that in Ch1-2, two of the AD cases contain larger numbers of cells than any of the control cases. B. Matched samples from A were processed using Northern (RNA) blotting to show decreased expression of NGF-R mRNA within the nucleus basalis (Ch4 cell group) in AD. NA1, NA2: normal aged controls; AD1, AD2: AD patients. Compare the intensity of NGF-R mRNA hybridization for AD1 and AD2 with the cell count values shown in A. 5 μg of poly A$^+$ RNA was loaded into each lane, size-fractionated by gel electrophoresis, transferred to Nytran membrane, and hybridized with ^{32}P-labeled human NGF-R cDNA insert and rodent CHOB cDNA-containing plasmid. Numbers on the left indicate size in kilobases.

ing, because these cell groups project to the hippocampal formation, a structure which is heavily affected by pathology in the disease. However, a recent detailed morphological study also did not detect significant decreases in neuronal number in Ch1 or Ch2 in the disease (Vogels et al., 1989), suggesting the possibility that the Ch1 and Ch2 cell groups are spared from the degenerative changes which occur within Ch4 in the disease. Further studies correlating the abundance of NGF-R mRNA in the basal forebrain with the pathological status of cortical target zones may provide insight into the temporal relationship between degenerative changes in the cortex and altered gene expression in the basal forebrain.

Both our in situ hybridization results and Northern analysis clearly show decreased levels of NGF-R mRNA as compared with normal aged individuals in the nucleus basalis (Ch4 cell group). These results do not agree with the findings of Goedert et al. (1989), who reported no gross change in basal forebrain NGF-R mRNA levels in AD using RNA blotting. However, recent immunocytochemical studies have also detected loss of NGF-R immunoreactive neurons within the nucleus basalis in the disease (Hefti and Mash, 1989; Mufson et al., 1989b). It is unclear whether the loss of NGF-R mRNA which we have observed in this study is due to the actual death of basal forebrain neurons, or reflects a loss of detectable NGF-R mRNA hybridization which coincides with the transition to an atrophic state. A growing body of morphometric data suggests that the majority of nucleus basalis neurons are not lost in the disease, but instead exhibits decreased cell size (Vogels et al., 1990). However, NGF can also induce NGF-R gene expression within neurons which do not contain detectable levels of NGF-R mRNA, as has been demonstrated in the rodent CNS, with recruitment of NGF-R mRNA-positive cells following infusion of the growth factor into the forebrain (see below; Higgins et al., 1989). Thus, the loss of NGF-R mRNA-positivity within basal forebrain neurons which we have observed in AD may be reversible by exogenous application of the ligand. Atrophic basal forebrain cholinergic neurons may lose most of their NGF receptors in AD, as evidenced by loss of NGF-R mRNA hybridization, but still maintain the capacity for NGF-R re-expression following exposure to NGF.

NGF induction of basal forebrain gene expression in the adult rat: a model for growth factor-mediated protection from neuronal degeneration

The majority of basal forebrain cholinergic neurons in the rat also contain receptors for NGF, and NGF-R mRNA has been localized within the basal forebrain in this species (Buck et al., 1987; Ayer-LeLievre et al., 1988; Ernfors et al., 1988; Gibbs et al., 1989; Koh et al., 1989). NGF-R mRNA and protein is also found in other neuronal cell groups in the adult rat CNS (Koh et al., 1989). One mechanism by which NGF may mediate its biological effects on basal forebrain neurons is by influencing the expression of its own receptor. Studies in the peripheral nervous system and in cultured neurons suggest that NGF positively regulates the expression of its own receptor (Rohrer and Barde, 1982; Bernd and Greene, 1984; Taniuchi et al., 1986; Heumann et al., 1987; Hartikka and Hefti, 1988), such that levels of the NGF-R are a sensitive indicator to the morphological integrity of responsive neurons. Thus, NGF induces NGF-R mRNA leading to neuronal hypertrophy, while decreased NGF-R mRNA levels reflect growth factor deprivation, resulting in neuronal atrophy and ultimately cell death.

If the atrophy and loss of basalis neurons during normal aging is due to decreases in the trophic responsivity of these cells, than levels of NGF and its receptor should be reduced in senescent rodents. A number of events could contribute to decreased levels of the NGF-R in the basal forebrain, such as a loss of NGF in target regions or defective retrograde transport of the receptor complex (Johnson et al., 1987). Several of these possibilities have been examined in rodent experiments. For example, 28 month old Fischer 344 rats show decreased NGF mRNA and protein levels in the hippocampal formation compared to young animals (Larkfors et al., 1987). In the basal forebrain, decreased numbers of NGF-R immunopositive neurons have been observed in 30 month old Long-Evans rats, and this decrease is associated with spatial memory impairment in these animals (Koh and Loy, 1988). Diminished NGF-R immunostaining of the cell bodies and primary dendrites of basal forebrain neurons have been observed in 24–27 month old Sprague Dawley rats (Gomez-Pinilla et al., 1989). Defects in the retrograde transport of ^{125}I-labeled NGF from the hippocampus to the basal forebrain have also been observed in aged rats (Koh et al., submitted). Decreased NGF-R immunoreactivity is also associated with normal aging in the human basal forebrain (Hefti and Mash, 1989). Collectively, these data suggest that the loss of NGF responsivity of basal forebrain neurons is a normal feature of the aging process, similar but less severe than the changes in NGF-R gene expression observed in AD (Higgins and Mufson, 1989).

We have examined the cellular and molecular effects of NGF treatment on basal forebrain neuronal subpopulations which have been shown to contain NGF-R immunoreactive neurons in the adult rat brain. This study forms part of a larger experimental series aimed at examining the capacity of adult NGF-responsive neurons to initiate trophic responses during periods of cellular stress which may accompany the aging process. NGF-responsive basal forebrain neurons of the rat CNS form a continuum extending through the medial septum, vertical and horizontal limbs of the nucleus of the diagonal band, and the nucleus basalis magnocellularis (Springer et al., 1987; Dawbarn et al., 1988; Koh et al., 1989). Co-localization studies in the rat, monkey and human have demonstrated that the majority of NGF-R immunoreactive neurons within these cell groups are cholinergic, containing markers of cholinergic function such as ChAT (Hefti et al., 1986; Kordower et al., 1988; Batchelor et al., 1990). For our experiments, we have determined the extent to which NGF can increase NGF-R gene expression within presumptive cholinergic neurons that normally express NGF-R in the adult. We have also addressed the possibility that vehicle-induced lesions may cause increased NGF-R mRNA expression within forebrain neurons which are normally NGF-responsive in the adult, as damage-induced expression of NGF-R immunoreactivity has been previously demonstrated in the rodent CNS (Gage et al., 1989a). In order to determine whether cholinergic neurons were a primary target of the hypertrophy caused by NGF infusion, we examined ChAT mRNA expression within these same basal forebrain neuronal populations.

Intraparenchymal infusion of NGF into the basal forebrain increases NGF-R mRNA and protein levels, NGF-R mRNA-positive cell number, and cell size, throughout the basal forebrain continuum (Higgins et al., 1989). For example, in situ hybridization shows increased NGF-R mRNA hybridization intensity and cell number, as well as hypertrophy of NGF-R mRNA-positive neurons, within the nucleus basalis on the side of the brain which received chronic infusion of NGF as compared to the non-infused side (Fig. 4). Quantitative studies showed that chronic infusion of NGF produced approximately a 1.5-fold average increase in the number of NGF-R mRNA-positive neurons throughout the NGF-R neuronal continuum versus vehicle-infused or non-infused sides (Higgins et

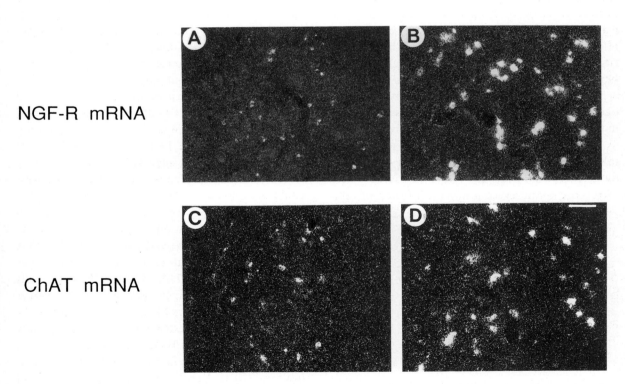

Fig. 4. NGF induction of NGF-R and ChAT mRNAs in the nucleus basalis magnocellularis of Meynert. The NGF infusion site was located within rostral portions of the nucleus. Darkfield photomicrographs of ^{35}S-labeled RNA probe hybridization. NGF-R mRNA hybridization in the (A) non-infused side and (B) NGF-infused side of the same tissue section. ChAT mRNA hybridization in the (C) non-infused and (D) NGF-infused side of the same tissue section. Magnification is the same for all of the figures. Bar = 75 μM. (Adapted, with permission, from Higgins et al., 1989.)

al., 1989). Measurements of cell diameter, determined from immunocytochemically-stained material, showed an average 2-fold increase in cell diameter produced by NGF infusion (Higgins et al., 1989).

In order to provide further confirmation that NGF induction of NGF-R mRNA and neuronal hypertrophy were occurring within cholinergic neurons, we hybridized adjacent tissue sections collected from 4 animals with a probe for ChAT mRNA. Fig. 4C and D show increases in ChAT mRNA expression and neuronal hypertrophy within nucleus basalis neurons following NGF infusion. The magnitude of increased ChAT mRNA abundance within hypertrophied neurons produced by NGF treatment appears qualitatively similar to that observed with NGF-R mRNA (Fig. 4A, B). However, cell counts within the medial septum, nucleus of the diagonal band and nucleus basalis in 4 animals showed no significant increases in ChAT mRNA-positive cell number produced by NGF infusion (non-infused side: 378 + 22 cells/animal; NGF-infused: 368 + 26 cells/animal; $P > 0.25$).

These results show that administration of exogenous NGF into the adult brain causes increases in the number of NGF-R mRNA-positive neurons, as well as hypertrophy of NGF-R and ChAT mRNA-positive neurons, within NGF-responsive basal forebrain neuronal subpopulations. These effects are not observed following infusion of vehi-

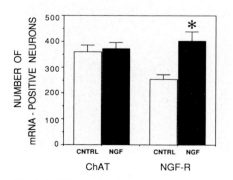

Fig. 5. NGF treatment increases the number of NGF-R mRNA-positive neurons, but does not affect the number of ChAT mRNA-positive neurons within the basal forebrain of the adult rat (* $P < 0.005$).

cle, suggesting that NGF-R gene induction and the accompanying hypertrophic response mediated by NGF receptors are a specific consequence of NGF-induced trophic changes within these cell groups in the adult CNS. In addition, no increases in ChAT-positive cell number were observed following NGF treatment, suggesting the possibility that NGF-R mRNA was induced within cholinergic neurons which initially did not contain detectable levels of NGF-R mRNA (Fig. 5).

Altered expression of the amyloid precursor protein (APP) gene in aging and Alzheimer's disease

The amyloid β/A4-protein is a major constituent of neuritic (senile) plaque and cerebrovascular amyloid deposits is Alzheimer's disease (Glenner and Wong, 1984a, b; Masters et al., 1985). Although a direct causal link between aberrant β/A4-protein accumulation and AD has not yet been proven, one possible mechanism of plaque formation may be differential amyloid expression in the disease. Increased expression of total amyloid precursor protein (APP) mRNA has been observed in the basal forebrain and hippocampal formation in AD (Cohen et al., 1988; Higgins et al., 1988; Palmert et al., 1988), suggesting a mechanism by which pathological deposits of the β/A4-protein could accumulate in the disease. At least five different APP mRNA transcripts are expressed in human brain. In addition to the original APP sequence of 695 amino acids, longer APP cDNA clones have been isolated, corresponding to larger precursor proteins of 714, 751 and 770 amino acids (Kitaguchi et al., 1988; Ponte et al., 1988; Tanzi et al., 1988; Golde et al., 1990). APP-751 and APP-770 share an inserted 168 nucleotide motif which encodes a novel 56 – 57 amino acid domain with identity to the Kunitz family of serine protease inhibitors (KPI: Kunitz Protease Inhibitor), and APP-770 contains an additional 19 amino acids with homology to the MRC OX-2 antigen. A shorter KPI-containing form of the APP molecule has also been cloned (De Sauvage and Octave,

1989). This amyloid precursor-related protein (APRP) encodes a 563 amino acid protein which contains the protease inhibitor domain present in APP-751 and APP-770, but lacks the β/A4 sequence and the hydrophobic transmembrane domain present in all of the other precursors, and thus may represent a secreted form of the precursor (De Sauvage and Octave, 1989). The presence of KPI-containing APP molecules which contain the β/A4 sequence has fueled speculation that aberrant proteolysis of APP may be a primary cause of amyloid deposition in AD, and that overexpression of a KPI-containing form (APP-751 or APP-770) of the APP molecule may either be directly responsible for amyloid pathology, or may constitute a CNS response to aberrant proteolysis of the non-inserted form of APP.

The secreted counterparts of APP-695 and APP-751 affect cell growth at physiologically relevant concentrations (Saitoh et al., 1989). In addition, APP-751 has been shown to be identical with protease nexin II, a molecule which has been shown to inhibit protease activity associated with growth factors such as NGF (Oltersdorf et al., 1989; Van Nostrand et al., 1989). Residues 1-28 of the β/A4 molecule may also have direct "neurotrophic" activity, because this peptide appears to prolong cell survival in explanted rat hippocampal cultures (Whitson et al., 1989), although these effects are only observed at concentrations which are several orders of magnitude higher than those required for cell survival with other growth factors such as NGF (Hosang and Shooter, 1987). The 105 amino acid carboxyl terminal portion of membrane-bound forms of the APP molecule has been shown to have neurotoxic effects in NGF-primed PC12 cells and in explanted rat hippocampal neurons (Yankner et al., 1989; see Neve et al., this volume), effects which may help to explain the widespread cell death which occurs in AD. This latter phenomenon is consistent with recent observations on the processing of membrane forms of the APP molecule, which suggest that the amino terminal portion of the precursor is "shed" from the cytoplasmic membrane, leaving behind the membrane-bound β/A4 fragment and the intracellular portion of the molecule (Oltersdorf et al., 1989; Rumble et al., 1989; Saitoh et al., 1989; Weidemann et al., 1989). In addition, the cloning of APRP-563 suggests that primary secreted forms of the precursor may exist, which lack the hydrophobic transmembrane domain and thus do not encode the β/A4 protein sequence (De Sauvage and Octave, 1989).

Accumulation of protease inhibitor-containing APP transcripts in the basal forebrain of behaviorally-impaired aged rats

In the context of human studies which have suggested that differential APP gene expression may be a feature of AD, we decided to investigate the possibility that changes in APP gene expression may occur as a consequence of aging in the rodent CNS. A subpopulation of aged rats show behavioral deficits which may mimic some of the learning and memory impairments associated with aging and AD (Gage et al., 1989b). Our working hypothesis is that altered levels of APP transcripts within basal forebrain cholinergic neurons may be associated with cellular atrophy and the accompanying behavioral deficits. Because the cholinergic-cortical pathway is dependent upon NGF for its survival during development, and during times of stress in the adult, we predict that a loss of NGF-responsiveness may be correlated with differential APP gene expression in aged animals. Developmental and cell culture studies show that APP mRNA is preferentially induced by NGF (Mobley et al., 1988; Schubert et al., 1989), and thus loss of NGF-responsiveness may be similar to that seen in AD: increased expression of KPI-containing forms of APP mRNA coupled with decreased expression of APP-695. We predict that administration of NGF to aged animals should act to reverse differential APP expression associated with the aging process.

In order to examine cellular changes in APP gene expression which may accompany aging in the rodent basal forebrain, we used in situ hybridization with both human and rat ^{35}S-tailed oligonucleotides for discrimination of KPI-inserted (APP-751/APP-770/APRP-563) from non-inserted (APP-695) forms of APP mRNA (Higgins et al., 1990). Spatial memory was tested in a water maze task. Increases in KPI-containing forms of APP mRNA were observed in basal forebrain NGF-responsive cell groups including the medial septum, ventral pallidum/diagonal band complex and the nucleus basalis magnocellularis in aged (25 month old) Sprague-Dawley rats versus young (9 month old) control animals. Quantitative analysis of hybridization intensity showed that the nucleus basalis in behaviorally-characterized aged rats showed increases in the ratio of KPI-inserted to APP-695 mRNA (Fig. 6), and this phenomenon was correlated with deficits of spatial memory. The increased expression of KPI-containing transcripts is neuroanatomically-specific, because other neuronal cell types, such as cerebral cortical, amygdaloid, and cerebellar Purkinje cells, showed similar levels of inserted forms of APP mRNA in all aged and young rats. Thus, both our studies in the rodent basal forebrain and other studies in human cortical

regions suggest that the ratio of KPI-inserted to the non-inserted form of APP mRNA is increased both in normal aging and in AD. To our knowledge, these are the first results linking a molecule which may be responsible for a major pathology of AD, with a related functional deficit in an animal model. However, it still remains unclear how changes in APP gene expression or protein processing contributes to amyloid deposition in AD (Selkoe, 1989).

Evidence for increased expression of a specific APP transcript in Alzheimer's disease

In situ hybridization studies have previously localized both total APP mRNA and various forms of APP mRNA to neurons in the human brain (Bahmanyar et al., 1987; Goedert, 1987; Higgins et al., 1988; Neve et al., 1988), and increased levels to total APP message in the disease have been observed in several brain regions (Cohen et al., 1988; Higgins et al., 1988). APP mRNA levels appear to be increased within the nucleus basalis in AD (Cohen et al., 1988). In the study of Palmert et al. (1988), increased expression of APP message in AD was attributed to APP-695, because total APP mRNA levels were elevated and no change was observed in KPI-inserted forms of the mRNA. However, because no direct measurement of APP-695 was made in this study, which relied solely on the use of in situ hybridization to examine total and inserted forms of APP (APP-751, APP-770, APRP-563), it is still unclear as to which form, if any, of APP mRNA is changed within basal forebrain neuronal populations in the disease. In contrast to reports of increased levels of APP-695 mRNA in AD, a number of studies, using transcript-specific probes which directly recognize both the non-inserted (APP-695) and KPI-containing forms of APP mRNA in both Northern (RNA) blotting and in situ hybridization experiments, have documented decreased levels of APP-695 and an increase in the ratio of KPI-containing APP mRNAs to APP-695 in AD. For example, Johnson et al. (1988, 1989) have shown decreased levels of APP-695 relative to inserted

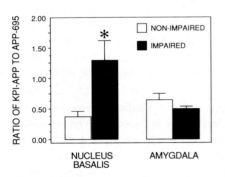

Fig. 6. Quantification of grain density measurements from in situ hybridization data shows that the ratio of KPI-containing APP mRNA to APP-695 mRNA hybridization is increased in the nucleus basalis of aged rats with behavioral impairments (mean ± S.E.M.; $P < 0.05$; non-impaired: 0.37 ± 0.09; impaired: 1.29 ± 0.33; n = 3 animals). In contrast, similar ratios of APP transcripts are found in the lateral nucleus of the amygdala in impaired versus non-impaired aged rats ($P > 0.25$; non-impaired: 0.64 ± 0.11; impaired: 0.50 ± 0.04; n = 3 animals). (Adapted, with permission, from Higgins et al., 1990.)

forms of APP in the neocortex and hippocampal formation in the disease. In addition, increased levels of a specific KPI-containing APP mRNA (i.e., APP-770) have been shown to be increased globally in the human brain in AD (Tanaka et al., 1988). In contrast to these studies showing small but reproducible shifts in the ratios of APP mRNAs in AD, more recent studies examining the relative abundance of APP-695, APP-714, APP-750 and APP-770 mRNAs have yielded equivocal results (Golde et al., 1990; Koo et al., 1990a), suggesting that differential APP gene expression may not be an important contributing factor for amyloid deposition in the disease.

In order to more thoroughly investigate the possibility that differential APP gene expression may contribute to amyloid deposition in AD, we undertook a detailed study of the expression of APP-695, APP-751, APP-770 and APRP-563 mRNAs in a variety of brain regions using a combination of RNA slot blotting, in situ hybridization and the reverse transcription – polymerase chain reaction (Neve et al., 1990). Although an increase in the ratio of KPI-containing APP transcripts to APP-695 message was observed in several different brain regions, the most dramatic changes in APP mRNA levels in AD cases relative to normal aged controls were observed with APRP-563. As mentioned previously, this transcript contains the KPI motif, but lacks the carboxyl terminal portion of the molecule which contains the β/A4 sequence, and may represent a secreted form of the precursor (De Savauge and Octave, 1989). Significant increases in APRP-563 mRNA levels were observed in the nucleus basalis, parahippocampal gyrus and occipitotemporal cortex, but not in the hippocampal formation, striatum, or visual cortex using RNA slot blotting methods (Fig. 7). Detailed in situ hybridization studies in the nucleus basalis showed that increased expression of APRP-563 was obvious both within magnocellular neurons (Fig. 8), as well as smaller cells which may represent a glial cell type (Neve et al., 1990). Further experiments may help to define the role of APRP-563 in aberrant processing of

APP precursor molecules, or whether this phenomemon may represent a secondary compensatory response to increased amyloidoises in the disease.

Is amyloid deposition correlated with altered APP gene expression in the basal forebrain?

If NGF deprivation leads to alterations in the expression of the APP gene in the basal forebrain, then a possible pathological consequence of reduced growth factor levels may be aberrant processing of APP molecule(s) leading to increased amyloid deposits in cortical regions. Thus, the β/A4 amyloid which is deposited in neocortical and hippocampal regions in AD may originate from basal forebrain neurons which normally provide cholinergic innervation to these structures. The possibility that amyloid deposits may occur within terminal projection fields is supported by a recent study showing fast anterograde axonal transport of the APP molecule within neurons (Koo et al., 1990b). However, previous studies would argue against basal forebrain neurons being a source for amyloid deposits in cortex. There appears to be no

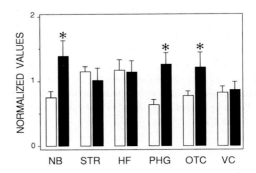

Fig. 7. Increased levels of amyloid precursor-related protein (APRP) 563 mRNA in Alzheimer's disease. RNA slot blotting shows that APRP-563 mRNA is increased in a variety of brain regions in AD. Significant (* $P < 0.05$) increases in APRP-563 message were found in the nucleus basalis (NB), parahippocampal gyrus (PHG) and occipitotemporal cortex (OTC), but not in the striatum (STR), hippocampal formation (HF) or primary visual cortex (VC). Normal aged cases are indicated by open bars and AD cases by closed bars. Data were normalized to hybridization with a control probe (see text for details).

A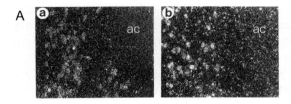

B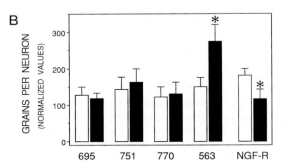

Fig. 8. In situ hybridization shows that APRP-563 mRNA levels are increased within magnocellular neurons of the nucleus basalis in Alzheimer's disease. *A.* Darkfield photomicrographs showing in situ hybridization of APRP-563 mRNA in the intermediate division (Ch4id) of the nucleus basalis in (a) a normal aged individual, and (b) an AD case. ^{35}S-probe hybridization is located within magnocellular neurons adjacent to the anterior commissure (ac) in both cases, but note that a new population of presumptive glial cells is also showing hybridization in the anterior commissure of the AD case. Magnification bar = 150 μM. *B.* Grain density measurements showing increased APRP-563 mRNA hybridization in the nucleus basalis in AD, as compared with the levels of APP-695, APP-751 and APP-770. In contrast, note that NGF-R mRNA levels are reduced per neuron in the AD cases. Measurements were made from large (> 50 μM diameter) profiles of presumptive magnocellular cholinergic neurons in both normal aged (open bars) and AD cases (closed bars) using APP transcript-specific probes (* $P < 0.05$).

simple anatomical correlation between the cortical projection zones of basal forebrain cholinergic neurons and the distribution of neuritic plaques in cortex. Although a preliminary study suggested that the pattern of loss of basal forebrain neurons within the complex subnuclear organization of the nucleus basalis correlated with the distribution of amyloid pathology in cortical target regions (Arendt et al., 1985), more recent studies have not

revealed such a simple relationship (Etienne et al., 1986). Basal forebrain neurons are prone to neurofibrillary tangle formation in AD, but the basal forebrain does not contain the density of amyloid plaques that is present in cortical regions in the disease (Arendt et al., 1988), arguing against these neurons providing an abundant local source of extracellular β/A4 protein. In spite of a lack of correlation between the distribution of neuritic plaques and the organization of basal forebrain neurons and their projection fields, recent immunocytochemical studies using antibodies directed against the APP molecule have revealed the presence and widespread distribution of amyloid deposits not previously visualized by traditional methods (Hyman et al., 1989). Thus, the issue of the neuroanatomical distribution of amyloid deposits in AD may have to be reevaluated in view of recent, more sensitive methodological findings.

One issue which needs to be addressed in the context of the discovery of differential APP gene expression in AD is whether NGF may selectively induce a specific form of APP mRNA. The APP promoter contains AP-1 binding sites (TRE), which can be activated by *c-fos* (complexed with *c-jun*), an "immediate early" gene product whose expression is induced by NGF (Milbrandt, 1988). In addition, putative NGF-responsive elements (NRE) have been identified within promoter regions of NGF-inducible genes (Changelian et al., 1989; Thompson and Ziff, 1989), and it is possible that such regulatory sequences may be present within the promoter of the APP gene. More specifically, several pieces of evidence suggest that NGF selectively induces expression of APP-695 mRNA. First, treatment of PC12 cells with NGF specifically induces the expression of APP-695 protein concomitant with differentiation to a neuronal phenotype (Schubert et al., 1989). Second, the developmental profile of APP expression shows that APP-695 mRNA accounts for most of the APP expressed during the period of maximal NGF-responsiveness within the developing basal forebrain (Mobley et al., 1988). Third, APP gene expression parallels that of ChAT activity during this time period, and NGF injection in the developing and adult rodent basal forebrain increases APP gene expression (Mobley et al., 1988). These studies argue strongly for a model in which NGF specifically induces a form of the APP molecule that lacks the protease inhibitor motif (e.g., APP-695), and suggest that diminished NGF responsivity is associated with an accumulation of KPI-containing APP mRNAs (Fig. 9).

In order to determine how NGF regulates differential APP gene expression in the adult CNS, we have begun to examine changes in the levels of specific APP transcripts using the NGF infusion model described above. The development of recent RT-PCR methods has allowed us the opportunity to quantify relative changes in the levels of different APP mRNA species using the same set of oligonucleotide primers for RT-PCR in brain RNA samples from infused versus non-infused animals. In situ hybridization shows that NGF treatment increases total APP mRNA levels, possibly as a consequence of the basal forebrain neuronal hyper-

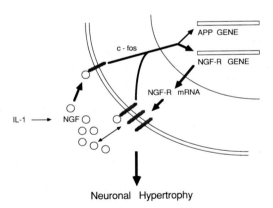

Fig. 9. Schematic depiction showing NGF induction of trophic gene expression in a basal forebrain neuron. NGF binds to the NGF-R and induces expression of NGF-R mRNA, leading to increased numbers of receptors available for binding to NGF. This positive feedback loop results in neuronal hypertrophy. It is unclear what second messengers may mediate NGF induction of gene expression, but they may include "immediate early" genes such as c-fos (Milbrandt, 1988). In addition, NGF appears to preferentially induce APP-695 mRNA as compared to the KPI-containing forms of APP mRNA. Interleukin-1 (IL-1) and other factors acting to increase NGF levels may be important for initiation of this molecular cascade.

trophy which occurs following exogenous application of the trophic factor. Preliminary RT-PCR studies show that this increase in APP message is caused by an increase in the ratio of APP-695 to APP-751 and/or APRP-563 mRNA (data not shown). Eventually, using competitive RT-PCR for quantitative mRNA analysis (Wang et al., 1989), it will be possible to determine whether this shift in the ratio of APP transcripts represents an increase in APP-695 or a decrease in APP-751/APRP-563 message levels.

Trophic regulation of basal forebrain gene expression in aging and Alzheimer's disease

We have presented evidence that the trophic state of basal forebrain neurons is reflected by the expression of genes related to NGF responsiveness, as exemplified by induction of NGF-R and ChAT mRNAs, as well as differential expression of the APP gene. Whether NGF-mediated regulation of APP gene expression is responsible for amyloid deposition in normal aging in the human or in Alzheimer's disease still remains unclear. However, our data support the following model (Fig. 9). NGF is released from cortical structures during development and causes basal forebrain neuronal hypertrophy, presumably mediated by increased NGF-R gene expression, which leads to increased expression of other transcripts such as ChAT, as well as specific induction of APP-695. Obviously some basal level of NGF-R must be present on a subpopulation of neurons which do not initially contain detectable levels of NGF-R mRNA or protein, as the number of NGF-R mRNA-positive neurons is increased following NGF infusion (Fig. 5). In contrast, we predict that defective NGF-mediated regulation in the aged CNS will be reflected by decreased levels of NGF-R mRNA, and an increase in the ratio of KPI-containing forms of APP transcripts to APP-695 mRNA in the basal forebrain. More specifically, we have documented that increases in KPI-containing forms of APP mRNA in AD can be accounted for by APRP-563, which lacks the $\beta/A4$ sequence, suggesting a more complicated scenario than simple over-expression of precursors encoding the $\beta/A4$ protein (Neve et al., 1990). In addition, this increase in APRP-563 mRNA is not limited to the subset of NGF-responsive basal forebrain neurons, but appears to be a more widespread finding in a number of brain regions in the disease. Thus, increased APP mRNA levels in the disease cannot solely be caused by altered NGF regulation, but must also or solely be due to other factor(s) which affect differential expression of the APP gene.

The hypothetical model presented in Fig. 9 provides several avenues for further experimentation. If reduced NGF levels are responsible for age-related changes in basal forebrain gene expression, than how is NGF expression normally regulated in the adult CNS? To answer this question, it will be necessary to determine which molecules are responsible for induction of NGF or related growth factor expression in the adult CNS. For example, interleukin-1β (IL-1β) appears to play a role in the induction of NGF expression in the PNS following sciatic nerve transection (Taniuchi et al., 1988). IL-1β also appears to induce APP gene expression in cultured human endothelial cells (Goldgaber et al., 1989), and IL-1β immunoreactivity is increased in AD brain compared to controls (Griffin et al., 1989). Thus, it is possible that IL-1β and other cytokines released as part of an immune response in the CNS may both regulate NGF levels, as well as inducing expression of APP mRNA, either directly or acting through an intermediate such as NGF. Future experiments examining the precise intercellular and intracellular mechanisms regulating growth factor expression, neuronal atrophy, and amyloidogenesis should resolve this complex molecular cascade.

Acknowledgements

The authors would like to thank Dr. Joseph Rogers for collaborative support on the human APP studies, Dr. Harold Civin for neuropathological evaluation, Dr. Moses V. Chao for the human NGF-R cDNA clone, Dr. A.S. Whitehead for synthesizing the APP oligonucleotides, and Dorothy Herrera and Nancy Dimmick for photographic assistance.

This work was supported by a Mallinckrodt Scholar Award, the Rochester Alzheimer's disease project (AG03644) and NIH grant NS26845 to G.A.H., the Pew Foundation to G.A.H., F.H.G. and R.L.N., NIH grant HD18658 to R.L.N., the American Health Assistance Foundation to E.J.M., and the J.D. French Foundation, NIH AG06088, the Office of Naval Research, and the California State DHHS to F.H.G.

References

Arendt, T., Bigl, V., Tennstedt, A. and Arendt, A. (1985) Neuronal loss in different parts of the nucleus basalis is related to neuritic plaque formation in cortical areas in Alzheimer's disease. *Neuroscience,* 14: 1 – 14.

Arendt, T., Taubert, G., Bigl, V. and Arendt, A. (1988) Amyloid deposition in the nucleus basalis of Meynert complex: a topographic marker for degenerating cell clusters in Alzheimer's disease. *Acta Neuropathol.,* 75: 226 – 232.

Ayer-Lelievre, L., Olson, L., Ebendal, T., Seiger, A. and Persson, H. (1988) Expression of the β-nerve growth factor gene in hippocampal neurons. *Science,* 240: 1339 – 1341.

Bahmanyar, S., Higgins, G.A., Goldgaber, D., Lewis, D.A., Morrison, J.H., Wilson, M.C., Shankar, S.K. and Gajdusek, D.C. (1987) Localization of amyloid-β-protein messenger RNA in brains from patients with Alzheimer's disease. *Science,* 237: 77 – 80.

Bartus, R.T., Dean, R.L., Beer, B. and Lippa, A.S. (1982) The cholinergic hypothesis of geriatric memory dysfunction. *Science,* 217: 408 – 417.

Batchelor, P.E., Armstrong, D.M., Blaker, S.N. and Gage, F.H. (1990) Nerve growth factor receptor and choline acetyltransferase co-localization in neurons within the rat forebrain: response to fimbria-fornix transection. *J. Comp. Neurol.,* in press.

Bernd, P. and Greene, L.A. (1984) Association of ^{125}I-nerve growth factor with PC12 pheochromocytoma cells. *J. Biol. Chem.,* 259: 15509 – 15516.

Buck, C.R., Martinez, H.J., Black, I.B. and Chao, M.V. (1987) Developmentally regulated expression of the nerve growth factor receptor gene in the periphery and brain. *Proc. Natl. Acad. Sci. U.S.A.,* 84: 3060 – 3063.

Changelian, P.S., Feng, P., King, T.C. and Milbrandt, J. (1989) Structure of the NGFI-A gene and detection of upstream sequences responsible for its transcriptional induction by nerve growth factor. *Proc. Natl. Acad. Sci. U.S.A.,* 86: 377 – 381.

Cohen, M.L., Golde, T.E., Usiak, M.F., Younkin, L.H. and Younkin, S.G. (1988) In situ hybridization of nucleus basalis neurons shows increased β-amyloid mRNA in Alzheimer disease. *Proc. Natl. Acad. Sci. U.S.A.*, 85: 1227 – 1231.

Coyle, J.T., Price, D.L. and DeLong, M.R. (1983) Alzheimer's disease: a disorder of cortical cholinergic innervation. *Science*, 219: 1184 – 1190.

De Sauvage, F. and Octave, J.-N. (1989) A novel mRNA of the A4 amyloid precursor gene coding for a possibly secreted protein. *Science*, 245: 651 – 653.

Ernfors, P., Hallbook, F., Ebendal, T., Shooter, E.M., Radeke, M.J., Misko, T.P. and Persson, H. (1988) Development and regional expression of β-nerve growth factor mRNA in the chick and rat. *Neuron*, 1: 983 – 996.

Etienne, P., Robitaille, Y., Wood, P., Gauthier, S., Nair, N.P.V. and Quirion, R. (1986) Nucleus basalis neuronal loss, neuritic plaques and choline acetyltransferase activity in advanced Alzheimer's disease. *Neuroscience*, 19: 1279 – 1291.

Gage, F.H., Batchelor, P., Chen, K.S., Chin, D., Deputy, S., Rosenberg, M.B., Higgins, G.A., Koh, S., Fischer, W. and Björklund, A. (1989a) NGF-receptor re-expression and NGF-mediated cholinergic neuronal hypertrophy in the damaged adult neostriatum. *Neuron*, 2: 1177 – 1184.

Gage, F.H., Tuszynski, M.H., Chen, K.S., Fagan, A. and Higgins, G.A. (1989b) Nerve growth factor function in the central nervous system. In: M. Bothwell (Ed.), *Trophic Factors in the Central Nervous System,* Springer-Verlag, Berlin, in press.

Gibbs, R.B., McCabe, J.T., Buck, C.R., Chao, M.V. and Pfaff, D.W. (1989) Expression of NGF receptor in the rat forebrain detected with in situ hybridization and immunohistochemistry. *Mol. Brain Res.*, 6: 275 – 287.

Glenner, G.G. and Wong, C.W. (1984a) Alzheimer's disease: initial report of the purification and characterization of a novel cerebrovascular amyloid protein. *Biochem. Biophys. Res. Comm.*, 120: 885 – 890.

Glenner, G.G. and Wong, C.W. (1984b) Alzheimer's disease and Down's syndrome: sharing of a unique cerebrovascular amyloid fibril protein. *Biochem. Biophys. Res. Comm.*, 122: 1131 – 1135.

Goedert, M. (1987) Neuronal localization of amyloid beta protein precursor mRNA in normal human brain and in Alzheimer's disease. *EMBO J.*, 6: 3627 – 3632.

Goedert, M., Fine, A., Hunt, S.P. and Ullrich, A. (1986) Nerve growth factor in peripheral and central rat tissue and in the human nervous system: lesion effects in the rat brain and levels in Alzheimer's disease. *Mol. Brain Res.*, 1: 85 – 92.

Goedert, M., Fine, A., Dawbarn, D., Wilcock, G.K. and Chao, M. (1989) Nerve growth factor receptor mRNA distribution in human brain: normal levels in basal forebrain in Alzheimer's disease. *Mol. Brain Res.*, 5: 1 – 7.

Golde, T.E., Estus, S., Usiak, M., Younkin, L.H. and Younkin, S.G. (1990) Polymerase chain reaction amplification of β amyloid protein precursor mRNAs: identification

of a novel alternatively spliced form and analysis of expression in Alzheimer's disease. *Neuron*, 4: 253 – 267.

Goldgaber, D., Lerman, M.T., McBride, O.W., Saffiot, U. and Gajdusek, D.C. (1987) Characterization and chromosomal localization of a cDNA encoding brain amyloid of Alzheimer's disease. *Science*, 235: 877 – 880.

Goldgaber, D., Harris, H.W., Hla, T., Maciag, T., Donnelly, R.J., Jacobsen, J.S., Vitek, M.P. and Gajdusek, D.C. (1989) Interleukin 1 regulates synthesis of amyloid β-protein precursor in human endothelial cells. *Proc. Natl. Acad. Sci. U.S.A.*, 86: 7606 – 7610.

Gomez-Pinilla, F., Cotman, C.W. and Nieto-Sampedro, M. (1989) NGF receptor immunoreactivity in aged rat brain. *Brain Res.*, 479: 255 – 262.

Griffin, W.S.T., Stanley, L.C., Ling, C., White, L., MacLeod, V., Perrot, L.J., White, C.L. and Araoz, C. (1989) Brain interleukin 1 and S-100 immunoreactivity are elevated in Down syndrome and Alzheimer disease. *Proc. Natl. Acad. Sci. U.S.A.*, 86: 7611 – 7615.

Hartikka, J. and Hefti, F. (1988) Development of septal cholinergic neurons in culture: plating density and glial cells modulate the effects of NGF on survival, fiber growth, and expression of transmitter-specific enzymes. *J. Neurosci.*, 8: 2967 – 2985.

Hefti, F. and Mash, D.C. (1989) Localization of nerve growth factor receptors in the normal human brain and in Alzheimer's disease. *Neurobiol. Aging*, 10: 75 – 87.

Hefti, F. and Weiner, W.J. (1986) Nerve growth factor and Alzheimer's disease. *Ann. Neurol.*, 20: 275 – 281.

Hefti, F., Hartikka, J., Salvatierra, A., Weiner, W.J. and Mash, D.C. (1986) Localization of nerve growth factor receptors in cholinergic neurons of the human basal forebrain. *Neurosci. Lett.*, 69: 37 – 41.

Henke, H. and Lang, W. (1983) Cholinergic enzymes in neocortex, hippocampus, and basal forebrain of non-neurological and senile dementia of Alzheimer-type patients. *Brain Res.*, 267: 281 – 291.

Heumann, R., Korsching, S. and Thoenen, H. (1987) Changes of nerve growth factor synthesis in non-neuronal cells in response to sciatic nerve transection. *J. Cell Biol.*, 104: 1623 – 1631.

Higgins, G.A. and Mufson, E.J. (1989) NGF-receptor gene expression is decreased in the nucleus basalis in Alzheimer's disease. *Exp. Neurol.*, 106: 222 – 236.

Higgins, G.A., Lewis, D.A., Goldgaber, D., Gajdusek, D.C., Morrison, J.H. and Wilson, M.C. (1988) Differential regulation of amyloid-β-protein mRNA expression within hippocampal neuronal subpopulations in Alzheimer's disease. *Proc. Natl. Acad. Sci. U.S.A.*, 85: 1297 – 1301.

Higgins, G.A., Koh, S., Chen, K.S. and Gage, F.H. (1989) NGF induction of NGF-receptor gene expression and cholinergic neuronal hypertrophy in the basal forebrain of the adult rat. *Neuron*, 3: 247 – 256.

Hohn, A., Leibrock, J., Bailey, K. and Barde, Y.-A. (1990)

254

Identification and characterization of a novel member of the nerve growth factor/brain-derived neurotrophic factor family. *Nature,* 344: 339 – 341.

Hosang, M. and Shooter, E.M. (1987) The internalization of nerve growth factor by high-affinity receptors on pheochromocytoma PC12 cells. *EMBO J.,* 6: 1197 – 1202.

Hyman, B.T., Van Hoesen, G.W., Masters, C.L. and Beyreuther, K. (1989) Aβ amyloid protein immunoreactivity in neurofibrillary tangles and terminal zones of the hippocampal formation in Alzheimer's disease. *Soc. Neurosci. Abstr.,* 19: 1378.

Johnson, D., Lanahan, A., Buck, C.R., Seghal, A., Morgan, C., Merecer, E., Bothwell, M. and Chao, M.V. (1986) Expression and structure of the human NGF receptor. *Cell,* 47: 545 – 554.

Johnson, E.M., Taniuchi, M., Clark, H.B., Springer, J.E., Koh, S., Tayrien, M.W. and Loy, R. (1987) Demonstration of the retrograde transport of nerve growth factor receptor in the peripheral and central nervous system. *J. Neurosci.,* 7: 923 – 929.

Johnson, S.A., Pasinetti, G.M., May, P.C., Ponte, P.A., Cordell, B. and Finch, C.E. (1988) Selective reduction of mRNA for the β-amyloid precursor protein that lacks a Kunitz-type protease inhibitor motif in cortex of Alzheimer's brains. *Exp. Neurol.,* 102: 264 – 268.

Johnson, S.A., Rogers, J. and Finch, C.E. (1989) APP-695 transcript prevalence is selectively reduced during Alzheimer's disease in cortex and hippocampus but not in cerebellum. *Neurobiol. Aging,* 10: 267 – 272.

Kang, J., Lemaire, H.G., Unterbeck, A., Salbaum, J.M., Masters, C.L., Grzechik, D.H., Multhaup, G., Beyreuther, K. and Muller-Hill, B. (1987) The precursor of Alzheimer's disease amyloid A4 protein resembles a cell surface receptor. *Nature,* 325: 733 – 736.

Kitaguchi, N., Takahashi, Y., Tokushima, Y., Shiojiri, S. and Ito, H. (1988) Novel precursor of Alzheimer's disease amyloid protein shows protease inhibitor activity. *Nature,* 331: 530 – 532.

Koh, S. and Loy, R. (1988) Age-related loss of nerve growth factor sensitivity in rat basal forebrain neurons. *Brain Res.,* 440: 396 – 401.

Koh, S., Oyler, G.A. and Higgins, G.A. (1989) Localization of NGF-R mRNA and protein in the adult rat brain. *Exp. Neurol.,* 106: 209 – 221.

Koo, E.H., Sisodia, S.S., Cork, L.C., Unterbeck, A., Bayney, R.M. and Price, D.L. (1990a) Differential expression of amyloid precursor protein mRNAs in cases of Alzheimer's disease and in aged non-human primates. *Neuron,* 2: 97 – 104.

Koo, E.H., Sisodia, S.S., Archer, D.R., Martin, L.J., Weidemann, A., Beyreuther, K., Fischer, P., Masters, C.L. and Price, D.L. (1990b) Precursor of amyloid protein in Alzheimer disease undergoes fast anterograde axonal transport. *Proc. Natl. Acad. Sci. U.S.A.,* 87: 1561 – 1565.

Kordower, J.H., Bartus, R.T., Bothwell, M., Schatteman, G. and Gash, D.M. (1988) Nerve growth factor receptor immunoreactivity in the non-human primate (*Cebus apella*): distribution, morphology and colocalization with cholinergic enzymes. *J. Comp. Neurol.,* 277: 465 – 486.

Larkfors, L., Ebendahl, T., Whittemore, S.R., Persson, H., Hoffer, B. and Olson, L. (1987) Decreased levels of nerve growth factor (NGF) and its messenger RNA in the aged rat brain. *Mol. Brain Res.,* 3: 55 – 60.

Maisonpierre, P.C., Belluscio, L., Squinto, S., Ip, N.Y., Furth, M.E., Lindsay, R.M. and Yancopoulos, G.D. (1990) Neurotrophin 3: a neurotrophic factor related to NGF and BDNF. *Science,* 247: 1446 – 1451.

Masters, C.L., Simms, G., Weinman, N.A., Multhaup, G., MacDonald, B.L. and Beyreuther, K. (1985) Amyloid plaque core protein in Alzheimer disease and Down syndrome. *Proc. Natl. Acad. Sci. U.S.A.,* 82: 4245 – 4249.

Mesulam, M.-M., Mufson, E.J., Levey, A.I. and Wainer, B.H. (1983) Cholinergic innervation of the cortex by the basal forebrain: cytochemistry and cortical connections of the septal area, diagonal band nuclei basalis (substantia innominata) and hypothalamus in the rhesus monkey. *J. Comp. Neurol.,* 214: 170 – 197.

Milbrandt, J. (1988) Nerve growth factor rapidly induces *c-fos* mRNA in PC12 rat pheochromocytoma cells. *Proc. Natl. Acad. Sci. U.S.A.,* 83: 4789 – 4793.

Mobley, W.C., Rutkowski, J.L., Tennekoon, G.I., Gemski, J., Buchanan, K. and Johnston, M.V. (1986) Nerve growth factor increases choline acetyltransferase activity in developing basal forebrain neurons. *Mol. Brain Res.,* 1: 53 – 62.

Mobley, W.C., Neve, R.L., Prusiner, S.B. and McKinley, M.P. (1988) Nerve growth factor increases mRNA levels for the prion protein and the β-amyloid protein precursor in developing hamster brain. *Proc. Natl. Acad. Sci. U.S.A.,* 85: 9811 – 9815.

Mufson, E.J., Bothwell, M., Hersh, L. and Kordower, J.H. (1989a) Nerve growth factor receptor immunoreactive profiles in the normal aged human basal forebrain: colocalization with cholinergic neurons. *J. Comp. Neurol.,* 285: 196 – 217.

Mufson, E.J., Bothwell, M. and Kordower, J.H. (1989b) Loss of nerve growth factor receptor-containing neurons in Alzheimer's disease: a quantitative analysis across subregions of the basal forebrain. *Exp. Neurol.,* 105: 221 – 232.

Neve, R.L., Finch, E.A. and Dawes, L.R. (1988) Expression of the Alzheimer amyloid precursor gene transcripts in the human brain. *Neuron,* 1: 669 – 676.

Neve, R.L., Rogers, J. and Higgins, G.A. (1990) The Alzheimer amyloid precursor-related transcript lacking the β/A4 sequence is specifically increased in Alzheimer disease brain, in press.

Oltersdorf, T., Fritz, L.C., Schenk, D.B., Lieberburg, I., Johnson-Wood, K.L., Beattie, E.C., Ward, P.J., Blacher, R.W., Dovey, H.F. and Sinha, S. (1989) The secreted form of the Alzheimer's precursor protein with the Kunitz domain is protease nexin II. *Nature,* 341: 144 – 147.

Palmert, M.R., Golde, T.E., Cohen, M.L., Kovacs, D.M., Tanzi, R.E., Gusella, J.F., Usiak, M.F., Younkin, L.H. and Younkin, S.G. (1988) Amyloid protein precursor messenger RNAs: differential expression in Alzheimer's disease. *Science,* 241: 1080 – 1084.

Ponte, P., Gonzalez-Dewhitt, P., Schilling, J., Miller, J., Hsu, D., Greenberg, B., Davis, K., Wallace, W., Lieberburg, I., Fuller, F. and Cordell, B. (1988) A new A4 amyloid mRNA contains a domain homologous to serine protease inhibitors. *Nature,* 331: 525 – 527.

Robakis, N.K., Ramakrishna, N., Wolfe, G. and Wisniewski, H.M. (1987) Molecular cloning and characterization of a cDNA encoding the cerebrovascular and the neuritic plaque amyloid peptides. *Proc. Natl. Acad. Sci. U.S.A.,* 84: 4190 – 4194.

Rumble, B. et al. (1989) Amyloid A4 protein and its precursor in Down's syndrome and Alzheimer's disease. *N. Engl. J. Med.,* 320: 1446 – 1452.

Saitoh, T., Sundsma, M., Roch, J.-M., Kimura, N., Cole, G., Schubert, D., Oltersdorf, T. and Schenk, D.B. (1989) Secreted form of amyloid β protein precursor is involved in the growth regulation of fibroblasts. *Cell,* 58: 615 – 622.

Salbaum, J.M., Weidemann, A., Lemaire, H.-G., Masters, C.L. and Beyreuther, K. (1988) The promoter of Alzheimer's disease amyloid A4 precursor gene. *EMBO J.,* 7: 2807 – 2813.

Schatteman, G.C., Gibbs, L., Lanahan, A.A., Claude, P. and Bothwell, M. (1988) Expression of NGF receptor in the developing and adult primate central nervous system. *J. Neurosci.,* 8: 860 – 873.

Schubert, D., Jin, L-W., Saitoh, T. and Cole, G. (1989) The regulation of amyloid β protein precursor secretion and its modulatory role in cell adhesion. *Neuron,* 3: 689 – 694.

Selkoe, D.J. (1989) Biochemistry of altered brain proteins. In: W.M. Cowan (Ed.), *Annu. Rev. Neurosci.,* 12: 463 – 490.

Shelton, D.L. and Reichardt, L.F. (1986) Studies on the expression of the β-nerve growth factor (NGF) gene in the central nervous system: levels and regional distribution of NGF mRNA suggest that NGF functions as a trophic factor for several distinct populations of neurons. *Proc. Natl. Acad. Sci. U.S.A.,* 83: 2714 – 2718.

Smith, G. (1988) Animal models of Alzheimer's disease: experimental cholinergic denervation. *Brain Res.,* 472: 103 – 118.

Springer, J.E., Koh, S., Tayrien, M.W. and Loy, R. (1987) Basal forebrain magnocellular neurons stain for nerve growth factor receptor: correlation with cholinergic cell bodies and effects of axotomy. *J. Neurosci. Res.,* 17: 111 – 118.

Tanaka, S., Nakamura, S., Ueda, K., Kameyama, M., Shiojiri, S., Takahashi, Y, Kitaguchi, N. and Ito, H. (1988) Three types of amyloid protein precursor mRNA in human brain: their differential expression in Alzheimer's disease. *Biochem. Biophys. Res. Commun.,* 157: 472 – 479.

Taniuchi, M., Clark, H.B. and Johnson, E.M. (1986) Induction of nerve growth factor receptor in Schwann cells after axotomy. *Proc. Natl. Acad. Sci. U.S.A.,* 83: 4094 – 4098.

Tanzi, R.E., Gusella, J.F., Watkins, P.C., Bruns, G.A.P., St. George-Hyslop, P., Van Keuren, M.L., Patterson, D., Pagan, S., Kurnit, D.M. and Neve, R.L. (1987) Amyloid-β-protein gene: cDNA mRNA distribution, and genetic linkage near the Alzheimer locus. *Science,* 235: 880 – 884.

Tanzi, R.E., McClatchey, A.I., Lamperti, E.D., Villa-Komaroff, L., Gusella J.F. and Neve R.L. (1988) Protease inhibitor domain encoded by an amyloid protein precursor mRNA associated with Alzheimer's disease. *Nature,* 331: 528 – 530.

Thompson, M.A. and Ziff, E.B. (1989) Structure of the gene encoding Peripherin, an NGF-regulated neuronal-specific type III intermediate filament protein. *Neuron,* 2: 1043 – 1053.

Van Nostrand, W.E., Wagner, S.L., Suzuki, M., Choi, B.H., Farrow, J.S., Cotman, C.W. and Cunningham, D. (1989) Protease nexin-II, a potent antichymotrypsin, shows identity to amyloid-β-protein precursor. *Nature,* 341: 546 – 548.

Vogels, O.J.M., Broere, C.A.J., Ter Laak, H.J., Ten Donkelaar Niewenhuys, R. and Schulte, B.P.M. (1990) Cell loss and shrinkage in the nucleus basalis Meynert complex in Alzheimer's disease. *Neurobiol. Aging,* 11: 3 – 14.

Wang, A.M., Doyle, M.V. and Mark, D.F. (1989) Quantitation of mRNA by the polymerase chain reaction. *Proc. Natl. Acad. Sci. U.S.A.,* 86: 9717 – 9721.

Weidemann, A., Koning, G., Bunke, D., Fischer, P., Salbaum, J.M., Masters, C.L. and Beyreuther, K. (1989) Identification, biogenesis, and localization of precursors of Alzheimer's disease A4 amyloid protein. *Cell,* 57: 115 – 126.

Whitehouse, P.J., Price, D.L., Struble, R.G., Clark, A.W., Coyle, J.T. and DeLong, M.R. (1982) Alzheimer's disease and senile dementia: loss of neurons in the basal forebrain. *Science,* 215: 1237 – 1239.

Whitson, J.S., Selkoe, D.J. and Cotman, C.W. (1989) Amyloid β protein enhances the survival of hippocampal neurons in vitro. *Science,* 243: 1488 – 1490.

Wion, D., LeBert, M. and Bracket, P. (1988) mRNAs of β amyloid precursor protein and prion protein are regulated by NGF in PC12 cells. *Int. J. Dev. Neurosci.,* 6: 387 – 393.

Yankner, B.A., Dawes, L.R., Fisher, S., Villa-Komaroff, L., Oster-Granite, M.L. and Neve, R.L. (1989) Neurotoxicity of a fragment of the amyloid precursor associated with Alzheimer's disease. *Science,* 245: 417 – 420.

P. Coleman, G. Higgins and C. Phelps (Eds.)
Progress in Brain Research, Vol. 86
© 1990 Elsevier Science Publishers B.V. (Biomedical Division)

CHAPTER 21

Genetics and biology of the Alzheimer amyloid precursor

Rachael L. Neve[1,4], Linda R. Dawes[1], Bruce A. Yankner[2,4], Larry I. Benowitz[3,5], William Rodriguez[3,5], and Gerald A. Higgins[6,7]

Departments of [1]Pediatrics, [2]Neuropathology and [3]Psychiatry, Harvard Medical School, [4]Children's Hospital, Boston, MA; [5]McLean Hospital, Belmont, MA; and [6]Department of Neurobiology and Anatomy, University of Rochester, Rochester, NY; and [7] National Institute on Aging, Baltimore, MD 21224, U.S.A.

Introduction

Alzheimer's disease (AD) is a progressive neurodegenerative disorder characterized by gradual loss of memory, reasoning, orientation, and judgement (Katzman, 1983). A striking aspect of the neuropathology of this disease is deposition of the proteinaceous material amyloid in the walls of the cerebral microvasculature and in the core of extracellular neuritic plaques (Terry et al., 1981; Glenner, 1983a, b). Similar amyloid deposits occur in the brains of older Down syndrome (DS) patients (Malamud, 1972) and, to a much lesser degree, in association with the normal aging process. The first clue to the identity of amyloid was revealed when its principal constituent was isolated and proved to be a 4.2 kilodalton (kDa) polypeptide from which the amino acid sequence was obtained (Glenner and Wong, 1984a, b; Masters et al., 1985). Several groups subsequently were able to use this amino sequence information to isolate, by reverse genetics, cDNAs encoding the precursor of this protein (Goldgaber et al., 1987; Kang et al., 1987; Robakis et al., 1987; Tanzi et al., 1987a).

This isolation of the gene for the precursor of the Alzheimer's disease amyloid peptide has made it possible to begin dissecting at a molecular level the processes whereby this normal protein may become altered in Alzheimer's disease. The finding that the principal component of the pathological amyloid deposit is encoded by only a portion of the precursor suggested the possibility that amyloid deposits in Alzheimer's disease may result from either an abnormal expression or a posttranslational modification of a normal molecular constituent. This possibility was strengthened by the finding that the gene encoding the amyloid protein precursor (APP) is found on chromosome 21 (Goldgaber et al., 1987; Kang et al., 1987; Robakis et al., 1987; Tanzi et al., 1987a), and hence may be the cause of the amyloid deposits common to Down syndrome and Alzheimer's disease. Additional studies, however, revealed that the APP gene is distinct from the genetic defect on chromosome 21 responsible for familial Alzheimer's disease (Tanzi et al., 1987b; Van Broeckhoven et al., 1987) and that the APP gene is not duplicated in sporadic or familial Alzheimer's disease (Podlisney et al., 1987; St. George-Hyslop et al., 1987; Tanzi et al., 1987c).

These data provide strong evidence that the amyloid protein precursor gene is not the site of the defect that leads to the neurodegeneration characteristic of Alzheimer's disease, Down syndrome and to a lesser degree the normal aging process. However, this does not rule out the possibility that changes in the levels of APP RNA, and/or aberrant processing of the normal protein product may play a role in the progress of the disease. The sequence of events which leads to the deposition of the small self-aggregating amyloid peptide in Alzheimer's disease is not known. A key question concerns the causal relationship of amyloid to the pathology of the disease. In the following pages, we will describe our work in which we have begun dissecting at a molecular level the processes whereby the normal precursor of the amyloid polypeptide may become altered in Alzheimer's disease. Hypotheses regarding the role of amyloid precursor gene expression in the progress of Alzheimer's disease and Down syndrome, and the functional consequences of the molecular transformation which the amyloid precursor undergoes in these diseases, are presented.

Expression of the amyloid precursor gene transcripts

Characterization of additional APP mRNAs

We screened complementary cDNA libraries constructed from non-neural tissues to determine whether the messenger RNA encoding APP in these tissues is identical to that expressed in brain, and we identified a second APP mRNA (Tanzi et al., 1988; also reported by Kitaguchi et al., 1988; Ponte et al., 1988), that encodes an additional internal domain with a sequence characteristic of a Kunitz-type serine protease inhibitor (Fig. 1). Kitaguchi et al. (1988) showed that this new domain functions as an active trypsin inhibitor. They also found a third APP cDNA containing not only the protease inhibitor domain but also a further contiguous sequence of 19 amino acids that has

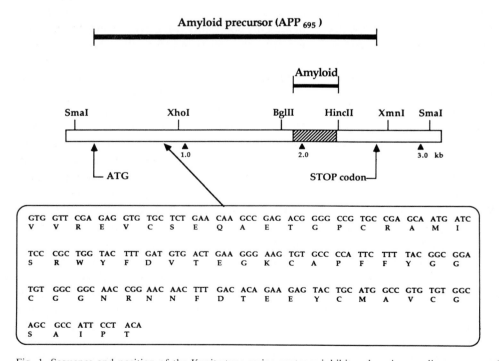

Fig. 1. Sequence and position of the Kunitz-type serine protease inhibitor domain-encoding segment of the APP-751 mRNA.

been noted by Weidemann et al. (1989) to show homology to the MRC OX-2 antigen (Clark et al., 1985). Genomic analysis suggests that the protease inhibitor domain as well as the 19 amino acid domain, arose from 2 extra exons within the APP gene, which are alternatively spliced to generate 3 mRNA species. These 3 mRNA species will hereafter be referred to as APP-695, APP-751 (containing the protease inhibitor domain), and APP-770 (containing the protease inhibitor and an additional 19 residues).

We utilized oligonucleotide probes specific for APP-695 and APP-751/770 to characterize the tissue specificity of their expression (Neve et al., 1988). The design of the oligonucleotide probes is shown in Fig. 2. The 40 base oligonucleotide specific for APP-695 encompasses 20 bases on either side of the potential splice junction sites in the APP-751/770 RNA, and therefore represents 40 contiguous bases in RNAs lacking the protease inhibitor domain. The 40 base oligonucleotide specific for APP-751/770 mRNAs is homologous to a relatively non-conserved portion of the nucleotide sequence encoding the protease inhibitor domain.

RNA blot analysis using these oligonucleotides revealed differences in the distribution of the RNAs in tissues. A survey of 12 fetal tissues showed that, while APP-751/770 is expressed in all

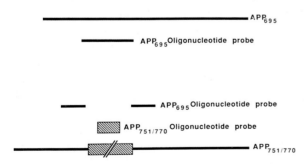

Fig. 2. Schematic diagram showing the design of APP RNA-specific oligonucleotide probes. The sequence of the APP-695 specific oligonucleotide is 5′CTGGCTGCTGTTGTAGGAAG-TCGAACCAGGTTTCCACAGA3′. The sequence of the APP-751/770 specific oligonucleotide is 5′CTTCCCTTCAGT-CACATCAAAGTACCAGCGGAGATCAT3′.

tissues examined, APP-695 is selectively expressed in nervous tissue. Hybridization of the APP-695 specific probe to cerebellum, brain and spinal cord, but not to meninges or other non-neural tissues was observed. Hybridizations with additional oligonucleotide probes differentiating between APP-751 and APP-770 indicated that both APP mRNAs are ubiquitously expressed, but that the abundance of APP-770 is several-fold lower than that of APP-751 in all tissues examined.

Expression of APP mRNAs in the human brain

Hybridization of an APP cDNA, which detects all APP mRNAs characterized thus far, to human fetal and adult human brain region RNAs (Fig. 3A, B) revealed striking developmental and regional patterns of expression. The APP cDNA hybridized intensely to RNA from most regions surveyed in a 19-week fetal brain. In the adult human brain, on the other hand, expression of APP RNAs showed a striking regional variation, exhibiting greatest abundance in associative regions of the neocortex, specifically in Brodmann areas A10, A20/21, A40 and A44. Use of oligonucleotide probes to distinguish the APP mRNAs showed that this regional variation was due to the expression of APP-695. The ubiquitously expressed APP-751/770 transcript was expressed homogeneously across brain regions (Tanzi et al., 1988). In contrast, APP-695 expression was highest in the association cortex (Neve et al., 1988). Notably, the contrast between APP-695 and APP-751/770 mRNA levels is greatest in the hippocampus, where the APP-695 transcript is almost undetectable by RNA blot analysis. Quantitative analysis revealed that the relative abundance of APP-695 RNA compared to APP-751/770 RNA in hippocampus, frontal cortex (A10) and inferior temporal cortex (A20) was 0.6, 1.4 and 1.2, respectively. The preferential increase in APP-695 mRNA in associative neocortex relative to primary sensory cortex is intriguing in that this regional variation parallels the regional distribution of neurofibrillary tangles found in visual cortices of Alzheimer's disease brains (Lewis et al., 1987).

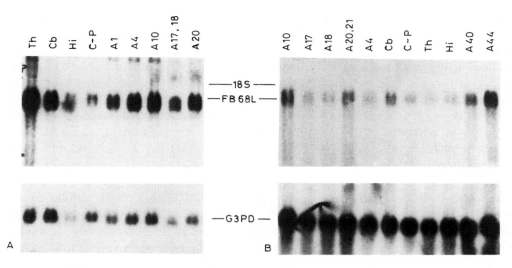

Fig. 3. RNA blot analysis of APP expression in human fetal and adult brain subregions. RNA was isolated, electrophoresed on agarose-formaldehyde gels, transferred to Biotrans membrane, and hybridized with labeled probe as described (Neve et al., 1986). *A*. Hybridization of the APP cDNA FB68L (Tanzi et al., 1987a) to 19-week fetal brain subregion RNAs. *B*. Hybridization of FB68L to adult brain subregion RNAs. Th, thalamus; Cb, cerebellum; Hi, hippocampus; C-P, caudate-putamen; A1, primary somatosensory area; A4, motor cortex; A10, frontal pole; A17/18, striate and extrastriate cortex; A20, temporal associative cortex; A40, posterior perisylvian cortex; A44, anterior perisylvian cortex. Each Northern blot was also hybridized with a cDNA for glyceraldehyde-3-phosphate dehydrogenase as a control (shown below FB68L hybridization).

Moreover, earlier studies have postulated a greater number of neuritic plaques and cerebrovascular amyloid deposits in association than in primary sensory areas (Mandybar, 1975; Morimatsu et al., 1975; Vinters and Gilbert, 1983).

In situ hybridization of the oligonucleotides to sections of adult human brain revealed a quantitative rather than a qualitative difference in their patterns of expression (Neve et al., 1988). Within the cortex, the overall pattern of hybridization for each probe reflected the laminar distribution of pyramidal neurons in the cortex, which varies among regions according to their cytoarchitecture. This pattern of distribution roughly parallels that of neocortical senile plaques (Pearson et al., 1985). APP-695 RNA levels were higher than those of APP-751/770, particularly in associative regions of the cortex, in agreement with the results of the RNA blot analyses. Both RNAs revealed an identical pattern of distribution in the hippocampus: RNA levels were high in the pyramidal cell layer of

Ammon's horn, and modest in the densely packed granule cells of the dentate gyrus.

APP gene expression in Down syndrome and Alzheimer's disease

In situ hybridization shows that all 3 APP mRNAs have a similar distribution in the normal aged human hippocampal formation and neocortex. Similarly, in situ hybridization shows that both APP-695 and APP-751/770 have similar regional and cellular patterns of distribution in brains from patients with Down syndrome and Alzheimer's disease. However, RNA blot analyses of a developmental series of Down syndrome brains reveal significant age-related changes in the relative expression of APP mRNAs in Down syndrome versus normal brain. A comparison of APP-695 and APP-751/770 expression in normal and Down syndrome fetal brain (Fig. 4A) revealed that, while the APP-695 transcript is expressed normally at higher levels than is APP-751/770 in

19-week fetal brain (as confirmed with in situ hybridization, Fig. 4*B*), both RNAs are increased several-fold relative to normal in 19-week Down syndrome fetal brain (DS/normal ratios: APP-695, 4.6-fold; APP-751/770, 3.8-fold). This result is particularly striking in light of the fact that APP expression is not increased more than 1.5-fold over normal in numerous non-neuronal DS tissues that were examined. Thus, several-fold amplification of APP mRNA expression in Down syndrome is confined to the brain.

Studies of regional expression of APP mRNAs in older Down syndrome brains reveal differential patterns of relative expression of the APP RNAs in DS brain compared to normal (Neve et al., 1988). In association areas of neocortex, levels of APP-695 mRNA appear to be decreased in aged Down syndrome brain compared to normal. This decrease is seen as early as 6 months postnatally

(G. Higgins and R. Neve, unpublished data), even though APP-695 is clearly overexpressed in DS fetal cortex compared to normal. In addition, in the hippocampal formation and caudate-putamen of aged Down syndrome brain, the abundance of APP-751/770 mRNA is markedly greater than that of APP-695 mRNA when compared to the normal adult or young Down syndrome brain (Higgins et al., 1988a). Fig. 5, which shows in situ hybridization of the oligonucleotide probes to Down syndrome adult hippocampus, illustrates this point. Detailed in situ hybridization studies of this region indicate that the increased levels of APP-751/770 mRNA seen in DS hippocampus on Northern blots are partly due to heightened levels of expression specifically in CA1 pyramidal cells of aged DS brains (G. Higgins and R. Neve, unpublished data). Moreover, the similarly increased APP-751/695 ratio in caudate observed on RNA blots is

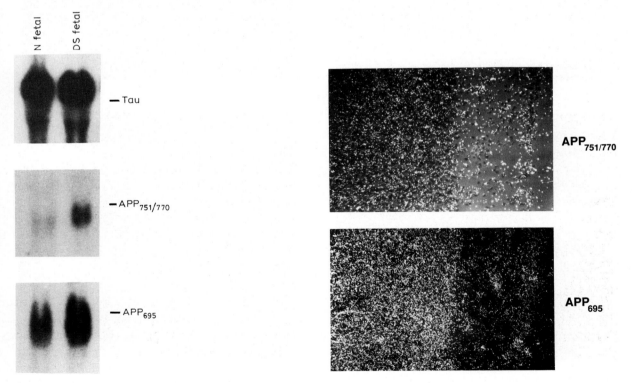

Fig. 4. Expression of APP RNAs in normal and Down syndrome fetal brain. *A*. RNA blot hybridization analysis. *B*. In situ hybridization of oligonucleotide probes specific for APP-695 and APP-751/770 to human 19 – 20 week temporal cortex. Details of the hybridization are described by Neve et al. (1988).

shown by in situ hybridization studies to be due to increased expression of APP-751/770 within the magnocellular neurons of the nucleus basalis of Meynert (G. Higgins and R. Neve, unpublished data).

Hybridizations of the APP-specific oligonucleotides to RNA from normal and AD cerebellum, a region relatively spared in Alzheimer's disease, show that both transcripts are present at approximately normal levels in AD cerebellum (Neve et al., 1988). However, in AD frontal cortex, which is severely affected by the disease, the level of APP-751/770 is near normal, while the APP-695 transcript appears to be selectively lost. Quantitative analyses revealed that the average ratio of APP-695 mRNA levels between normal and AD

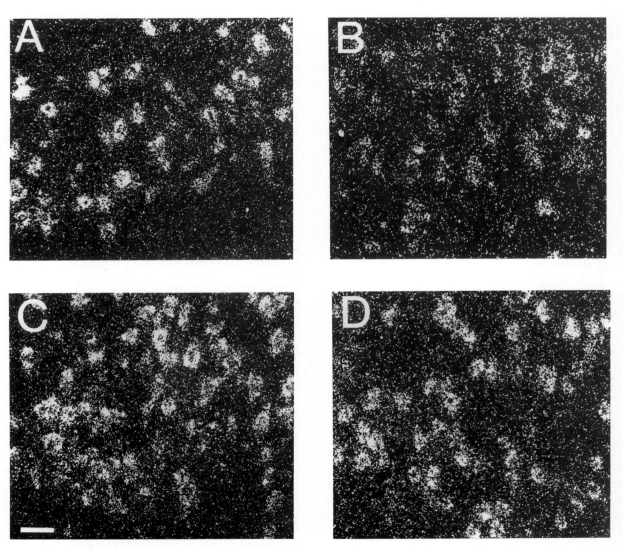

Fig. 5. In situ hybridization of (A, B) APP-695 and (C, D) APP-751/770 mRNAs in the hippocampal formation of a 40 year old male with Down syndrome. Darkfield photomicrographs with ^{35}S-labeled oligonucleotides show that the ratio of APP-751/770 to APP-695 mRNA is increased in (B, D) CA1 relative to (A, C) CA3 pyramidal neurons in this individual. Magnification bar = 100 μm.

cortex was 3.5; for APP-751/770 it was 1.5. The loss of APP-695 mRNA in AD neocortex may be due to death of the neurons that normally express the APP-695 transcript, or to decreased expression of this transcript in affected regions of the AD brain. In situ hybridization analyses suggest that the former explanation is primary. The level of APP-751/770 could appear relatively unaffected in AD if the cells expressing this transcript are spared, or if the transcript is overexpressed to the extent that, despite loss of cells expressing APP-751/770 RNA, a significant level of the message remains. In this case, in situ hybridization results indicate that the latter explanation seems to primarily account for the data.

Distribution of amyloid precursor protein in the brain

We used antibodies raised against portions of the APP to map its normal distribution in the human brain and to gain further insights into the events that lead to amyloid deposition. Antibodies raised against distinct domains of APP reacted with proteins having apparent molecular sizes of 65, 67 and 132 kDa on Western blots of human brain homogenates. An antibody directed against a region within the protease inhibitor domain showed an additional band just below the 65 kDa band that is presumably specific for APP-751.

Immunocytochemistry in sections through the normal human brain revealed punctate concentrations of the protein in pyramidal cells of the neocortex, particularly in associative regions, and intense staining in the CA1 pyramidal cells of the hippocampus. Fig. 6 shows that the staining has a discrete, vesicular appearance, with granules scattered throughout the soma up to the apical dendrite. An antibody to the carboxyterminal end of the APP molecule stained both cell bodies and the neuropil, whereas antibodies to the other domains of APP displayed staining primarily of the cell soma. The antibody directed against the APP-751/770 protease inhibitor domain showed astrocytic staining, consistent with the previous

finding that the mRNA for this form of APP is abundant in non-neural tissues (Neve et al., 1988; Tanzi et al., 1988).

By electron microscopy, the punctate distribution of APP coincided with dense concentrations of the protein in secondary lysosomes. In the hippocampus of Alzheimer's disease subjects, the density of anti-APP antibody staining in pyramidal cells of Sommer's sector (CA1) was markedly increased, and was marked by atrophy of many of these cells. Within these neurons, APP immunoreactivity appeared within enlarged intracellular organelles, which presumably reflect fused lysosomes. Even in one case with a clinical picture consistent with possible AD but no neuropathological findings, the abnormally dense deposition of APP and atrophy in CA1 pyramidal neurons were still seen.

Role of APP abundance in the disease process

Our immunohistochemical studies, which reveal an increase in density of APP in pyramidal cells of the CA1 region of the hippocampus in brains of subjects diagnosed as having AD, parallel the results of our RNA studies, which show an increase specifically of APP-751/770 RNA in this region. It is significant that these neurons are known to be at risk in AD, and the data raise the possibility that the dense concentration of APP in these neurons and in other affected areas may account for the accumulation of amyloid polypeptide in neuritic plaques. A shift in the level of one of the APP mRNAs, or of the ratio of the different forms, may play a role in the disease process. Two reports utilizing in situ hybridization with APP probes recognizing all 3 APP transcripts add additional evidence that differential APP mRNA expression does occur in AD hippocampus (Higgins et al., 1988b) and in AD nucleus basalis (Cohen et al., 1988) compared to normal. Higgins et al. (1988b) demonstrated that whereas neurons of the dentate gyrus and cornu Ammonis (CA) fields contain a 2.5-times greater APP hybridization signal than neurons of the subiculum and entorhinal cortex in

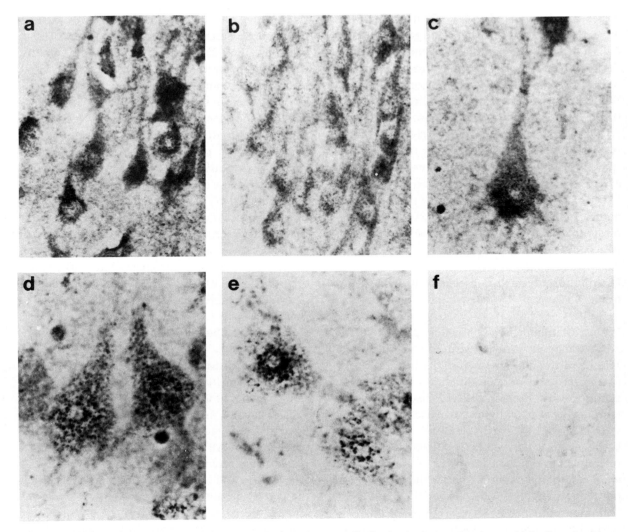

Fig. 6. The reaction product of the anti-APP antibody has a punctate distribution in the somata of pyramidal cells and a fainter, granular appearance in the background neuropil. (*a*) In the hippocampal complex, pyramidal cells of the CA1 region (Sommer's sector) show denser staining than CA3 pyramidal cells (*b*). In other parts of the cortex, immunoreactivity is likewise concentrated in intracellular organelles of pyramidal cells (a giant Betz cell from layer 5 of the motor cortex is shown in *c*; magnification for $a - c$ is × 400). At higher magnification, the punctate nature of the immunoreactivity within intracellular organelles is evident in the hippocampal Sommer's sector neuron shown in (*d*) and in the less densely stained pyramidal cell of the hilus shown in (*e*), in which these organelles are clustered around the nucleus. CA1 neurons stained with neutral serum show little specific staining (*f*). $d - f$ photographed at × 1000.

normal brain, the levels of APP RNA in CA3 (a region relatively unaffected in AD) and parasubiculum are equivalent in AD brain. This suggests that neurons of the subicular complex and entorhinal cortex, which are sensitive to the pathological consequences of AD (Hyman et al., 1986), may express elevated levels of APP in the disease. Cohen et al. (1988) reported that nucleus basalis neurons from AD patients consistently hybridized with more APP probe than those from controls. This increase in APP expression was proposed to be correlated with the severe neuronal degeneration in nucleus basalis of AD patients (Whitehouse et al., 1982). Careful in situ hybridization analysis of the level and pattern of expression of the APP transcripts in the associative cortex and subcortical regions of normal and affected brains may shed some light on the participation of the APP gene products in the process of neuronal degeneration in Alzheimer's disease, Down syndrome and normal aging.

Neurotoxicity of the carboxyterminus of the amyloid precursor

The sequence of events leading to the deposition of the small, pathological amyloid polypeptide derived from the normal precursor protein in Alzheimer's disease is not known, nor is it clear which of the precursors is implicated. A key question concerns the relationships of amyloid to the pathology of Alzheimer's disease. Is the generation of this polypeptide instrumental in causing the degeneration of nerve cells in the diseased or aged brain, or is it merely a final marker of cell death? As a first step in answering this question, we sought to create a situation in which neuronal cells were specifically expressing the amyloid polypeptide, or a portion of APP from which the amyloid peptide could easily be derived.

We designed 3 recombinant constructs containing different segments of APP-695 in the retroviral expression vector DO (Korman et al., 1987). The recombinant AS1 carried the entire APP-695 coding sequence, whereas the recombinants AB1 and AD1 both initiated just upstream of the methioning immediately preceding the amyloid peptide-encoding portion of the precursor. AB1 comprises the last 105 amino acids of APP, whereas AD1 terminates just downstream of the amyloid-encoding sequence. AB1 and AD1 were designed with the goal of creating transfectants that constitutively synthesized the pathological amyloid polypeptide without upstream sequences; AB1, unlike AD1, also carries the full carboxyterminus of APP.

These constructs were transfected into PC12 cells. Although all of the transfected PC12 cells were similar to controls while in the undifferentiated state, differences appeared when the cells were induced to differentiate into neuronal type cells with nerve growth factor (NGF). The AB1 transfectant, but not the other transfectants or non-transfected controls, degenerated upon exposure to NGF. Degeneration was greatest during the period in which maximal process outgrowth normally occurs, i.e., 5 – 8 days. Conditioned medium from AB1 transfectants caused death of neurons in primary cultures derived from embryonic rat hippocampus, whereas conditioned medium from controls and from the other transfectants had no effect on the neurons. We were able to immunoabsorb the neurotoxicity from the AB1 conditioned medium with an antibody directed against the first 15 amino acids of the amyloid peptide. These data suggest that the AB1 fragment of the amyloid precursor, containing the carboxyterminal 105 amino acids, is toxic.

It is intriguing that the neurotoxicity we see in culture results from the presence of a portion of the precursor that includes not only the amyloid polypeptide sequence but also all of the coding sequence carboxyterminal to it. The construct AD1, which includes little more than the amyloid polypeptide sequence alone, did not cause neurodegenerative effects when transfected into PC12 cells. The initial event in the generation of the amyloid peptide in Alzheimer's disease and Down syndrome may involve the formation of this approximately 100 amino acid intermediate from the precursor.

References

Clark, M.J., Gagnon, J., Williams, A.F. and Barclay, A.N. (1985) MRC OX-2 antigen: a lymphoid/neuronal glycoprotein with a structure like a single immunoglobulin light chain. *EMBO J.,* 4: 113 – 118.

Cohen, M.L., Golde, T.E., Usiak, M.F., Younkin, L.H. and Younkin, S.G. (1988) In situ hybridization of nucleus basalis neurons shows increased β-amyloid mRNA in Alzheimer

266

disease. *Proc. Natl. Acad. Sci. U.S.A.,* 85: 1227 – 1231.

Glenner, G. (1983a) Alzheimer's disease: the commonest form of amyloidosis. *Arch. Pathol. Lab. Med.,* 107: 281 – 282.

Glenner, G.G. (1983a) Alzheimer's disease: multiple cerebral amyloidosis. In: R. Katzman (Ed.), *Banbury Report 15: Biological Aspects of Alzheimer's Disease,* Cold Spring Harbor Laboratory, Cold Spring Harbor, NY, pp. 137 – 144.

Glenner, G.G. and Wong, C.W. (1984a) Alzheimer's disease: initial report of the purification and characterization of a novel cerebrovascular amyloid protein. *Biochem. Biophys. Res. Commun.,* 120: 885 – 890.

Glenner, G.G. and Wong, C.W. (1984b) Alzheimer's disease and Down's syndrome: sharing of a unique cerebrovascular amyloid protein. *Biochem. Biophys. Res. Commun.,* 122: 1131 – 1135.

Goldgaber, D., Lerman, M.I., McBride, W., Saffioti, U. and Gajdusek, D.C. (1987) Characterization and chromosomal localization of a cDNA encoding brain amyloid of Alzheimer's disease. *Science,* 235: 877 – 880.

Higgins, G.A., Dawes, L.R. and Neve, R.L. (1988a) Expression of amyloid-β-protein precursor (APP) mRNA transcripts in Down syndrome and Alzheimer's disease. *Soc. Neurosci. Abstr.,* 14: 637.

Higgins, G.A., Lewis, D.A., Bahmanyar, S., Goldgaber, D., Gajdusek, D.C., Young, W.G., Morrison, J.H. and Wilson, M.C. (1988b) Differential regulation of amyloid-β-protein mRNA expression within hippocampal neuronal subpopulations in Alzheimer disease. *Proc. Natl. Acad. Sci. U.S.A.,* 85: 1297 – 1301.

Hyman, B.T., Van Hoesen, G.W., Kromer, L.J. and Damasio, A.R. (1986) Perforant pathway changes and the memory impairment of Alzheimer's disease. *Ann. Neurol.,* 20: 472 – 481.

Kang, J., Lemaire, H.-G., Unterbeck, A., Salbaum, M.J., Masters, C.L., Grzeschik, K.H., Multhaup, G., Beyreuther, K. and Muller-Hill, B. (1987) The precursor of Alzheimer's disease amyloid A4 protein resembles a cell surface receptor. *Nature,* 325: 733 – 736.

Katzman, R. (Ed.) (1983) *Banbury Report 15: Biological Aspects of Alzheimer's Disease,* Cold Spring Harbor Laboratory, Cold Spring Harbor, NY.

Kitaguchi, N., Takahashi, Y., Tokushima, Y., Shiojiri, S. and Ito, H. (1988) Novel precursor of Alzheimer's disease amyloid A4 protein resembles a cell surface receptor. *Nature,* 331: 530 – 532.

Korman, A.J., Frantz, J.D., Strominger, R.C. and Mulligan, R.C. (1987) Expression of human class II major histocompatibility complex antigens using retrovirus vectors. *Proc. Natl. Acad. Sci. U.S.A.,* 84: 2150 – 2154.

Lewis, D.A., Campbell, M.J., Terry, R.D. and Morrison, J.H. (1987) Laminar and regional distributions of neurofibrillary tangles and neurites plaques in Alzheimer's disease: a quantitative study of visual and auditory cortices. *J. Neurosci.,* 7: 1799 – 1808.

Malamud, N. (1972) Neuropathology of organic brain syndromes associated with aging. In: C.M. Gaitz (Ed.), *Aging and the Brain,* 3rd ed., Plenum, New York, pp. 63 – 87.

Mandybar, T.I. (1975) The incidence of cerebral amyloid angiopathy in Alzheimer's disease. *Neurology,* 25: 120 – 126.

Masters, C.L., Simms, G., Weinman, N.A., Multhaup, G., McDonald, B.L. and Beyreuther, K. (1985) Amyloid plaque core protein in Alzheimer's disease and Down syndrome. *Proc. Natl. Acad. Sci. U.S.A.,* 82: 4245 – 4249.

Morimatsu, M. et al. (1975) Senile degenerative brain lesions and dementia. *J. Am. Geriatr. Soc.,* 23: 390 – 406.

Neve, R.L., Harris, P., Kosik, K.S., Kurnit, D.M. and Donlon T.D. (1986) Identification of cDNA clones for the human microtubule associated protein tau and chromosomal localization of the genes for tau and microtubule associated protein 2. *Mol. Brain Res.,* 1: 271 – 280.

Neve, R.L., Finch, E.A. and Dawes, L.R. (1988) Expression of the Alzheimer amyloid precursor gene transcripts in the human brain. *Neuron,* 1: 669 – 677.

Pearson, R.C.A., Esiri, M.M., Hiorns, R.W., Wilcock, G.K. and Powell, T.P.S. (1985) Anatomical correlates of the distribution of the pathological changes in the neocortex in Alzheimer's disease. *Proc. Natl. Acad. Sci. U.S.A.,* 82: 4531 – 4534.

Podlisney, M.B., Lee, G. and Selkow, D.J. (1987) Gene dosage of the amyloid beta precursor protein in Alzheimer's disease. *Science,* 238: 669 – 671.

Ponte, P., Gonzalez-DeWhitt, P., Schilling, J., Miller, J., Hsu, D., Greenberg, B., Davis, K., Wallace, W., Lieberburg, I., Fuller, F. and Cordell, B. (1988) A new A4 amyloid mRNA contains a domain homologous to serine protease inhibitors. *Nature,* 331: 525 – 527.

Robakis, N.K., Ramakrinshna, N., Wolfe, G. and Wisniewski, H.M. (1987) Molecular cloning and characterization of a cDNA encoding the cerebrovascular and the neurite plaque amyloid peptides. *Proc. Natl. Acad. Sci. U.S.A.,* 84: 4190 – 4194.

St. George-Hyslop, P.H., Tanzi, R.E., Polinkski, R.J., Neve, R.L., Pollen, D., Drachman, D., Growdon, J. Cupples, L.A., Nee, L., Myers, R.H., O'Sullivan, D., Watkins, P.C., Amos, J.A., Deutsch, C.K., Bodfish, J.W., Kinsbourne, M., Feldman, R.G., Bruni, A., Amaducci, L., Foncin, J.-F. and Gusella, J.F. (1987) Absence of duplication of chromosome 21 genes in familial and sporadic Alzheimer's disease. *Science,* 238: 664 – 666.

Tanzi, R.E., Gusella, J.F., Watkins, P.C., Bruns, G.A.P., St. George-Hyslop, P., Van Keuren, M.L., Patterson, D.D., Pagan, S., Kurnit, D.M. and Neve, R.L. (1987a) Amyloid beta-protein gene: cDNA, mRNA distribution and genetic linkage near the Alzheimer locus. *Science,* 235: 880 – 884.

Tanzi, R.E., St. George-Hyslop, P.H., Haines, J.L., Polinsky, R.J., Nee, L., Foncin, J.-F., Neve, R.L., McClatchey, A.I., Conneally, P.M. and Gusella, J.F. (1987b) The genetic defect in familial Alzheimer's disease is not tightly linked to the amyloid beta protein gene. *Nature,* 329: 156 – 157.

Tanzi, R.E., Bird, E.D., Latt, S.A. and Neve, R.L. (1987c) The amyloid beta protein is not duplicated in brains from patients with Alzheimer's disease. *Science,* 238: 666 – 669.

Tanzi, R.E., McClatchey, A.I., Lamperti, E.D., Villa-Komaroff, L., Gusella, J.F. and Neve, R.L. (1988) Protease inhibitor domain encoded by an amyloid protein precursor mRNA associated with Alzheimer's disease. *Nature,* 331: 528 – 530.

Terry, R.D., Peck, A., DeTeresa, R., Schechter, R. and Horoupian, D.S. (1981) Some morphometric aspects of the brain in senile dementia of the Alzheimer type. *Ann. Neurol.,* 10: 184 – 192.

Van Broeckhoven C., Genthe, A.M., Vandeberghe, A., Horsthemke, B., Backhovens, H., Raeymaekers, P., Van Hul, W., Wehnert, A., Gheuens, J., Gras, P., Bruyland, M.,

Martin, J.J. and Salbaum, M. (1987) Failure of familial Alzheimer's disease to segregate with the A4-amyloid gene in several European families. *Nature,* 329: 153 – 155.

Vinters, H.V. and Gilbert, J.J. (1983) Cerebral amyloid angiopathy: incidence and complications in the aging brain. II. The distribution of amyloid vascular changes. *Stroke,* 14: 924 – 928.

Weidemann, A., König, G., Bunke, D., Fischer, P., Salbaum, J.M., Masters, C.L. and Beyreuther, K. (1989) Identification, biogenesis, and localization of precursors of Alzheimer's disease A4 amyloid protein. *Cell,* 57: 115 – 126.

Whitehouse, P.J., Price, D.L., Struble, R.G., Clark, A.W., Coyle, J.T. and DeLong, M.R. (1982) Alzheimer's disease and senile dementia: loss of neurons in the basal forebrain. *Science,* 215: 1237 – 1239.

P. Coleman, G. Higgins and C. Phelps (Eds.)
Progress in Brain Research, Vol. 86
© 1990 Elsevier Science Publishers B.V. (Biomedical Division)

CHAPTER 22

Receptor-effector coupling by G-proteins: implications for neuronal plasticity

Allen M. Spiegel

Molecular Pathophysiology Branch, National Institute of Diabetes, Digestive and Kidney Diseases, National Institutes of Health, Bethesda, MD 20892, U.S.A.

G-proteins: general features of structure and function

G-proteins involved in signal transduction are members of a guanine nucleotide-binding protein superfamily that includes cytoskeletal proteins such as tubulin, soluble proteins (initiation and elongation factors involved in protein synthesis), and low molecular weight GTP-binding proteins such as the *ras* p21 protooncogenes and *ras*-related proteins (Gilman, 1987; Iyengar and Birnbaumer, 1987; Spiegel, 1987). Members of the G-protein subset of the GTP-binding protein superfamily share certain general features in common with other members of the GTP-binding protein superfamily: (1) all GTP-binding proteins bind guanine nucleotides with high affinity and specificity, and possess intrinsic GTPase activity that modulates interactions between the GTP-binding protein and other elements; and (2) GTP-binding proteins serve as substrates for ADP-ribosylation by bacterial toxins; this covalent modification disrupts normal function.

G-proteins share other features that distinguish them from other GTP-binding proteins. These features include: (1) association with the cytoplasmic surface of the plasma membrane (*ras* p21 and some other low molecular weight GTP-binding proteins are also associated with the cytoplasmic membrane surface); (2) function as

receptor-effector couplers; and (3) heterotrimeric structure (see Fig. 1). G-proteins contain α, β, and γ subunits, each distinct gene products. The latter two subunits are tightly, but non-covalently linked in a $\beta\gamma$ complex. α Subunits bind guanine nucleotide, serve as toxin substrates, confer specificity in receptor-effector coupling, and directly modulate effector activity. Upon activation by GTP, α subunits are thought to dissociate from the $\beta\gamma$ complex (see Fig. 2). The latter is required for G-protein receptor interaction, can inhibit G-protein activation by blocking α subunit dissociation, and may in some cases directly regulate effector activity.

Receptors coupled to G-proteins share a common overall topographic structure (Fig. 1). Hydrophobicity plots of the amino acid sequences predicted by cDNAs encoding G-protein-coupled receptors suggest that a "generic" receptor consists of a single polypeptide chain that spans the plasma membrane 7 times (O'Dowd et al., 1989). The amino-terminus, containing sites for N-linked glycosylation and three loops are located extracellularly, whereas the carboxy-terminus and three other loops are cytoplasmically oriented. The latter are presumably involved in coupling to G-protein. The ligand binding site (at least for monoamines) has been localized to the putative transmembrane domains. Examples of receptors whose sequences conform to this general pattern

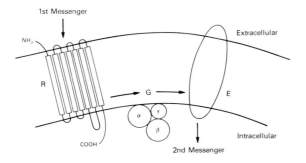

Fig. 1. Schematic diagram of generic G-protein-coupled receptor and effector. Extracellular "first messengers" interact with specific receptors (R) that are transmembrane glycoproteins. The receptor's putative 7 membrane-spanning domains, extracellular amino-terminus and 3 loops, and intracellular 3 loops plus carboxy-terminus are indicated. Activation of receptor by first messenger leads to interaction with, and activation of, the heterotrimeric G-protein (G) associated with the cytoplasmic surface of the membrane. The G-protein in turn interacts with, and regulates, an effector (E) that generates an intracellular signal. Effectors may be transmembrane glycoproteins (e.g., adenylyl cyclase).

include: (a) photon receptors such as rhodopsin and the cone opsins; (b) monoamine neurotransmitter receptors such as α and β-adrenergic, dopaminergic, muscarinic cholinergic and serotoninergic; and (c) peptide neurotransmitter receptors such as substance K.

Effectors regulated by G-proteins include enzymes of second messenger metabolism and ion channels. Some of these are clearly transmembrane proteins (e.g., adenylyl cyclase), but others (e.g., cGMP phosphodiesterase) are peripheral membrane proteins, and for others the structure has yet to be elucidated.

Specific features of G-protein structure and function

Molecular cloning provides evidence for a minimum of nine distinct α subunit genes, including G_s, G_o, G_{i1}, G_{i2}, G_{i3}, G_{t1}, G_{t2} (Gilman, 1987; Iyengar and Birnbaumer, 1987; Spiegel, 1987), G_{olf} (Jones and Reed, 1989), and $G_{x(z)}$ (Fong et al., 1988; Lochrie and Simon, 1988; Mat-

suoka et al., 1988). Further diversity is created by alternative splicing leading to the expression of 4 forms of G_s (Bray et al., 1986). At least 2 distinct genes each exist for both β and γ subunits. The expression of certain α subunits is highly restricted, e.g., G_{t1} and G_{t2} are found in photoreceptor rod and cone cells, respectively, and G_{olf} only in olfactory neuroepithelium, whereas others such as G_s and G_{i2} are expressed ubiquitously. In brain, G_o (comprising about 1% of total membrane protein) and G_{i1} are the most abundant G-proteins (Gierschik et al., 1986). G_{i2} is particularly abun-

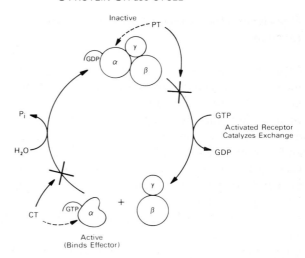

Fig. 2. The G-protein GTPase cycle. The α subunits of G-proteins in their basal (inactive) state contain tightly bound GDP, and are associated with the $\beta\gamma$ complex. Interaction with an activated receptor catalyzes exchange of bound GDP for ambient GTP. Binding of GTP leads to dissociation of G-protein from receptor, and of α subunit from $\beta\gamma$. GTP-bound α interacts with and regulates the effector. Whether the $\beta\gamma$ complex also directly regulates certain effector activities is not clear. The intrinsic GTPase activity of the α subunit leads to hydrolysis of bound GTP to GDP. This "turns off" the α subunit; the latter dissociates from effector and reassociates with $\beta\gamma$ to reenter the GTPase cycle. Bacterial toxins transfer ADP-ribose from NAD to G-protein α subunits. Pertussis toxin (PT) leads to uncoupling of its G-protein substrates from receptors. This blocks signal transduction by preventing exchange of GTP for GDP. Cholera toxin (CT) acts on G_s to reduce its intrinsic rate of GTPase activity. This causes more long-lived G-protein (and thereby, effector) activation.

dant in glial cells. G_{i3}, in contrast, is present at very low concentration in brain, but has been localized by immunohistochemistry to discrete regions such as the substantia nigra and the hippocampus (Cortes et al., 1988). In situ hybridization performed with specific probes for G-protein α subunits shows a widespread distribution for G_s and G_{i2}, but more discrete localization for G_o and G_{i1} (see Brann et al., 1987, for detailed description). G_z, by mRNA hybridization studies, is preferentially expressed in brain; the protein itself has not yet been visualized.

Immunohistochemistry of retina performed with specific antibodies against α subunits of G_o and rod G_t, and against the common β subunit illustrates the discrete localization of specific G-proteins (Fig. 3). G_t is found exclusively in the rod photoreceptor layer, whereas G_o is found in the inner and outer plexiform layers and the ganglion cell layer (Lad et al., 1987). The β subunit, as expected, colocalizes with each of the α subunits. At the ultrastructural level, G_o has been found to be associated with the cytoplasmic face of the plasma membrane lining cell bodies and neurites but not at synapses (Gabrion et al., 1989). Additional immunoreactivity was noted in vesicular structures

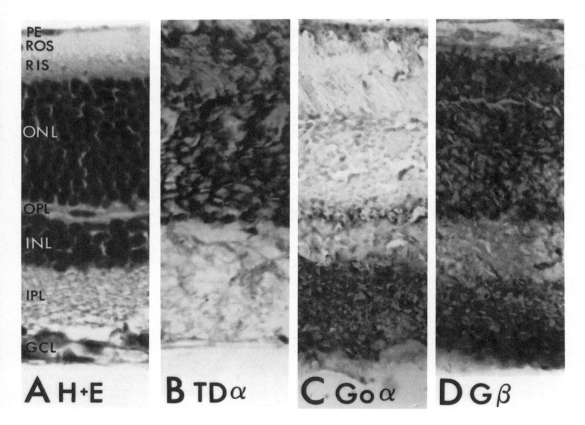

Fig. 3. *A*. Hematoxylin and eosin (H + E) stained section of rat retina; laminae from top (outer surface) to bottom (inner surface) are: pigment epithelium (PE); receptor cell layers: outer segments (ROS), inner segments (RIS), and outer nuclear layer (ONL); outer plexiform layer (OPL), location of synaptic contacts between photoreceptor cells and bipolar cells; inner nuclear layer (INL), location of bipolar cell bodies; inner plexiform layer (IPL), location of synaptic contacts between bipolar cells and ganglion cells; and ganglion cell layer (GCL). *B*. Section stained for G_t (TD)-α immunoreactivity. Labeling is evident throughout the photoreceptor layers. *C*. Section stained for G_o-α immunoreactivity. Labeling primarily in OPL, IPL and GCL. *D*. Section stained for G-β immunoreactivity. The pattern of labeling is the sum of that for G_t and G_o α subunits. (From Lad et al., 1987.)

within the cytoplasm.

The specificity of G-protein interactions with receptors and effectors has been defined in very few cases (see Table I). Studies involving reconstitution of purified receptors and G-proteins in phospholipid vesicles showed that β-adrenergic receptors couple, in decreasing order of efficiency, to $G_s > G_i >> G_t$, and that for rhodopsin, the selectivity of coupling is $G_t = G_i >> G_s$ (Cerione et al., 1985). Similar studies involving G-protein effector interaction indicated that only G_s can activate adenylyl cyclase (G_s also appears to stimulate another effector, a Ca^{2+} channel), and that G_t uniquely activates retinal cGMP phosphodiesterase (see Roof et al., 1985, for example). The endogenous G-proteins coupled to most other receptors and effectors, however, remain to be identified. Many G-protein-coupled receptors (D_2-dopaminergic for example; Senogles et al., 1987), and a variety of effectors, including adenylyl cyclase (inhibition), certain Ca^{2+} (inhibition) and K^+ (stimulation) channels, and phospholipase C in cell types such as neutrophils (e.g., f-Met-Leu-Phe receptor) are regulated by one or more pertussis toxin-sensitive G-proteins (Gilman, 1987; Iyengar and Birnbaumer, 1987; Spiegel, 1987). Since, not only both forms of G_t,

but also G_{i1}, G_{i2}, G_{i3}, and G_o are pertussis toxin-sensitive G-proteins, demonstration of an effect of pertussis toxin on receptor or effector regulation does not uniquely identify the relevant endogenous G-protein. In most cells, phospholipase C is regulated by a pertussis toxin-insensitive G-protein. $G_{z(x)}$ may play this role, but definitive evidence is lacking. Phospholipase A_2 activity may also be regulated by one or more G-proteins, perhaps by the $\beta\gamma$ complex. The latter has also been suggested to stimulate a K^+ channel, but recent evidence suggests this is an indirect effect (Kim et al., 1989).

The primary sequences of G-protein α and β subunits have been highly conserved during evolution. Among mammalian species, amino acid sequence is > 95% identical. Conservation among vertebrates, and even invertebrates such as *Drosophila* (M. Forte, personal communication), is > 80%. This high degree of conservation of structure accounts for cross-reactivity of antibodies raised against mammalian G-proteins with other vertebrate (see Fig. 4) and invertebrate G-proteins. Within a given species, α subunit subtypes may differ only slightly in sequence, e.g., human G_{i1} and G_{i2} are 88% identical. Yet even these slight differences between subtypes are con-

TABLE I

Receptor-effector coupling by G-proteins

Receptors	G-proteins	Effectors
Opsins	G_t-rod, G_t-cone	cGMP-PDE
Odorant (?)	G_{olf}	A. cyclase (stim.)
β-adrenergic	G_s	A. cyclase (stim.)
		Ca^{2+} channel (stim.)
α_2-adrenergic	G_{i1}*, G_{i2}*, G_{i3}*, G_o*	A. cyclase (inhib.)*
M_2 muscarinic		Ca^{2+} channel (inhib.)*
		K^+ channel (stim.)*
f-Met-Leu-Phe		PLC (stim.)*
α_1-adrenergic	?	PLC (stim.)
M_1 muscarinic		
?	$G_{z(x)}$	?
?	?	PLA_2 (stim.)**

* pertussis toxin-sensitive. **Direct modulation by $\beta\gamma$ (?).

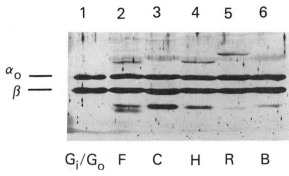

α_o ——
β ——

G_i/G_o F   C   H   R   B

Fig. 4. Immunoblot of brain membranes from several vertebrate species with a 1 : 100 dilution of crude antiserum RV/3 raised against purified bovine brain G_i/G_o. Lane *1*: 1 μg purified bovine brain G_i/G_o. Lanes *2 – 6*: membranes (150 μg/lane) from whole frog brain (F), from chicken forebrain (C), and from human (H), rat (R) and bovine (B) cerebral cortex. The positions of immunoreactive G_o-α and β subunits are indicated. Unique patterns of non-specific bands are also evident in each lane. (From Gierschik et al., 1986.)

served in different species, e.g., bovine G_{i1} is identical to human G_{i1}, rat and mouse G_{i2} more closely resemble human G_{i2} than does human G_{i1}. This evolutionary conservation strongly suggests, but does not prove, that different G-protein subtypes may not be merely "isotypes" with identical function, but rather that each may subserve distinct functions.

Molecular biologic approaches should help clarify the specificity of receptor-effector coupling by G-proteins. For example, recombinant proteins expressed in *E. coli* corresponding to all three forms of G_i-α (but not G_o) proved capable of stimulating a cardiac K$^+$ channel (Yatani et al., 1988). Immunochemical techniques, particularly antisera raised against synthetic peptides corresponding to predicted sequences of G-protein subunits (Goldsmith et al., 1987, 1988a, b), have also been helpful in identifying and localizing G-protein subtypes. Antisera directed against the C-terminal decapeptide of G-protein α subunits, a region known to be involved in receptor interaction (West et al., 1985; Sullivan et al., 1987), have been shown to recognize native G-proteins and to block receptor, but not effector, interaction (Cerione et al., 1988).

Altered signal transduction due to changes in receptor-effector coupling by G-proteins

Increased understanding at the molecular level of mechanisms of signal transduction has led to the appreciation that cellular response to external signals is modulated not merely by quantitative changes in the extracellular "first messengers," but also by quantitative and qualitative changes in the transduction apparatus. Substantial evidence exists for modulation of G-protein-coupled receptors (O'Dowd et al., 1989). Although a detailed description of receptor alterations is beyond the scope of this chapter, one aspect deserves mention here.

Desensitization is a general term applied to reduced cellular response to continued presence of agonist. In one form, termed homologous, response is diminished only to the specific agonist added, and not to other agonists that bind to distinct receptors. This implies a receptor-specific alteration. Recent evidence (O'Dowd et al., 1989) indicates that a specific enzyme (termed β-adrenergic receptor kinase although it will modify many receptor types) specifically phosphorylates the agonist-bound form of the receptor. In a reaction analogous to that catalyzed by rhodopsin kinase, cytoplasmic domains of the receptor are phosphorylated with resultant reduction in ability to couple to G-protein. This mechanism may well account for the homologous form of desensitization.

In heterologous desensitization, the presence of a given agonist leads to reduced response to multiple agonists that bind to distinct receptors. This may involve a change distal to the receptor itself, e.g., at a point of convergence of input from multiple receptors such as the G-protein. Covalent modifications of G-proteins are known to occur (Gilman, 1987; Spiegel, 1987); as mentioned earlier, bacterial toxins catalyze ADP-ribosylation of α subunits with important functional consequences. Also, phosphorylation of α subunits has been demonstrated in vitro, but the physiologic relevance of these modifications is not clear.

Quantitative changes in G-proteins may account for some aspects of heterologous desensitization. Adipocytes from rats infused with an adenosine analog show reduced response not only to A_1 adenosine agonists, but also to PGE_1 (Parsons and Stiles, 1987). Decreased G_i- and increased G_s-α subunits were found in adipocyte membranes from "desensitized" rats. Chronic treatment of cultured neuronal cells with agents that inhibit cAMP formation, e.g., morphine, leads to adenylyl cyclase "supersensitivity." This change may result from reciprocal changes in G_s and G_i, as noted for adipocytes from adenosine-infused rats, and may represent a general cellular adaptation to "inhibitory" agonists. Such changes could account for increased enzyme response after drug withdrawal, and as such could account for some aspects of addiction (Thomas and Hoffman, 1987). In at least one study, however, chronic morphine treatment of rats led to increased pertussis toxin substrate (G_o?) in the locus coeruleus (Nestler et al., 1989).

Genetic changes in G-proteins can profoundly alter signal transduction. Mutants of the S49 mouse lymphoma cell line may be totally lacking α_s or may contain single amino acid substitutions (Sullivan et al., 1987). The resultant phenotype is completely resistant to agonists for receptors coupled to G_s. A human genetic disorder termed pseudohypoparathyroidism (PHP) was initially described as resistance to parathyroid hormone. In one form, PHP type Ia, affected subjects are in fact resistant to multiple agonists that act by stimulating cAMP formation. In addition, such individuals show characteristic constitutional features including short stature, obesity, and mild mental retardation. An approximate 50% reduction in α_s protein and mRNA (Carter et al., 1987) may be the basis for target organ resistance (and mental dysfunction) in PHP Ia. So-called learning mutants in *Drosophila* have been shown to involve transduction components including enzymes of cAMP formation and degradation, adenylyl cyclase and cAMP phosphodiesterase, respectively. With the cloning of cDNAs encoding *Drosophila* G-protein subunits (M. Forte, personal communication), powerful genetic studies on the function of these proteins should be feasible.

Normal differentiation and development are also associated with important changes in G-proteins. A major increase in the amount of G_o in brain occurs postnatally in rats (Milligan et al., 1987; Asano et al., 1988). Differentiation of NG108-15 neuroblastoma X glioma hybrid cells in culture is accompanied by morphologic changes (neuritic extension) as well as a significant increase in G_o but not G_i (Mullaney and Milligan, 1989). Increased G_o may account for acquisition of response of certain ion channels to opiate agonists.

G-proteins may also represent an important site of action for various drugs. A report that lithium acts by uncoupling G-proteins from receptors (Avissar et al., 1988) requires confirmation. Chronic ethanol has been reported to cause a form of heterologous desensitization. This may be due to reduction in α_s mRNA and protein (Mochly-Rosen et al., 1988). Hormones that act by mechanisms not directly linked to G-proteins may nonetheless indirectly affect G-protein function. Steroids such as glucocorticoids are known to exert "permissive" effects on other agents such as β-adrenergic catecholamines. Recent studies suggest that glucocorticoids may regulate G_s (increased) and G_i (decreased) α subunit mRNA expression in rat brain (Saito et al., 1989).

Other studies, some preliminary, suggest that G-proteins could be the site of defects in neuropsychiatric disease and senescence. Chronic membrane depolarization (with veratridine) of cultured neuroblastoma cells led to increased levels of G_o (Luetje and Nathanson, 1988). Also, a pertussis toxin-sensitive G-protein has been implicated in long-term potentiation in the hippocampus (Goh and Pennefather, 1989). These studies raise the possibility that altered G-proteins could underly changes in neuronal function that occur with aging. Studies on peripheral cells, primarily leukocytes, suggest that age-related reduction in β-adrenergic responsiveness in man may be due to a defect in coupling of receptor to effector

(Feldman, 1986). In contrast, enhanced adenylyl cyclase stimulation by D_1 dopaminergic agonist in homogenates of caudate nucleus from schizophrenic subjects was attributed to increased receptor-effector coupling (Memo et al., 1983). The dramatic increase in our understanding of the molecular mechanisms of receptor-effector coupling by G-proteins should allow direct evaluation of these and other observations on the relevance of G-proteins to normal and abnormal neuronal function and plasticity.

References

Asano, T., Kamiya, N., Semba, R. and Kato, K. (1988) Ontogeny of the GTP-binding protein G_o in rat brain and heart. *J. Neurochem.*, 51: 1711–1716.

Avissar, S., Schreiber, G., Danon, A. and Belmaker, R.H. (1988) Lithium inhibits adrenergic and cholinergic increases in GTP binding in rat cortex. *Nature*, 331: 440–442.

Brann, M.R., Collins, R.M. and Spiegel, A. (1987) Localization of mRNAs encoding the α-subunits of signal-transducing G-proteins within rat brain and among peripheral tissues. *FEBS Lett.*, 222: 191–198.

Bray, P., Carter, A., Simons, C., Guo, V., Puckett, C., Kamholz, J., Spiegel, A. and Nirenberg, M. (1986) Human cDNA clones for four species of G-α_s signal transduction protein. *Proc. Natl. Acad. Sci. U.S.A.*, 83: 8893–8897.

Carter, A., Bardin, C., Collins, R., Simons, C., Bray, P. and Spiegel, A. (1987) Reduced expression of multiple forms of the α subunit of the stimulatory GTP-binding protein in pseudohypoparathyroidism type Ia. *Proc. Natl. Acad. Sci. U.S.A.*, 84: 7266–7269.

Cerione, R.A., Staniszewski, C., Benovic, J.L., Lefkowitz, R.J., Caron, M.G., Gierschik, P., Somers, R., Spiegel, A.M., Codina, J. and Birnbaumer, L. (1985) Specificity of the functional interactions of the β-adrenergic receptor and rhodopsin with guanine nucleotide regulatory proteins reconstituted in phospholipid vesicles. *J. Biol. Chem.*, 260: 1493–1500.

Cerione, R.A., Spencer, K., Rajaram, R., Unson, C., Goldsmith, P. and Spiegel, A. (1988) An antibody directed against the carboxyl-terminal decapeptide of the α subunit of the retinal GTP-binding protein, transducin. *J. Biol. Chem.*, 263: 9345–9352.

Cortes, R., Hofkelt, T., Schalling, M., Goldstein, M., Goldsmith, P., Spiegel, A., Unson, C. and Walsh, J. (1988) Antiserum raised against residues 159–168 of the guanine nucleotide-binding protein G_{i3}-α reacts with ependymal cells and some neurons in the rat brain containing cholecystokinin- or cholecystokinin- and tyrosine 3-

hydroxylase-like immunoreactivities. *Proc. Natl. Acad. Sci. U.S.A.*, 85: 9351–9355.

Feldman, R.D. (1986) Physiological and molecular correlates of age-related changes in the human β-adrenergic receptor system. *Fed. Proc.*, 45: 48–50.

Fong, H.K.W., Yoshimoto, K.K., Eversole-Cire, P. and Simon, M.I. (1988) Identification of a GTP-binding protein α subunit that lacks an apparent ADP-ribosylation site for pertussis toxin. *Proc. Natl. Acad. Sci. U.S.A.*, 85: 3066–3070.

Gabrion, J., Brabet, P., Nguyen Than Dao, B., Homburger, V., Dumuis, A., Sebben, M., Rouot, B. and Bockaert, J. (1989) Ultrastructural localization of the GTP-binding protein G_o in neurons. *Cell. Signal.*, 1: 107–123.

Gierschik, P., Milligan, G., Pines, M., Goldsmith, P., Codina, J., Werner, K. and Spiegel, A. (1986) Use of specific antibodies to quantitate the guanine nucleotide-binding protein G_o in brain. *Proc. Natl. Acad. Sci.U.S.A.*, 83: 2258–2262.

Gilman, A. (1987) G proteins: transducers of receptor-generated signals. *Annu. Rev. Biochem.*, 56: 615–549.

Goh, J.W. and Pennefather, P.S. (1989) A pertussis toxin-sensitive G protein in hippocampal long-term potentiation. *Science* 244: 980–983.

Goldsmith, P., Gierschik, P., Milligan, G., Unson, C.G., Vinitsky, R., Malech, H. and Spiegel, A. (1987) Antibodies directed against synthetic peptides distinguish between GTP-binding proteins in neutrophil and brain. *J. Biol. Chem.*, 262: 14683–14688.

Goldsmith, P., Backlund, P.S., Jr., Rossiter, K., Carter, A., Milligan, G., Unson, C.G. and Spiegel, A. (1988a) Purification of heterotrimeric GTP-binding proteins from brain: identification of a novel form of G_o. *Biochemistry*, 27: 7085–7090.

Goldsmith, P., Rossiter, K., Carter, A., Simonds, W., Unson, C.G., Vinitsky, R. and Spiegel, A. (1988b) Identification of the GTP-binding protein encoded by G_{i3} complementary DNA. *J. Biol. Chem.*, 263: 6476–6479.

Iyengar, R. and Birnbaumer, L. (1987) Signal transduction by G-proteins. In: *ISI Atlas of Science: Pharmacology*, 1: 213–221.

Jones, D.T. and Reed, R.R. (1989) G_{olf}: an olfactory neuron specific-G protein involved in odorant signal transduction. *Science*, 244: 790–795.

Kim, D., Lewis, D.L., Graziadei, L., Neer, E.J., Bar-Sagi, D. and Clapham, D.E. (1989) G-protein $\beta\gamma$-subunits activate the cardiac muscarinic K^+-channel via phospholipase A_2. *Nature*, 337: 557–560.

Lad, R.P., Simons, C., Gierschik, P., Milligan, G., Woodard, C., Griffo, M., Goldsmith, P., Ornberg, R., Gerfen, C.R. and Spiegel, A. (1987) Differential distribution of signal-transducing G-proteins in retina. *Brain Res.*, 423: 237–246.

Lochrie, M.A. and Simon, M.I. (1988) G protein multiplicity in eukaryotic signal transduction systems. *Biochemistry*, 27: 4957–4965.

Luetje, C.W. and Nathanson, N.M. (1988) Chronic membrane depolarization regulates the level of the guanine nucleotide binding protein $G_o\alpha$ in cultured neuronal cells. *J. Neurochem.,* 50: 1775 – 1782.

Matsuoka, M., Itoh, H., Tohru, K. and Kaziro,Y. (1988) Sequence analysis of cDNA and genomic DNA for a putative pertussis toxin-insensitive guanine nucleotide-binding regulatory protein α subunit. *Proc. Natl. Acad. Sci. U.S.A.,* 85: 5384 – 5388.

Memo, M., Kleinman, J.E. and Hanbauer, I. (1983) Coupling of dopamine D_1 recognition sites with adenylate cyclase in nuclei accumbens and caudatus of schizophrenics. *Science,* 221: 1304 – 1307.

Milligan, G., Streaty, R.A., Gierschik, P., Spiegel, A.M. and Klee, W.A. (1987) Development of opiate receptors and GTP-binding regulatory proteins in neonatal rat brain. *J. Biol. Chem.,* 262: 8626 – 8630.

Mochly-Rosen, D., Chang, F., Cheever, L., Kim, M., Diamond, I. and Gordon, A.S. (1988) Chronic ethanol causes heterologous desensitization of receptors by reducing α_s messenger RNA. *Nature,* 333: 848 – 850.

Mullaney, I. and Milligan, G. (1989) Elevated levels of the guanine nucleotide binding protein, G_o, are associated with differentiation of neuroblastoma X glioma hybrid cells. *FEBS Lett.,* 244: 113 – 118.

Nestler, E.J., Erdos, J.J., Terwilliger, R., Duman, R.S. and Tallman, J.F. (1989) Regulation of G-proteins by chronic morphine in the rat locus coeruleus. *Brain Res.,* 476: 230 – 239.

O'Dowd, B.F., Lefkowitz, R.J. and Caron, M.G. (1989) Structure of the adrenergic and related receptors. *Annu. Rev. Neurosci.,* 12: 67 – 83.

Parson, W.J. and Stiles, G.L. (1987) Heterologous desensitization of the inhibitory A_1 adenosine receptor-adenylate cyclase system in rat adipocytes. *J. Biol. Chem.,* 262: 841 – 847.

Roof, D.J., Applebury, M.L. and Sternweis, P.C. (1985) Relationships within the family of GTP-binding proteins isolated from bovine central nervous system. *J. Biol. Chem.,* 260: 16242 – 16249.

Saito, N., Guitart, X., Hayward, M., Tallman, J.F., Duman, R.S. and Nestler, E.J. (1989) Corticosterone differentially regulates the expression of $G_{s\alpha}$ and $G_{i\alpha}$ messenger RNA and protein in rat cerebral cortex. *Proc. Natl. Acad. Sci. U.S.A.,* 86: 3906 – 3910.

Senogles, S.E., Benovic, J.L., Amlaiky, N., Unson, C., Milligan, G., Vinitsky, R., Spiegel, A.M. and Caron, M.G. (1987) The D_2-dopamine receptor of anterior pituitary is functionally associated with a pertussis toxin-sensitive guanine nucleotide binding protein. *J. Biol. Chem.,* 262: 4860 – 4867.

Spiegel, A. (1987) Signal transduction by guanine nucleotide binding proteins. *Mol. Cell. Endocrinol.,* 49: 1 – 16.

Sullivan, K.A., Miller, R.T., Masters, S.B., Beiderman, B., Heideman, W. and Bourne, H.R. (1987) Identification of receptor contact site involved in receptor-G protein coupling. *Nature,* 330: 758 – 760.

Thomas, J.M. and Hoffman, B.B. (1987) Adenylate cyclase supersensitivity: a general means of cellular adaptation to inhibitory agonists? *Trends Pharmacol. Sci.,* 8: 308 – 311.

West, R.E., Jr., Moss, J., Vaughan, M., Liu, T. and Liu, T.-Y. (1985) Pertussis toxin-catalyzed ADP-ribosylation of transducin. Cysteine 347 is the ADP-ribose acceptor site. *J. Biol. Chem.,* 260: 14428 – 14430.

Yatani, A., Mattera, R., Codina, J., Graf, R., Okabe, K., Padrell, E., Iyengar, R., Brown, A.M. and Birnbaumer, L. (1988) The G protein-gated atrial K^+ channel is stimulated by three distinct G_i α-subunits. *Nature,* 336: 680 – 682.

P. Coleman, G. Higgins and C. Phelps (Eds.)
Progress in Brain Research, Vol. 86
© 1990 Elsevier Science Publishers B.V. (Biomedical Division)

CHAPTER 23

Regulation of immediate early genes in brain: role of NMDA receptor activation

Paul F. Worley, Andrew J. Cole, David W. Saffen and Jay M. Baraban

Departments of Neuroscience, Neurology, Psychiatry and Behavioral Sciences, Johns Hopkins University School of Medicine, Baltimore, MD 21205, U.S.A.

A fundamental goal of neurobiology is to understand the basic mechanisms that underlie neural plasticity. Recent evidence suggests that cell surface receptor stimulation regulates expression of genes that may in turn be involved in long-term alterations of cellular behavior. For example, growth factor stimulation of fibroblasts, which causes cell growth and division, rapidly induces transcription of a set of genes that has been characterized by molecular biological techniques (Cochran et al., 1983; Lau and Nathans, 1985, 1987). These genes are referred to as cellular immediate early genes (IEGs) by analogy with viral genes involved in early stages of viral replication. Several IEGs code for known or presumed transcription factors and include *c-fos* (Franza et al., 1988), *c-jun* (Rauscher et al., 1988; Ryder and Nathans 1988), *jun-B* (Ryder et al., 1988), *zif/*268 (Christy et al., 1988) (also termed NGFI-A (Milbrandt, 1987), Egr-1 (Sukhatme et al., 1988) and Krox-24 (Lemaire et al., 1988)). Identification of these genes as possible transcription factors supports the notion that these genes may translate brief cell surface receptor activation into long-term changes in cellular physiology.

The genomic effect of cell-surface receptor activation has also been examined in neural cells. Acetylcholine, acting at nicotinic receptors, rapidly induces transcription of *c-fos* in cultured PC12 cells (Greenberg et al., 1986). NGF stimulation of these cells, which induces differentiation, causes rapid transcription of NGFI-A as well as *c-fos* (Milbrandt, 1987). Parallels between fibroblast and neural systems suggest that receptor stimulation of transcription factor genes may underlie aspects of synaptic plasticity.

A possible role for receptor-mediated gene activation in synaptic plasticity is enticing since synaptically released neurotransmitters are involved in the induction of plasticity (Nicoll et al., 1988) and since RNA and protein synthesis during or shortly after stimulation are required to maintain plasticity (Montarolo et al., 1986). Evidence that *c-fos* like immunoreactivity and mRNA are rapidly induced in brain neurons by pharmacologically-induced seizures (Morgan et al., 1987) supports this notion and suggested that other IEGs may also be induced by seizures. To evaluate this possibility, we assayed IEG mRNAs in rat brain at various intervals after pentylenetetrazol-induced seizures. In our initial screen, we found that mRNA levels for *c-fos, zif/*268, *jun-B* and *c-jun* increase within minutes after seizure onset (Fig. 1), reach maximal levels by 30 min and return to near basal levels by 2 h (Saffen et al., 1988). Northern analysis of RNA from different brain regions demonstrates coordinate increases in mRNA of these genes in neocortex and hippocampus with less consistent increases in cerebellum. In situ hybridization autoradiography demonstrates that IEG mRNA is

278

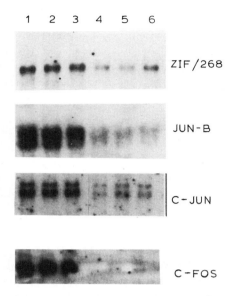

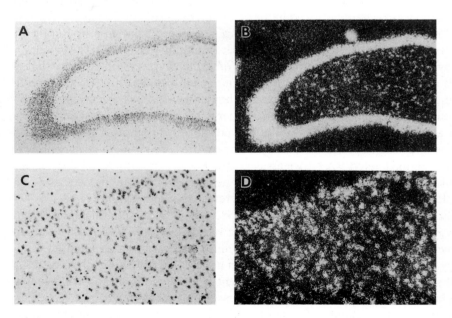

Fig. 1. Northern blot analysis of *zif*/268, *jun-B, c-jun* and *c-fos* mRNA levels in rat hippocampus 30 min after a maximal electroconvulsive shock induced seizure (lanes *1 – 3*) versus control hippocampus (lanes *4 – 6*). Methods according to Saffen et al. (1988).

increased in neurons of the hippocampus, pyriform cortex and neocortex (Fig. 2). Seizures induced by other methods including bicuculline, picrotoxin and maximal electroconvulsive shock (MECS) were also effective in stimulating IEG mRNA increases. In characterizing seizure-induced IEGs, we find MECS preferable to pharmacologically induced seizures since MECS is more reliable, less frequently lethal, and the stimulus onset is precisely defined.

Growth factor stimulated IEG mRNA increases in fibroblasts are transient but can be prolonged and potentiated by protein synthesis inhibitors (Lau and Nathans, 1987). This effect of protein synthesis inhibition indicates that IEG transcription is independent of new protein synthesis and suggests that IEG products exert negative feedback regulation at the level of transcription. To assess these characteristics of IEGs in vivo, we determined the effect of protein synthesis inhibitors on basal and seizure-induced IEG mRNA levels in brain. Cycloheximide (20 mg/kg i.p.), a potent

Fig. 2. Autoradiographic localization of *zif*/268 mRNA to neurons of the dentate gyrus and pyriform cortex of rat brain 60 min after pentylenetetrazol-induced seizures. Photomicrographs (magnification: × 140) of dentate gyrus (*A* and *B*) and pyriform cortex (*C* and *D*) stained with toluidine blue after development of photographic emulsion. Bright field (*A* and *C*); dark field (*B* and *D*).

protein synthesis inhibitor, was administered to rats 30 min prior to MECS. Forebrain RNA was prepared 4 h later from these animals and compared to RNA prepared from animals treated with cycloheximide alone (no MECS), MECS alone and control animals. Northern analysis demonstrates that cycloheximide alone increases basal levels of *c-fos* and *zif*/268 (Fig. 3). Furthermore, cycloheximide potentiates and prolongs the seizure-induced IEG mRNA response. In situ hybridization demonstrates enhanced mRNA levels due to combined MECS and cycloheximide in neocortex and hippocampus, most notable over dense clusters of neurons (Fig. 4). We also note that the effect of cycloheximide alone on mRNA levels is most robust in the neocortex and is comparatively less pronounced in the dentate gyrus. Identical results were also obtained with the protein synthesis inhibitor anisomycin (100 mg/kg i.p.) confirming the role of protein synthesis inhibition in IEG

superinduction in brain. These findings indicate that adult brain neurons are capable of mounting a rapid and complex genomic response to stimulation with marked similarities to the genomic response of growth factor-stimulated fibroblasts.

To determine if electrical activation of neurons is necessary for seizures to induce increases in IEG mRNA levels, we blocked sodium channel activity with tetrodotoxin prior to a seizure and assayed IEGs mRNA levels by in situ hybridization. When sufficient tetrodotoxin was infused into the hippocampus to block synaptic transmission (2 μl of 1 mM tetrodotoxin), a subsequent seizure failed to increase *zif*/268 mRNA levels in the injected hippocampus while other regions exhibited typical *zif*/268 mRNA increases (Fig. 5). This observation indicates that sodium channel activity is involved in seizure-induced IEG increases.

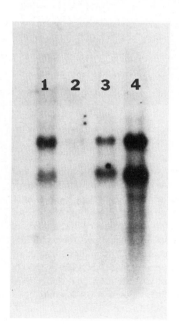

Fig. 3. Northern blot analysis of effect of cycloheximide and MECS on *zif*/268 and *c-fos* mRNA levels in rat forebrain. 10 μg of RNA from: naive control, lane 2; 30 min after MECS, lane *1*; 4.5 h after cycloheximide (20 mg/kg i.p.), lane *3*; 4.5 h after cycloheximide (20 mg/kg i.p.) and 4 h after MECS, lane *4*. Upper and lower bands are *zif*/268 and *c-fos* mRNA respectively.

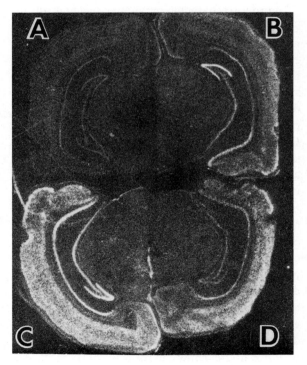

Fig. 4. In situ hybridization demonstrating effect of cycloheximide (20 mg/kg i.p.) and MECS on rat forebrain *zif*/268 mRNA levels. Brains from 4 animals were cut in half along the midline and then embedded together in one tissue block. *A*. Naive control; *B*. 30 min after MECS; *C*. 4.5 h after cycloheximide and 4 h after MECS; *D*. 4.5 h after cycloheximide.

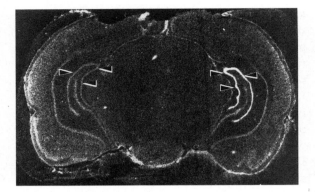

Fig. 5. In situ hybridization demonstrating effect of tetrodotoxin on seizure induced *zif*/268 mRNA levels. Tetrodotoxin was injected into the left hippocampus prior to inducing a seizure with pentylenetetrazol (50 mg/kg i.p.). Note reduced levels of *zif*/268 mRNA in the tetrodotoxin treated granule cell layer (arrows) relative to the non-injected hippocampus (right).

In order to characterize synaptic mechanisms involved in regulating IEGs in brain, we monitored mRNA levels in hippocampal granule cells after excitatory stimulation via perforant path (pp) afferents (Cole et al., 1989). The pp-granule cell synapse has been extensively characterized since it demonstrates long-term potentiation of synaptic potentials following specific stimuli (Bliss and Lynch, 1988). This paradigm therefore provides the opportunity to examine the association of IEG activation with specific synaptic stimuli as well as with neuronal plasticity. Standard in vivo stimulation and recording techniques were used (McNaughton et al., 1978; Bliss et al., 1983). Stimulation of the pp evokes a population excitatory post-synaptic potential (EPSP) and population spike (PS) recorded from the dorsal dentate gyrus. Continuous low-frequency stimulation (0.1 Hz, 60 min) at an intensity sufficient to elicit both EPSP and near maximal PS responses did not alter mRNA levels of *zif*/268, *c-fos*, *c-jun* or *jun-B* in the dentate gyrus (Fig. 6) (n = 9). Additionally, 50 Hz stimulus trains lasting 1 sec and repeated at 0.1 Hz for 15 min had no effect on IEG levels in the dentate gyrus (n = 3). By contrast, brief high-frequency trains (twelve 20 msec trains at 500 Hz repeated at 0.1 Hz) reproducibly induced

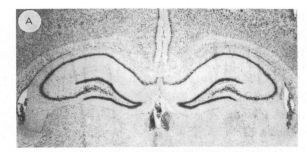

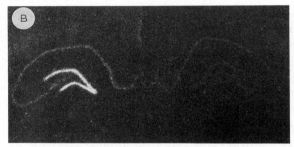

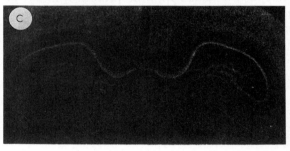

Fig. 6. High-frequency stimulation of the perforant path induces increases in *zif*/268 mRNA in granule cell neurons. *A*. Rat dorsal hippocampus (magnification: × 5). Tissue section is stained with Cresyl violet and demonstrates the molecular and granule cell layers of the dentate gyrus. Perforant path afferents synapse on granule cell dendrites in the molecular layer. (*B* and *C*): Autoradiograms of ^{35}S-labeled *zif*/268 riboprobe in situ hybridization to rat dorsal hippocampus following in vivo orthodromic stimulation of granule cells via perforant path afferents. *B*. 1 h after a high-frequency pp stimulus composed of twelve 20 msec bursts of monophasic pulses (50 μsec) at 500 Hz repeated at 0.1 Hz. The intensity of the individual pulses were sufficient to elicit a maximal PS response at 0.1 Hz (60 V). In 14 of 15 preparations (data pooled from animals sacrificed 30 and 60 min after stimulation), hybridization was unilaterally increased in the dentate gyrus ipsilateral to the stimulating electrode (left side). *C*. Low-frequency stimulation. Synaptic responses to single stimuli were monitored every 10 sec (0.1 Hz) throughout a 1 h recording period prior to sacrifice. Hybridization remained at basal levels in 9 of 9 preparations. Methods in Cole et al. (1989).

increases in *zif/268* mRNA levels in the granule cell layer of the dentate gyrus (14 of 15 animals). Increased levels of *zif/268* mRNA appear over granule cell neurons.

Since kindling stimuli induce *c-fos* like immunoreactivity (Dragunow and Robertson, 1987) and since seizure activity increases IEG mRNA levels (Saffen et al., 1988), we monitored spontaneous and induced electrical activity during and immediately following the high-frequency stimuli and detected no after-discharges or spontaneous bursts. Several other lines of evidence indicate that the induction of *zif/268* mRNA levels by the high-frequency pp stimulus is qualitatively different from induction by seizures. Unlike seizures, which increase *zif/268* mRNA levels throughout the dentate gyri bilaterally, *zif/268* mRNA increases following the high-frequency pp stimulus, are strictly unilateral and appear more intense in the dorsal as compared with the ventral hippocampus. In contrast to seizures which induce coordinate increases in *zif/268*, *c-jun*, *jun-B* and *c-fos* mRNAs, the high-frequency pp stimulus is somewhat selective for *zif/268* (14 of 15 animals) since mRNA levels for *c-jun* and *jun-B* were detectably increased in only half and *c-fos* was increased in only a quarter of the same animals. Another difference between IEG mRNA induction by seizures and high-frequency pp stimuli, to be described below, is their respective dependencies on NMDA receptor activation. Despite these differences, levels of *zif/268* mRNA induced by high-frequency stimuli are typically similar to those induced in the dentate gyrus by pharmacological or MECS seizures (see Fig. 8).

Since *zif/268* mRNA levels most closely correlated with high-frequency pp stimulation, we focused on characterizing this response. As noted earlier, the time course of IEG mRNA increases following a stimulus is very transient in most systems (Lau and Nathans, 1987; Saffen et al., 1988). *zif/268* mRNA levels following a high-frequency pp stimulus train display a similar pattern as they are increased by 15 min (2 of 3 animals), maximal at 30 min and return to basal

levels by 3 h (n = 6).

Cortical and hippocampal injury also induce rapid increases in mRNA levels of *c-fos*, *c-jun*, *jun-B* and *zif/268* (manuscript in preparation). Penetration of the dentate gyrus with a large-bore probe such as the 23-gauge stimulating electrode induces coordinate increases in IEG mRNA levels throughout the entire ipsilateral dentate gyrus that remain elevated for 24 h. By contrast, we find no evidence of injury-induced IEG increases in the dentate gyrus when penetrated with a fine bore glass microelectrode used for electrical recordings (9 of 9 animals). These observations, in conjunction with the frequency dependence of the synaptic pp-granule cell *zif/268* mRNA response, distinguish injury from synaptically induced IEG mRNA increases.

As noted previously, the pp-granule cell synapse displays long-term potentiation after specific synaptic stimuli. The high-frequency pp stimuli used in the preceding experiments are reported to reliably induce long-term potentiation (McNaughton et al., 1978; Bliss et al., 1983). We observed greater than 50% potentiation of the PS amplitude in response to submaximal low-frequency stimuli in 12 of the 14 animals assayed for IEG mRNA levels (Fig. 7). By contrast, no long-lasting potentiation was detected following either the 0.1 Hz or 50 Hz stimuli. Since long-term potentiation by high-frequency stimulation of the pp-granule cell synapse is blocked by NMDA receptor antagonists (Errington et al., 1987), we determined the effect of these antagonists on high-frequency pp stimulus-induced *zif/268* mRNA increases. (+)MK-801 (1 mg/kg i.p.), a non-competitive NMDA antagonist (Wong et al., 1986) that blocks pp-granule cell LTP (Abraham and Mason, 1988), also blocks high-frequency pp stimulus-induced increases in *zif/268* mRNA (n = 5 of 6 preparations; Fig. 8). By contrast, the relatively less active NMDA antagonist (−)MK-801 (1 mg/kg i.p.) (Wong et al., 1986) failed to block this *zif/268* mRNA response (n = 2). A role for NMDA receptor activation in inducing *zif/268* mRNA is further supported by blockade of the *zif/268* mRNA

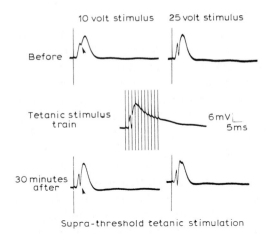

10 volt stimulus   25 volt stimulus

Before

Tetanic stimulus
train   6 mV
                                     5ms

30 minutes
after

Supra-threshold tetanic stimulation

Fig. 7. Electrical recordings from the dentate gyrus demonstrating long-term potentiation. Perforant path stimulation evokes a broad up-going EPSP and superimposed PS (arrow). Prior to the tetanic stimulus train (described in Fig. 6), PS evoked by 25 V stimulus is larger than the PS evoked by a 10 V stimulus (top row). By contrast, 30 min after the stimulus train, the amplitude of a PS evoked by a 10 V stimulus is increased and is nearly identical to that evoked by a 25 V stimulus.

response by CGS-19755 (n = 3 of 3; 10 mg/kg i.p.), a competitive NMDA antagonist (Lodge et al., 1988; Murphy et al., 1988). Evidence for specificity of action of these NMDA antagonists is provided by the observation that CGS-19755 (15 mg/kg i.p.) or (+)MK-801 (10 mg/kg i.p.) fail to block MECS-induced increases in *zif*/268 mRNA (Fig. 8; n = 3 and 2, respectively).

To further evaluate the association between synaptic plasticity and *zif*/268 mRNA levels, we determined the effect on *zif*/268 mRNA levels of experimental manipulations known to modulate the induction of LTP. The induction of LTP in the pp-granule cell synapse is blocked by coincident stimulation of the contralateral dentate gyrus (Douglas et al., 1982). This blockade is believed to be due to stimulation of a crossed synaptic pathway that inhibits granule cell activation. LTP is blocked if the inhibitory pathway is activated immediately before the pp-granule cell stimulus but not if their order is reversed. Using this paradigm,

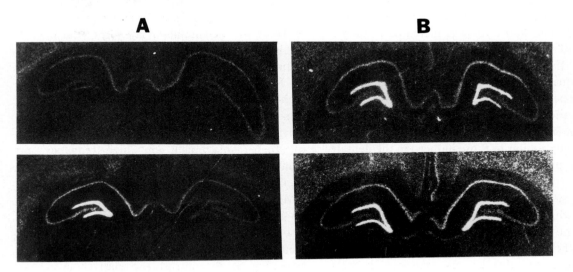

Fig. 8. High-frequency stimulus-induced increases in *zif*/268 mRNA are blocked by NMDA antagonists. *Zif*/268 in situ autoradiograms. *A*. 30 min after a high-frequency pp stimulus as in Fig. 6. Animals were pretreated 1 h before the pp stimulus with either (+)MK-801 (upper panel) or (−)MK-801 (lower panel) (1 mg/kg i.p.). (+)MK-801 blocked the high-frequency pp stimulus-induced increase in *zif*/268 probe hybridization in 5 of 6 preparations while (−)MK-801 failed to block the effect in 2 of 2 preparations. *B*. 30 min after MECS. Animals were pretreated for 1 h with either (+)MK-801 (10 mg/kg) (upper panel) or an identical volume of solvent (ethanol) (lower panel). (+)MK-801 failed to block MECS induced increases in *zif*/268 mRNA (n = 3).

we observed that *zif/268* mRNA increases are blocked if the contralateral dentate hilus is stimulated before, but not after, the pp-granule cell synapse (Fig. 9). Stimulation of the dentate gyrus alone had no effect on *zif/268* mRNA levels in the contralateral dentate gyrus. These observations indicate that both excitatory and inhibitory synaptic mechanisms regulating the induction of LTP also regulate *zif/268* mRNA increases.

Another characteristic of LTP that we examined for its role in regulating *zif/268* mRNA levels is the threshold phenomenon. High-frequency pp stimuli must exceed a defined intensity threshold in order to reliably induce LTP (McNaughton et al., 1978; Bliss et al., 1983). The intensity threshold is thought to represent the minimum NMDA receptor activation necessary to induce LTP (Nicoll et al., 1988). Accordingly, we examined the effec-

tiveness of pp stimuli with intensities either above or below this LTP threshold. Consistent with previous descriptions of the intensity threshold, we observed LTP in 8 of 13 preparations in which the stimulus intensity was just above threshold and in 2 of 6 preparations in which subthreshold intensities were administered. In these same animals, *zif/268* increases occurred in 1 of 6 (subthreshold) and 6 of 13 (threshold) preparations. These data, in conjunction with data from the suprathreshold stimulus intensity group (14 of 15 with increased *zif/268* mRNA levels) or low-frequency stimulus group (0 of 9 with increased *zif/268* mRNA levels) described previously, indicate a direct relation between the intensity of the stimulus and the incidence of increased *zif/268* mRNA levels (Cole et al., 1989). Furthermore, the minimum stimulus intensity necessary to induce *zif/268* mRNA in-

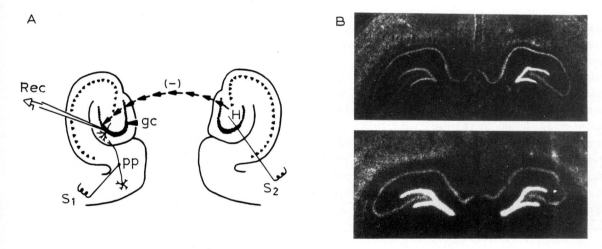

Fig. 9. Inhibitory projections from the contralateral dentate hilus block high-frequency pp stimulus-induced increases in *zif/268* mRNA in the dentate gyrus. *A*. Schematic horizontal section through the rat forebrain illustrating electrode positions and crossed inhibitory input. Standard stimulating (S_1) and recording (Rec) electrodes were positioned in the perforant path and ipsilateral dentate gyrus. The intensity of the S_1 stimulus was adjusted to evoke a maximum PS response at 0.1 Hz (60 V). A second bipolar stimulating electrode (S_2) was placed in the contralateral dentate hilus and the intensity adjusted such that an S_2 stimulus delivered 10 msec prior to S_1 blocked the orthodromically evoked PS (from 60 V to 80 V). At these defined intensities, high-frequency stimulus trains as described in Fig. 6 were delivered to both S_1 and S_2. LTP is blocked if S_2 immediately precedes S_1 but not if their order is reversed (Douglas et al., 1982). *B*. In situ autoradiograms of *zif/268* ^{35}S-riboprobe hybridization to the dorsal hippocampus 30 min after high-frequency pp stimulation. In the top panel, S_2 immediately preceded S_1 while in the bottom panel S_1 immediately preceded S_2. In 3 of 4 preparations in which S_2 preceded S_1, *zif/268* mRNA levels in the orthodromically stimulated dentate gyrus remained at basal levels (top; left dentate gyrus). By contrast, if S_1 preceded S_2, typical increases in *zif/268* mRNA were induced by the high-frequency pp stimulus (bottom; left dentate gyrus). Penetration of the dentate hilus with the S_2 electrode enhanced *zif/268* mRNA levels in the ipsilateral dentate gyrus in all preparations (top and bottom; right dentate gyri).

creases is similar to that required to induce LTP.

Despite the similarities between induction of LTP and *zif*/268 mRNA increases, there were preparations demonstrating LTP but in which increases in *zif*/268 mRNA were not detected. Even though NMDA receptor activation appears necessary for both phenomena, this discordance suggests that there may be distinct mechanisms involved in their respective inductions. On this point, it may be significant that induction of LTP involves dendrites of the post-synaptic neuron while regulation of mRNA levels occurs at the cell soma.

In summary, the major findings of these studies are: (1) IEG mRNA levels are dynamically regulated in brain by neuron activating stimuli; (2) immediate early genes may be selectively regulated by specific stimuli; (3) synaptic NMDA receptor activation is involved in the rapid regulation of *zif*/268 mRNA levels by high-frequency pp stimuli; (4) convergent inhibitory synaptic inputs coordinately modulate LTP and *zif*/268 mRNA increases; and (5) the intensity of synaptic stimuli necesssary to increase *zif*/268 mRNA levels is similar to that required to induce LTP.

Since *zif*/268 appears to code for a transcription factor (Milbrandt, 1987; Christy et al., 1988; Lemaire et al., 1988; Sukhatme et al., 1988), its association with synaptic plasticity makes it an appealing candidate for a "plasticity gene". Our studies indicate that LTP and *zif*/268 mRNA are activated in parallel. Whether or not *zif*/268 plays a direct role in the induction of LTP, an understanding of the cellular processes leading from membrane NMDA receptor activation to *zif*/268 mRNA regulation will add significantly to our understanding of neuronal plasticity.

Acknowledgements

We thank Drs. B. Christy, K. Ryder, T. Nakabeppu and D. Nathans for use of the IEG clones. We thank Darla Lawrence for superb secretarial assistance.

This research was supported by grants to J.M.B. from the Lucille P. Markey Charitable Trust, the Sloan Foundation, the Blades Center for Research in Alcoholism, and the National Institute for Drug Abuse. A.J.C. was supported by an American Academy of Neurology Neuropharmacology fellowship, and by an Epilepsy Foundation of America research fellowship; D.W.S. by a postdoctoral fellowship from the Monsanto Corp.; and P.F.W. by a Physician Scientist Award, and a grant from the Klingenstein Foundation.

References

Abraham, W.C. and Mason, S.E. (1988) Effects of the NMDA receptor/channel antagonists CPP and MK-801 on hippocampal field potentials and long-term potentiation in anesthestized rats. *Brain Res.*, 462: 40–46.

Bliss, T.V.P. and Lynch, M.A. (1988) Long-term potentiation of synaptic transmission in the hippocampus: properties and mechanisms. In: *Long-Term Potentiation: from Biophysics to Behavior*, Alan Liss, New York, pp. 3–72.

Bliss, T.V.P., Goddard, G.V. and Riives, M. (1983) Reduction of long-term potentiation in the dentate gyrus of the rat following selective depletion of monoamines. *J. Physiol., (Lond.)*, 334: 475–491.

Christy, B.A., Lau, L.F. and Nathans, D. (1988) A gene activated in mouse 3T3 cells by serum growth factors encodes a protein with "zinc finger" sequences. *Proc. Natl. Acad. Sci. U.S.A.*, 85: 7857–7861.

Cochran, B.H., Keffel, A.C. and Stiles, C.D. (1983) Molecular cloning of gene sequences regulated by platelet-derived growth factor. *Cell*, 33: 939–947.

Cole, A.J., Saffen, D.W., Baraban, J.M. and Worley, P.F. (1989) Rapid increase of an immediate early gene mRNA in hippocampal neurons by synaptic NMDA receptor activation. *Nature*, 340: 474–476.

Douglas, R.M., Goddard, G.V. and Riives, M. (1982) Inhibitory modulation of long-term potentiation: evidence for a post-synaptic locus of control. *Brain Res.*, 240: 259–272.

Dragunow, M. and Robertson, H.A. (1987) Kindling stimulation induces *c-fos* protein(s) in granule cells of the rat dentate gyrus. *Nature*, 329: 441–442.

Errington, M.L., Lynch, M.A. and Bliss, T.V.P. (1987) Long-term potentiation in the dentate gyrus: induction and increased glutamate release are blocked by D-aminophosphonovalerate. *Neuroscience*, 20: 279–284.

Franza, B.R., Jr., Rauscher, III, F.J., Josephs, S.F. and Curran, T. (1988) The *fos* complex and *fos*-related antigens recognize sequence elements that contain AP-1 binding sites. *Science*, 239: 1150–1153.

Greenberg, M.E., Ziff, E.B. and Greene, L.A. (1986) Stimulation of neuronal acetylcholine receptors induces rapid gene transcription. *Science,* 234: 80 – 83.

Lau, L.F. and Nathans, D. (1985) Identification of a set of genes expressed during the G_0/G_1 transition of cultured mouse cells. *EMBO J.,* 4: 3145 – 3151.

Lau, L.F. and Nathans, D. (1987) Expression of a set of growth-related immediate early genes in BALB/c 3T3 cells: coordinate regulation with *c-fos* or *c-myc. Proc. Natl. Acad. Sci. U.S.A.,* 84: 1182 – 1186.

Lemaire, P., Revelant, O., Bravo, R. and Charnay, P. (1988) Two mouse genes encoding potential transcription factors with identical DNA-binding domains are activated by growth factors in cultured cells. *Proc. Natl. Acad. Sci. U.S.A.,* 85: 4691 – 4695.

Lodge, D., Davies, S.N., Jones, M.G. et al. (1988) A comparison between the in vivo and in vitro activity of five potent and competitive NMDA antagonists. *Br. J. Pharmacol.,* 95: 957 – 965.

McNaughton, B.L., Douglas, R.M. and Goddard, G.V. (1978) Synaptic enhancement in fascia dentata: cooperativity among coactive afferents. *Brain Res.,* 157: 227 – 293.

Milbrandt, J. (1987) A nerve growth factor-induced gene encodes a possible transcriptional regulatory factor. *Science,* 238: 797 – 799.

Montarolo, P.G., Goelet, P., Castellucci, V.F., Morgan, J., Kandel, E.R. and Schacher, S. (1986) A critical period for macromolecular synthesis in long-term heterosynaptic facilitation in *Aplysia. Science,* 234: 1249 – 1254.

Morgan, J.I., Cohen, D.R., Hempstead, J.L. and Curran, T. (1987) Mapping patterns of *c-fos* expression in the central nervous system after seizure. *Science,* 237: 192 – 197.

Murphy, D.E., Hutchison, A.J., Hurt, S.D., Williams, M. and Sills, M.A. (1988) Characterization of the binding of [^{3}H]-CGS 19755: a novel *N*-methyl-D-aspartate antagonist with nanomolar affinity in rat brain. *Br. J. Pharmacol.,* 95: 932 – 938.

Nicoll, R.A., Kauer, J.A. and Malenka, R.C. (1988) The current excitement in long-term potentiation. *Neuron,* 1: 97 – 103.

Rauscher, III, F.J., Cohen, D.R., Curran, T., Bos, T.J., Vogt, P.K., Bohmann, D., Tijan, R. and Franza, B.R. (1988) *Fos*-associated protein p39 is the product of the *jun* proto-oncogene. *Science,* 240: 1010 – 1016.

Ryder, K. and Nathans, D. (1988) Induction of protooncogene *c-jun* by serum growth factors. *Proc. Natl. Acad. Sci. U.S.A.,* 85: 8464 – 8467.

Ryder, K., Lau, L.F. and Nathans, D. (1988) A gene activated by growth factors is related to the oncogene *v-jun. Proc. Natl. Acad. Sci. U.S.A.,* 85: 1487 – 1491.

Saffen, D.W., Cole, A.J., Worley, P.F., Christy, B.A., Ryder, K. and Baraban, J.M. (1988) Convulsant-induced increase in transcription factor messenger RNAs in rat brain. *Proc. Natl. Acad. Sci. U.S.A.,* 85: 7795 – 7799.

Sukhatme, V.P., Cao, X., Chang, L.C., Tsai-Morris, C-H., Stamenkovich, D., Ferreira, P.C.P., Cohen, D.R., Edwards, S.A., Shows, T.B., Curran, T., Le Beau, M.M. and Adamson, E.D. (1988) A zinc finger-encoding gene coregulated with *c-fos* during growth and differentiation, and after cellular depolarization. *Cell,* 53: 37 – 43.

Wong, E.H.F., Kemp, J.A., Priestley, T., Knight, A.R., Woodruff, G.N. and Iversen, L.L. (1986) The anticonvulsant MK-801 is a potent *N*-methyl-D-aspartate antagonist. *Proc. Natl. Acad. Sci. U.S.A.,* 83: 7104 – 7108.

P. Coleman, G. Higgins and C. Phelps (Eds.)
Progress in Brain Research, Vol. 86
© 1990 Elsevier Science Publishers B.V. (Biomedical Division)

CHAPTER 24

Inducible proto-oncogenes of the nervous system: their contribution to transcription factors and neuroplasticity

James I. Morgan and Tom Curran

Departments of Neuroscience and Molecular Oncology, Roche Institute of Molecular Biology, Roche Research Center, Nutley, NJ 07110, U.S.A.

Stimulation of neurons results in the execution of a highly organized cellular response that is dictated, ultimately, by the phenotype of the neuron. Historically much attention has been focused upon the rapid events that follow upon neuronal excitation and generally involve second messenger-mediated modifications of existing substrates. These cellular responses occur within fractions of a second to a few minutes and include modulation of ion channel function, alterations in neurotransmitter release, changes in the activity of neurotransmitter synthetic enzymes and post-translational modification of cytoskeletal and membrane components. These processes do not have a requirement for de novo protein synthesis. This situation may be contrasted with what has now been recognized to be a long-term response to neuronal stimulation. Many studies have established that excitation results in adaptive and plastic alterations within the neuron that either require ongoing protein synthesis or that lead to alterations in gene expression (see for example Agranoff, 1976; Goelet et al., 1986; Montarolo et al., 1987). This has led to the important conclusion that mechanisms must exist to couple extracellular stimuli to gene transcription (Goelet et al., 1986; Curran and Morgan, 1987). Recently, the molecular details of stimulus-transcription coupling in neurons have begun to be elucidated. In particular we will emphasize the contributions played by the products of the *fos* and *jun* proto-oncogenes.

Excitation of cells results in the rapid transcriptional activation of a number of genes, some of which are believed to orchestrate the long-term response to stimulation (Cochran et al., 1983; Goelet et al., 1986; Morgan and Curran, 1986; Curran and Morgan, 1987; Lau and Nathans, 1987; Lim et al., 1987; Morgan et al., 1987). Many of these genes are induced even in the presence of protein synthesis inhibitors (Cochran et al., 1983; Lim et al., 1987; Curran, 1988), indicating that their transcriptional activation is a direct consequence of stimulation. In several regards the properties of these rapidly induced genes are like those of the immediate-early genes of some eukaryotic viruses. That is, they are both expressed in the absence of de novo protein synthesis and their products appear immediately upon infection/stimulation of a cell. For this reason the rapidly inducible genes of eukaryotic cells are often referred to as immediate-early genes (Curran and Morgan, 1987; Lau and Nathans, 1987). Since the immediate-early genes of viruses regulate the expression of early genes, thereby controlling the cycle of infectivity, the eukaryotic counterparts are considered to constitute a cellular immediate-early response to stimulation which, by analogy, is believed to orchestrate the long-term response (see Fig. 1).

Many, although by no means all, of the

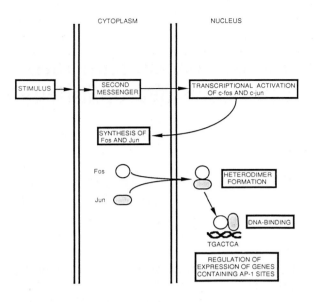

ROLE OF Fos IN STIMULUS-RESPONSE COUPLING

Fig. 1. A schematic representation of the activation of the immediate-early gene cascade and its putative consequences for the regulation of target gene expression.

immediate-early genes encode nuclear proteins (Curran and Morgan, 1987; Lau and Nathans, 1987; Cohen and Curran, 1988; Sukhatme et al., 1988). We have proposed that these proteins should be viewed as nuclear third messengers in a stimulus-transcription coupling cascade (Curran and Morgan, 1987). In particular, the properties of two rapidly inducible genes, *fos* and *jun*, fulfill most of the criteria for nuclear third messengers. First, these genes are transiently induced by a range of biological stimuli (Lau and Nathans, 1987; Curran, 1988). That is, their products (Fos and Jun) accumulate rapidly within the cell nucleus in response to stimulation but are then quickly eliminated. Second, the rise in *c-fos* and *c-jun* expression is independent of protein synthesis and precedes alterations in transcriptional activity of many other genes. That is, the temporal relationship between cell stimulation, the rise in *c-fos* and *c-jun* transcription and the altered expression of

further genes is consistent with the notion that Fos and Jun link excitation to these later events. Finally, as we will outline below, Fos and Jun are components of a nucleoprotein complex that is capable of regulating transcription from identified genes. Thus we suggest that the rapid induction of *c-fos* and *c-jun* leads to the transient accumulation of Fos-Jun nucleoprotein complexes that directly modulate the transcriptional activity of genes required for the adaptive response of neurons. The repertoire of potential target genes influenced by Fos-Jun is likely to be dictated by the phenotype of the neuron so that not all genes possessing the recognition sequence for the complex will necessarily be affected.

Both *c-fos* and *c-jun* belong to families of genes that are rapidly induced in many cell types by a diverse array of stimulants (Curran, 1988; Cohen and Curran, 1988; Nakabeppu et al., 1988; Ryder et al., 1988). Fos and Jun associate with one another to form heterodimers that bind specifically to the DNA consensus recognition sequence for transcription factor AP-1 (Rauscher et al., 1988a, b, c). This sequence is present in regulatory elements of a number of genes where it is essential for both basal and stimulated transcription (Angel et al., 1987; Distel et al., 1987; Lee et al., 1987a, b; Piette and Yaniv, 1987; Franza et al., 1988; Rauscher et al., 1988b, c). Transcription factor AP-1 was originally defined as a DNA binding activity present in HeLa cell nuclear extracts. Subsequently AP-1 was shown to comprise at least Fos and Jun as well as several Fos- and Jun-related polypeptides (Bohmann et al., 1987; Rauscher et al., 1988b). It is now accepted that one member of the Fos family associates with one member of the Jun family, with all of the variations of the heterodimeric complexes (tested to date) being able to bind to the AP-1 DNA recognition sequence (Nakabeppu et al., 1988; Rauscher et al., 1988a, b, c; Cohen et al., 1989; Gentz et al., 1989). Thus AP-1 is unlikely to be a single molecular entity, but rather a series of heterodimers composed of the products of the *fos* and *jun* gene families. It is unclear at present whether these various AP-1 complexes have the same activity upon gene transcription, although it would appear biologically wasteful to have generated such diversity to achieve the same function.

Recent investigations have revealed some of the molecular details underlying the interactions between Fos and Jun as well as between the protein complex and its DNA target. Both Fos and Jun possess a structurally-related functional domain that is essential for their dimerization. The dimerization regions of both proteins are predicted to form amphipathic alpha helices and contain a heptad repeat of leucine residues termed a "leucine zipper" (Landschulz et al., 1988; Gentz et al., 1989). This situation results in the leucine residues being present on the same face of the helix at every other turn. The evidence suggests that the helical domains of Fos and Jun associate in a parallel coiled-coil structure with the hydrophobic leucine residues of one helix being aligned with their counterparts in the other protein (Gentz et al., 1989). It is this configuration that serves to stabilize the protein-protein interaction. DNA binding does not reside in the leucine-zipper domain but rather in regions of basic amino acids that are located on the amino terminal side of the zipper. Both Fos and Jun possess regions essential for binding of the heterodimer to its DNA target. In a generalized model it is envisaged that Fos and Jun each provide a half site for DNA binding. Thus the formation of mutant heterodimers in which one partner lacks a DNA binding domain but where both have intact leucine-zippers results in complexes that cannot associate with the DNA target (Gentz et al., 1989). Furthermore, Jun, unlike Fos, can homodimerize. The resulting Jun-Jun homodimer can bind to DNA, since it possesses two half sites for binding, but the affinity is much lower than that of the Fos-Jun heterodimer for the same DNA sequence (Rauscher et al., 1988a). Thus the composition of the AP-1 complex does determine whether, and with what affinity, the AP-1 target sequence is bound.

The *fos* gene can be induced by a diverse array of stimulants that utilize different second messenger pathways. In cultures of neuronal cells, depolarizing conditions (Morgan and Curran, 1986), agents that activate voltage-dependent calcium channels (Morgan and Curran, 1986), neurotransmitters (Greenberg et al., 1986) and neurotrophic factors (Curran and Morgan, 1985) can all induce *c-fos* expression. These various agents utilize several second messenger systems that include modulation of the levels of intracellular calcium, cyclic AMP and protein kinase C activity (Morgan and Curran, 1989). That is, the induction of *c-fos* is a stereotypic response of cells to stimulation. The limitations on the induction must reside with the phenotype of the cell. Here one has trivial considerations such as whether a given cell has a receptor for a particular stimulant molecule or a specific ion channel. However, there are more complex issues regarding the efficiency of coupling of given second messenger systems to *c-fos*. For instance, in PC12 cells, nerve growth factor (NGF) is a potent inducer of *c-fos* while phorbol esters, presumably acting via the protein kinase C pathway, are weak inducers. In contrast, the phenotypically related cell line, SY5Y, has exactly the opposite properties, NGF being a weak, and phorbol ester a strong, inducer of *fos* (Morgan and Curran, 1989). From the perspective of the nervous system, the calcium-dependent induction of *fos* is one of the more relevant situations where the recruitment of this gene occurs. In PC12 cells, membrane depolarization by elevation of the extracellular potassium concentration or administration of veratridine both result in a calcium-dependent induction of *c-fos* (Morgan and Curran, 1986). NGF, in contrast, does not require extracellular calcium to induce *c-fos* and, unlike depolarizing agents, NGF induction of *c-fos* is not blocked by dihydropyridine calcium channel blockers (Morgan and Curran, 1986). Further pharmacological analyses have indicated that calcium gains entry to the PC12 cell via L-type voltage-sensitive calcium channels. Subsequently, calmodulin-dependent mechanisms appear to be essential for coupling the elevated calcium to *fos* induction (Morgan and Curran, 1986).

Since a great deal of biochemical and pharmacological information has been amassed in PC12 cells with regard to *fos* induction it has permitted molecular genetic analyses to be carried out in this cell line. These studies have revealed that different stimulants and intracellular second messenger pathways have requirements for distinct DNA elements in the 5' regulatory region of *fos*. For instance, growth factors such as NGF have an absolute requirement for a short nucleotide sequence located approximately 300 bp upstream of the transcription start site (Treisman, 1985; Gilman, 1988; Sheng et al., 1988). In contrast, the calcium-dependent inducers require a short stretch of DNA 60 bp upstream of transcription start (Gilman, 1988; Sheng et al., 1988). That is, there is a mechanistic dichotomy, at the level of DNA regulatory elements, between the various signalling pathways. Interestingly, we have shown a post-translational distinction between the calcium-dependent and -independent pathways, with Fos showing less post-translational modification following induction with the former class of agents (Curran and Morgan, 1986). Whether, these differentially modified forms of Fos have distinct biological activities is unknown at present, however, it does demonstrate that transcriptional activation of *c-fos* can be separated from the post-translation modification of its product.

The study of *c-fos* expression in cultured neuronal cells naturally led to investigations of the proto-oncogene in the CNS itself. The results of these lines of research were both rewarding and confusing in that they revealed a much higher level of organizational complexity at the molecular genetic and biochemical levels than had been expected from studies on cultured neuronal cells and fibroblasts. Stimulation of the nervous system in rodents by pharmacological (Morgan et al., 1987), electrical (Dragunow and Robertson, 1987; Sagar et al., 1988), surgical (White and Gall, 1987) and physiological (Hunt et al., 1987; Sagar et al., 1988) means have all been shown to result in an induction of *c-fos*. Furthermore, it has been possible to

localize the cells elaborating Fos by immunocytochemistry. This has suggested the application of Fos-mapping to investigate pathways of neuronal activation in vivo and to identify the cellular targets for neuroactive substances in the CNS.

In those instances where it was investigated, neural stimulation also resulted in an induction of *c-jun* and *jun-B*. Thus, both components of the AP-1 complex are induced in the mammalian brain. This is confirmed by our studies where we have established that there is a large increase in AP-1 DNA binding activity in brain extracts after pentylenetetrazole seizures. The increases in AP-1 binding activity persist for 6 – 8 h in the mouse and rat brain after seizure, despite the fact that there is no more *fos* mRNA present after 4 h. Furthermore, preincubation of the brain extracts with a Fos antiserum completely removed the AP-1 binding activity, demonstrating that the AP-1 complexes contained proteins that were recognized by antibodies directed against Fos. This spurred us to examine the levels of Fos in the brain by immunoblot analysis.

Unstimulated mouse brain contains very low levels of Fos. However, an additional immunoreactive band is evident in the blots that has an apparent molecular weight of 35 kDa. We assume this protein to be a Fos-related antigen and have termed it Fra-35K. This implies that as the same antiserum is used for both immunocytochemistry and immunoblotting the immunoreactive nuclei evident in untreated brain contain Fra-35K rather than Fos. Following administration of pentylenetetrazole, or indeed other agents that increase neuronal activity, there is a rapid appearance of Fos in the nervous system. However, there is also a dramatic increase in two major immunoreactive bands of molecular weights 35 and 46 kDa respectively. The 35 kDa band is indistinguishable from the Fra-35K seen in unstimulated brain. Thus we term the bands Fra-35K and Fra-46K. Following stimulation, Fos, like its mRNA, rises to a peak and then declines rapidly and is essentially gone by 4 h post-treatment. The two Fra's in contrast, rise with a delay and persist for much longer periods, which may be in excess of 8 h in some situations. Indeed, it is as though there is a cascade of these various proteins with waves of the proteins appearing and disappearing in a staggered manner. Thus Fos appears first, followed by Fra-46K and then Fra-35K, with each decaying away in order.

With these results it is now possible to begin to interpret the increased AP-1 binding activity observed in brain following seizure. We, and others, have established that *c-fos, c-jun* and *jun-B* mRNAs increase immediately following seizure activity. In our hands *c-fos* and *jun-B* mRNAs are induced, accumulate and disappear within 2 − 3 h after treatment. In contrast elevated levels of *c-jun* mRNA are present for significantly longer periods of time. Thus, we infer that Jun may be elaborated over a longer time-frame than either Fos or Jun-B and is probably a constitutive component of the AP-1 complexes following seizure. At the earlier time points following administration of PTZ, we presume neurons to elaborate Jun and Jun-B both of which can form heterodimers with Fos (Nakabeppu et al., 1988). At intermediate and later times, Fos levels decline but there is a large increase in the concentrations of the two Fra's. Since AP-1 DNA binding activity is absorbed by anti-Fos antibodies at times when no Fos is present we conclude that one or more of the Fra's must be present in the complexes. In fact, if the brain extracts are subjected to AP-1 oligo-affinity purification followed by analysis by immunoblotting, all of the Fra species are found bound to the DNA. That is, at later times Fos-Jun and Fos-Jun-B heterodimers have been replaced, in the same neurons, by Fra-Jun dimers. Since we do not have any reagents to determine directly the levels of the Jun and Jun-like proteins we cannot make quantitative estimates of the relative contributions of each type of complex.

The data suggest that neuronal stimulation results in a cascade of events involving transcriptional activation of members of the *fos* and *jun* gene families (see Fig. 2). The products of these genes associate in heterodimeric complexes that are capable of binding to the AP-1 DNA consensus recognition sequence. Because of the temporal differences in expression of the various proteins involved in AP-1 complexes both the level and composition of the heterodimers must alter with time after stimulation. Thus, at any one time, an individual neuron must harbour a mixture of AP-1 protein complexes and the quantitative and qualitative composition of these must vary over time.

The above situation raises the question of the function of these different AP-1 complexes. It is assumed, on the basis of biological economy, that not all the variations of the AP-1 complex have the same activity. Thus two possibilities are suggested. First, it is known that the DNA recognition sequence for AP-1 has a number of naturally-occurring variations in enhancers. Therefore, it is possible that the various complexes can discriminate these fine differences in DNA sequence. This would provide a mechanism that

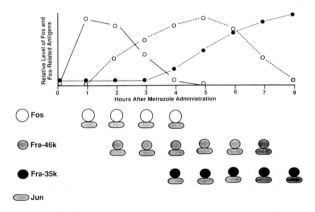

Fig. 2. The AP-1 cascade in the nervous system. The upper panel shows the average content of Fos, Fra-46K and Fra-35K in the brains of mice at various times after administration of pentylenetetrazole. The results were determined by quantitative densitometry of a series of 4 separate immunoblots. The lower part of the figure is a schematic representation of the AP-1 complexes at these various times and serves to highlight the fact that not only the average content of AP-1 increases following seizure but also that the composition of these complexes changes with time. Since we have no antibodies that are useful for studying Jun or its relatives in immunoblots we are unable to ascertain their contributions directly.

could regulate the expression of groups of genes in a staggered manner. Second, since all of the AP-1 complexes appear to bind the AP-1 consensus DNA sequence one could argue that they have essentially identical affinities for the target but bring about different consequences for transcription. Some, for instance, being positive regulators and yet others negative regulators. It is possible that some of the complexes may associate with their target DNA sequence with no overt activity but block access of positively transactivating complexes. By combining these different potential activities a complex pattern of transcriptional regulation may be constructed. Indeed, as *fos* contains a potential AP-1 binding site in its 5' non-transcribed flank it is quite conceivable that these gene products feedback on themselves or other members of their family. In this context it should be remarked that repeated administration of PTZ, while causing seizures, does not fully reinduce *fos*. This attenuation is maximal at a time when no Fos is present in brain but when large amounts of the two Fra's are present. Therefore, it is possible that the Fra's, which accumulate subsequent to Fos, could serve to repress further *fos* expression.

While there is much evidence documenting the induction of *fos* and *jun*, both in cell lines and in vivo, very little is known concerning the identity of endogenous genes that are responding to AP-1. It has been one of our goals to identify putative target genes in the mammalian CNS. An initial premise was that target genes should be activated in those regions of the brain where *fos* expression is highest following PTZ seizures. Further, the temporal changes in transcription of these genes should occur in a manner appropriate for the appearance of Fos and Fra. A survey of the literature revealed that the expression of a number of genes altered in the hippocampus in a number of seizure paradigms, the most experimentally tractable and plausible candidate being preproenkephalin. The hippocampus, and in particular the dentate gyrus, is amongst the first neural structures to become Fos-positive following PTZ (Morgan et al., 1987). Furthermore, it is a well defined structure that can

be readily dissected for analysis. The preproenkephalin gene has been cloned and its promoter analysed and found to contain a regulatory element that has an AP-1-like sequence (Comb et al., 1986). Following PTZ seizures in the hippocampus of rat we observed a maximal rise in *c-fos*, *c-jun* and *jun-B* mRNAs within half an hour. The preproenkephalin mRNA, however, does not become elevated for 1 h. That is, there is a lag between *fos* expression and increased preproenkephalin expression. This would be consistent with Fos (and Jun) having to be synthesized before preproenkephalin transcription is enhanced. However, this is nothing more than an appropriate temporal correlation. Recently we have assayed the activity of the preproenkephalin promoter fused to a reporter gene (pENK-CAT; kindly provided by Dr. M. Comb) by transient cotransfection. In the recipient cell line the pENK-CAT has a very low level of basal transcription. Cotransfection of the construction with an expression vector encoding either Fos or Jun results in either no (Fos) or a small (Jun) increase in transcription from pENK-CAT. However, cotransfection of the reporter with both the Fos and Jun vectors results in a large stimulation of transcription. Thus the co-expression of Fos and Jun results in the positive activation of the intact preproenkephalin promoter. The small effect with Jun is also consistent with its known biology. As mentioned above, Jun can homodimerize and bind with low affinity to the AP-1 sequence; we believe that the small transcriptional effect of the Jun vector can be attributed to the inefficient action of the Jun homodimer.

What these final series of experiments suggest is that the immediate-early genes, as exemplified by the *fos* and *jun* gene families, may play a role in neuronal homeostasis. The enkephalins are released as a consequence of neuronal stimulation and are replenished, under normal circumstances, by the basal transcription and translation from the preproenkephalin gene. Following a period of stimulation that exceeds a threshold where secretion would outstrip synthesis we would contend that the immediate-early cascade is recruited. This would result in a period of enhanced transcription from the preproenkephalin gene in order to replenish the neuropeptide. In other words there exists an interrelationship between stimulus-secretion and stimulus-transcription coupling in the mammalian nervous system.

References

Agranoff, B.W. (1976) In memory and protein synthesis. *Sci. Am.*, 216: 115 – 122.

Angel, P.M., Imagawa, M., Chiu, R., Stein, B., Imbra, R.J., Rahmsorf, H.J., Jonat, C., Herrlich, P. and Karin, M. (1987) Phorbolester-inducible genes contain a common *cis* element recognized by a TPA-modulated *trans*-acting factor. *Cell*, 49: 729 – 739.

Bohmann, D., Bos, T.J., Admon, A., Nishimura, T., Vogt, P.K. and Tjian, R. (1987) Human proto-oncogene *c-jun* encodes a DNA-binding protein with structural and functional properties of transcription factor AP-1. *Science*, 238: 1386 – 1392.

Cochran, B.H., Reffel, A.C. and Stiles, C.D. (1983) Molecular cloning of gene sequences regulated by platelet-derived growth factor. *Cell*, 33: 939 – 947.

Cohen, D.R. and Curran, T. (1988) *fra-1*: a serum inducible cellular immediate-early gene that encodes a *fos*-related antigen. *Mol. Cell. Biol.*, 8: 2063 – 2069.

Cohen, D.R., Ferreira, P.C.P., Gentz, R., Franza, B.R., Jr. and Curran, T. (1989) The product of a *fos*-related gene *fra-1* binds cooperatively to the AP-1 site with *jun*: transcription factor AP-1 is comprised of multiple protein complexes. *Genes Dev.*, 3: 173 – 184.

Comb, M., Birnberg, N.C., Seasholtz, A., Herbert, E. and Goodman, H.M. (1986) A cyclic AMP-and phorbol ester-inducible DNA element. *Nature*, 232: 353 – 356.

Curran, T. (1988) The *fos* oncogene. In: E.P. Reddy, A.M. Skalka and T. Curran (Eds.), *The Oncogene Handbook*, Elsevier, Amsterdam, pp. 307 – 325.

Curran, T. and Morgan, J.I. (1985) Superinduction of *c-fos* by nerve growth factor in the presence of peripherally active benzodiazepines. *Science*, 229: 1265 – 1268.

Curran, T. and Morgan, J.I. (1986) Barium modulates *c-fos* expression and post-translational modification. *Proc. Natl. Acad. Sci. U.S.A.*, 83: 8521 – 8524.

Curran, T. and Morgan, J.I. (1987) Memories of *fos*. *BioEssays*, 7: 255 – 258.

Distel, R.J., Ro, H.-S., Rosen, B.S., Groves, D.L. and Spiegelman, B.M. (1987) Nucleoprotein complexes that regulate gene expression in adipocyte differentiation: direct participation of *c-fos*. *Cell*, 49: 835 – 844.

Dragunow, M. and Robertson, H.A. (1987) Kindling stimula-tion induces *c-fos* protein(s) in granule cells of the rat dentate gyrus. *Nature*, 329: 441 – 442.

Franza, B.R., Jr., Rauscher, III, F.J., Josephs, S.F. and Curran, T. (1988) The Fos complex and Fos-related antigens recognize sequence elements that contain AP-1 binding sites. *Science*, 239: 1150 – 1153.

Gentz, R., Rauscher, III, F.J., Abate, C. and Curran, T. (1989) Fos and Jun dimerize through a parallel leucine zipper that juxtaposes DNA-binding domains. *Science*, 243: 1695 – 1699.

Gilman, M.Z. (1988) The *c-fos* serum response element responds to protein kinase C-dependent and -independent signals but not to cyclic AMP. *Genes Dev.*, 2: 394 – 402.

Goelet, P., Castellucci, V.F., Schacher, S. and Kandel, E.R. (1986) The long and short of long-term memory – a molecular framework. *Nature*, 322: 419 – 422.

Greenberg, M.E., Ziff, E.G. and Greene, L.A. (1986) Stimulation of neuronal acetylcholine receptors induces rapid gene transcription. *Science*, 234: 80 – 83.

Hunt, S.P., Pini, A. and Evan, G. (1987) Induction of *c-fos*-like protein in spinal cord neurons following sensory stimulation. *Nature*, 328: 632 – 634.

Landschulz, W.M., Johnson, P.F., Adashi, E.Y., Graves, B.J. and McKnight, S.L. (1988) The leucine zipper: a hypothetical structure common to a new class of DNA-binding proteins. *Science*, 240: 1759 – 1764.

Lau, L.F. and Nathans, D. (1987) Expression of a set of growth-related immediate-early genes in BALB/C 3T3 cells: coordinate regulation with *c-fos* or *c-myc*. *Proc. Natl. Acad. Sci. U.S.A.*, 84: 1182 – 1186.

Lee, W., Haslinger, A., Karin, M. and Tjian, R. (1987a) Two factors that bind and activate the human metallothionein II$_A$ gene in vitro also interact with the SV40 promoter and enhancer regions. *Nature*, 325: 368 – 372.

Lee, W., Mitchell, P. and Tjian, R. (1987b) Purified transcription factor AP-1 interacts with TPA-inducible enhancer elements. *Cell*, 49: 741 – 752.

Lim, R.W., Varnum, B.C. and Herschman, H.R. (1987) Cloning of tetradecanoyl phorbol ester induced "primary response" sequences and their expression in density-arrested Swiss 3T3 cells and a TPA non-proliferative variant. *Oncogene*, 1: 263 – 270.

Montarolo, P.G., Goelet, P., Castellucci, V.F., Morgan, J., Kandel, E.R. and Schacher, S. (1987) A critical period of macromolecular synthesis in long-term heterosynaptic facilitation in *Aplysia*. *Science*, 239: 1249 – 1255.

Morgan, J.I. and Curran, T. (1986) Role of ion flux in control of *c-fos* expression. *Nature*, 322: 552 – 555.

Morgan, J.I. and Curran, T. (1989) *fos* and the immediate-early response in the central nervous system. In: N.H. Colburn (Ed.), *Genes and Signal Transduction in Multistage Carcinogenesis*, Marcel Dekker, New York and Basel, pp. 377 – 390.

Morgan, J.I., Cohen, D.R., Hempstead, J.L. and Curran, T.

294

(1987) Mapping patterns of c-fos expression in the central nervous system after seizure. *Science,* 237: 192 – 197.

Nakabeppu, Y., Ryder, K. and Nathans, D. (1988) DNA-binding activities of three murine *jun* proteins: stimulation by *fos. Cell,* 55: 907 – 915.

Piette, J. and Yaniv, M. (1987) Two different factors bind to the a-domain of the polyoma virus enhancer, one of which also interacts with the SV-40 and c-fos enhancers. *EMBO J.,* 6: 1331 – 1337.

Rauscher, III, F.J., Cohen, D.R., Curran, T., Bos, T.J., Vogt, P.K., Bohmann, D., Tjian, R. and Franza, B.R., Jr. (1988c) Fos-associated protein p39 is the product of the *jun* proto-oncogene. *Science,* 240: 1010 – 1016.

Rauscher, III, F.J., Sambucetti, L.C., Curran, T., Distel, J. and Spiegelman, B.N. (1988b) Common DNA-binding site for Fos protein complexes and transcription factor AP-1. *Cell,* 52: 471 – 480.

Rauscher, III, F.J., Voulalas, P.J., Franza, B.R., Jr. and Curran, T. (1988a) Fos and Jun bind cooperatively to the AP-1 site: reconstitution in vitro. *Genes Dev.,* 2: 1687 – 1699.

Ryder, K., Lau, L.F. and Nathans, D. (1988) A gene activated by growth factors related to the oncogene *v-jun. Proc. Natl.*

Acad. Sci. U.S.A., 85: 1487 – 1491.

Sagar, S.M., Sharp, F.R. and Curran, T. (1988) Expression of c-fos protein in brain: a novel method of neuroanatomic metabolic mapping at the cellular level. *Science,* 240: 1328 – 1331.

Sheng, M., Dougan, S.T., McFadden, G. and Greenberg, M.E. (1988) Calcium and growth factor pathways of c-fos transcriptional activation require distinct upstream regulatory sequences. *Mol. Cell. Biol.,* 8: 2787 – 2796.

Sukhatme, V.P., Cao, X., Chang, L.C., Tsai-Morris, C.H., Stamenkovich, D., Ferreira, P.C.P., Cohen, D.R., Edwards, S.A., Shows, T.B., Curran, T., LeBeau, M.M. and Adamson, E.D. (1988) A zinc-finger encoded gene coregulated with c-fos during growth and differentiation and after cellular depolarization. *Cell,* 53: 37 – 43.

Treisman, R. (1985) Transient accumulation of c-fos RNA following serum stimulation requires a conserved 5′ element and c-fos 3′ sequences. *Cell,* 42: 889 – 902.

White, J.D. and Gall, C.M. (1987) Differential regulation of neuropeptide and proto-oncogene mRNA content in the hippocampus following recurrent seizures. *Mol. Brain Res.,* 3: 21 – 29.

Gene Expression during Normal and Abnormal Neuronal Growth

P. Coleman, G. Higgins and C. Phelps (Eds.)
Progress in Brain Research, Vol. 86
© 1990 Elsevier Science Publishers B.V. (Biomedical Division)

CHAPTER 25

Neuronal responses to injury and aging: lessons from animal models

Donald L. Price[1,2,3,4], Edward H. Koo[1,2,3], Sangram S. Sisodia[1,2], Lee J. Martin[1,2], Vassilis E. Koliatsos[1,2,3], Nancy A. Muma[1,2], Lary C. Walker[1,2] and Linda C. Cork[1,2,5]

Neuropathology Laboratory[1], the Departments of [2]Pathology, [3]Neurology and [4]Neuroscience, and the Division of Comparative Medicine[5], Johns Hopkins University School of Medicine, Baltimore, MD, U.S.A.

Alzheimer's disease (AD), the most common type of adult-onset dementia, is characterized by a variety of brain abnormalities, including degeneration of certain populations of nerve cells, alterations in the neuronal cytoskeleton, and the abnormal deposition of amyloid within brain parenchyma. Pathogenetic processes that lead to these brain abnormalities are difficult to study in humans. Recently, investigators have begun to utilize animal models to examine some of the mechanisms that cause cellular/molecular alterations in transmitter systems, cytoskeletal elements, and APP. These investigations have helped to clarify issues related to the lesions that occur in aged humans and individuals with AD.

Introduction

The complex brain abnormalities of AD involve: degeneration of certain neuronal circuits in brain (Kemper, 1983; Price et al., 1986); perturbations of cytoskeletal elements, particularly in perikarya and distal axons (Anderton et al., 1982; Polinsky, 1984; Brion et al., 1985; Perry et al., 1985; Wischik et al., 1985, 1988a, b; Cork et al., 1986; Grundke-Iqbal et al., 1986; Joachim et al., 1987b; Wolozin and Davies, 1987; Goedert et al., 1988; Love et al., 1988; Kosik, 1989); and alterations in APP that give rise to the deposition of the β-amyloid protein (β/A4) in senile plaques and blood vessels (congophilic angiopathy) (Glenner, 1983; Masters et al., 1985b; Wong et al., 1985; Goldgaber et al., 1987; Kang et al., 1987; Robakis et al., 1987a; Tanzi et al., 1987, 1988; Kitaguchi et al., 1988; Ponte et al., 1988; Selkoe, 1989). The dynamics of these structural/chemical abnormalities are difficult to study in human tissues. Therefore, investigators have begun to use animal models to

delineate some of the mechanisms by which neurons are affected by injury and disease. In this review, we briefly discuss the neuropathological, neurobiological, and molecular abnormalities that occur in the brains of individuals with AD, and we then illustrate the usefulness of animal models in studies of cellular/molecular abnormalities involving transmitter circuits, cytoskeletal elements, and APP.

Alzheimer's disease

Neuronal circuits affected in AD

Basal forebrain cholinergic neurons, which innervate amygdala, hippocampus, and neocortex, are affected in virtually all cases of AD (Price, 1986). These cells develop neurofibrillary tangles (NFT) (Arendt et al., 1988), and their distal axons/nerve terminals contribute neurites to some senile plaques (Armstrong et al., 1986). Cholinergic markers are reduced in target fields of basal forebrain cholinergic neurons (Francis et al.,

1985). In one study (Perry et al., 1982), a discrepancy was noted between the number of cells in the nucleus basalis and the magnitude of reductions in cortical ChAT activity. Thus, at some stage in this degenerative process, it is possible that viable cholinergic neurons may no longer exhibit normal levels of cholinergic markers.

Monoaminergic systems, including cells in the locus coeruleus, raphe complex and ventral tegmental area, show evidence of neuronal degeneration in some cases of AD (Bondareff et al., 1981; Curcio and Kemper, 1984; Mann et al., 1987). Monoaminergic axons and terminals may become enlarged and form neurites in plaques (Berger et al., 1980; Powers et al., 1988), and monoaminergic markers may be reduced in cortex (D'Amato et al., 1987). Reductions in numbers of neurons of the locus coeruleus may correlate with the presence of depression in AD (Zubenko and Moossy, 1988; Zweig et al., 1988).

Pyramidal neurons in hippocampus and in entorhinal cortex consistently develop NFT, Hirano bodies, and granulovacuolar degeneration (Jamada and Mahraein, 1968; Ball, 1977; Kemper, 1983, 1984; Hyman et al., 1986, 1988; Van Hoesen and Damasio, 1987; Powers et al., 1988); eventually, these cells degenerate.

Neocortical neurons, particularly pyramidal neurons, may become atrophic and exhibit NFT (Terry et al., 1981; Kemper, 1984; Pearson et al., 1984; Rogers and Morrison, 1985; Lewis et al., 1987; Morrison et al., 1987; Van Hoesen and Damasio, 1987; Hansen et al., 1988). Smaller cortical neurons utilizing neuropeptides (corticotropin-releasing factor (CRF) or somatostatin) also degenerate (Davies et al., 1980; Rossor et al., 1980; Bissette et al., 1985; Roberts et al., 1985; De Souza et al., 1986), and axons/terminals/dendrites of these cells contribute neurites to plaques (Armstrong et al., 1985; Morrison et al., 1985; Struble et al., 1987; Powers et al., 1987). Somatostatin receptors are reduced (Beal et al., 1985), but CRF receptors may be increased (De Souza et al., 1986). Other peptidergic neurons in neocortex may also contribute neurites to plaques (Kulmala, 1985a, b;

Chan-Palay et al., 1986a, b; Chan-Palay, 1987; Struble et al., 1987).

Cytoskeletal abnormalities

NFT, argyrophilic, intracytoplasmic inclusions in nerve cells, are made up of accumulations of paired helical filaments (PHF) and straight filaments (15 nm in diameter) (Kidd, 1963; Anderton et al., 1982; Brion et al., 1985; Perry et al., 1985, 1987a; Cork et al., 1986; Guiroy et al., 1987; Joachim et al., 1987b; Mori et al., 1987; Wolozin and Davies, 1987). After cell death, these filamentous aggregates persist as extracellular "ghosts" or "tombstones" (Terry, 1963; Wisniewski et al., 1976, 1984; Wischik et al., 1985; Kosik, 1989). The relative insolubility of these filaments has made it difficult to perform traditional protein chemical analyses. Immunocytochemistry and limited biochemical studies have shown that NFT are associated with amino acid sequences derived from: tau; A68; microtubule-associated protein 2; phosphorylated 200-kiloDalton (kDa) polypeptide neurofilament subunit (NF-H); ubiquitin; and, possibly, APP (Anderton et al., 1982; Kosik et al., 1984; Brion et al., 1985; Dickson et al., 1985; Masters et al., 1985a; Perry et al., 1985, 1987a, b; Sternberger et al., 1985; Cork et al., 1986; Goldman and Yen, 1986; Grundke-Iqbal et al., 1986; Kosik et al., 1986; Miller et al., 1986; Wise, 1986; Wood et al., 1986; Gambetti et al., 1987; Guiroy et al., 1987; Joachim et al., 1987a, b; Mori et al., 1987; Wolozin and Davies, 1987; Goedert et al., 1988; Love et al., 1988; Wischik et al., 1988a, b).

Abnormal neurites, associated with deposits of β/A4, are a principal component of plaques. These distended axons, nerve terminals, and dendrites are enlarged with accumulated PHF/straight filaments; they show immunoreactivities for neurofilament proteins, tau, A68, PHF, and ubiquitin (Anderton et al., 1982; Kosik et al., 1984, 1986; Brion et al., 1985; Dickson et al., 1985; Masters et al., 1985a; Perry et al., 1985, 1987a, b; Sternberger et al., 1985; Armstrong et al., 1986; Cork et al., 1986; Goldman and Yen, 1986;

Grundke-Iqbal et al., 1986; Miller et al., 1986; Wise, 1986; Wood et al., 1986; Gambetti et al., 1987; Guiroy et al., 1987; Joachim et al., 1987a, b; Kowall and Kosik, 1987; Mori et al., 1987; Wolozin and Davies, 1987; Goedert et al., 1988; Love et al., 1988; Wischik et al., 1988a, b).

Amyloidogenesis

β/A4, a 4-kDa peptide, is the major component of the extracellular amyloid fibrils in plaques and around blood vessels (Masters et al., 1985a; Wong et al., 1985; Selkoe et al., 1987; Castaño and Frangione, 1988; Selkoe, 1989; Price et al., 1989). β/A4 is a truncated form of APP, a membrane-spanning glycoprotein (Dyrks et al., 1988) encoded by a gene located on chromosome 21 (Goldgaber et al., 1987; Kang et al., 1987; Robakis et al., 1987b; Tanzi et al., 1987). The original 695-residue APP lacks a protease inhibitor domain (APP-695) (Kang et al., 1987), but alternative transcripts (APP-751 and APP-770) code for domains that show homology with proteins in the family of Kunitz protease inhibitors (KPI) (Kitaguchi et al., 1988; Ponte et al., 1988; Tanzi et al., 1988). These mRNAs have tissue-specific distributions (Kitaguchi et al., 1988; Ponte et al., 1988; Tanzi et al., 1988): APP-695 is expressed predominantly in the brain and increases during development (Ponte et al., 1988; Koo et al., 1990b); and APP-751 and APP-770 are expressed in the adult brain as well as in a variety of other organs (Kitaguchi et al., 1988; Ponte et al., 1988; Tanzi et al., 1988). APP-695 and APP-751/770 are actively transcribed by neurons (Bahmanyar et al., 1987; Goedert, 1987; Cohen et al., 1988; Higgins et al., 1988; Koo et al., 1988, 1990a; Palmert et al., 1988). Although β/A4 is readily visualized by immunocytochemistry in the brain in cases of AD, patterns of APP isoforms in human brain have been difficult to demonstrate. However, studies of non-human primates have demonstrated APP in neuronal cell bodies, proximal dendrites, and axons (Martin et al., 1989).

Investigations of the expression of APP mRNAs in brains of individuals with AD have yielded disparate results: RNA blotting studies have shown decreased levels of APP-695 mRNA (Johnson et al., 1988; Neve et al., 1988) and increased levels of APP-770 mRNA (Tanaka et al., 1988); in situ hybridization experiments have demonstrated a selective increase in APP-695 expression in neurons of the nucleus basalis and locus coeruleus, but not in cortical neurons (Palmert et al., 1988). Using an assay based on RNase digestion and S_1 nuclease protection, the relative levels of APP-695 and APP-751/770 mRNAs can be measured within a single sample of RNA. These studies suggest that the relative ratios of APP-751/770:APP-695 mRNAs increase in cases of AD and in age-matched controls (Koo et al., 1990b). These lines of evidence suggest that levels of gene expression alone may not be the principal determinants of amyloidogenesis and focus attention on other processes, including abnormal proteolysis that occurs in proximity to sites of amyloid deposition.

Animal models

Studies of both simple and complex animal model systems have provided new information concerning age- and disease-associated alterations in the biology of transmitters markers, cytoskeletal constituents, and APP.

Transection/ligation of axons in the peripheral and central nervous systems

Simple model systems are very useful for investigations of the biology of neuronal responses to injury. Following axonal injury, the proximal and distal stumps of transected axons become enlarged due to the accumulation of constituents carried by anterograde (proximal side) transport, whereas the distal stump undergoes Wallerian degeneration. The regenerative response of neuronal perikarya is associated with a series of characteristic morphological and biochemical alterations, particularly with regard to transmitter markers and cytoskeletal elements (Hendry, 1976; Price et al., 1984; Hoffman et al., 1985, 1987; Rosenfeld et al., 1987; Goldstein et al., 1988; Koo et al., 1988). This highly reproducible model has been used to study a variety of issues. For example, because APP is a membrane-associated glycoprotein, it appeared likely that this protein may be carried by fast axonal transport, as are other neuronal glycoproteins. Studies of a paradigm of nerve ligation with several immunodetection techniques demonstrated the anterograde transport of APP within peripheral nerves (Koo et al., 1989, 1990b). In brains of individuals with AD, neuronal APP may be delivered to nerve terminals, where abnormal proteolytic processes lead to amyloid deposition within plaques.

The axotomy model can also be used to examine alterations in the regulation of genes important in neurotransmission and cytoskeletal biology. Following crush of rat superior cervical ganglia axons, sympathetic neurons show reversible reductions in levels of tyrosine hydroxylase mRNA (Koo et al., 1988), indicating that the induced decrements in tyrosine hydroxylase enzyme activity are correlated with altered levels of gene expression. Similar alterations in choline acetyltransferase (ChAT) gene expression could explain the postulated reduction of ChAT activity in neurons of the nucleus basalis in cases of AD (Perry et al., 1982). Axotomy is also associated with reductions in neurofilament gene expression (Hoffman et al., 1987; Koo et al., 1989), increased levels of phosphorylated neurofilaments in perikarya (Rosenfeld et al., 1987), and the amount of neurofilament protein entering axons (Hoffman et al., 1985; Tetzlaff et al., 1988). Because transported neurofilament proteins are a major determinant of axonal caliber (Hoffman et al., 1987), decreased levels of neurofilament proteins entering axons are reflected in reductions in axonal caliber (Hoffman et al., 1985). Some of these alterations in neurofilament biology also have been detected in neurons in AD brains.

In the central nervous system, transection of axons in the fimbria-fornix leads to alteration in the properties of medial septal neurons in the basal forebrain cholinergic system. Reductions occur in the size of perikarya and in levels of ChAT immunoreactivity; some perikarya develop abnormal accumulations of phosphorylated neurofilaments. Eventually, some neurons appear to degenerate (Koliatsos et al., 1989). Some of these abnormalities resemble those that occur in basal forebrain cholinergic neurons in AD (Perry et al., 1982; Price, 1986; Price et al., 1987). Thus, transection of the fimbria-fornix provides a model for investigations of degenerative processes involving transmitter-specific pathways in the central nervous system. This model in both rodents and non-human primates should prove very useful for examining the efficacy of human recombinant nerve growth factor in promoting the survival of injured cholinergic nerve cells (Will and Hefti, 1985; Hefti, 1986; Gage et al., 1988; Hagg et al., 1988; Rosenberg et al., 1988; Phelps et al., 1989; Whittemore et al., 1989; Montero and Hefti, 1988).

Behavioral and brain abnormalities in aged non-human primates

Rhesus monkeys are relatively close phylogenetically to humans and have a potential lifespan of > 30 years (Tigges et al., 1988) (equivalent to humans of 90 years of age). With age (> 20 years), non-human primates exhibit a decline in performance on memory tasks examining visual recognition, spatial learning, habit formation, and visuospatial manipulations (Bartus et al., 1983; Presty et al., 1986, 1987; Brickson et al., 1987). As these macaques develop age-associated abnormalities in behavior (Presty et al., 1987; Walker et al., 1988b), they also show some of the neuropathological features that may occur in aged humans, as well as in all subjects with AD (Selkoe et al., 1987; Walker et al., 1988a). The distributions and severities of these lesions vary in different animals of the same age (Struble et al., 1985; Walker et al., 1988b), and it is likely that neuropathological/neurochemical abnormalities underlie some of the behavioral deficits that occur in these animals (Brickson et al., 1987; Presty et al., 1987; Walker et al., 1988b).

The brains of older macaques contain a variety of structural lesions: abnormal patterns of cytoskeletal antigens in some nerve cells; alterations in axons/nerve terminals to form neurites; atrophy and, perhaps, degeneration of neurons; and deposits of amyloid in plaques and around blood vessels. Our studies of age-associated brain abnormalities of non-human primates have led us to outline a hypothetical scenario for the structural alterations that occur in aged non-human primates (Fig. 1).

One of the earliest age-associated alterations of neurons is the appearance of axonal abnormalities and neurites visualized by immunocytochemistry for phosphorylated neurofilaments and transmitter markers, including acetylcholinesterase, ChAT,

dopamine β-hydroxylase, tyrosine hydroxylase, and 5-hydroxytryptamine (Struble et al., 1982, 1984, 1985; Kitt et al., 1984, 1985; Walker et al., 1985, 1987, 1988b). Some of these abnormal axons/nerve terminals form neurites in plaques. These abnormalities may be related to age-associated decrements in certain transmitter markers (Wenk et al., 1989; Wagster et al., 1990).

The cortices of some monkeys contain extracellular deposits of amyloid at the end of the second decade (Struble et al., 1985). Because old monkeys develop senile plaques, they provide a useful model for the study of structural and chemical abnormalities associated with amyloidogenesis. In monkey, APP-695 mRNA has been identified and has 100% amino acid identity with the human APP-695 (Berman-Podlisny et al., 1988). By Northern blotting, APP-751/770 mRNAs can be identified with probes complementary to the human sequence and have molecular weights comparable to human transcripts. APP-695 and APP-751/770 transcripts are present in monkey cortex and are expressed in similar patterns. For example, APP mRNAs are detected in

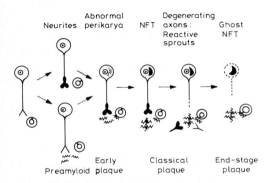

Fig. 1. Hypothetical sequence for the development of some of the structural abnormalities that appear in the brains of aged non-human primates. The vector of temporal evolution procedes from left to right. In normal neurons, transcription and translation occur in perikarya; a variety of proteins are then translocated to target sites by fast and slow transport. For example, APP is rapidly transported in axons, whereas cytoskeletal elements (neurofilament proteins, tau, tubulin, etc.) are transported slowly. Note small blood vessel. The initial age-associated structural abnormalities are still uncertain. Early manifestations of disease appear to be the formation of neurites (i.e., enlarged distal axons and nerve terminals) and the appearance of preamyloid deposits, detected with newly available antibodies to β/A4. The cellular source of amyloid is not known: some investigators believe that β/A4 is derived from APP synthesized in neurons and transported to axons and nerve terminals; others suggest that APP and β/A4 are derived from the bloodstream or from endothelial cells. Early plaques show both neurites and amyloid. APP- and phosphorylated neurofilament-immunoreactive neurites are observed in a subset of plaques that exhibit β/A4 immunoreactivity. Some APP-immunoreactive neurites are capped by deposits of β/A4. The

presence of APP-like immunoreactivity in neuronal perikarya, axons, and some neurites within β/A4-containing plaques provides indirect evidence for a possible neuronal source of some of the amyloid deposited in brains of these aged animals. As the degenerative process continues, axons may degenerate. Some plaque neurites are degenerating elements, whereas others may be reactive sprouts. One source of parenchymal β/A4 may be abnormally processed neurite-derived APP. β/A4 associated with the membrane does not appear to self-assemble into fibrils, and it is likely that self-assembly of amyloid fibrils will only occur when the β/A4 fragment is liberated from neuronal membranes. A cascade of local events involving interactions between degenerating distal neurites, APP isoforms, and other cellular constituents, such as proteases and their inhibitors, presumably play significant roles in the deposition of parenchymal β/A4. At later stages, some neurons develop abnormalities in perikarya, including the presence of tau, phosphorylated neurofilaments, and A68 immunoreactivities. Some cells become atrophic, and NFT develop in a few cells. The final stage of disease is marked by evidence of neuronal degeneration, leaving behind "ghost" tangles and end-stage plaques.

pyramidal neurons of hippocampus, in neurons of the dentate gyrus, and in pyramidal neurons in layers III and V of neocortex. In monkeys 4–35 years of age, the ratios of these transcripts did not change with age. The finding that APP-751/770: APP-695 ratios in brains of monkeys do not change between the first through the fourth decade suggests that relative levels of APP with or without KPI domains are unlikely to be directly related to the deposition of amyloid. Rather, as noted above, it appears more likely that the parenchymal deposition of amyloid may result from local processing of APP. We have observed that APP is transported within axons (Koo et al., 1989, 1990a), and APP-like immunoreactivity is detected in some neurites of plaques (Martin et al., 1989). These neurites are sometimes decorated by a rim of β/A4 immunoreactivity (Martin et al., 1989). Thus, we hypothesize a scenario whereby APP accumulating in these abnormal neurites may be associated with a cascade of events involving interactions between APP-751/770 and APP-695 and other cellular constituents, such as proteases or protease inhibitors, including α-antichymotrypsin (ACT) (Abraham et al., 1989), that alter the processing of APP to form β/A4 in the brain parenchyma. β/A4 not associated with the membrane is highly insoluble (Wong et al., 1985) and spontaneously self-assembles (Masters et al., 1985a) into amyloid fibrils (Castaño et al., 1986; Kirschner et al., 1990). Therefore, the proteolysis of APP results in the release of β/A4 into the neuropil, where it is likely to occur at or near sites of amyloid deposits in brain. Studies of aged non-human primates favor a neuronal origin for parenchymal deposits of β/A4 (Table I). However, it should be emphasized that evidence for a neuronal origin for β/A4 is indirect and does not exclude other sources of amyloid (i.e., APP) derived, in part, from other cells in brain or from the serum (Table I). One interpretation of our findings is that amyloid deposits in the parenchyma may be related to APP derived from neurons, whereas amyloid deposits in blood vessels may arise from other sources. Clearly, more information is needed concerning these processes; studies designed to parallel our investigations of non-human primates will be necessary to clarify the evolution of brain abnormalities that occur in aged humans, older subjects with Down's syndrome, and individuals with AD.

TABLE I

Possible sources of β/A4 in aged non-human primates

Systemic origin	Neuronal origin
APP mRNA and isoforms in some systemic organs	APP mRNAs and isoforms present in neurons
β/A4 deposits outside brain parenchyma (meningeal arteries)	APP transported to distal nerve terminals
Amyloid in capillary walls at centers of some plaques	β/A4 deposited in brain (gray matter, not white matter)
Several circulating proteins (i.e., ACT, etc.) closely associated with β/A4 in plaques	Parenchymal amyloid has an anatomical (laminar) distribution
	APP-positive neurites in proximity to β/A4 deposits plaques)
	Poor correlation between plaques and vascular amyloid

Conclusion

New approaches to investigations of animal models of injury/disease of neurons can provide important information concerning the molecular and cellular processes that lead to age-associated brain abnormalities. These model systems are not only useful for studying pathogenetic mechanisms but should prove very helpful in designing and testing novel biological approaches, including the use of growth factors (Phelps et al., 1989), to prevent or ameliorate disease processes that occur in degenerative disorders of the brain.

Acknowledgements

The authors thank Drs. Axel Unterbeck, Konrad Beyreuther, Dennis J. Selkoe, Carmela R. Abraham and Huntington Potter for helpful discussions.

This work was supported by grants from the U.S. Public Health Service (NIH AG 03359, AG 05146, NS 17079, NS 20471) and funds from The Robert L. and Clara G. Patterson Trust and the American Health Assistance Foundation. Dr. Price is the recipient of a Javits Neuroscience Investigator Award (NIH NS 10580). Drs. Price, Muma, and Koo are recipients of a Leadership and Excellence in Alzheimer's Disease (LEAD) award (NIA AG 07914).

References

Abraham, C.R., Selkoe, D.J., Potter, H., Price, D.L. and Cork, L.C. (1989) α_1-Antichymotrypsin is present together with the β-protein in monkey brain amyloid deposits. *Neuroscience,* 32: 715 – 720.

Anderton, B.H., Breinburg, D., Downes, M.J., Green, P.J., Tomlinson, B.E., Ulrich, J., Wood, J.N. and Kahn, J. (1982) Monoclonal antibodies show that neurofibrillary tangles and neurofilaments share antigenic determinants. *Nature,* 298: 84 – 86.

Arendt, T., Taubert, G., Bigl, V. and Arendt, A. (1988) Amyloid deposition in the nucleus basalis of Meynert complex: a topographic marker for degenerating cell clusters in Alzheimer's disease. *Acta Neuropathol. (Berl.),* 75: 226 – 232.

Armstrong, D.M., LeRoy, S., Shields, D. and Terry, R.D. (1985) Somatostatin-like immunoreactivity within neuritic plaques. *Brain Res.,* 338: 71 – 79.

Armstrong, D.M., Bruce, G., Hersh, L.B. and Terry, R.D. (1986) Choline acetyltransferase immunoreactivity in neuritic plaques of Alzheimer brain. *Neurosci. Lett.,* 71: 229 – 234.

Bahmanyar, S., Higgins, G.A., Goldgaber, D., Lewis, D.A., Morrison, J.H., Wilson, M.C., Shankar, S.K. and Gajdusek, D.C. (1987) Localization of amyloid β protein messenger RNA in brains from patients with Alzheimer's disease. *Science,* 237: 77 – 79.

Ball, M.J. (1977) Neuronal loss, neurofibrillary tangles and granulovacuolar degeneration in the hippocampus with ageing and dementia. A qualitative study. *Acta Neuropathol. (Berl.),* 37: 111 – 118.

Bartus, R.T., Dean, R.L. and Beer, B. (1983) An evaluation of drugs for improving memory in aged monkeys: implications for clinical trials in humans. *Psychopharmacol. Bull.,* 19: 168 – 184.

Beal, M.F., Mazurek, M.F., Tran, V.T., Chattha, G., Bird, E.D. and Martin, J.B. (1985) Reduced numbers of somatostatin receptors in the cerebral cortex in Alzheimer's disease. *Science,* 229: 289 – 291.

Berger, B., Tassin, J.P., Rancurel, G. and Blanc, G. (1980) Catecholaminergic innervation of the human cerebral cortex in presenile and senile dementia – histochemical and biochemical studies. In: E. Usdin, T.L. Sourkes and M.B.H. Youdim (Eds.), *Enzymes and Neurotransmitters in Mental Disease,* Wiley, Chichester, pp. 317 – 328.

Berman-Podlisny, M., Tolan, D. and Selkoe, D. (1988) The monkey homolog of the β-amyloid precursor protein of Alzheimer's disease: isolation of cDNAs and detection of precursor protein. *Soc. Neurosci. Abstr.,* 14: 896.

Bissette, G., Reynolds, G.P., Kilts, C.D., Widerlöv, E. and Nemeroff, C.B. (1985) Corticotropin-releasing factor (CRF)-like immunoreactivity in senile dementia of the Alzheimer type. *JAMA,* 254: 3067 – 3069.

Bondareff, W., Mountjoy, C.Q. and Roth, M. (1981) Selective loss of neurones of origin of adrenergic projection to cerebral cortex (nucleus locus coeruleus) in senile dementia. *Lancet,* i: 783 – 784.

Brickson, M., Bachevalier, J., Watermeier, L.S., Walker, L.C., Struble, R.G., Price, D.L., Mishkin, M. and Cork, L.C. (1987) Performance of aged rhesus monkeys on a visuospatial task. *Soc. Neurosci. Abstr.,* 13: 1627.

Brion, J.P., Van Den Bosch de Aguilar, P. and Flament-Durand, J. (1985) Senile dementia of the Alzheimer type: morphological and immunocytochemical studies. In: J. Traber and W.H. Gispen (Eds.), *Senile Dementia of the Alzheimer Type,* Springer-Verlag, Berlin, pp. 164 – 174.

Castaño, E.M. and Frangione, B. (1988) Biology of disease. Human amyloidosis, Alzheimer disease and related disorders. *Lab. Invest.,* 58: 122 – 132.

Castaño, E.M., Ghiso, J., Prelli, F., Gorevic, P.D., Migheli, A. and Frangione, B. (1986) In vitro formation of amyloid fibrils from two synthetic peptides of different lengths homologous to Alzheimer's disease β-protein. *Biochem. Biophys. Res. Commun.,* 141: 782 – 789.

Chan-Palay, V. (1987) Somatostatin immunoreactive neurons in the human hippocampus and cortex shown by immunogold/silver intensification on vibratome sections: coexistence with neuropeptide Y neurons, and effects in Alzheimer-type dementia. *J. Comp. Neurol.,* 260: 201 – 223.

Chan-Palay, V., Köhler, C., Haesler, U., Lang, W. and Yasargil, G. (1986a) Distribution of neurons and axons immunoreactive with antisera against neuropeptide Y in the normal human hippocampus. *J. Comp. Neurol.,* 248: 360 – 375.

Chan-Palay, V., Lang, W., Heasler, U., Köhler, C. and Yasargil, G. (1986b) Distribution of altered hippocampal neurons and axons immunoreactive with antisera against neuropeptide Y in Alzheimer's-type dementia. *J. Comp. Neurol.*, 248: 376–394.

Cohen, M.L., Golde, T.E., Usiak, M.F., Younkin, L.H. and Younkin, S.G. (1988) In situ hybridization of nucleus basalis neurons shows increased β-amyloid mRNA in Alzheimer disease. *Proc. Natl. Acad. Sci. U.S.A.*, 85: 1227–1231.

Cork, L.C., Sternberger, N.H., Sternberger, L.A., Casanova, M.V., Struble, R.G. and Price, D.L. (1986) Phosphorylated neurofilament antigens in neurofibrillary tangles in Alzheimer's disease. *J. Neuropathol. Exp. Neurol.*, 45: 56–64.

Curcio, C.A. and Kemper, T. (1984) Nucleus raphe dorsalis in dementia of the Alzheimer type: neurofibrillary changes and neuronal packing density. *J. Neuropathol. Exp. Neurol.*, 43: 359–368.

D'Amato, R.J., Zweig, R.M., Whitehouse, P.J., Wenk, G.L., Singer, H.S., Mayeux, R., Price, D.L. and Snyder, S.H. (1987) Aminergic systems in Alzheimer's disease and Parkinson's disease. *Ann. Neurol.*, 22: 229–236.

Davies, P., Katzman, R. and Terry, R.D. (1980) Reduced somatostatin-like immunoreactivity in cerebral cortex from cases of Alzheimer disease and Alzheimer senile dementia. *Nature*, 288: 279–280.

De Souza, E.B., Whitehouse, P.J., Kuhar, M.J., Price, D.L. and Vale, W.W. (1986) Reciprocal changes in corticotropin-releasing factor (CRF)-like immunoreactivity and CRF receptors in cerebral cortex of Alzheimer's disease. *Nature*, 319: 593–595.

Dickson, D.W., Kress, Y., Crowe, A. and Yen, S-.H. (1985) Monoclonal antibodies to Alzheimer neurofibrillary tangles. 2. Demonstration of a common antigenic determinant between ANT and neurofibrillary degeneration in progressive supranuclear palsy. *Am. J. Pathol.*, 120: 292–303.

Dyrks, T., Weidemann, A., Multhaup, G., Salbaum, J.M., Lemaire, H-.G., Kang, J., Müller-Hill, B., Masters, C.L. and Beyreuther, K. (1988) Identification, transmembrane orientation and biogenesis of the amyloid A4 precursor of Alzheimer's disease. *EMBO J.*, 7: 949–957.

Francis, P.T., Palmer, A.M., Sims, N.R., Bowen, D.M., Davison, A.N., Esiri, M.M., Neary, D., Snowden, J.S. and Wilcock, G.K. (1985) Neurochemical studies of early-onset Alzheimer's disease. Possible influence on treatment. *N. Engl. J. Med.*, 313: 7–11.

Gage, F.H., Armstrong, D.M., Williams, D.R. and Varon, S. (1988) Morphological response of axotomized septal neurons to nerve growth factor. *J. Comp. Neurol.*, 269: 147–155.

Gambetti, P., Autilio-Gambetti, L., Manetto, V. and Perry, G. (1987) Composition of paired helical filaments of Alzheimer's disease as determined by specific probes. *Banbury Rep.*, 27: 309–320.

Glenner, G.G. (1983) Alzheimers disease: multiple cerebral amyloidosis. Biological aspects of Alzheimer's disease. *Banbury Rep.*, 15: 137–144.

Goedert, M. (1987) Neuronal localization of amyloid beta protein precursor mRNA in normal human brain and in Alzheimer's disease. *EMBO J.*, 6: 3627–3632.

Goedert, M., Wischik, C.M., Crowther, R.A., Walker, J.E. and Klug, A. (1988) Cloning and sequencing of the cDNA encoding a core protein of the paired helical filament of Alzheimer disease: identification as the microtubule-associated protein tau. *Proc. Natl. Acad. Sci. U.S.A.*, 85: 4051–4055.

Goldgaber, D., Lerman, M.I., McBride, O.W., Saffiotti, U. and Gajdusek, D.C. (1987) Characterization and chromosomal localization of a cDNA encoding brain amyloid of Alzheimer's disease. *Science*, 235: 877–880.

Goldman, J.E. and Yen, S-.H. (1986) Cytoskeletal abnormalities in neurodegenerative diseases. *Ann. Neurol.*, 19: 209–223.

Goldstein, M.E., Weiss, S.R., Lazzarini, R.A., Shneidman, P.S., Lees, J.F. and Schlaepfer, W.W. (1988) mRNA levels of all three neurofilament proteins decline following nerve transection. *Mol. Brain Res.*, 3: 287–292.

Grundke-Iqbal, I., Iqbal, K., Quinlan, M., Tung, Y-.C., Zaidi, M.S. and Wisniewski, H.M. (1986) Microtubule-associated protein tau. A component of Alzheimer paired helical filaments. *J. Biol. Chem.*, 261: 6084–6089.

Guiroy, D.C., Miyazaki, M., Multhaup, G., Fischer, P., Garruto, R.M., Beyreuther, K., Masters, C.L., Simms, G., Gibbs, C.J., Jr. and Gajdusek, D.C. (1987) Amyloid of neurofibrillary tangles of Guamanian parkinsonism-dementia and Alzheimer disease share identical amino acid sequence. *Proc. Natl. Acad. Sci. U.S.A.*, 84: 2073–2077.

Hagg, T., Manthorpe, M., Vahlsing, H.L. and Varon, S. (1988) Delayed treatment with nerve growth factor reverses the apparent loss of cholinergic neurons after acute brain damage. *Exp. Neurol.*, 101: 303–312.

Hansen, L.A., DeTeresa, R., Davies, P. and Terry, R.D. (1988) Neocortical morphometry, lesion counts, and choline acetyltransferase levels in the age spectrum of Alzheimer's disease. *Neurology*, 38: 48–54.

Hefti, F. (1986) Nerve growth factor promotes survival of septal cholinergic neurons after fimbrial transections. *J. Neurosci.*, 6: 2155–2162.

Hendry, I.A. (1976) Effects of axotomy on the trans-synaptic regulation of enzyme activity in adult rat superior cervical ganglia. *Brain Res.*, 107: 105–116.

Higgins, G.A., Lewis, D.A., Bahmanyar, S., Goldgaber, D., Gajdusek, D.C., Young, W.G., Morrison, J.H. and Wilson, M.C. (1988) Differential regulation of amyloid-β-protein mRNA expression within hippocampal neuronal subpopulations in Alzheimer's disease. *Proc. Natl. Acad. Sci. U.S.A.*, 85: 1297–1301.

Hoffman, P.N., Thompson, G.W., Griffin, J.W. and Price, D.L. (1985) Changes in neurofilament transport coincide temporally with alterations in the caliber of axons in regenerating motor fibers. *J. Cell Biol.*, 101: 1332–1340.

Hoffman, P.N., Cleveland, D.W., Griffin, J.W., Landes,

P.W., Cowan, N.J. and Price, D.L. (1987) Neurofilament gene expression: a major determinant of axonal caliber. *Proc. Natl. Acad. Sci. U.S.A.*, 84: 3472 – 3476.

Hyman, B.T., Van Hoesen, G.W., Kromer, L.J. and Damasio, A.R. (1986) Perforant pathway changes and the memory impairment of Alzheimer's disease. *Ann. Neurol.*, 20: 472 – 481.

Hyman, B.T., Van Hoesen, G.W., Wolozin, B.L., Davies, P., Kromer, L.J. and Damasio, A.R. (1988) Alz-50 antibody recognizes Alzheimer-related neuronal changes. *Ann. Neurol.*, 23: 371 – 379.

Jamada, M. and Mehraein, P. (1968) Verteilungsmuster der senilen Veränderungen in Gehirn. Die Beteiligung des limbischen Systems bei hirnatrophischen Prozessen des Seniums und bei Morbus Alzheimer. *Arch. Psychiatr. Z. Neurol.*, 211: 308 – 324.

James, A.E., Jr., Burns, B., Flor, W.F., Strecker, E-.P., Merz, T., Bush, M. and Price, D.L. (1975) Pathophysiology of chronic communicating hydrocephalus in dogs (*Canis familiaris*): experimental studies. *J. Neurol. Sci.*, 24: 151 – 178.

Joachim, C.L., Morris, J.H., Kosik, K.S. and Selkoe, D.J. (1987a) Tau antisera recognize neurofibrillary tangles in a range of neurodegenerative disorders. *Ann. Neurol.*, 22: 514 – 520.

Joachim, C.L., Morris, J.H., Selkoe, D.J. and Kosik, K.S. (1987b) Tau epitopes are incorporated into a range of lesions in Alzheimer's disease. *J. Neuropathol. Exp. Neurol.*, 46: 611 – 622.

Johnson, S.A., Pasinetti, G.M., May, P.C., Ponte, P.A., Cordell, B. and Finch, C.E. (1988) Selective reduction of mRNA for the β-amyloid precursor protein that lacks a Kunitz-type protease inhibitor motif in cortex for Alzheimer brains. *Exp. Neurol.*, 102: 264 – 268.

Kang, J., Lemaire, H-.G., Unterbeck, A., Salbaum, J.M., Masters, C.L., Grzeschik, K-.H., Multhaup, G., Beyreuther, K. and Müller-Hill, B. (1987) The precursor of Alzheimer's disease amyloid A4 protein resembles a cell-surface receptor. *Nature*, 325: 733 – 736.

Kemper, T.L. (1983) Organization of the neuropathology of the amygdala in Alzheimer's disease. Biological aspects of Alzheimer's disease. *Banbury Rep.*, 15: 31 – 35.

Kemper, T.L. (1984) Neuroanatomical and neuropathological changes in normal aging and in dementia. In: M.L. Albert (Ed.), *Clinical Neurology of Aging*, Oxford University Press, New York, pp. 9 – 52.

Kidd, M. (1963) Paired helical filaments in electron microscopy of Alzheimer's disease. *Nature*, 197: 192 – 193.

Kirschner, D.A., Abraham, C. and Selkoe, D.J. (1990) X-ray diffraction from intraneuronal paired helical filaments and extraneuronal amyloid fibers in Alzheimer disease indicates cross-β conformation. *Proc. Natl. Acad. Sci. U.S.A.*, in press.

Kitaguchi, N., Takahashi, Y., Tokushima, Y., Shiojiri, S. and Ito, H. (1988) Novel precursor of Alzheimer's disease amyloid protein shows protease inhibitory activity. *Nature*, 331: 530 – 532.

Kitt, C.A., Price, D.L., Struble, R.G., Cork, L.C., Wainer, B.H., Becher, M.W. and Mobley, W.C. (1984) Evidence for cholinergic neurites in senile plaques. *Science*, 226: 1443 – 1445.

Kitt, C.A. Struble, R.G., Cork, L.C., Mobley, W.C., Walker, L.C., Joh, T.H. and Price, D.L. (1985) Catecholaminergic neurites in senile plaques in prefrontal cortex of aged non-human primates. *Neuroscience*, 16: 691 – 699.

Koliatsos, V.E., Applegate, M.D., Kitt, C.A., Walker, L.C., DeLong, M.R. and Price, D.L. (1989) Aberrant phosphorylation of neurofilaments accompanies transmitter-related changes in rat septal neurons following transection of the fimbria-fornix. *Brain Res.*, 482: 205 – 218.

Koo, E.H., Hoffman, P.N. and Price, D.L. (1988) Levels of neurotransmitter and cytoskeletal mRNAs during nerve regeneration in sympathetic ganglia. *Brain Res.*, 449: 361 – 363.

Koo, E.H., Sisodia, S.S., Archer, D.R., Martin, L.J., Beyreuther, K., Weidemann, A. and Price, D.L. (1989) Amyloid precursor protein (APP) undergoes fast anterograde transport. *Soc. Neurosci. Abstr.*, 15: 23.

Koo, E.H., Sisodia, S.S., Archer, D.R., Martin, L.J., Weidemann, A., Beyreuther, K., Fischer, P., Masters, C.L. and Price, D.L. (1990a) Precursor of amyloid protein in Alzheimer disease undergoes fast anterograde axonal transport. *Proc. Natl. Acad. Sci. U.S.A.*, 87: 1561 – 1565.

Koo, E.H., Sisodia, S.S., Cork, L.C., Unterbeck, A., Bayney, R.M. and Price, D.L. (1990b) Differential expression of amyloid precursor protein mRNAs in cases of Alzheimer's disease and in aged non-human primates. *Neuron*, 2: 97 – 104.

Kosik, K.S. (1989) Minireview: the molecular and cellular pathology of Alzheimer neurofibrillary lesions. *J. Gerontol. Biol. Sci.*, 44: B55 – B58.

Kosik, K.S., Duffy, L.K., Dowling, M.M., Abraham, C., McCluskey, A. and Selkoe, D.J. (1984) Microtubule-associated protein 2: monoclonal antibodies demonstrate the selective incorporation of certain epitopes into Alzheimer neurofibrillary tangles. *Proc. Natl. Acad. Sci. U.S.A.*, 81: 7941 – 7945.

Kosik, K.S., Joachim, C.L. and Selkoe, D.J. (1986) Microtubule-associated protein τ (tau) is a major antigenic component of paired helical filaments in Alzheimer disease. *Proc. Natl. Acad. Sci. U.S.A.*, 83: 4044 – 4048.

Kowall, N.W. and Kosik, K.S. (1987) Axonal disruption and aberrant localization of tau protein characterize the neuropil pathology of Alzheimer's disease. *Ann. Neurol.*, 22: 639 – 643.

Kulmala, H.K. (1985a) Some enkephalin- or VIP-immunoreactive hippocampal pyramidal cells contain neurofibrillary tangles in the brains of aged humans and persons with Alzheimer's disease. *Neurochem. Pathol.,* 3: 41 – 51.

Kulmala, H.K. (1985b) Immunocytochemical localization of enkephalin-like immunoreactivity in neurons of human hippocampal formation: effects of aging and Alzheimer's disease. *Neuropathol. Appl. Neurobiol.,* 11: 105 – 115.

Lewis, D.A., Campbell, M.J., Terry, R.D. and Morrison, J.H. (1987) Laminar and regional distributions of neurofibrillary tangles and neuritic plaques in Alzheimer's disease: a quantitative study of visual and auditory cortices. *J. Neurosci.,* 7: 1799 – 1808.

Love, S., Saitoh, T., Quijada, S., Cole, G.M. and Terry, R.D. (1988) Alz-50, ubiquitin and tau immunoreactivity of neurofibrillary tangles, Pick bodies and Lewy bodies. *J. Neuropathol. Exp. Neurol.,* 47: 393 – 405.

Mann, D.M.A., Yates, P.O. and Marcyniuk, B. (1987) Dopaminergic neurotransmitter systems in Alzheimer's disease and in Down's syndrome at middle age. *J. Neurol. Neurosurg. Psychiatry,* 50: 341 – 344.

Martin, L.J., Cork, L.C., Koo, E.H., Sisodia, S.S., Weidemann, A., Beyreuther, K., Masters, C. and Price, D.L. (1989) Localization of amyloid precursor protein (APP) in brains of young and aged monkeys. *Soc. Neurosci. Abstr.,* 15: 23.

Masters, C.L., Multhaup, G., Simms, G., Pottgiesser, J., Martins, R.N. and Beyreuther, K. (1985a) Neuronal origin of a cerebral amyloid: neurofibrillary tangles of Alzheimer's disease contain the same protein as the amyloid of plaque cores and blood vessels. *EMBO J.,* 4: 2757 – 2763.

Masters, C.L., Simms, G., Weinman, N.A., Multhaup, G., McDonald, B.L. and Beyreuther, K. (1985b) Amyloid plaque core protein in Alzheimer disease and Down syndrome. *Proc. Natl. Acad. Sci. U.S.A.,* 82: 4245 – 4249.

Miller, C.C.J., Brion, J-.P., Calvert, R., Chin, T.K., Eagles, P.A.M., Downes, M.J., Flament-Durand, J., Haugh, M., Kahn, J., Probst, A., Ulrich, J. and Anderton, B.H. (1986) Alzheimer's paired helical filaments share epitopes with neurofilament side arms. *EMBO J.,* 5: 269 – 276.

Montero, C.N. and Hefti, F. (1988) Rescue of lesioned septal cholinergic neurons by nerve growth factor: specificity and requirement for chronic treatment. *J. Neurosci.,* 8: 2986 – 2999.

Mori, H., Kondo, J. and Ihara, Y. (1987) Ubiquitin is a component of paired helical filaments in Alzheimer's disease. *Science,* 235: 1641 – 1644.

Morrison, J.H., Rogers, J., Scherr, S., Benoit, R. and Bloom, F.E. (1985) Somatostatin immunoreactivity in neuritic plaques of Alzheimer's patients. *Nature,* 314: 90 – 94.

Morrison, J.H., Lewis, D.A., Campbell, M.J., Huntley, G.W., Benson, D.L. and Bouras, C. (1987) A monoclonal antibody to non-phosphorylated neurofilament protein marks the vulnerable cortical neurons in Alzheimer's disease. *Brain Res.,* 416: 331 – 336.

Neve, R.L., Finch, E.A. and Dawes, L.R. (1988) Expression of

the Alzheimer amyloid precursor gene transcripts in the human brain. *Neuron,* 1: 669 – 677.

Palmert, M.R., Golde, T.E., Cohen, M.L., Kovacs, D.M., Tanzi, R.E., Gusella, J.F., Usiak, M.F., Younkin, L.H. and Younkin, S.G. (1988) Amyloid protein precursor messenger RNAs: differential expression in Alzheimer's disease; *Science,* 241: 1080 – 1084.

Pearson, R.C.A., Esiri, M.M., Hiorns, R.W., Wilcock, G.K. and Powell, T.P.S. (1985) Anatomical correlates of the distribution of the pathological changes in the neocortex in Alzheimer disease. *Proc. Natl. Acad. Sci. U.S.A.,* 82: 4531 – 4534.

Perry, G., Rizzuto, N., Autilio-Gambetti, L. and Gambetti, P. (1985) Paired helical filaments from Alzheimer disease patients contain cytoskeletal components. *Proc. Natl. Acad. Sci. U.S.A.,* 82: 3916 – 3920.

Perry, G., Friedman, R., Shaw, G. and Chau, V. (1987a) Ubiquitin is detected in neurofibrillary tangles and senile plaque neurites of Alzheimer disease brains. *Proc. Natl. Acad. Sci. U.S.A.,* 84: 3033 – 3036.

Perry, G., Mulvihill, P., Manetto, V., Autilio-Gambetti, L. and Gambetti, P. (1987b) Immunocytochemical properties of Alzheimer straight filaments. *J. Neurosci.,* 7: 3736 – 3738.

Perry, R.H., Candy, J.M., Perry, E.K., Irving, D., Blessed, G., Fairbairn, A.F. and Tomlinson, B.E. (1982) Extensive loss of choline acetyltransferase activity is not reflected by neuronal loss in the nucleus of Meynert in Alzheimer's disease. *Neurosci. Lett.,* 33: 311 – 315.

Phelps, C.H., Gage, F.H., Growdon, J.H., Hefti, F., Harbaugh, R., Johnston, M.V., Khachaturian, Z.S., Mobley, W.C., Price, D.L., Raskind, M., Simpkins, J., Thal, L.J. and Woodcock, J. (1989) Potential use of nerve growth factor to treat Alzheimer's disease. *Neurobiol. Aging,* 10: 205 – 207.

Polinsky, R.J. (1984) Multiple system atrophy. Clinical aspects, pathophysiology, and treatment. *Neurol. Clin.,* 2: 487 – 498.

Ponte, P., Gonzalez-DeWhitt, P., Schilling, J., Miller, J., Hsu, D., Greenberg, B., Davis, K., Wallace, W., Lieberburg, I., Fuller, F. and Cordell, B. (1988) A new A4 amyloid mRNA contains a domain homologous to serine proteinase inhibitors. *Nature,* 331: 525 – 527.

Powers, R.E., Walker, L.C., DeSouza, E.B., Vale, W.W., Struble, R.G., Whitehouse, P.J. and Price, D.L. (1987) Immunohistochemical study of neurons containing corticotropin-releasing factor in Alzheimer's disease. *Synapse,* 1: 405 – 410.

Powers, R.E., Struble, R.G., Casanova, M.F., O'Connor, D.T., Kitt, C.A. and Price, D.L. (1988) Innervation of human hippocampus by noradrenergic systems: normal anatomy and structural abnormalities in aging and in Alzheimer's disease. *Neuroscience,* 25: 401 – 417.

Presty, S.K., Watermeier, L.S., Cork, L.C., Price, D.L., Struble, R.G., Walker, L.C., Bachevalier, J. and Mishkin, M. (1986) Further behavioral evidence of widespread cerebral dysfunction in aged rhesus monkeys *(Macaca mulatta)*. *Soc. Neurosci. Abstr.,* 12: 1312.

Presty, S.K., Bachevalier, J., Walker, L.C., Struble, R.G., Price, D.L., Mishkin, M. and Cork, L.C. (1987) Age differences in recognition memory of the rhesus monkey *(Macaca mulatta)*. *Neurobiol. Aging,* 8: 435 – 440.

Price, D.L. (1986) New perspectives on Alzheimer's disease. *Annu. Rev. Neurosci.,* 9: 489 – 512.

Price, D.L., Koo, E.H. and Unterbeck A. (1989) Cellular and molecular biology of Alzheimer's disease. *BioEssays,* 10: 69 – 74.

Price, D.L., Griffin, J.W., Hoffman, P.N., Cork, L.C. and Spencer, P.S. (1984) The response of motor neurons to injury and disease. In: P.J. Dyck, P.K. Thomas, E.H. Lambert and R. Bunge (Eds.), *Peripheral Neuropathy, Vol. I,* W.B. Saunders, Philadelphia, PA, pp. 732 – 759.

Price, D.L., Altschuler, R.J., Struble, R.G., Casanova, M.F., Cork, L.C. and Murphy, D.B. (1986) Sequestration of tubulin in neurons in Alzheimer's disease. *Brain Res.,* 385: 305 – 310.

Price, D.L., Cork, L.C., Struble, R.G., Kitt, C.A., Walker, L.C., Powers, R.E., Whitehouse, P.J. and Griffin, J.W. (1987) Dysfunction and death of neurons in human degenerative neurological diseases and in animal models. *Ciba Found. Symp.,* 126: 30 – 48.

Robakis, N.K., Ramakrishna, N., Wolfe, G. and Wisniewski, H.M. (1987a) Molecular cloning and characterization of a cDNA encoding the cerebrovascular and the neuritic plaque amyloid peptides. *Proc. Natl. Acad. Sci. U.S.A.,* 84: 4190 – 4194.

Robakis, N.K., Wisniewski, H.M., Jenkins, E.C., Devine-Gage, E.A., Houck, G.E., Yau, X-.L., Ramakrishna, N., Wolfe, G., Silverman, W.P. and Brown, W.T. (1987b) Chromosome 21q21 sublocalisation of gene encoding beta-amyloid peptide in cerebral vessels and neuritic (senile) plaques of people with Alzheimer disease and Down syndrome. *Lancet,* i, 384 – 385.

Roberts, G.W., Crow, T.J. and Polak, J.M. (1985) Location of neuronal tangles in somatostatin neurones in Alzheimer's disease. *Nature,* 314: 92 – 94.

Rogers, J. and Morrison, J.H. (1985) Quantitative morphology and regional and laminar distributions of senile plaques in Alzheimer's disease. *J. Neurosci.,* 5: 2801 – 2808.

Rosenberg, M.B., Friedmann, T., Robertson, R.C., Tuszynski, M., Wolff, J.A., Breakefield, X.O. and Gage, F.H. (1988) Grafting genetically modified cells to the damaged brain: restorative effects of NGF expression. *Science,* 242: 1575 – 1581.

Rosenfeld, J., Dorman, M.E., Griffin, J.W., Gold, B.G., Sternberger, L.A., Sternberger, N.H. and Price, D.L. (1987) Distribution of neurofilament antigens after axonal injury. *J. Neuropathol. Exp. Neurol.,* 46: 269 – 282.

Rossor, M.N., Emson, P.C., Mountjoy, C.Q., Roth, M. and Iversen, L.L. (1980) Reduced amounts of immunoreactive somatostatin in the temporal cortex in senile dementia of Alzheimer type. *Neurosci. Lett.,* 20: 373 – 377.

Selkoe, D.J. (1989) Biochemistry of altered brain proteins in Alzheimer's disease. *Annu. Rev. Neurosci.,* 12: 463 – 490.

Selkoe, D.J., Bell, D.S., Podlisny, M.B., Price, D.L. and Cork, L.C. (1987) Conservation of brain amyloid proteins in aged mammals and humans with Alzheimer's disease. *Science,* 235: 873 – 877.

Sternberger, N.H., Sternberger, L.A. and Ulrich, J. (1985) Aberrant neurofilament phosphorylation in Alzheimer disease. *Proc. Natl. Acad. Sci. U.S.A.,* 82: 4274 – 4276.

Struble, R.G., Cork, L.C., Whitehouse, P.J. and Price, D.L. (1982) Cholinergic innervation in neuritic plaques. *Science,* 216: 413 – 415.

Struble, R.G., Kitt, C.A., Walker, L.C., Cork, L.C. and Price, D.L. (1984) Somatostatinergic neurites in senile plaques of aged non-human primates. *Brain Res.,* 324: 394 – 396.

Struble, R.G., Price, D.L., Jr., Cork, L.C. and Price, D.L. (1985) Senile plaques in cortex of aged normal monkeys. *Brain Res.,* 361: 267 – 275.

Struble, R.G., Powers, R.E., Casanova, M.F., Kitt, C.A., Brown, E.C. and Price, D.L. (1987) Neuropeptidergic systems in plaques of Alzheimer's disease. *J. Neuropathol. Exp. Neurol.,* 46: 567 – 584.

Tanaka, S., Nakamura, S., Ueda, K., Kameyama, M., Shiojiri, S., Takahashi, Y., Kitaguchi, N. and Ito, H. (1988) Three types of amyloid protein precursor mRNA in human brain: their differential expression in Alzheimer's disease. *Biochem. Biophys. Res. Commun.,* 157: 472 – 479.

Tanzi, R.E., Gusella, J.F., Watkins, P.C., Bruns, G.A.P., St George-Hyslop, P., Van Keuren, M.L., Patterson, D., Pagan, S., Kurnit, D.M. and Neve, R.L. (1987) Amyloid β protein gene: cDNA, mRNA distribution, and genetic linkage near the Alzheimer locus. *Science,* 235: 880 – 884.

Tanzi R.E., McClatchey, A.I., Lampert, E.D., Villa-Komaroff, L., Gusella, J.F. and Neve, R.L. (1988) Protease inhibitor domain encoded by a amyloid protein precursor mRNA associated with Alzheimer's disease. *Nature,* 331: 528 – 530.

Terry, R.D. (1963) The fine structure of neurofibrillary tangles in Alzheimer's disease. *J. Neuropathol. Exp. Neurol.,* 22: 629 – 642.

Terry, R.D., Peck, A., DeTeresa, R., Schechter, R. and Horoupian, D.S. (1981) Some morphometric aspects of the brain in senile dementia of the Alzheimer type. *Ann. Neurol.,* 10: 184 – 192.

Tetzlaff, W., Graeber, M.B., Bisby, M.A. and Kreutzberg, G.W. (1988) Increased glial fibrillary acidic protein synthesis in astrocytes during retrograde reaction of the rat facial nucleus. *Glia,* 1: 90 – 95.

Tigges, J., Gordon, T.P., McClure, H.M., Hall, E.C. and Peters, A. (1988) Survival rate and life span of rhesus monkeys at the Yerkes Regional Primate Research Center. *Am. J. Primatol.,* 15: 263 – 273.

308

Van Hoesen, G.W. and Damasio, A.R. (1987) Neural correlates of cognitive impairment in Alzheimer's disease. In: V.B. Mountcastle (Ed.), *Handbook of Physiology, Section 1: The Nervous System, Vol. V, Higher Functions of the Brain, Part 2*, American Physiological Society, Bethesda, MD, pp. 871 – 898.

Wagster, M.V., Whitehouse, P.J., Walker, L.C., Kellar, K.J. and Price, D.L. (1990) Laminar organization and age-related loss of cholinergic receptors in temporal neocortex of rhesus monkey. *J. Neurosci.,* in press.

Walker, L.C., Kitt, C.A., Struble, R.G., Schmechel, D.E., Oertel, W.H., Cork, L.C. and Price, D.L. (1985) Glutamic acid decarboxylase-like immunoreactive neurites in senile plaques. *Neurosci. Lett.,* 59: 165 – 169.

Walker, L.C., Kitt, C.A., Schwam, E., Buckwald, B., Garcia, F., Sepinwall, J. and Price, D.L. (1987) Senile plaques in aged squirrel monkeys. *Neurobiol. Aging,* 8: 291 – 296.

Walker, L.C., Kitt, C.A., Cork, L.C., Struble, R.G., Dellovade, T.L. and Price, D.L. (1988a) Multiple transmitter systems contribute neurites to individual senile plaques. *J. Neuropathol. Exp. Neurol.,* 47: 138 – 144.

Walker, L.C., Kitt, C.A., Struble, R.G., Wagster, M.V., Price, D.L. and Cork, L.C. (1988b) The neural basis of memory decline in aged monkeys. *Neurobiol. Aging,* 9: 657 – 666.

Wenk, G.L., Pierce, D.J., Struble, R.G., Price, D.L. and Cork, L.C. (1989) Age-related changes in multiple neurotransmitter systems in the monkey brain. *Neurobiol. Aging,* 10: 11 – 19.

Whittemore, S.R., Holets, V.R. and Levy, D.J. (1989) Transplantation of a hippocampal, NGF-secreting, temperature-sensitive cell line into adult rats with fimbria-fornix lesions spares cholinergic septal neurons. *Mol. Neurobiol. Neuropharmacol.,* 9: 85.

Will, B. and Hefti, F. (1985) Behavioural and neurochemical effects of chronic intraventricular injections of nerve growth factor in adult rats with fimbria lesions. *Behav. Brain Res.,* 17: 17 – 24.

Wischik, C.M., Crowther, R.A., Stewart, M. and Roth, M. (1985) Subunit structure of paired helical filaments in Alzheimer's disease. *J. Cell Biol.,* 100: 1905 – 1912.

Wischik, C.M., Novak, M., Edwards, P.C., Klug, A., Tichelaar, W. and Crowther, R.A. (1988a) Structural characterization of the core of the paired helical filament of Alzheimer disease. *Proc. Natl. Acad. Sci. U.S.A.,* 85: 4884 – 4888.

Wischik, C.M., Novak, M., Thogersen, H.C., Edwards, P.C., Runswick, M.J., Jakes, R., Walker, J.E., Milstein, C., Roth, M. and Klug, A. (1988b) Isolation of a fragment of tau derived from the core of the paired helical filament of Alzheimer disease. *Proc. Natl. Acad. Sci. U.S.A.,* 85: 4506 – 4510.

Wise, P.M. (1986) Changes in the central nervous system and neuroendocrine control of reproduction in males and females. In: L. Mastroianni Jr. and C.A. Paulsen (Eds.), *Aging, Reproduction, and the Climacteric,* Plenum, New York, pp. 81 – 95.

Wisniewski, H.M., Narang, H.K. and Terry, R.D. (1976) Neurofibrillary tangles of paired helical filaments. *J. Neurol. Sci.,* 27: 173 – 181.

Wisniewski, H.M., Merz, P.A. and Iqbal, K. (1984) Ultrastructure of paired helical filaments of Alzheimer's neurofibrillary tangle. *J. Neuropathol. Exp. Neurol.,* 43: 643 – 656.

Wolozin, B. and Davies, P. (1987) Alzheimer-related neuronal protein A68: specificity and distribution. *Ann. Neurol.,* 22: 521 – 526.

Wong, C.W., Quaranta, V. and Glenner, G.G. (1985) Neuritic plaques and cerebrovascular amyloid in Alzheimer disease are antigenically related. *Proc. Natl. Acad. Sci. U.S.A.,* 82: 8729 – 8732.

Wood, J.G., Mirra, S.S., Pollock, N.J. and Binder, L.I. (1986) Neurofibrillary tangles of Alzheimer disease share antigenic determinants with the axonal microtubule-associated protein tau (τ). *Proc. Natl. Acad. Sci. U.S.A.,* 83: 4040 – 4043.

Zubenko, G.S. and Moossy, J. (1988) Major depression in primary dementia: clinical and neuropathologic correlates. *Arch. Neurol.,* 45: 1182 – 1186.

Zweig, R.M., Ross, C.A., Hedreen, J.C., Steele, C., Cardillo, J.E., Whitehouse, P.J., Folstein, M.F. and Price, D.L. (1988) The neuropathology of aminergic nuclei in Alzheimer's disease. *Ann. Neurol.,* 24: 233 – 242.

P. Coleman, G. Higgins and C. Phelps (Eds.)
Progress in Brain Research, Vol. 86
© 1990 Elsevier Science Publishers B.V. (Biomedical Division)

CHAPTER 26

GAP-43 as a marker for structural plasticity in the mature CNS

Larry I. Benowitz[1,3,5,*], Nora I. Perrone-Bizzozero[1,5], Rachael L. Neve[2,3,4] and William Rodriguez[5]

Departments of [1] Psychiatry, [2] Pediatrics and [3] Program in Neuroscience, Harvard Medical School, and [4]Children's Hospital, Boston, MA; and [5]Mailman Research Center, McLean Hospital, Belmont, MA, U.S.A.

Introduction

Although most of the major events of brain development are completed shortly after birth (Jacobson, 1978), more subtle changes in the structural organization of the nervous system continue to occur later in life. Such changes have been demonstrated experimentally as a consequence of prolonged sensory stimulation or deprivation (Greenough and Bailey, 1988), drug treatments (Benes et al., 1985), brain lesions that induce a reactive growth of processes in remaining neurons (Cotman and Nieto-Sampedro, 1984), and even relatively brief behavioral or physiological stimuli (Greenough and Bailey, 1988). An understanding of the cellular and molecular processes that underlie such instances of plasticity is essential for untangling the mystery of how learning occurs; how and where memories are stored; and how the nervous system responds, or fails to respond, to acute injury, normal atrophy, and to pathological processes, as in Alzheimer's or Huntington's disease.

In the following sections, we will describe the involvement of one particular protein in mediating plasticity in the nervous system. This protein was

discovered independently in several laboratories, which implicated it in a range of phenomena that include neuronal regeneration and development, growth cone motility, signal transduction, phospholipid metabolism, calmodulin-binding, and synaptic potentiation. Accordingly, a variety of names were assigned to it, including GAP-43, 48K4.8 (or GAP-48), B-50, F1, pp46, protein 4, and P-57 (neuromodulin). The recognition that these all represent the same molecule (reviewed in Benowitz and Routtenberg, 1987) generated a good deal of excitement that this protein might provide insights for understanding the neurobiology of synaptic development and plasticity. For the sake of simplicity, we will refer to this protein throughout as GAP-43, though it should be acknowledged that much of what is known about it comes from laboratories investigating its properties under other guises.

GAP-43 in the development and regeneration of neuronal connections

To investigate biological underpinnings of plasticity in the vertebrate nervous system, we began about 10 years ago to examine an example of structural growth and synaptogenesis that had already been well-characterized at the cellular and physiological levels. Unlike higher vertebrates, fish and

* Current address: Department of Neurosurgery, Harvard Medical School, Children's Hospital, Boston, MA 02115, U.S.A.

amphibia retain the capacity to regenerate damaged pathways of the central nervous system throughout life. One instance of this, which happens to offer a number of experimental advantages, is the regeneration of the goldfish optic nerve. Following damage to the nerve, massive changes begin to appear in the retinal ganglion cells (enlargement of the soma, translocation of the nucleus, proliferation of ribosomes); regenerating optic axons begin to grow out within a few days, reach their targets in the midbrain optic tectum in about two weeks, and begin forming synapses with the appropriate post-synaptic cells after a delay of several days (reviewed in Grafstein, 1986). By injecting radioactive precursors into the eye and then examining the pattern of labeled proteins transported down the growing axons, we were able to identify a group of proteins associated with various stages of the regenerative process. The most striking change noted in these studies was a 100-fold increase in the synthesis of a highly acidic protein that is associated with the nerve terminal membrane, and which had an apparent molecular size of 44 – 48 kDa (Benowitz et al., 1981, 1983; Benowitz and Lewis, 1983). Studies by Skene and Willard (1981a, b) produced identical findings in the regenerating optic nerve of the toad, and also demonstrated high levels of this protein in other developing and regenerating systems, but not in nerves that fail to regenerate. Based on these observations, this protein was given the name GAP-43, a Growth-Associated Protein with an apparent size of 43 kDa (later studies showed that this protein migrates anomalously on SDS gels and has a true size of 24 kDa).

A proliferation of further studies showed that GAP-43 is a ubiquitous, developmentally-regulated phosphoprotein associated with the nerve terminal membrane. GAP-43 is expressed at high levels by all neurons as soon as they begin growing processes in culture (Fig. 1; Perrone-Bizzozero et al., 1986) and by pheochromocytoma cells induced to differentiate by nerve-growth factor (NGF) (Van Hooff et al., 1986; Karns et al., 1987; Federoff et al., 1988). The protein is abundant along the entire length of axons as they are elongating, becomes increasingly restricted to growth cones and immature synapses as development proceeds, then disappears abruptly from most nerve terminals (Meiri et al., 1986, 1988; Oestreicher and Gispen, 1986; Goslin et al., 1988; McGuire et al., 1988; Moya et al., 1988, 1989). In growth cones, GAP-43 is a major constituent of the membrane (De Graan et al., 1985; Katz et al., 1985; Skene et al., 1986), whereas in mature presynaptic membranes, its concentration is 1 – 2 orders of magnitude lower, though it is still quite evident (Zwiers et al., 1980; Nelson and Routtenberg, 1985; Jacobson et al., 1986).

The time at which GAP-43 levels decline coincides with the end of the so-called *critical period* or *sensitive period* of development, at which time the pattern of neuronal connections becomes relatively fixed, and less amenable to being altered by physiological activity. In the regenerating goldfish optic pathway, for example, physiological manipulations that impede the normal transmission of information down the optic nerve will alter the precise pattern of the retinotectal projection if applied within the first month or so after the optic

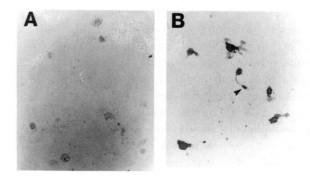

Fig. 1. GAP-43 is expressed by neurons during differentiation. Quiescent neurons from the embryonic rat cortex do not extend axons or dendrites and fail to express GAP-43 when maintained in culture with a hormone supplement but no serum (*A*). When serum is added, neurons begin to extend processes and show strong GAP-43 immunoreactivity (dark reaction product in *B*; arrow points to a growth cone). Cells were stained using a monospecific antibody for GAP-43 (Perrone-Bizzozero et al., 1986; K.L. Moya, N.I. Perrone-Bizzozero, P.J. Apostolides, L.I. Benowitz, unpublished observations).

nerve has returned, but will be ineffective if applied afterwards (Schmidt, 1985). This sensitive period coincides with the time in which GAP-43 levels remain elevated in the regenerated optic fibers before returning to low baseline levels (Benowitz and Schmidt, 1987). Likewise, in developing mammalian sensory pathways, levels of GAP-43 and its mRNA are high throughout the period of synaptic organization, then decline sharply. This has been shown for the rat brain as a whole (Jacobson et al., 1986; McGuire et al., 1988) and for specific pathways in which the critical period has been established, including the hamster retinotectal projection (Moya et al., 1988, 1989), the cat striate cortex (McIntosh et al., 1988; Neve and Bear, 1988; Benowitz et al., 1989a), and the hamster pyramidal tract (Kalil and Skene, 1986). It is quite possible that GAP-43 may itself contribute to the capacity of the nerve terminal membrane to change its functions or structure in response to the impingent activity pattern, a possibility that is reinforced by the physiological and biochemical findings reviewed below.

GAP-43 may link physiological activity to changes in nerve terminal structure

Protein phosphorylation has long been thought to play a role in bringing about the rapid changes in the function and structure of the nerve terminal that occur in response to various stimuli (Kandel and Schwartz, 1982; Nestler and Greengard, 1984; Gispen and Routtenberg, 1986). GAP-43 is in fact one of the most abundant phosphoproteins of the growth cone membrane (De Graan et al., 1985; Katz et al., 1985; Meiri et al., 1986; Skene et al., 1986), where its phosphorylation can be regulated by calcium and phospholipids (Fig. 2; Meiri et al., 1988; Van Hooff et al., 1988). While some evidence suggests that GAP-43 phosphorylation in growth cones and mature synapses may also be regulated by other factors (Katz et al., 1985; Pisano et al., 1988; Simkowitz et al., 1989), the protein kinase C-mediated phosphorylation on serine 41 is particularly well-established (Coggins and Zwiers, 1988; Schrama et al., 1988).

One likely role for GAP-43 in the synapse is in

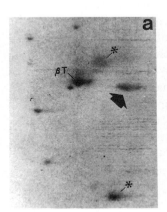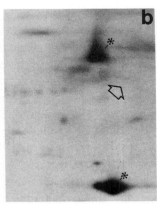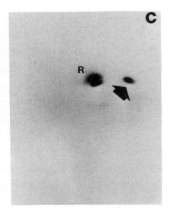

Fig. 2. GAP-43 is one of the principal proteins transported to developing nerve endings, but levels decline in most neurons shortly after birth. In the visual system of the hamster, GAP-43 is one of the major proteins that is synthesized in the retinal ganglion cells and conveyed (by rapid axonal transport) to growth cones and immature synapses up through the first week after birth (dark arrow in *a*). After the second postnatal week, it becomes undetectable (open arrow in *b*). By labeling synaptic membranes from the neonate rat with radioactive ATP, GAP-43 is seen to be one of the major nerve-terminal phosphoproteins (closed arrow in *c*). Asterisks in *a* and *b* show proteins which, unlike GAP-43, *increase* during development. R and βT point to two reference proteins in the gels (from Moya et al., 1988; and unpublished observations).

the modulation of phospholipid metabolism. Two of the major signal transduction pathways of the nerve terminal membrane involve phospholipid metabolism and the regulation of free calcium levels. Changes in intracellular free calcium can result either from an influx of extracellular calcium or from the release of calcium from intracellular stores in the endoplasmic reticulum. The latter release mechanism is regulated by the binding of inositol triphosphate (IP_3), which is generated from the receptor-mediated hydrolysis of phosphatidylinositol 4,5-bisphosphate (PIP_2) by the enzyme phospholipase C. This hydrolysis also gives rise to a second important intracellular signal, diacylglycerol (DAG), which directly activates protein kinase C (Nishizuka, 1983; Berridge and Irvine, 1984). In purifying GAP-43, it was discovered that it is tightly associated both with its own kinase, protein kinase C, as well as with phosphatidylinositol phosphate (PIP) kinase, the enzyme responsible for the formation of PIP_2 from the precursor PIP (Jolles et al., 1980). Phosphorylation of GAP-43 was shown to inhibit the activity of PIP kinase, thus limiting the amount of PIP_2 available for hydrolysis to form DAG and IP_3 (and hence limiting both the activation of protein kinase C and the release of calcium from the endoplasmic reticulum; see Jolles et al., 1980). Conversely, antibodies to GAP-43 result in an activation of the PIP kinase and an increase in PIP_2 levels (Oestreicher et al., 1983). One consequence of this pathway is that the phosphorylation of GAP-43 would be self-limiting, since decreased diacylglycerol levels resulting from less PIP_2 would decrease the activity of protein kinase C. However, this mechanism could have other physiological effects on the nerve terminal membrane, since many key events are regulated by calcium-calmodulin and calcium-phospholipid dependent kinases.

A second possible way in which GAP-43 phosphorylation may regulate the properties of the nerve terminal membrane is through its association with calmodulin. The protein calmodulin binds calcium, and this complex in turn interacts with a variety of molecules, including various enzymes, to regulate their function. Unlike other proteins that bind to calmodulin only in the *presence* of calcium, GAP-43 has the unique property of binding calmodulin in the *absence* of calcium (Alexander et al., 1987). It has been proposed that one role of GAP-43 might be to sequester calmodulin locally at certain sites of the nerve terminal membrane. When calcium levels rise, calmodulin would then be released to activate other molecules, such as the calcium-calmodulin-dependent kinases. The association of GAP-43 with calmodulin occurs only when GAP-43 is in the dephosphorylated state (Alexander et al., 1987). Hence, at the same time as GAP-43 phosphorylation would decrease the activity of the PIP kinase, it would also have the effect of liberating calmodulin.

From another perspective, calmodulin could be seen as acting upon GAP-43. Calmodulin binding decreases the rate of phosphorylation of GAP-43 by protein kinase C (Alexander et al., 1987) and would therefore influence other downstream effects of GAP-43, including the regulation of PIP metabolism. The ultimate consequence of these events for the physiological state of the membrane is presently unknown. Nevertheless, these findings suggest that at least one way in which GAP-43 regulates the functions and/or structure of the nerve terminal is by coordinating the activity of the major kinase systems of the membrane.

Changes in the phosphorylation state of GAP-43 can be brought about by a number of physiological signals. In isolated synaptosomes, neurons growing in culture, or in hippocampal slices, changes in GAP-43 phosphorylation can be induced by phorbol esters (which substitute for diacylglycerol to activate protein kinase C), or by membrane depolarization, as would happen following the invasion of the nerve terminal by action potentials (Meiri et al., 1988; Schrama et al., 1988; Dekker et al., 1989). Phosphorylation of GAP-43 in turn correlates with increases in transmitter release (Dekker et al., 1989), suggesting that the protein could participate in regulating either ion fluxes (e.g., decreasing K^+ efflux or increasing Ca^{2+} influx) in the nerve ending, vesicle translocation, or vesicle fusion. The latter possibility is particularly intriguing since it might likewise be important for membrane addition during growth. In any event, the fact that GAP-43 phosphorylation occurs in response to physiological signals indicates that the protein is in a position to transduce patterns of activity into changes in the structure or function of the membrane.

The role of GAP-43 in synaptic potentiation

An important link between synaptic plasticity and signal transduction is the finding that changes in GAP-43 phosphorylation take place in synapses that show a long-term enhancement of their firing properties. Such long-term enhancement (or long-term potentiation), which can be demonstrated most readily in the hippocampus, has been widely studied as a model for the synaptic changes that may take place during learning. When the perforant pathway projection (from the entorhinal cortex to the dentate gyrus) is briefly stimulated at a high frequency, the firing properties of the activated synapses show a long-lasting increase in their subsequent responsiveness (Bliss and Lømo, 1973). The intensity and duration of the enhanced responsiveness correlates closely with the increased phosphorylation of GAP-43 (Akers and Routtenberg, 1985; Nelson and Routtenberg, 1985; Melchers et al., 1988). Underlying this change is a translocation of protein kinase C from the cytosol to the synaptic membrane, where it may bind to GAP-43 and other substrate proteins and cause a persistent increase in their phosphorylation (Akers et al., 1986).

Although events mediated by protein kinase C are important for the *persistence* of long-term potentiation, the *initiation* of this phenomenon requires the activation of the NMDA class of glutamate receptors, which are predominantly *post-synaptic* (Collingridge and Bliss, 1987). This activation must then somehow feed information back to the pre-synaptic membrane, where GAP-43 phosphorylation occurs. Although the nature of this feedback mechanism is unknown, evidence that it is likely to occur comes from the findings

that LTP causes a long-lasting increase in the release of the transmitter glutamate from perforant pathway synapses, which is *pre-synaptic* (Bliss et al., 1986), and that blockade of the *post-synaptic* NMDA receptors, using the specific antagonist aminophosphovalerate (APV), blocks the *pre-synaptic* phosphorylation of GAP-43 (Linden et al., 1988). The involvement of GAP-43 with synaptic development would suggest that the phosphorylation changes seen during LTP might be related to structural changes in pre-synaptic elements of the perforant pathway projection (Nelson and Routtenberg, 1985); conversely, the changes in GAP-43 phosphorylation that accompany LTP may afford insights into the role that the protein plays in transducing physiological stimuli during synaptic development (e.g., membrane turnover; Benowitz and Routtenberg, 1987).

GAP-43 is involved in structural remodeling in the adult CNS

Further evidence that GAP-43 participates in structural changes in the mature brain comes from studies implicating this protein in known examples of synaptic remodeling. One well-characterized instance of such remodeling is the reactive synaptogenesis that occurs in the hippocampal formation following lesions of the perforant pathway. These lesions remove the input from the entorhinal cortex onto the outer dendritic segments of the dentate granule cells. This induces other afferents to the dentate gyrus to sprout collateral branches which form synapses onto denervated portions of the granule cell dendrites (Cotman and Nieto-Sampedro, 1984). By immunocytochemistry, we find that the sprouting of the commissural-associational fibers, i.e., the projection that arises from the pyramidal cells of the hilus and CA3 regions of the hippocampus, is accompanied by massive increases in GAP-43 levels which persist for up to a month (Fig. 3; Benowitz et al., 1990; Norden et al., 1988). A somewhat surprising aspect of this reactive sprouting is that other axonal projections of the same hilar and CA3 neurons, such

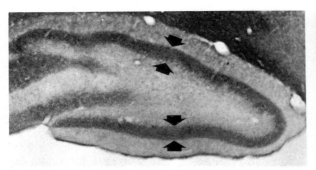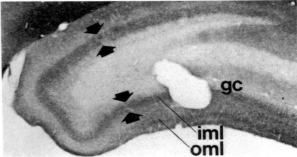

Fig. 3. GAP-43 is involved in the formation of new synapses in the adult central nervous system. After damaging the projections from the rat entorhinal cortex to the dentate gyrus, other neurons that project to the latter region sprout axon collaterals and form new synapses on dendritic segments denervated by the lesion (Cotman and Nieto-Sampedro, 1984). Following unilateral surgery, the intensity of GAP-43 immunostaining is considerably greater in the expanded inner molecular layer (iml, bounded by dark arrows) of the dentate gyrus ipsilateral to the lesion (left) than on the control side (right). Other abbreviations: oml, outer molecular layer of the dentate gyrus; gc, granule cell layer. (Adapted from Benowitz et al., 1990.)

as those to the *contralateral* dentate gyrus, also show significant increases in GAP-43. This implies that a neuron induced to remodel some of its terminals indiscriminately alters the pattern of proteins transported down to its other branches as well, which may have the fortuitous (and perhaps maladaptive) consequence of restructuring *all* of its connections. Another instance of this lack of selectivity is seen after peripheral nerve injury. Following injury to a peripheral nerve, the pseudounipolar neurons of the dorsal root ganglion undergo a series of changes that culminates in the regeneration of the damaged axon. This regeneration is marked by massive increases in the levels of GAP-43 (and its mRNA) synthesized in the ganglionic neuron and transported down to the regenerating nerve endings (Skene and Willard, 1981a, b; Redshaw and Bisby, 1984; Hoffman, 1989). Recent studies also point to a massive increase in the levels of protein transported down the non-regenerating *central* branch of these neurons (Schreyer and Skene, 1988; Woolf et al., 1990; Erzurumlu et al., 1989). If centrally-directed GAP-43 is associated with structural remodeling in the dorsal horn or dorsal column nuclei, this could alter the representation of sensory information at all higher levels of the neuraxis, and might help explain, for example, hyperalgesia following peripheral nerve damage.

One other instance of GAP-43 increasing in the mature nervous system comes from post-mortem studies on individuals who had sustained a stroke prior to the time of death. Levels of GAP-43 mRNA are considerably increased in the vicinity of the infarct, suggesting that neurons projecting to the damaged area may have begun to sprout collateral branches (Ng et al., 1988). This possibility is reinforced by the aforementioned studies of sprouting in the rat hippocampal formation.

Distribution of GAP-43 in the adult nervous system

The previous sections have reviewed evidence linking GAP-43 with changes in synaptic structure and function. Given this background, it seems possible that those neurons that continue to have high levels of the protein throughout life may retain the capacity to alter their synaptic relationships in response to physiological stimuli (Benowitz and Routtenberg, 1987; Nelson et al., 1987). In all species examined to date (rat, mouse, hamster, cat, rhesus monkey, human), the picture that emerges is that GAP-43 and its mRNA are abundant throughout the neuraxis at early stages of development, then become increasingly restricted to the forebrain shortly after birth, and remain concentrated almost exclusively in higher integrative areas, rather than in primary sensory and motor regions (Nelson et al., 1987; Neve et al., 1987, 1988; Benowitz et al., 1988, 1989a; Dani et al., 1988; McGuire et al., 1988; McIntosh et al., 1988; Moya et al., 1989; studies in preparation with P.J. Apostolides, D. Armstrong, L. Benowitz, M. Cynader, J. Dani, R. Erzurumlu, J. Gossels, S. Haber, S. Jhaveri, H. Kinney, G. Prusky, L. Rava, W. Rodriguez, S. Roffler-Tarlov). Nowhere are the regional differences as dramatic, however, as in the human brain. As in other species, GAP-43 and its mRNA are high in all parts of the fetal human brain, but in the adult nervous system they are almost entirely absent from most of the brain stem, primary sensory areas of the forebrain (e.g., striate and peristriate cortex, postcentral gyrus), and motor areas (e.g., the precentral gyrus). However, GAP-43 continues to be abundant in certain synaptic endings of the hippocampus, associative and limbic areas of the neocortex (e.g., frontal, perisylvian, and inferior temporal cortex) and a few limbic and integrative subcortical structures (e.g., amygdala, caudate-putamen) (Fig. 4; Neve et al., 1987, 1988; Benowitz et al., 1989b).

By in situ hybridization, we have found that the small pyramidal cells that lie within layer II of associative areas of the neocortex, along with the CA3 pyramidal cells of the hippocampus, express the highest levels of GAP-43 mRNA (Fig. 5; Neve et al., 1988). These results are intriguing from the neurobehavioral perspective, since brain-damaged patients who have had injuries restricted to sensory and motor areas of the brain will not suffer major losses in intellectual abilities or mental associations, whereas patients with lesions of the hippocampus and non-somatosensory-specific areas of the neocortex will. Moreover, the observation that it is the layer II pyramidal cells that synthesize highest levels of GAP-43 is also quite interesting; it has long been suspected that plasticity underlying information storage is likely to involve locally-projecting neurons, such as the layer II cells, rather than neurons involved in the initial receipt of in-

formation (e.g., layer IV stellate cells) or long-distance communication with other parts of the brain (e.g., the larger pyramidal cells of layers III and V), where changes would have a non-specific effect on all input – output relationships. By immunocytochemistry, highest levels of the protein are seen in the marginal layer (i.e., layer I) and within layer VI of the same cortical areas that have high levels of the mRNA, consistent with the known projections of layer II pyramidal cells.

In the hippocampus, the protein is most abundant in the dendritic fields of the CA1 region and in the dentate gyrus molecular layer, as would be predicted from the presence of the mRNA in CA3 neurons (which project to the CA1 region via the Schaeffer collaterals) and in pyramidal cells of the entorhinal cortex that give rise to the perforant pathway. Although the hippocampus unquestionably plays a central role in the initial consolidation of memories, it is not likely to be a major repository of long-term memories; this is indicated by the relative preservation of information acquired prior to hippocampal injury (Squire and Zola-Morgan, 1988). We would like to imagine that the functional and structural reorganization underlying long-term memory storage take place within those synapses of particular associative neocortical laminae in which we have visualized highest levels of GAP-43.

Perspectives for aging and dementia

As mentioned in the introductory comments, structural remodeling is of relevance in the normal adult human brain and in pathological conditions for two reasons. First, normal information storage and its pathology might involve structural changes in specific synapses. Second, in response to normal atrophy, acute injury, or degenerative disorders, the loss of some neuronal connections or the development of abnormal foci of trophic activity could induce a reactive sprouting in other neurons. The evidence that GAP-43 may participate in both types of structural remodeling comes from studies showing that phosphorylation changes in the pro-

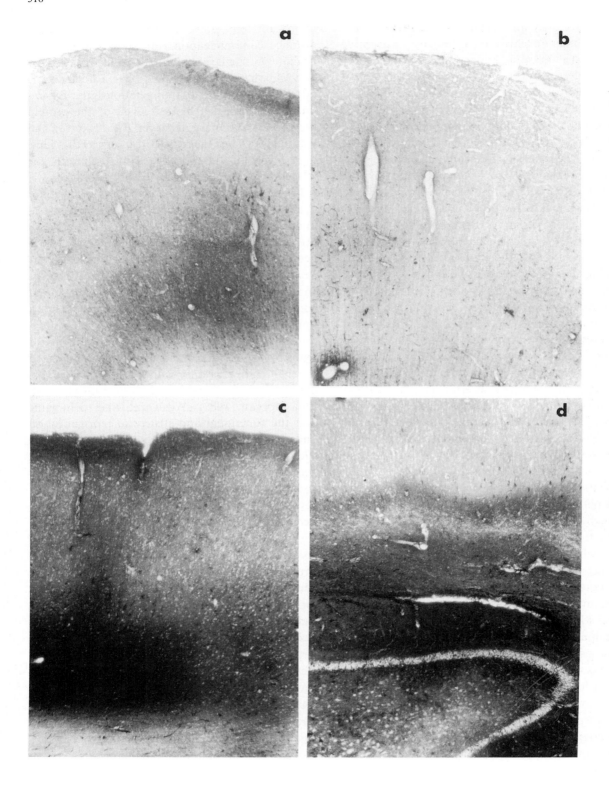

tein accompany the persistent changes in synaptic efficacy that take place during long-term potentiation, and the findings that levels of GAP-43 increase appreciably in known instances of synaptic growth. With aging, changes in the overall levels, distribution, or phosphorylation of GAP-43 could have severe consequences on memory, and longitudinal studies in the rat indicate that such changes

do occur (Lovinger et al., 1986; Oestreicher et al., 1987). In Alzheimer's disease, pathological changes occur more readily in associative areas of the neocortex and hippocampus than in sensory or motor areas, hence affecting those areas where GAP-43 is normally the highest. Alzheimer's disease is also marked by synaptic rearrangements in the dentate gyrus similar to those that follow entorhinal lesions in rats, and this rearrangement in Alzheimer's disease is likewise accompanied by changes in the pattern of GAP-43 immunostaining (J. Hamos, P.J. Apostolides, W. Rodriguez and L. Benowitz, unpublished observations). Cerebral infarcts are also likely to cause a reactive growth of nearby neurons, and increases in GAP-43 mRNA in such regions have been demonstrated (Ng et al., 1988). Such changes may be either restorative or maladaptive if inappropriate connections develop.

At the present time, GAP-43 would appear to be a well-validated marker for plasticity in the nervous system. Beyond this, a more detailed understanding of the role that this protein plays is likely to advance our comprehension of synaptic plasticity. As reviewed above, changes in the phosphorylation state of GAP-43 come about in response to physiological signals at the nerve terminal, persist in parallel with long-term synaptic potentiation, and are linked to specific biochemical changes in the synapse. However, the ultimate consequences of these changes on the function and structure of the nerve terminal membrane remain to be clarified. It will also be of considerable interest to understand how the expression of the GAP-43 gene is regulated, in order to understand better why certain neurons may be more plastic than others, and to suggest ways in which the gene might be turned on after injury to allow for some degree of functional restoration. Nevertheless, the convergent discoveries by many laboratories over the past ten years concerning GAP-43 have put us

GAP-43

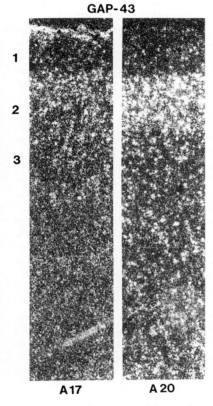

Fig. 5. GAP-43 is synthesized in locally-projecting pyramidal cells of the associative neocortex. By in situ hybridization, only low levels of GAP-43 messenger RNA are seen in primary sensory and motor areas, such as the striate cortex (Area 17, left); far greater levels are found in higher integrative areas, such as the inferior temporal cortex (Area 20, right), a region involved in higher-level visual associations, particularly within the small pyramidal cells of layer II. (Adapted from Neve et al., 1988.)

Fig. 4. GAP-43 is concentrated in higher integrative areas of the human brain. By immunocytochemistry, GAP-43 levels are found to be low in primary sensory areas of the brain (visual cortex, Brodmann area 17, shown in *a*) and in motor control areas (precentral gyrus, Brodmann area 4, in *b*), but are very high in associative regions of the neocortex (inferior temporal cortex, Brodmann area 20, in *c*) and the hippocampal formation (*d*). (Adapted from Benowitz et al., 1989b.)

318

in a better position to explore the next generation of questions on structural remodeling in the vertebrate central nervous system.

Acknowledgements

We are grateful for the support of the National Eye Institute (NIH EY 05690) and the National Institute of Neurological Diseases and Stroke (NIH NS 25830). We would also like to acknowledge other colleagues who have contributed to our research, including Paul Jon Apostolides, Edward Bird, Elizabeth Finch, Seth Finklestein, Elizabeth Franck, Jamie Gossels, James Hamos, Sonal Jhaveri, Ellen Lewis, Susan Lewis, Ken Moya, John Schmidt, Gerald Schneider, Victor Shashoua, David Wiener, Jonathan Winickoff, Clifford Woolf, Myong G. Yoon and Henk Zwiers.

References

Akers, R.F. and Routtenberg, A. (1985) Protein kinase C phosphorylates a 47 M_r protein directly related to synaptic plasticity. Brain Res., 334: 147–551.

Akers, R.F., Lovinger, D.M., Colley, P.A., Linden, D.J. and Routtenberg, A. (1986) Translocation of protein kinase C (PKC) activity may mediate hippocampal long-term potentiation. Science, 231: 587–589.

Alexander, K.A., Cimler, B.M., Meier, K.E. and Storm, D.R. (1987) Regulation of calmodulin binding to P-57. J. Biol. Chem., 263: 7544–7549.

Aloyo, V.J., Zwiers, H. and Gispen, W.H. (1983) Phosphorylation of B-50 protein by calcium-activated, phospholipid-dependent protein kinase and B-50 protein kinase. J. Neurochem., 41: 649–653.

Basi, G.S., Jacobson, R.D., Virag, I., Schilling, J. and Skene, J.H.P. (1987) Primary structure and transcriptional regulation of GAP-43, a protein associated with nerve growth. Cell, 49: 785–791.

Benes, F.M., Paskevich, P.A., Davidson, J. and Domesick, V.B. (1985) Synaptic rearrangements in medial prefrontal cortex of haloperidol-treated rats. Brain Res., 348: 15–20.

Benowitz, L.I. and Lewis, E.R. (1983) Increased transport of 44,000- to 49,000-Dalton acidic proteins during regeneration of the goldfish optic nerve: a two-dimensional gel analysis. J. Neurosci., 3: 2153–2163.

Benowitz, L.I. and Routtenberg, A. (1987) A membrane phosphoprotein associated with neural development, axonal regeneration, phospholipid metabolism, and synaptic plasticity. Trends Neurosci., 10: 527–532.

Benowitz, L.I. and Schmidt, J.T. (1987) Activity-dependent sharpening of the regenerating retinotectal projection in goldfish: relationship to the expression of growth-associated proteins. Brain Res., 417: 118–126.

Benowitz, L.I., Shashoua, V.E. and Yoon, M.G. (1981) Specific changes in rapidly transported proteins during regeneration of the goldfish optic nerve. J. Neurosci., 1: 300–307.

Benowitz, L.I., Yoon, M.G. and Lewis, E. (1983) Transported proteins in the regenerating optic nerve: regulation by interactions with the optic tectum. Science, 222: 185–188.

Benowitz, L.I., Apostolides, P.J., Perrone-Bizzozero, N.I., Finklestein, S.P. and Zwiers, H. (1988) Anatomical distribution of the growth-associated protein GAP-43/B-50 in the adult rat brain. J. Neurosci., 8: 339–352.

Benowitz, L.I., Perrone-Bizzozero, N.I., Finklestein, S.P. and Bird, E.D. (1989b) Localization of the growth-associated phosphoprotein GAP-43 in the human cerebral cortex. J. Neurosci., 9: 990–995.

Benowitz, L.I., Rodriquez, W.R., Prusky, G.T. and Cynader, M.S. (1989a) GAP-43 levels in cat striate cortex peak during the critical period. Neurosci. Abstr., 15: 796.

Benowitz, L.I., Rodriquez, W.R. and Neve, R.L. (1990) The pattern of GAP-43 immunostaining changes in the rat hippocampal formation during reactive synaptogenesis. Mol. Brain. Res., 8: 17–23.

Berridge, M.J. and Irvine, R.F. (1984) Inositol triphosphate, a novel second messenger in cellular signal transduction. Nature, 312: 315–321.

Bliss, T.V.P. and Lømo, T. (1973) Long-lasting potentiation of synaptic transmission on the dentate area of the anaesthetized rabbit following stimulation of the performant path. J. Physiol. (Lond.), 232: 331–356.

Bliss, T.V.P., Douglas, R.M., Errington, M.L. and Lynch, M.A. (1986) Correlation between long-term potentiation and release of endogenous amino acids from dentate gyrus of anaesthetized rats. J. Physiol. (Lond.), 377: 391–408.

Coggins, P.J. and Zwiers, H. (1988) Evidence for a single phosphorylation site in neuronal protein B-50. Neurosci. Abstr., 14: 1126.

Collingridge, G.L. and Bliss, T.V.P. (1987) NMDA receptors – their role in long-term potentiation. Trends Neurosci., 10: 288–293.

Cotman, C.W. and Nieto-Sampedro, M. (1984) Cell biology of synaptic plasticity. Science, 225: 1287–1294.

Dani, J.W., Gage, F.H., Benowitz, L.I. and Armstrong, D.M. (1988) Immunocytochemical localization of GAP-43 in the developing rat brain. Neurosci. Abstr., 14: 1125.

De Graan, P.N.E., Van Hooff, C.O.M., Tilly, B.C., Oestreicher, A.B., Schotman, P. and Gispen, W.H. (1985) Phosphoprotein B-50 in nerve growth cones from fetal rat brain. Neurosci. Lett., 61: 235–241.

Dekker, L.V., De Graan, P.N.E., Versteeg, D.H.G., Oestreicher, A.B. and Gispen, W.H. (1989) Phosphorylation of B-50 (GAP-43) is correlated with neurotransmitter release in rat hippocampal slices. *J. Neurochem.,* 52: 24 – 30.

Erzurumlu, R.S., Jhaveri, S., Moya, K.L. and Benowitz, L.I. (1989) Peripheral nerve regeneration induces elevated expression of GAP-43 in the brain stem trigeminal complex of adult hamsters. *Brain Res.,* 498: 135 – 139.

Federoff, H.J., Grabczyk, E. and Fishman, M.C. (1988) Dual regulation of GAP-43 gene expression by nerve growth factor and glucocorticoids. *J. Biol. Chem.,* 263: 19290 – 19295.

Gispen, W.H. and Routtenberg, A. (Eds.) (1986) *Progress in Brain Reseach, vol. 69,* Elsevier, Amsterdam.

Gispen, W.H., Leunissen, L.M., Oestreicher, A.B., Verkleij, A.J. and Zwiers, H. (1985) Pre-synaptic localization of B-50 phosphoprotein: the ACTH-sensitive protein kinase substrate involved in rat brain phosphoinositide metabolism. *Brain Res.,* 328: 381 – 385.

Goslin, K., Schreyer, D.J., Skene, J.H.P. and Banker, G. (1988) Development of neuronal polarity: GAP-43 distinguishes axonal from dendritic growth cones. *Nature,* 336: 672 – 674.

Grafstein, B. (1986) The retina as a regenerating organ. In: R. Adler and D.B. Farber (Eds.), *The Retina: a Model for Cell Biology Studies, part II,* Academic Press, New York, pp. 275 – 333.

Greenough, W.T. and Bailey, C.H. (1988) The anatomy of a memory: convergence of results across a diversity of tests. *Trends Neurosci.,* 11: 142 – 147.

Hoffman, P.N. (1989) Expression of GAP-43, a rapidly transported growth-associated protein, and class II beta tubulin, a slowly transported cytoskeletal protein, are coordinated in regenerating neurons. *J. Neurosci.,* 9: 893 – 897.

Jacobson, M. (1978) *Developmental Neurobiology,* 2nd ed., Plenum Press, New York.

Jacobson, R.D., Virag, I. and Skene, J.H.P. (1986) A protein associated with axon growth, GAP-43, is widely distributed and developmentally regulated in rat CNS. *J. Neurosci.,* 6: 1843 – 1855.

Jolles, J., Zwiers, H., Van Dongen, C., Schotman, P., Wirtz, K.W.A. and Gispen, W.H. (1980) Modulation of brain polyphosphoinositide metabolism by ACTH-sensitive protein phosphorylation. *Nature,* 286: 623 – 625.

Kalil, K. and Skene, J.H.P. (1986) Elevated synthesis of an axonally transported protein correlated with axon outgrowth in normal and injured pyramidal tracts. *J. Neurosci.,* 6: 2563 – 2570.

Kandel, E.R. and Schwartz, J.H. (1982) Molecular biology of learning: modulation of transmitter release. *Science,* 218: 433 – 443.

Karns, L.R., Ng, S-C., Freeman, J.A. and Fishman, M.C. (1987) Cloning of complementary DNA for GAP-43, a neuronal growth-related protein. *Science,* 23: 597 – 600.

Katz, F., Ellis, L. and Pfenninger, K.H. (1985) Nerve growth cones isolated from fetal rat brain. III. Calcium-dependent protein phosphorylation. *J. Neurosci.,* 5: 1402 – 1411.

Linden, D.J., Wong, K.L., Sheu, F-S. and Routtenberg, A. (1988) NMDA receptor blockade prevents the increase in protein kinase C substrate (protein F1) phosphorylation produced by long-term potentiation. *Brain Res.,* 458: 142 – 146.

Lovinger, D.M., Akers, R.F., Nelson, R.B., Barnes, C.A., McNaughton, B.L. and Routtenberg, A. (1985) A selective increase in phosphorylation of protein F1, a protein kinase C substrate, directly related to three day growth of long term synaptic enhancement. *Brain Res.,* 343: 137 – 143.

Lovinger, D.M., Barnes, C.A., Mizumori, S.J.Y., Chan, S.Y., Linden, D., Murakami, K., Sheu, F.-S. and Routtenberg, A. (1986) Protein F1, previously related to synaptic plasticity, exhibits decreased phosphorylation in senescent rat hippocampus. *Neurosci. Abstr.,* 13: 1168.

McGuire, C.B., Snipes, G.J. and Norden, J.J. (1988) Light-microscopic immunolocalization of the growth-associated protein GAP-43 in the developing brain. *Dev. Brain Res.,* 41: 277 – 291.

McIntosh, H., Parkinson, D., Willard, M. and Daw, N.W. (1988) Characteristics of cat GAP: a GAP-43-like protein in visual cortex. *Neurosci. Abstr.,* 14: 187.

Meiri, K., Pfenninger, K.H. and Willard, M. (1986) Growth-associated protein, GAP-43, a polypeptide that is induced when neurons extend axons is a component of growth cones and corresponds to pp46, a major polypeptide of a subcellular fraction enriched in growth cones. *Proc. Natl. Acad. Sci. U.S.A.,* 83: 3537 – 3541.

Meiri, K.F., Willard, M. and Johnson, M.I. (1988) Distribution and phosphorylation of the growth-associated protein GAP-43 in regenerating sympathetic neurons in culture. *J. Neurosci.,* 8: 2571 – 2581.

Melchers, B.P.C., De Graan, P.N.E., Schrama, L.H., Wadman, W.J., Lopes da Silva, F.H. and Gispen, W.H. (1988) Synaptic potentiation and membrane phosphoproteins. In: *Long-Term Potentiation; from Biophysics to Behavior,* Alan R. Liss, New York, pp. 307 – 327.

Moya, K.L., Benowitz, L.I., Jhaveri, S. and Schneider, G.E. (1988) Changes in rapidly transported proteins in developing hamster retinofugal axons. *J. Neurosci.,* 8: 4445 – 4454.

Moya, K.L., Jhaveri, S., Schneider, G.E. and Benowitz, L.I. (1989) Immunohistochemical localization of GAP-43 in the developing hamster retinofugal pathway. *J. Comp. Neurol.,* in press.

Nelson, R.B. and Routtenberg, A. (1985) Characterization of protein F1 (47 kDa, 4.5 pI): a kinase C substrate directly related to neural plasticity. *Exp. Neurol.,* 89: 213 – 224.

Nelson, R.B., Friedman, D.P., O'Neill, J.B., Mishkin, M. and Routtenberg, A. (1987) Gradients of protein kinase C substrate phosphorylation in primate visual system peak in visual memory storage areas. *Brain Res.,* 416: 387 – 392.

Nestler, E. and Greengard, P. (1984) *Protein Phosphorylation in the Nervous System,* Wiley, New York.

Neve, R.L. and Bear, M.F. (1988) Postnatal changes in gene expression in kitten visual cortex and the effects of dark-

320

rearing. *Neurosci. Abstr.,* 14: 187.

Neve, R.L., Perrone-Bizzozero, N.I., Finklestein, S.P., Zwiers, H., Bird, E., Kurnit, D.M. and Benowitz, L.I. (1987) The neuronal growth-associated protein GAP-43 (B-50, F1): neuronal specificity, developmental regulation and regional distribution of the human and rat mRNAs. *Mol. Brain Res.,* 2: 177 – 183.

Neve, R.L., Finch, E.A., Bird, E.D. and Benowtiz, L.I. (1988) The growth-associated protein GAP-43 (B-50, F1) is expressed selectively in associative regions of the adult human brain. *Proc. Natl. Acad. Sci. U.S.A.,* 85: 3638 – 3642.

Ng, S-C., De la Monte, S.M., Conboy, G.L., Karns, L.R. and Fishman, M.C. (1988) Cloning of human GAP-43: growth association and ischemic resurgence. *Neuron,* 1: 133 – 139.

Nishizuka, Y. (1983) Phospholipid degradation and signal translation for protein phosphorylation. *Trends Biochem. Sci.,* 8: 13 – 16.

Norden, J.J., Woltjer, R. and Steward, O. (1988) Changes in the immunolocalization of the growth- and plasticity-associated protein GAP-43 during lesion-induced sprouting in the rat dentate gyrus. *Neurosci. Abstr.,* 14: 116.

Oestreicher, A.B. and Gispen, W.H. (1986) Comparison of the immunocytochemical distribution of the phosphoprotein B-50 in the cerebellum and hippocampus of immature and adult rat brain. *Brain Res.,* 375: 267 – 279.

Oestreicher, A.B., Van Dongen, C.J., Zwiers, H. and Gispen, W.H. (1983) Affinity purified anti B-50 protein antibody: interference with the function of the phosphoprotein in synaptic plasma membranes. *J. Neurochem.,* 41: 331 – 340.

Oestreicher, A.B., Dekker, L.V., Bloemen, R.J., Keur, S., Schrama, L.H. and Gispen, W.H. (1987) The neuron-specific phosphoprotein B-50: age-dependent changes in distribution in the rat brain. *J. Neurochem.,* 48 (Suppl.): S155.

Perrone-Bizzozero, N.I., Finklestein, S.P. and Benowitz, L.I. (1986) Synthesis of a growth-associated protein by embryonic rat cerebrocortical neurons in vitro. *J. Neurosci.,* 6: 3721 – 3730.

Pisano, M.R., Hegazy, M.G., Reimann, E.M. and Dokas, L.A. (1988) Phosphorylation of the pre-synaptic membrane-bound protein B-50 (GAP-43) by casein kinase II. *Neurosci. Abstr.,* 14: 1127.

Redshaw, J.D. and Bisby, M.A. (1984) Proteins of fast axonal transport in the regenerating hypoglossal nerve of the rat. *Can. J. Physiol. Pharmacol.,* 62: 1387 – 1393.

Schmidt, J.T. (1985) Formation of retinotopic connections: selective stabilization by an activity-dependent mechanism. *Cell. Mol. Neurobiol.,* 5: 65 – 84.

Schrama, L.H., De Graan, P.N.E., Dekker, L.V., Oestreicher, A.B., Nielander,H., Schotman, P. and Gispen, W.H. (1988)

Functional significance and localization of phosphosite(s) in the neuron-specific protein B-50/GAP-43. *Neurosci. Abstr.,* 14: 478.

Schreyer, D.J. and Skene, J.H.P. (1988) GAP-43 induction in regenerating dorsal root ganglion cells: an analysis of sorting in axonal transport. *Neurosci. Abstr.,* 14: 803.

Simkowitz, P., Ellis, L. and Pfenninger, K.H. (1989) Membrane proteins of the nerve growth cone and their developmental regulation. *J. Neurosci.,* 9: 1004 – 1017.

Skene, J.H.P. and Willard, M. (1981a) Changes in axonally transported proteins during axon regeneration in toad ganglion cells. *J. Cell Biol.,* 89: 86 – 95.

Skene, J.H.P. and Willard, M. (1981b) Axonally transported proteins associated with axon growth in rabbit central and peripheral nervous system. *J. Cell Biol.,* 89: 96 – 103.

Skene, J.H.P., Jacobson, R.D., Snipes, G.J., McGuire, C.B., Norden, J.J. and Freeman, J.A. (1986) A protein induced during nerve growth (GAP-43) is a major component of growth-cone membranes. *Science,* 233: 783 – 786.

Snipes, G.J., McGuire, C.B., Chan, S., Costello, B.R., Norden, J.J., Freeman, J.A. and Routtenberg, A. (1987) Evidence for the coidentification of GAP-43, a growth-associated protein, and F1, a plasticity-associated protein. *J. Neurosci.,* 7: 4066 – 4075.

Squire, L.R. and Morgan-Zola, S. (1988) Memory: brain systems and behavior. *Trends Neurosci.,* 11: 170 – 175.

Van Hooff, C.O.M., De Graan, P.N.E., Boonstra, J., Oestreicher, A.B., Schmidt-Michels, M.H. and Gispen, W.H. (1986) Nerve growth factor enhances the level of the PKC substrate B-50 in pheochromocytoma PC 12 cells. *Biochem. Biophys. Res. Commun.,* 139: 644 – 651.

Van Hooff, C.O.M., De Graan, P.N.E., Oestreicher, A.B. and Gispen, W.H. (1988) B-50 phosphorylation and polyphosphoinositide metabolism in nerve growth cone membranes. *J. Neurosci.,* 8: 1789 – 1795.

Verhaagen, J., Oestreicher, A.B., Edwards, P.M., Veldman, H., Jennehens, F.G.I. and Gispen, W.H. (1988) Light- and electron-microscopical study of phosphoprotein B-50 following denervation and reinnervation of the rat soleus muscle. *J. Neurosci.,* 8: 1759 – 1766.

Woolf, C.J., Reynolds, M.L., Molander, C., O'Brien, C., Lindsay, R.M. and Benowitz, L.I. (1990) The growth-associated protein GAP-43 appears in rat dorsal root ganglion cells and in the dorsal horn of the rat spinal cord following peripheral nerve injury. *Neuroscience,* 34: 465 – 478.

Zwiers, H., Schotman, P. and Gispen, W.H. (1980) Purification and some characteristics of an ACTH-sensitive protein kinase and its substrate protein in rat brain membranes. *J. Neurochem.,* 34: 1689 – 1699.

P. Coleman, G. Higgins and C. Phelps (Eds.)
Progress in Brain Research, Vol. 86
© 1990 Elsevier Science Publishers B.V. (Biomedical Division)

CHAPTER 27

Increased expression of the major embryonic α-tubulin mRNA, Tα1, during neuronal regeneration, sprouting, and in Alzheimer's disease

Freda D. Miller[a], and James W. Geddes[b]

[a]*Department of Anatomy and Cell Biology, University of Alberta, Edmonton, Canada T6G 2H7, and* [b]*Division of Neurosurgery, University of California, Irvine, CA 92717, U.S.A.*

Introduction

Normal growth and morphological differentiation of mammalian neurons involve a complex interplay between extrinsic influences and intrinsic neuronal genetic mechanisms. Developing neurons express a battery of genes that are involved, sequentially, in commitment, migration, process outgrowth and synaptogenesis. In the mature nervous system, with a few notable exceptions such as the olfactory system (Graziadei et al., 1980), neurons neither develop de novo nor migrate to new positions. However, new process outgrowth and synaptogenesis occur in response to neural trauma or pathology (for a review see Cotman et al., 1981), and may be ongoing phenomena in the normal animal (Purves et al., 1986). The molecular mechanisms underlying this type of structural plasticity, and the extraneuronal cues that regulate it remain largely undefined.

Our approach to this problem has been: (a) to identify genes that are associated with process outgrowth in developing neurons (Miller et al., 1987a); (b) to determine whether these same genes are recruited during the regeneration and sprouting of mature neurons; and (c) to define the factors that regulate the expression of these genes. Four mRNAs have been identified that are highly

enriched in the embryonic nervous system and not in the adult, and that are expressed in neurons following terminal mitosis and cell migration. At least three of these developmentally-regulated mRNAs are expressed by regenerating peripheral neurons (F.D. Miller, unpublished results), suggesting that the molecular mechanisms underlying morphological differentiation may be similar in developing and mature neurons.

One of the initially-identified mRNAs encodes an α-tubulin isotype referred to as Tα1 in the rat (Lemischka et al., 1981), Mα1 in the mouse (Lewis et al., 1985), and bα1 in the human (Cowan et al., 1983). In mammals, both α- and β-tubulin isotypes are encoded by large multigene families (Cleveland and Sullivan, 1985; Sullivan, 1988). Although several members of these families are pseudogenes, at least 6 different α-tubulin genes (Villasante et al., 1986), and 5 different β-tubulin genes (Wang et al., 1986) are expressed in the mouse. Two α-tubulin mRNAs (Ginzburg et al., 1981; Lemischka et al., 1981), termed T26 and Tα1, are expressed in rat brain. A third mouse α-tubulin mRNA, Mα4, which has no known rat homologue, is also expressed in the post-natal brain (Villasante et al., 1986).

In this review, we summarize studies examining expression of Tα1 and T26 α-tubulin mRNAs in

322

developing and mature neurons of the rat. These studies demonstrate that abundant expression of Tα1 mRNA is specifically associated with process outgrowth in developing and regenerating central neurons, whereas expression of T26 mRNA is constitutive in all neural cell types (Miller et al., 1987b, 1989). Tα1 α-tubulin mRNA is also up-regulated after lesions of the entorhinal cortex in both injured and uninjured neurons (Geddes et al., 1990), and during contralateral sprouting of sympathetic neurons of the superior cervical ganglion (Mathew and Miller, 1990). Finally, we have observed that bα1 α-tubulin mRNA, the human homologue of Tα1 is expressed at elevated levels in the hippocampus of patients with Alzheimer's disease (AD). Thus, expression of Tα1 α-tubulin mRNA is associated with the growth or remodeling of both developing and mature neurons. Induction and aberrant regulation of this growth-associated mRNA may contribute to some of the cytoskeletal abnormalities observed in neuropathological disorders such as Alzheimer's disease.

α-Tubulin genes are differentially regulated during neuronal development

Developing mammalian neurons synthesize large quantities of α- and β-tubulin monomers as building blocks for the microtubules that are essential to neuronal growth and differentiation. This is reflected in the expression of high levels of total α-tubulin mRNA in embryonic versus adult neurons (Miller et al., 1987a). Two members of the mammalian α-tubulin multigene family, referred to as Tα1 (Lemischka et al., 1981) and T26 (Ginzburg et al., 1981), are expressed in the embryonic rat nervous system. We have compared the expression of these 2 α-tubulin mRNAs during neural development by Northern blot and in situ hybridization analyses, using probes specific to unique sequences in each mRNA (Miller et al., 1987b).

Levels of Tα1 α-tubulin mRNA (Fig. 1) are highest in the developing brain at embryonic day 16 (E16) and post-natal day 1 (P1), when extensive morphological differentiation occurs; Tα1 mRNA

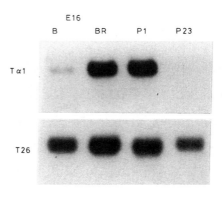

Fig. 1. Expression of Tα1 and T26 α-tubulin mRNAs in the developing embryonic and neonatal brain. Aliquots (2 μg) of poly (A)+ RNA prepared from embryonic day 16 body (E16 B), embryonic day 16 brain (E16 BR), post-natal day 1 brain (P1), and post-natal day 23 brain (P23) were separated by electrophoresis, blotted to nitrocellulose, and hybridized with probes specific to the 3′ untranslated regions of Tα1 or T26 α-tubulin mRNAs as previously described (Miller et al., 1987b).

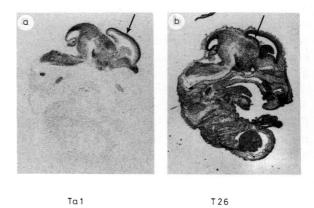

Fig. 2. Distribution of Tα1 and T26 α-tubulin mRNAs in E16 embryos. mRNA was detected by in situ hybridization to sagittal sections of E16 embryos: representative autoradiographs are shown. a. Hybridization with a 3′ untranslated region RNA probe specific to Tα1 mRNA. Note the intense hybridization to the developing neuroaxis and the lack of hybridization to the rest of the body. Levels of Tα1 mRNA are particularly high in the cortical plate (arrow). b. Hybridization with a 3′ untranslated region oligonucleotide probe specific to T26 mRNA. In situ hybridization demonstrates widespread hybridization to a variety of tissues, with a somewhat higher degree of hybridization to ventricular zones of the developing brain, such as that seen around the lateral ventricle (arrow). (Modified from Miller et al., 1987b.)

levels decrease dramatically by post-natal day 23 (P23), when neuronal development is largely complete. In contrast, levels of T26 α-tubulin mRNA in the brain decline only 2-fold over the same developmental period. In situ hybridization of E16 embryos (Fig. 2) revealed that Tα1 mRNA is localized specifically to the embryonic nervous system, and is not detectable in non-neuronal tissues. Within the developing nervous system, Tα1 mRNA is enriched in neurons that are actively undergoing neurite extension, such as those of the developing cortical plate. In contrast, T26 mRNA is relatively homogeneously expressed throughout the developing embryo and nervous system, with some enrichment in proliferative zones of the brain.

The correlation between Tα1 α-tubulin mRNA expression and neurite extension has also been observed in PC12 cells treated with nerve growth factor (NGF) (Miller et al., 1987b). Levels of Tα1 α-tubulin mRNA increase at least 2-fold within 12 h after NGF treatment, while T26 mRNA levels remain unchanged for up to 24 h. Similar results were observed in primary cultures of embryonic cortical neurons (M. Durand, F. Miller and R. Milner, unpublished results). Tα1 α-tubulin mRNA is expressed at the highest levels in primary cortical neurons during process extension, whereas T26 α-tubulin mRNA levels remain constant in these cultured neurons.

Tα1 α-tubulin mRNA is specifically reinduced during regeneration of mature motor neurons

Most vertebrate motoneurons respond to axonal injury by undergoing a series of well-defined morphological changes, including axonal regeneration and formation of functional synapses with muscle targets. Regeneration of motoneurons involves the increased synthesis of tubulin protein (Tetzlaff et al., 1988) and net production of new microtubules, which are integral components of the regenerating axon. To determine whether patterns of tubulin isotype expression that occur in developing neurons are reinduced in regenerating

motoneurons, we examined the expression of Tα1 and T26 α-tubulin mRNAs following unilateral injury of the facial nerve (Miller et al., 1989). Facial motoneurons of adult rats were unilaterally crushed, and coronal sections through the facial nuclei were hybridized with a probe specific to Tα1 α-tubulin mRNA at 1–49 days following axotomy (Fig. 3). Tα1 mRNA was rapidly induced in axotomized motoneurons of the facial nerve: increased levels of mRNA were detectable 4 h after a lesion was made 1.5 cm distal to the neuronal cell bodies. Tα1 α-tubulin mRNA increased to peak levels between 3 and 7 days, and declined slowly 14–21 days following crush (reinnervation of facial muscles was established between 10 and 15 days post-crush, as assayed by the return of vibrissal activity). Seven weeks post-axotomy, Tα1 mRNA hybridization was similar in control and operated neurons. In contrast, levels of T26 α-tubulin mRNA in facial nuclei did not change following axotomy, as determined by Northern blot and in situ hybridization analyses. These results show that Tα1 α-tubulin mRNA was rapidly and specifically reinduced during regeneration of mature facial motoneurons, was maintained at high levels during the period of axonal growth, and was subsequently down-regulated at the time of target contact, in a manner reminiscent of neuronal development.

Tα1 α-tubulin mRNA also increased in response to facial nerve transection, a procedure that is unlikely to result in target reinnervation. Resection of the facial nerve led to an increase in abundance of Tα1 mRNA comparable to crushed, successfully-regenerating motoneurons (Miller et al., 1989). Seven weeks following transection, however, Tα1 mRNA remained elevated relative to crushed or control neurons. This suggests that lack of contact with an appropriate target can prolong the genetic growth response, as indicated by Tα1 mRNA expression.

Induction of Tα1 α-tubulin mRNA following axonal injury is not confined just to regenerating facial motoneurons. It also occurs in spinal cord motoneurons following crush or ligation of the

324

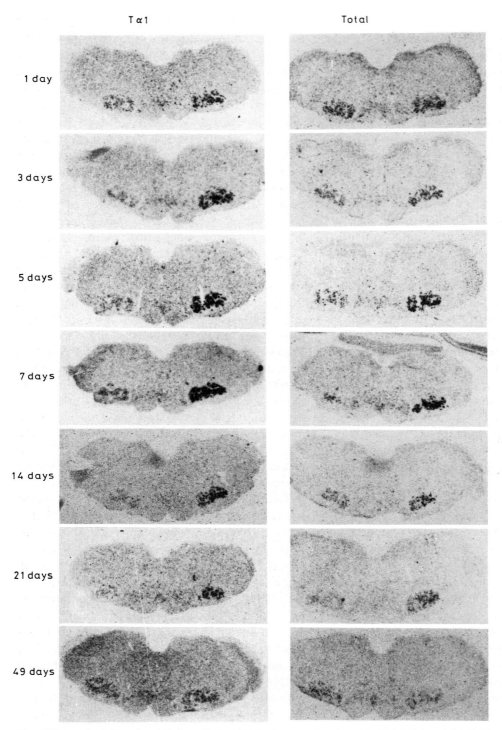

Fig. 3. Expression of total and Tα1 α-tubulin mRNAs in control and axotomized facial nuclei following unilateral crush axotomy of the facial nerve. Representative autoradiographs are shown of alternate coronal sections through the facial nuclei of operated rats hybridized to ^{35}S-labeled probes specific to the 3′-untranslated region of Tα1 and the coding region of total α-tubulin mRNA at 1, 3, 5, 7, 14, 21 and 49 days following axotomy. In all photographed sections, the cell bodies of neurons on the operated side are situated to the right of the midline. Scale bar: 1 mm. (From Miller et al., 1989.)

sciatic nerve (Miller et al., 1989), in axotomized sympathetic neurons of the superior cervical ganglion (Mathew and Miller, 1990), and in transected sensory neurons arising in dorsal root ganglia (T.C. Mathew and F. Miller, unpublished observations). Therefore, induction of Tα1 α-tubulin mRNA occurs during axonal regeneration in both the peripheral and central nervous systems.

Sprouting of hippocampal neurons involves increased expression of Tα1 α-tubulin mRNA

The molecular programs underlying neuronal sprouting remain undefined, but may involve a selective reactivation of developmental mechanisms (Cotman and Nieto-Sampedro, 1984). To test this hypothesis, we analyzed the expression of Tα1 α-tubulin mRNA in the rat hippocampus following unilateral lesions of the entorhinal cortex (Geddes et al., 1990). Within 1 day following a lesion, increased levels of Tα1 mRNA were observed by in situ hybridization in the ipsilateral hippocampus, in dentate granule cells, polymorphic hilar neurons, and pyramidal neurons of the CA3 and CA1 regions. Peak levels of Tα1 mRNA were observed 3 – 5 days following the lesion, and levels decreased by 14 days post-lesion. The time course of expression of Tα1 α-tubulin mRNA correlates well with previous studies on sprouting, remodeling, and synapse turnover triggered by entorhinal cell loss (Cotman and Anderson, 1988). The hilar neurons, which exhibit increased Tα1 α-tubulin mRNA, extends axonal collaterals to the denervated dentate gyrus, and are known to sprout following lesion of the entorhinal cortex. A second group of uninjured neurons (granule cells of the dentate gyrus, pyramidal neurons in CA1 and CA3) also induce Tα1 mRNA, possibly as part of a dendritic sprouting response to the loss of entorhinal input.

In addition to the increased Tα1 α-tubulin mRNA in the ipsilateral hippocampus, we observed elevated levels in cortical neurons located proximal to the lesion site (Fig. 4). These neurons could be inducing Tα1 mRNA as a result of dendritic or axonal injury and/or could be responding to a localized increase in factor(s) produced at the site of the injury. But other, less localized mechanisms are apparently operative, since we also detected increased Tα1 α-tubulin mRNA in the contralateral hippocampus. The stimulus leading to induction of Tα1 mRNA and remodeling of neurons in the contralateral hippocampus (Hoff et al., 1981) is unknown, but is possibly transneuronal in nature. Nonetheless, these studies indicate that the neuronal response to entorhinal cell loss may be more widespread than previously suspected.

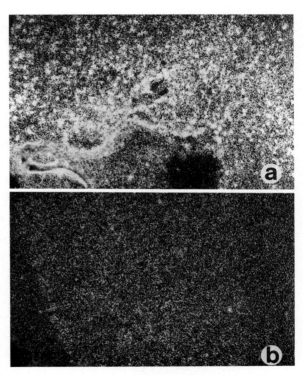

Fig. 4. Expression of Tα1 α-tubulin mRNA in cortical neurons following electrolytic lesion of the entorhinal cortex. Horizontal sections through the ipsilateral (*a*) and contralateral (*b*) cortex near the site of the lesion were hybridized to a probe specific for Tα1 α-tubulin mRNA. Hybridized sections were coated with emulsion for autoradiography, developed, and photographed under darkfield illumination. Both photographs were exposed and developed under identical conditions. Ipsilateral and contralateral neurons were photographed on the same section.

bα1 α-tubulin mRNA, the human homologue of Tα1, is expressed at elevated levels in hippocampal neurons of Alzheimer's disease patients

Alzheimer's disease (AD) is a neurodegenerative disorder histologically characterized by neurofibrillary tangles, neuritic plaques, Hirano bodies, granulovacuolar degeneration, and dystrophic neurites (for a review, see Price, 1986). Although AD is commonly associated with neural degeneration, there is increasing evidence of neuronal sprouting in AD patients (Probst et al., 1983; Arendt, 1986; Braak et al., 1986; Geddes et al., 1986; Ihara, 1988). In fact, some of the cytoskeletal abnormalities characteristic of AD could be explained by inappropriate regulation of cytoskeletal mRNAs expressed during aberrant neuronal sprouting. To test this hypothesis, we measured bα1 α-tubulin mRNA, the human homologue of Tα1, in the hippocampus of individuals suffering from AD (Geddes et al., 1990). In situ hybridization of sections of hippocampal tissues from 5 AD patients and from 5 age-matched controls revealed that bα1 α-tubulin mRNA is consistently elevated in neurons of the

CA3 region of the hippocampus in AD (Figs. 5, 6). In most AD cases, we observed a similar increase in the granule cells of the dentate gyrus (Geddes et al., 1990). Grain counting revealed an average 3 – 4-fold increase in the amount of bα1 α-tubulin mRNA per pyramidal neuron in the CA3 region. There was, however, significant variability, with some CA3 neurons expressing control levels of bα1 mRNA, while others expressed levels 5-fold higher than controls.

Neurons of the entorhinal cortex are particularly vulnerable in AD (Hyman et al., 1984), and previous studies have shown that at least some aspects of the sprouting response to AD- or lesion-induced enthorhinal cell loss are similar (Geddes et al., 1986). This study supports that conclusion, and suggests that in the later stages of AD neurons may continue to sprout in response to ongoing neuronal loss. Alternatively, elevated bα1 mRNA may represent an aberrantly-regulated growth response possibly resulting either from lack of reinnervation of an appropriate target or from inappropriate environmental cues. Continued elevation of bα1 α-tubulin mRNA may ultimately be deleterious rather than beneficial. For example, tubulin immunoreactivity has been associated with

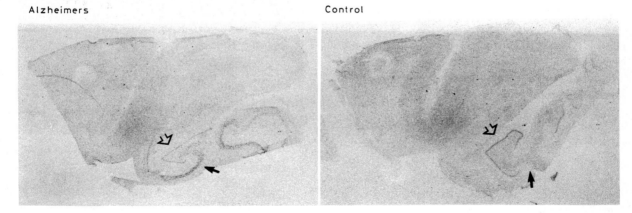

Fig. 5. Expression of bα1 α-tubulin mRNA, the human homologue of Tα1 α-tubulin mRNA, in human hippocampal sections. The human tissue was obtained at autopsy from a 76-year-old male patient with Alzheimer's disease, and from a 69-year-old male control patient. Representative autoradiographs are shown of sections hybridized to ^{35}S-labeled probes specific to the 3'-untranslated region of bα1 α-tubulin mRNA. Note the increased relative level of bα1 mRNA in the CA3 region (closed arrows) as compared to the dentate gyrus (open arrows) in the Alzheimer versus control patients.

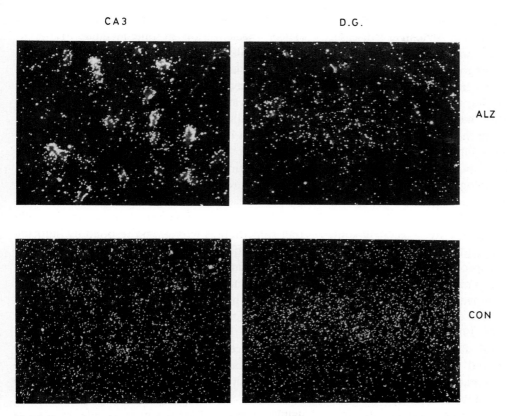

Fig. 6. Expression of bα1 α-tubulin mRNA in pyramidal neurons of the CA3 region and granule cells of the dentate gyrus (D.G.) in a 76-year-old male control patient (CON) and in a 79-year-old female patient with Alzheimer's disease (ALZ). Sections were hybridized with a probe specific for bα1 α-tubulin mRNA, coated with emulsion for autoradiography, developed, and photographed under darkfield illumination.

granulovacuolar degeneration, which is particularly evident in CA3 (Price et al., 1986).

The results of this study suggest that some of the embryonic markers observed in the AD brain are the consequence of a reinduction of developmental patterns of gene expression associated with neuronal sprouting. Previous studies consistent with a replay of developmental events in AD include the staining of tangles by vimentin, an intermediate filament protein associated with immature neurons and glial cells (Yen et al., 1983), and the presence of elevated levels of phosphomonoesters (Pettegrew et al., 1988) and of the ganglioside GM1 (Emory et al., 1987), both of which are elevated in the fetal brain. Im-

munocytochemical studies suggest that a highly modified, perhaps fetal, form of tau is abundant in the AD brain (Wolozin et al., 1988). Thus, inappropriate regulation of select growth-associated genes may contribute to the etiology of neuropathological disorders such as Alzheimer's disease.

Discussion

The studies described in this paper demonstrate that Tα1 α-tubulin mRNA is abundantly and specifically expressed during the development, regeneration, and sprouting of central mammalian neurons. They further demonstrate that bα1 α-tubulin mRNA, the human homologue of Tα1, is expressed at elevated levels in Alzheimer's disease, potentially as part of an aberrantly-regulated sprouting response to ongoing neuronal loss. The specific expression of one member of the α-tubulin multigene family during the growth of both developing and mature mammalian neurons supports the hypothesis that there is a intrinsic genetic growth program that is initially expressed during neuronal development, and that is subsequently recruited during morphological differentiation and remodeling of mature neurons. Inappropriate regulation of this growth program in neurodegenerative disorders may contribute, at least in some cases, to the observed neuropathology.

It is likely that the proposed "growth-associated" genetic response is multigenic in nature. We have observed that at least two other embryo-enriched mRNAs that are expressed in developing neurons (Miller et al., 1987a), are also induced during regeneration of facial motoneurons (F. Miller, W. Tetzlaff and L. Mah, unpublished observations) and sympathetic neurons of the superior cervical ganglion (T. Mathew and F. Miller, unpublished observations). Previous studies have also demonstrated that a class II β-tubulin mRNA is enriched in the nervous system and is specifically reinduced in regenerating sensory neurons (Hoffman and Cleveland, 1988), and that GAP-43 is expressed at elevated levels in developing (Meiri et al., 1986), as well as regenerating mammalian neurons (Skene and Willard, 1981).

In all of the growth paradigms that we have examined, a tight correlation exists between expression of Tα1 α-tubulin mRNA and the morphological growth or remodeling of mammalian neurons. The abundant expression of Tα1 α-tubulin mRNA during neuronal growth may reflect a specific requirement for the Tα1 α-tubulin isotype. For example, in the embryonic nervous system, Tα1 α-tubulin mRNA comprises greater than 95% of the total α-tubulin mRNA (Miller et al., 1987b), and must therefore encode the α-tubulin subunits for almost all of the axonal and dendritic microtubules. Alternatively, it may reflect specialization of one member of the α-tubulin multigene family as a means of increasing the available pool of α-tubulin for neurite extension. It may simply be easier to regulate two or more equivalent genes in a tissue-specific manner than a single gene, particularly when the protein serves both ubiquitous and cell type-specific functions.

The factors that induce Tα1 α-tubulin mRNA in mature neurons are ill-defined, but could involve both intrinsic and extrinsic cues. For example, it is possible that injured neurons "know" intrinsically that something is wrong, and respond by inducing growth-associated genes. However, it is equally possible that environmentally-produced factors or transneuronal cues are responsible for turning-on a growth response, particularly in the case of the hippocampal neurons that induce Tα1 mRNA following lesion of the entorhinal cortex. Maintenance of elevated Tα1 mRNA may also be an intrinsically determined event, or it may require contact with or production of factors by cells in the immediate vicinity of the growing neuron. We know, however, that appropriate guidance cues, as defined developmentally, are not essential, since ligated spinal cord motoneurons maintained Tα1 mRNA at elevated levels for at least 7 days post-lesion (Miller et al., 1989).

During successful neuronal regeneration, Tα1 α-tubulin mRNA remains elevated until the approximate time of functional reinnervation (Miller et al., 1989). It is likely that target — neuron interactions are at least partially responsible for turning off Tα1 mRNA expression following neuronal growth since resection of facial motoneurons prevents appropriate down-regulation. Contact and synaptogenesis with the original target is not, however, necessary: sprouting hippocampal neurons that form heterotypic contacts also down-regulate Tα1 mRNA.

There are a number of possible explanations why bα1 α-tubulin mRNA is elevated in the post-mortem AD hippocampus. Increased bα1 mRNA may be associated with the continued neuronal sprouting of spared neurons in response to ongoing neuronal loss. Alternatively, there may be a defect in the down-regulation of bα1 α-tubulin mRNA following neuronal sprouting due, at least partially, to lack of target neuron reinnervation. Finally, there may be an aberrant uncoupling of growth-associated genes like bα1 from neuronal growth in the diseased brain.

The correlation between abundant expression of Tα1 α-tubulin mRNA and neuronal growth makes Tα1 mRNA an ideal marker for the regeneration and sprouting of mature neurons. It will be of interest to identify the extrinsic cues that are responsible for up-regulating this growth-associated mRNA in the mature nervous system.

Acknowledgements

We wish to thank Lenna Mah and Suzanne Cooper for technical assistance; Robert Milner, Floyd Bloom, Chris Naus, Wolfram Tetzlaff, Carl Cotman, Chacko Mathew, and James Fawcett for their support and collaboration in some of these studies; Gerry Higgins, and Klaus-Armin Nave for frequent discussion and advice; and Richard Murphy and Robert Campenot for critical readings of the manuscript.

F.M. is a scholar of the A.H.F.M.R., and is supported by the M.R.C., and J.G. was an N.D.S.F. Science Scholar during the tenure of these studies, and is currently supported by the N.I.A. LEAD Grant AG0798.

References

Arendt, T., Zvegintseua, H.G. and Leontovich, T.A. (1986) Dendritic changes in the basal nucleus of Meynert and in the diagonal band nucleus in Alzheimer's disease − a quantitative golgi investigation. *Neuroscience,* 19: 1256−1278.

Braak, H., Braak, E., Grundke-Iqbal, I. and Iqbal, K. (1986) Occurrence of neuropil threads in the senile human brain and in Alzheimer's disease: a third location of paired helical filaments outside of neurofibrillary tangles and neuritic plaques. *Neurosci. Lett.,* 65: 351−355.

Cleveland, D.W. and Sullivan, K.F. (1985) Molecular biology and genetics of tubulin. *Annu. Rev. Biochem.,* 54: 331−365.

Cotman, C.W. and Anderson, K.J. (1988) Synaptic plasticity and functional stabilization in the hippocampal formation: possible role in Alzheimer's disease. *Adv. Neurol.,* 47: 313−335.

Cotman, C.W. and Nieto-Sampedro, M. (1984) Cell biology of synaptic plasticity. *Science,* 225: 1287−1294.

Cotman, C.W., Nieto-Sampedro, M. and Harris, E.W. (1981) Synapse replacement in the nervous system of adult vertebrates. *Physiol. Rev.,* 61: 684−784.

Cowan, N.J., Dobner, P.R., Fuchs, E.V. and Cleveland, D.W. (1983) Expression of human α-tubulin genes: interspecies conservation of 3' untranslated regions. *Mol. Cell. Biol.,* 1738−1745.

Emory, C.R. Ala, T.A. and Frey II, W.H. (1987) Ganglioside monoclonal antibody (A2B5) labels Alzheimer's neurofibrillary tangles. *Neurology,* 37: 768−772.

Geddes, J.W., Anderson, K.J. and Cotman, C.W. (1986) Senile plaques as aberrant sprout-stimulating structures. *Exp. Neurol.,* 94: 767−776.

Geddes, J.W., Wong, J., Choi, B.H., Kim, R.C., Cotman, C.W. and Miller, F.D. (1990) Increased expression of the embryonic form of a developmentally-regulated mRNA in Alzheimer's disease. *Neurosci. Lett.,* 109: 54−61.

Ginzburg, J., Behar, L., Givol, D. and Littauer, U.Z. (1981) The nucleotide sequence of rat α-tubulin: 3'-end characteristics and evolutionary conservation. *Nucleic Acids Res.,* 9: 2691−2697.

Graziadei, P.P.C., Karlan, M.S., Monti-Graziadei, G.A. and Bernstein, J.J. (1980) Neurogenesis of sensory neurons in the primate olfactory system after section of the *filia olfactoria. Brain Res.,* 186: 289−300.

Hoff, S.F., Scheff, S.W., Kwan, A.Y. and Cotman, C.W. (1981) A new type of lesion-induced synaptogenesis. I. Synaptic turnover in non-denervated zones of the dentate gyrus in young adult rats. *Brain Res.,* 222: 1−13.

Hoffman, P.N. and Cleveland, D.W. (1988) Neurofilament and tubulin expression recapitulates the developmental pattern during axonal regeneration: induction of a specific β-tubulin isotype. *Proc. Natl. Acad. Sci. U.S.A.,* 85: 4530−4533.

Hyman, B.T., Van Hoesen, G.W., Damasio, A.R. and Barnes, C.L. (1984) Alzheimer's disease: cell-specific pathology isolates the hippocampal formation. *Science,* 225: 1168−1170.

Ihara, Y. (1988) Massive somatodendritic sprouting of cortical neurons in Alzheimer's disease. *Brain Res.,* 459: 138−144.

Lemischka, I.R., Farmer, S., Racaniello, V.R. and Sharp, P.A. (1981) Nucleotide sequence and evolution of a mammalian α-tubulin mRNA. *J. Mol. Biol.,* 150: 101−120.

Lewis, S.A., Lee, M.G.-S. and Cowan, N.J. (1985) Five mouse α-tubulin isotypes and their regulated expression during development. *J. Cell Biol.,* 101: 852−861.

Mathew, T.C. and Miller, F.D. (1990) Increased expression of Tα1 α-tubulin mRNA during collateral and NGF-induced sprouting of sympathetic neurons. *Dev. Biol.,* 141: 84−92.

Meiri, K.F., Pfenninger, K.H. and Willard, M.B. (1986) Growth-associated protein, GAP-43, a polypeptide that is induced when neurons extend axons, is a component of growth cones and corresponds to pp46, a major polypeptide of a subcellular fraction enriched in growth cones. *Proc. Natl. Acad. Sci. U.S.A.,* 83: 3537–3541.

Miller, F.D., Naus, C.C.G., Higgins, G.A., Bloom, F.E. and Milner, R.J. (1987a) Developmentally regulated rat brain mRNAs: molecular and anatomical characterization. *J. Neurosci.,* 7: 2433–2444.

Miller, F.D., Naus, C.C.G., Durand, M., Bloom, F.E. and Milner, R.J. (1987b) Isotypes of α-tubulin are differentially regulated during neuronal maturation. *J. Cell Biol.,* 105: 3065–3073.

Miller, F.D., Tetzlaff, W., Bisby, M.A., Fawcett, J.W. and Milner, R.J. (1989) Rapid induction of the major embryonic α-tubulin mRNA, Tα1, during nerve regeneration in adult rats. *J. Neurosci.,* in press.

Pettegrew, J.W., Moosy, J., Withers, G., McKeag, D. and Panchalingam, K. (1988) ^{31}P nuclear magnetic resonance studies of Alzheimer brain. *J. Neuropathol. Exp. Neurol.,* 47: 235–248.

Price, D.L. (1986) New perspectives on Alzheimer's disease. *Annu. Rev. Neurosci.,* 9: 489–512.

Price, D.L., Altschuler, R.J., Struble, R.G., Casanova, M.F., Cork, L.C. and Murphy, D.B. (1986) Sequestration of tubulin in neurons in Alzheimer's disease. *Brain Res.,* 383: 305–310.

Probst, A., Basler, V., Bron, B. and Ulrich, J. (1983) Neuritic plaques in senile dementia of Alzheimer type A golgi analysis in the hippocampal region. *Brain Res.,* 268: 249–254.

Purves, D., Hadley, R.D. and Voyvodic, J.T. (1986) Dynamic changes in the dendritic geometry of individual neurons visualized over periods of up to three months in the superior cervical ganglion of living mice. *J. Neurosci.,* 6: 1051–1060.

Skene, J.H.P. and Willard, M. (1981) Axonally transported proteins associated with axon growth in rabbit central and peripheral nervous systems. *J. Cell Biol.,* 89: 96–105.

Sullivan, K.F. (1988) Structure and utilization of tubulin isotypes. *Annu. Rev. Cell. Biol.,* 4: 687–716.

Tetzlaff, W., Bisby, A. and Kreutzberg, G.W. (1988) Changes in cytoskeletal proteins in the rat facial nucleus following axotomy. *J. Neurosci.,* 8: 3181–3189.

Villasante, A., Wang, D., Dobner, P., Dolph, P., Lewis, S.A. and Cowan, N.J. (1986) Six mouse α-tubulin mRNAs encode five distinct isotypes: testis-specific expression of two sister genes. *Mol. Cell. Biol.,* 6. 2409–2419.

Wang, D., Villasante, A., Lewis, S.A. and Cowan, N.J. (1986) The mammalian β-tubulin repertoire: hematopoietic expression of a novel, heterologous β-tubulin isotype. *J. Cell Biol.,* 103: 1903–1910.

Wolozin, B., Scicutella, A. and Davies, P. (1988) Reexpression of a developmentally regulated antigen in Down syndrome and Alzheimer disease. *Proc. Natl. Acad. Sci. U.S.A.,* 85: 6202–6206.

Yen, S.H., Gaskin, F. and Fu, S.M. (1983) Neurofibrillary tangles in senile dementia of Alzheimers type share an antigenic determinant with intermediate filaments of the vimentin class. *Am. J. Pathol.,* 113: 373–381.

P. Coleman, G. Higgins and C. Phelps (Eds.)
Progress in Brain Research, Vol. 86
© 1990 Elsevier Science Publishers B.V. (Biomedical Division)

CHAPTER 28

Adhesion and the in vitro development of axons and dendrites

A. Prochiantz, A. Rousselet and B. Chamak

CNRS URA 1414, Département de Biologie, ENS, 46 rue d'Ulm, 75005 Paris, France

Introduction

Neuritogenesis is the focus of numerous in vitro studies aimed at the purification of molecules capable of regulating neurite elongation. Several soluble, membrane-bound and extracellular matrix-associated factors have been described. However, their modes of action remain obscure in many cases. In particular, it is difficult to understand the series of events which occur between the interaction of the factors with their neuronal receptors and the three-dimensional development of the neuritic arbor. In fact, in spite of the primary physiological importance of the development of neuronal shape, it is fair to say that it is still a poorly understood process.

One possible way towards a better understanding of this question is certainly to study the establishment of neuronal polarity and, in particular, the regulation of dendritic and axonal growth. Indeed, axons and dendrites are two separate neuronal compartments with specific biochemical, morphological and physiological characteristics (for review, see Lasek, 1988). In this short review of our work, we shall insist on the role of cell-cell and cell-substratum adhesion in the separate regulation of the growth of axons and dendrites.

The role of region-specific neuro-astroglial interactions in the expression of neuronal polarity

In 1984, we demonstrated that mesencephalic dopaminergic neurons cultured for 2 days on mesencephalic (homotopic) or striatal (heterotopic) astrocytes differed very much in shape (Denis-Donini et al., 1984). Briefly, compared to the single long and unbranched neurites observed in the heterotopic situation, the neuritic arbor of the dopaminergic neurons cultured on homotopic astrocytes appeared very complex. Indeed, in such homotopic neuro-astroglial cocultures, dopaminergic neurons had several primary neurites and branch points. Thus, we hypothesized that the growth of dendrites and axons was regulated separately and, more precisely, that specific neuro-astroglial interactions might play an important role in this regulatory process.

In order to investigate this possibility, we cultured mesencephalic and striatal neurons on pre-established monolayers of mesencephalic and striatal astrocytes (Chamak et al., 1987). After 2 days the cells were fixed and incubated with an antibody directed against the microtubule associated protein 2 (MAP2), a specific marker of the dendritic and somatic compartments (Matus et al.,

1981). Clearly, the number of MAP2 positive neurites was much higher in homotopic than in heterotopic neuro-astroglial cocultures. These results, suggesting that homotopic neuro-astroglial interactions augment the rate of growth of the dendritic arbor both in mesencephalic and in striatal neurons, were further confirmed by ultrastructural observations (Autillo-Touati et al., 1988).

The influence of astrocyte-conditioned media on neuronal shape and polarity

We studied the action of astrocyte-conditioned media on the shape of mesencephalic neurons. Mesencephalic neurons cultured in a chemically defined medium previously conditioned on monolayers of mesencephalic astrocytes (CM Gmes) were in majority multipolar. Conversely, mesencephalic neurons in striatal astrocyte conditioned medium (CM Gstr) were, in general, unipolar (Rousselet et al., 1988). As in the case of the neuro-astroglial cocultures, ultrastructural and immunocytochemical criteria allowed us to demonstrate that dendrite growth was strongly stimulated in the homotopic conditioned medium (Rousselet et al., 1990).

The mesencephalic conditioned medium was centrifuged at $100,000 \times g$, allowing us to separate an insoluble (P100) from a soluble (S100) fraction. The neurons cultured in the insoluble fraction were all monopolar; their unique neurite, long and unbranched, could be stained with an antibody directed against the axon-specific phosphorylated isoforms of the 200 kDa neurofilament subunit (Foster et al., 1987; Liem, personal communication). In the soluble fraction, all neurons were multipolar with well developed axons and dendrites. Analysis of the molecules present in the conditioned medium and in the two fractions revealed the presence of high quantities of matrix molecules. We thus hypothesized that soluble and insoluble complexes of extracellular matrix molecules could be involved in the separate regulation of axonal and dendritic initiation and elongation.

The influence of bound and soluble matrix molecules in the definition of neuronal polarity

The possibility that soluble and insoluble (substrate bound) forms of matrix molecules could differentially regulate the growth of dendrites and axons was directly investigated with purified laminin (LN) and fibronectin (FN). Mesencephalic neurons were plated on polyornithine (PORN), on polyornithine pre-coated with LN (bound LN, bLN) or FN (bFN), on polyornithine in the presence of soluble LN (sLN) or FN (sFN). The concentrations used were the following: 3.5, 1.2, 4.0 and 0.5 μg/ml for sFN, bFN, sLN and bLN, respectively (Chamak and Prochiantz, 1989a, b).

The use of morphological, ultrastructural and immunocytochemical criteria demonstrated that sLN and bFN stimulated axonal growth and inhibited dendrite elongation, whereas sFN and bLN allowed the two categories of neurite to elongate. However, it was interesting to note that, whenever dendrite growth seemed to be repressed, the rate of axonal elongation was doubled.

Adhesion, viscosity and neuronal polarity

In all conditions favouring axonal versus dendritic growth, we could measure a clear reduction of the apparent surfaces of the neuronal cell bodies (Autillo-Touati et al., 1988; Chamak and Prochiantz, 1989a, b; Rousselet et al., 1990). This suggested that the specific inhibition of dendrite initiation was associated with reduced attachment and spreading of the cells. Direct measurements of neuronal adhesion were performed which confirmed our hypothesis (Chamak and Prochiantz, 1989a, b; Rousselet et al., 1990). It was thus concluded that axons can initiate and elongate in low adhesion conditions, whereas dendrite initiation necessitates strong adhesion and spreading of the cell body.

The different sensitivity of axonal and dendritic growth toward adhesion was interpreted in term of fluid mechanics. If one assumes neurites behave as liquid cylinders developing within a liquid environment, the laws of Plateau predict the existence of a maximal theoretical length beyond which the cylinder will break. According to these laws, this maximum can only be surpassed if the viscosity of the liquid cylinder is increased (spider thread model) or if the adhesion between the two media is increased, thus decreasing surface tensions (the oil on water model). These questions have been thoroughly discussed by D'Arcy Thompson (1917).

As a consequence of such considerations, we postulated that the ability of axons to initiate in low adhesion conditions could relate to their high intrinsic viscosity, possibly explained by the presence of large amounts of polymerized tubulin (Chamak and Prochiantz, 1989a, b). In fact, ultrastructural studies clearly indicated that, compared to the initial segments of dendrites, axonal shafts contained a high per volume ratio of polymerized microtubules (Autillo-Touati et al., 1988). Moreover, the treatment of live cells with GTP and detergent demonstrated that the polymerized tubulin was much more stable in the axons than in the dendrites (Rousselet et al., 1990).

Spreading dendrites and jumping axons

We are now able to propose a model based on our experiments. This model proposes that dendrite initiation requires a strong adhesion and spreading of the neuronal soma and that this requirement is due to the low viscosity of the initial dendritic stump. In fact, ultrastructural studies strongly suggest that the cytoplasm and the dendroplasm have very similar compositions and properties. It could even be said that the initial dendritic segments are simple extensions of the neuronal soma. In contrast, the axon, thanks to its peculiar structure, is able to initiate and grow in low adhesion conditions. As illustrated in Fig. 1, dendrites would spread and axons would jump.

The jumping hypothesis is based on morphological observation, both at light and electron

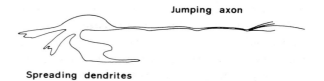

Fig. 1. Jumping axon and spreading dendrites.

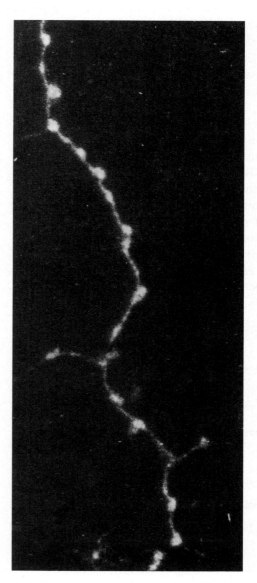

Fig. 2. Axonal segment immunostained with an anti neurofilament antibody. Magnification: × 2250.

microscopic levels. As seen in Fig. 2, where a 5-day-old axon has been stained with the axon-specific anti-neurofilament antibody, the growth of the axon has a fractal pattern. In fact, the axonal shaft is made of a series of straight segments (0.2 – 0.5 μm long), separated by "varicosities". When examined at the electron microscopic level, the straight segments are filled with fasciculated microtubules. These microtubules are, in general, not interrupted at the level of the "varicosities". However, when a directional change is made, it always occurs at the level of a "varicosity" where it is associated with an abrupt change in the orientation of the microtubule bundles (Rousselet et al., 1990).

The hypothetical jumping character of axonal growth is schematized in Fig. 3. In a generally poorly adhesive environment the axonal filopodia are able to search for an adhesion point. Once attached, they pull the axonal shaft, thus promoting the polymerization of the microtubules. Such an effect of mechanical traction on microtubule formation has been well established by Bray (1984). Then new filopodia are formed that search for another adhesion point. This explains why turning decisions are made at the level of these

"varicosities" which, if we are right, should be equivalent to the fibroblastic adhesion plaque. Indeed, between two plaques the axonal segment does not need to be firmly attached to the substratum.

Some implications of the model

The proposal that axonal initiation is clearly distinct from that of dendrites has several implications. The most important one being that an axon is an axon as soon as it is produced by the cell body. Indeed, the existence of undifferentiated neurites that would mature into axons or dendrites is, according to our model rather unlikely. This latter possibility (the existence of undecided neurites) has, however, been raised by other investigators on the basis of strong evidence and thus requires discussion (Dotti et al., 1988; Goslin and Banker, 1989).

A first point concerns the well known fact that axons often emerge from dendrites. If so, how is it possible to first have the axon going out (in the low adhesion conditions characteristic of the young embryo), and then the dendrites? Fig. 4 explains this apparent contradiction. In fact, the presence of the axonal initial stump on a dendrite does not mean that the dendrites grew first, it can simply reflect the deformation of the cell caused by cellular adhesion and dendrite growth.

Secondly, upon lesioning the axon can reform, starting from any other point in the cell, including from another proximal dendrite (Dotti and Banker, 1987; Hall et al., 1989). If we consider that,

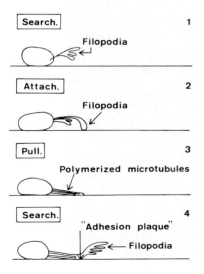

Fig. 3. The different steps of axonal elongation (hypothetical model).

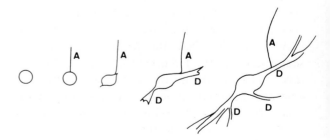

Fig. 4. Schematic representation of axonal and dendritic growth (A, axon; D, dendrite).

basically, there is no real difference between a proximal dendrite and the soma, the possibility for an axon, in a regenerative situation, to form from a dendrite is not surprising. In fact it has to, since dendrites are present. The only surprise is that axon initiation occurs in a region of the soma different from its initial localization. This, in fact, requires explanation, but does not go against our model which only says that the axon is different as soon as it goes out, but makes no prediction as to where it should be initiated.

A third point is the presence of the dendritic marker MAP2 in the immature axon, in the absence of dendritic trees. This phenomenon has been noted by several authors, including us (Caceres et al., 1986; Chamak et al., 1987). It has been interpreted as the sign that this initial neurite could be either an axon or a dendrite, the decision being made later and being accompanied by, among other things, a change in MAP2 targeting. We propose a much simpler explanation illustrated in Fig. 5. In the absence of dendrites MAP2 molecules diffuse passively into the axonal shaft. In an older neuron with axons and dendrites, the passively diffusing molecules, including MAP2 molecules, accumulate preferentially in the dendrites since, compared to that of the axons, their surface sections are much larger.

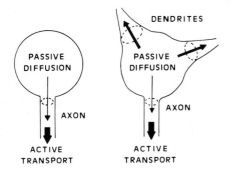

Fig. 5. Hypothetical representation of passive and active molecular fluxes.

Possible physiological significance of dendrite inhibition

If we now come back to our first observation, that is the enhanced dendrite growth observed in homotopic neuro-astroglial cultures, we can now interpret it in terms of preferential adhesion. This suggests the existence of region-specific and stage-specific isoforms of adhesion molecules, matrix components and adhesion receptors. In fact, the molecular basis for such an heterogeneity exists and the roles of these molecules as position antigens have been demonstrated in different systems (Leptin et al., 1987; Rabacchi et al., 1988). In so far as NCAM is concerned, it has certainly been demonstrated that embryonic development is associated with a decrease in sialic acid content (Edelman, 1986; Rutishauser and Goridis, 1986). According to our model, the fact that highly sialicated NCAM molecules are less adhesive than the mature forms could explain why, during development, dendrites do not develop until the axons have reached their targets.

It must also be remembered that a majority of brain neurons, after they have been generated in the germinal zone, leave this region and join their final location. During this migration period they are in an heterotopic situation and, accordingly, put out their axons, but have no true dendritic arbor. It is only after they have reached their normal position that they start to develop their dendritic tree. However, this dendritic elongation can remain rather modest until axon terminals have found their innervation fields. In fact, in the absence of dendrite growth the rate of axonal elongation is significantly increased, and therefore dendrite inhibition might have the critical function to reduce the time necessary for the axonal growth cone to reach its target, a likely source of trophic factor.

Conclusions: axonal and dendritic genetic programs

The problem of axonal and dendritic elongation is

not simply a question of neuritic shape, but also of intrinsic polarity. In fact, we presently foresee two main questions. The first one relates to the understanding of how vesicles and molecules are targeted toward axons or dendrites. The second question concerns the mechanism through which adhesion (as a primary signal) regulates the transcription of genes implied in the making of a specific type of neurite. Both questions, although raised at the unicellular level, relate to the general problem of the genetic control of animal form. It can thus be speculated that their solution will require the study of the roles of "developmental genes" in the economy of the developing cell.

Acknowledgements

We wish to thank Dr.J. Glowinski for his help and participation in several aspects of this work. The support of DRET 89-200 and Rhône-Poulenc Santé is also acknowledged.

References

Autillo-Touati, A., Chamak, B., Araud, D., Vuillet, J., Seite, R. and Prochiantz, A. (1988) Region-specific neuro-astroglial interactions: ultrastructural study of the in vitro expression of neuronal polarity. *J. Neurosci. Res.,* 19: 326 – 342.

Bray, D. (1984) Axonal growth in response to experimentally applied mechanical tension. *Dev. Biol.,* 102: 379 – 389.

Caceres, A., Banker, G. and Binder, L. (1986) Immunocytochemical localization of tubulin and microtubule associated protein 2 during the development of hippocampal neurons in culture. *J. Neurosci.,* 6: 714 – 722.

Chamak, B. and Prochiantz, A. (1989) Axones, dendrites et adhésion. *C.R. Acad. Sci.,* 308: 353 – 358.

Chamak, B. and Prochiantz, A. (1989) Influence of extracellular matrix proteins on the expression of neuronal polarity. *Development,* in press.

Chamak, B., Fellous, A., Glowinski, J. and Prochiantz, A. (1987) MAP2 expression and neurite outgrowth and branching are co-regulated through region-specific neuroastroglial interactions. *J. Neurosci.,* 7: 3163 – 3170.

D'Arcy Thompson (1917) *On Growth and Form.* Cambridge University Press.

Denis-Donini, S., Glowinski, J. and Prochiantz, A. (1984) Glial heterogeneity may define the three-dimensional shape of mesencephalic dopaminergic neurones. *Nature,* 307: 641 – 643.

Dotti, C.G. and Banker, G. (1987) Experimentally induced alteration in the polarity of developing neurons. *Nature,* 330: 254 – 256.

Dotti, C.G., Sullivan, C.A. and Banker, G.A. (1988) The establishment of polarity by hippocampal neurons in culture. *J. Neurosci.,* 8: 1454 – 1468.

Edelman, G.M. (1986) Cell adhesion molecules in the regulation of animal form and tissue pattern. *Annu. Rev. Cell Biol.,* 2: 81 – 116.

Foster, G.A., Dahl, D. and Lee, V. (1987) Temporal and topographic relationships between the phosphorylated and non-phosphorylated epitopes of the 200 kDa neurofilament protein during development in vitro. *J. Neurosci.,* 7: 2651 – 2663.

Goslin, K. and Banker, G. (1989) Experimental observations on the development of polarity by hippocampal neurons in culture. *J. Cell Biol.,* 108: 1507 – 1516.

Hall, G.F., Poulos, A. and Cohen, M.J. (1989) Sprouts emerging from the dendrites of axotomized lamprey central neurons have axon-like ultrastructure. *J. Neurosci.,* 9: 588 – 599.

Lasek, R.J. (1988) Studying the intrinsic determinants of neuronal form and function. In: R.J. Lasek and M.M. Black (Eds.), *Intrinsic Determinants of Neuronal Form and Function,* Alan Liss, New York, pp. 1 – 60.

Leptin, M., Aebersold, R. and Wilcox, M. (1987) *Drosophila* position-specific antigens resemble the vertebrate fibronectin-receptor family. *EMBO J.,* 6: 1037 – 1043.

Matus, A., Bernhardt, R. and Hugh-Jones, T. (1981) High molecular weight microtubules associated proteins are preferentially associated with dendritic microtubules in the brain. *Proc. Natl. Acad. Sci. U.S.A.,* 78: 3010 – 3014.

Rabacchi, S.A., Neve, R.L. and Dräger, U.C. (1988) Molecular cloning of the "dorsal eye antigen": homology to the high affinity laminin receptor. *Soc. Neurosci. Abstr.,* 14: 311.4.

Rousselet, A., Fetler, L., Chamak, B. and Prochiantz, A. (1988) Rat mesencephalic neurons in culture exhibit different morphological traits in the presence of media conditioned on mesencephalic or striatal astroglia. *Dev. Biol.,* 129: 495 – 504.

Rousselet, A., Autillo-Tovati, A., Arand, D. and Prochiantz, A. (1990) In vitro regulation of neuronal morphogenesis and polarity by astrocyte-derived factors. *Dev. Biol.,* 137: 33 – 45.

Rutishauser, U. and Goridis, C. (1986) NCAM: the molecule and its enetics. *Trends Genet.,* 2: 72 – 75.

SECTION VII

Finale

P. Coleman, G. Higgins and C. Phelps (Eds.)
Progress in Brain Research, Vol. 86
© 1990 Elsevier Science Publishers B.V. (Biomedical Division)

CHAPTER 29

A systems approach to aging, Alzheimer's disease, and spinal cord regeneration

Eugene Roberts

Department of Neurobiochemistry, Beckman Research Institute of the City of Hope, Duarte, CA 91010, U.S.A.

Introduction

With regard to normal and abnormal function, to a considerable extent neuroscientists still are lost in the labyrinths of the nervous system. This may be because the conceptual frameworks employed are inadequate. One must strive constantly to establish valid core positions from which to view meaningfully both phenomena of major human interest such as memory, consciousness, various aspects of normal and abnormal behavior, neurological disease, aging, etc., and the molecular and submolecular events that constantly are taking place at the levels of excitable membranes and genomic expression. However, it is difficult to view nervous system function at all pertinent levels. "There are so many realities that in trying to encompass them all one ends in darkness. That is why, when one paints a portrait, one must stop somewhere, in a sort of caricature. Otherwise there would be nothing left at the end" (Picasso, cited by Ashton, 1988).

Some general characteristics of living systems

All living systems are pattern-recognizing or generalizing entities, from single cells to complex human organizations. When a living system, unicellular or international, is presented with a new information pattern in its environment (external and internal), it is activated in a unique fashion. The types of impinging influences and their sequences, intensities, and rates of change result in an activation pattern that is likely to be different from any experienced previously. Even in well-controlled experiments in which single variables are manipulated, it is the change in the pattern of the environment which is the stimulus (stress, pressure, forcing function) for the system. Progress has been made recently toward establishing a universal law of generalization or pattern recognition that may be helpful in estimating the probability of whether or not an organism will react to a novel stimulus pattern in accordance with consequences associated with previously experienced stimulus patterns (Shepard, 1987; Ennis, 1988).

At all levels of observation, from genomic expression to freeway driving, *progressive disinhibition is coupled to increased variability generation in healthy organisms* (Roberts and Matthysse, 1970; Roberts, 1976, 1986a; Hikosaka and Wurtz, 1983). A released sytem, like a wound spring, has the tactical advantage over a driven one in that it does not have to overcome the inertia of start-up when it switches from an inactive or minimally active to a fully active state. Metaphorically, metabolically-generated energy is used to wind the biological springs. Ever-present tonically active inhibitory influences, together with phasically active ones, maintain barriers to physicochemical perturbations, so that the interactions within the system in Yin-Yang fashion produce asymmetric graded local changes. Transient signals are transduced by a variety of devices at hand to release processes that govern amounts and turnovers of substances, their locations, and their relations to each other.

Coupling exists between the driving force (pressure) and the generation of variability (information-processing capacity) among the subunits that participate in the nest of relations comprising the particular system being considered, i.e., healthy living systems have an expansible capacity for processing information in relation to demand. Paradoxical as it may seem initially, facile traverse of the adaptive functional range largely is made possible by diverse activities of inhibitory (attenuating and/or time-delaying) influences. In the central nervous system (CNS) inhibitory projection and local circuit neurons play crucial roles in information processing (Roberts, 1986a – c).

I surmise that increases in activities with increases in forcing function occur according to principles of non-linear dynamics. It would be expected according to the latter concept that with progressively increasing force parameter each living system considered would show three characteristic behaviors: smooth, periodic (oscillatory) and turbulent (chaotic). With full participation of inhibition and with tight coupling between degrees of disinhibition and variability generation, the region of smooth flow (efficiently adaptive behavior) would extend over a much greater range of force parameters than in their absence (Lorenz, 1963; Rössler, 1976; Mandell, 1983).

When healthy living systems are effectively stimulated, processes are released to operate at rates and for durations that enable them to react adaptively in a manner compatible with their individual behavioral repertoires. Cascades of processes are generated by actions of environmental factors that reduce transmembrane potential and/or interact with specific membrane receptors. Cascades of other processes are released by expression of genetic potential (Ames et al., 1986; Morgan et al., 1987; Saffen et al., 1988). When en-

vironmental pressures are increased, the number of such countercurrent cascades and their extents are increased in such a way that the probability of their meshing to give system-typical adaptive patterns tends to remain approximately constant. The relative constancies of structural, compositional, and functional features of cells, tissues, and organs in mature animals under various environmental conditions are indicative of the existence of remarkable biochemical and biophysical servomechanisms which coordinate a variety of complex biosynthetic and degradative pathways and which continuously adjust the rates of flow of substances between the organism and its environment, between extracellular and intracellular compartments of tissues, and between cytosol and organelles and among cytosolic aggregates (molecular ensembles) of individual cells (Schoenheimer, 1942; Roberts and Simonsen, 1962; Ratner, 1979; Goldberg et al., 1983; Goldberg and Walseth, 1985; Wheatley and Ingles, 1986).

Because several response options may be available even to the simplest cell in a particular instance, because the particular choices made among the options often are unpredictable, and because the exercise of options results in functional and structural changes of varying extents and durations, it may be said that creativity and memory exist in every living unit (Tam et al., 1986). Although increasing in levels of complexity, the operations of multicellular organisms in their environments are not different in basic principle from those of single cells.

Disease, aging, and the Tower of Babel

Disease in general

A normal system is one that can cycle freely through all of its operational modes, and its activities are aimed at maintaining this capacity. In pre-disease states, impediments may begin to arise in patterns of communication among various components of the particular system being observed. Tendencies to malfunction, which are undetectable in the resting or idling state, may appear when stress is applied. For example, a pre-diabetic state in an obese individual with a normal fasting blood sugar might be revealed by abnormal blood-sugar levels observed during a glucose tolerance test. A tendency to develop cardiac arrhythmia in an individual with a normal resting electrocardiogram may be detected during exercise on a treadmill. Hyperventilation may be required to elicit electroencephalographic evidence of a tendency to seizures. All of the above would be evidence, albeit in an extremely primitive form, of impediments in operational modes which are revealed under stress but which are inapparent at rest. Appropriate therapies at this point might be those which would improve inadequacies in intercellular and intracellular communications.

In the above instances, weight reduction in the pre-diabetic individual and the administration of small amounts of a calcium channel blocker and a suitable antiepileptic agent to the individuals with stress-revealed cardiac and cerebral abnormalities, respectively, might be sufficient to achieve the desired goals.

Disease may be said to occur when there is continued uncoupling between environmental pressures on a living system and its ability to adapt to them. If the individual with the cardiac problem posited above were to spend all his waking hours on a treadmill under conditions that elicited his arrhythmia, instead of just briefly during a stress test, he could be said to have cardiac disease in the same sense as if he had a similar arrhythmia during the activities of his normal day. A disease state differs from a pre-disease state in that uncoupling already has occurred and a chaotic state exists among the ordinarily coordinated and hierarchically nested metabolic and physiological cascades. I believe that such uncoupling represents a discontinuity, metaphorically a catastrophe (Thom, 1975), rather than being part of a phenomenological continuum. This would be as true of a paranoid schizophrenic in society as of a cancer cell in its host organism. Finding a therapeutic wedge at this stage is much more dif-

ficult than when it is possible to attempt to strengthen weak, but still functional, coupling mechanisms in the pre-disease condition.

Disease phenomena, at all levels from social to molecular, result in deculturation, i.e., disruption of meaningful communication channels between components of relevant members of interlocking systems, so that adaptive behaviors eventually are not possible and the organism literally crumbles, like a biological Tower of Babel. In view of the great complexity of the interactions in nested biological systems and the radiating effects of disease processes at any particular level, one should not be surprised to find changes in a myriad of measured parameters in a diseased organism. Presently it is not of much use to engage in "chicken-egg" discussions in most instances, with the exception of those disorders caused by known toxicants and infectious agents or those in which genetic mutations have been detected.

Limited as our knowledge may be, I believe a primary task in dealing with disease is to attempt to identify and ameliorate those processes that are rate-limiting. A common approach in attempting to improve functions in a poorly operational system is to keep the components "talking to each other." Experience shows that the self-organizing properties of biological systems often enable them to begin to function adaptively at all levels, from intercellular to international, once effective interactions are reinstituted.

Cellular and organismic aging

No one dies of old age per se. Aging is a progressive concatenation of disease processes occurring with the passage of time. The aging human organism — whether one looks at physiologic, biochemical, behavioral or pathological aspects — appears to follow a final common path. Options ordinarily available to achieve adaptive responses are precluded by degeneration of the body machinery. Even during the early normal adult period, degenerative changes are taking place to some extent, but are being compensated for by ac-

342

tivities of redundant elements and by adjustments in feedback and modulator systems. However, eventually pathologic changes become sufficiently extensive so that the latter activities are inadequate, the social behavior and physiological responses of severely affected individuals become maladaptive, and survival becomes dependent upon extensive use of artificial social and medical support systems until death ensues.

There is general agreement that with time losses occur in capacities of cells to transcribe essential DNA-coded information in a coordinated fashion, for reasons ranging from hits by cosmic rays, carcinogens and viruses, decreases in circulating levels of steroid hormones and other hormones and growth factors, failure of DNA repair processes, etc. (Kirkwood, 1989). The transcriptional imbalances lead to decreased adaptability and eventual loss of viability. Dying non-neural cells may be replaced by division of unaffected cells or by differentiation of stem cells. This is not possible for most neurons, which usually do not undergo mitosis in mature organisms. For the neuroendocrine system and the CNS, and, therefore, for the organism as a whole, the course would be downhill all of the way, only the rate of decline varying from one circumstance to another. For a neuron whose role is to receive, integrate, and transmit signals on a millisecond time scale as well as possibly to adapt to changing circumstances with plastic changes, e.g., glutamatergic or GABAergic neurons, it would be of little use to regenerate lost cell processes, reestablish synapses, etc., if it were no longer possible to produce a variety of essential components, such as K$^+$ channels, for example, that are necessary to perform its subtle and highly demanding role. The best strategy for the organism under the latter circumstances would be to make maximal use of remaining healthy redundant neurons and neural circuits and to keep them operational as long as possible.

Age-related disease processes accelerate greatly when reproduction ceases: imbalances between glucocorticoids and sex-related steroids may be critical

In complex organisms, degenerative processes associated with aging become most evident toward the conclusion of the reproductive period, e.g., cancer, autoimmune disorders, etc., and the dramatic case of the migrating salmon. It seemed reasonable to look for rate-limiting events among aspects of the neuroendocrine machinery, which controls homeostatic and integrative systems of the body. Sex steroids generally exert anabolic effects and glucocorticoids have catabolic effects at target sites. Although these substances exert effects from membrane to genomic expression, the most important long-range effects probably are on the latter. Adequately balanced availability of members of these classes of steroids, such as exists between 15 and 25 years of age in human beings of both sexes (Orentreich et al., 1984), probably is necessary to maintain properly orchestrated transcriptional responses to environmental pressures. A relative excess of glucocorticoids would favor catabolic or self-destruct programs (Sapolsky, 1990); excesses of sex steroids would favor inappropriately hypertrophic responses (Parker, 1989).

Specifically where to look comes from Shakespeare's concise characterization of what happens to a man from the sixth of his seven ages on to his final demise (from *As You Like It*):

. . .The sixth age shifts
Into the lean and slippered pantaloon,
With spectacles on nose and pouch on side,
His youthful hose well saved, a world too wide
For his shrunk shank; and his big manly voice,
Turning again toward childish treble, pipes
And whistles in his sound. Last scene of all,
That ends this strange eventful history,
Is second childishness, and mere oblivion,
Sans teeth, sans eyes, sans taste, sans everything.

Shakespeare, unparalleled genius of an observer

that he was, has seen clearly that in the aging male a loss in muscle mass and other androgen-related characteristics preceded frank signs of mental deterioration.

For as long as they have been known, androgens and estrogens have been administered to males and females, respectively, to retard one or another feature of aging. The literature on the subject is replete with less than satisfactory measurements and experimental designs. In those instances in which documentation was adequate, problems often arose that precluded prolonged use of the hormones. Endometrial bleeding, prostatic hypertrophy, and danger of carcinogenesis have been among the several danger signs along the road. Obviously, cybernetic control mechanisms of the organism were being overwhelmed by the exogenously imposed hormonal thrusts.

It was necessary to look elsewhere than to the sex hormones, for substances that might help to correct the progressive incoordinations of bodily systems with age. I considered the possibility of dehydroepiandrosterone (DHEA) and its sulfate (DHEAS), naturally occurring, largely adrenally-derived, precursors of androgens, which in turn are precursors for estrogens (Sonka, 1976; Roberts, 1986e; Parker, 1989). Among the major blood serum steroid classes, monotonic decreases after puberty in both sexes occur only in mean levels of the readily interconvertible dehydroepiandrosterone (DHEA) and dehydroepiandrosterone sulfate (DHEAS). The stimulated release of DHEA and DHEAS by ACTH is significantly reduced in the aging human organism and during prolonged acute stress (Parker and Odell, 1980; Parker et al., 1985; Parker, 1989). Cortisol levels and the stimulative ability of cortisol release by ACTH are hardly affected by age.

If the DHEA and DHEAS could penetrate to androgen- or estrogen-synthetic sites in the various tissues, conditions existing at such sites would determine quantities and rates of androgen and estrogen synthesis. Such hormone synthesis would be more likely to be subject to meaningful cybernetic controls. Administration of DHEA and DHEAS might not be nearly as intrusive physiologically as the administration of arbitrarily selected amounts of the sex hormones, themselves. The possibility exists that DHEA and DHEAS and/or intermediate metabolites on the way to androgens and estrogens also might react with membrane, cytosolic, and nuclear receptors and exert important effects at several levels of cellular function.

Focusing on the nervous system, we first found that low concentrations of DHEA and DHEAS enhanced neuronal and glial survival and differentiation and reduced astroglial proliferation rates in dissociated cultures of 14-day mouse embryo brain (Bologa et al., 1987; Roberts, 1987). DHEA and DHEAS showed convincing memory enhancing effects in *undertrained* young (2-month-old) mice whether administered intracerebroventricularly, subcutaneously or orally (Roberts et al., 1987; Flood et al., 1988). It then seemed worthwhile to determine whether or not administering DHEA and DHEAS to older animals would reverse any quantitatively measurable variables associated with aging.

Old mice and men have poorer memories than young ones. With age, many processes involved in memory formation, retention, and retrieval might be adversely affected. Flood and I undertook to determine whether or not the water-soluble DHEAS could improve impaired memory processes in aging mice (Flood and Roberts, 1988). Employing a footshock active avoidance paradigm, we found that middle-aged (18-month-old) and old (24-month-old) mice showed poorer retention of the task than young mice (2-month-old) in a paradigm in which the young mice showed excellent retention (Figs. 1, 2). However, when a single subcutaneous injection of DHEAS (20 mg/kg) was given within 2 min after training and the old and middle-aged mice were tested 1 week and 2 months later, respectively, the retention of the older groups was improved remarkably to the high levels observed in young mice. These results are compatible with the idea that inadequate availability of DHEA and/or DHEAS or of the variety of sex-related steroids derived from them (Sonka, 1976; Roberts, 1986e; Parker, 1989) could be rate-limiting in achievement of plastic changes required for retention of learning to take place.

Steroid hormones are known to form complexes with specific receptor proteins that regulate gene expression (Chouros et al., 1986; Litwack et al., 1986; Slater et al., 1986; Cordingley et al., 1987; Evans, 1988). These complexes also may be involved in post-transcriptional mechanisms of regulating gene expression, e.g., affecting translational efficiency, protein stability, etc. (Gupta et

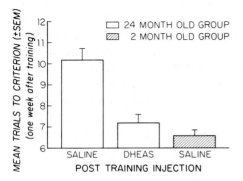

Fig. 1. Effects of subcutaneously injected DHEAS on memory retention in 24-month-old mice. Injections of test solutions were made within 2 min after initial training and testing was performed 1 week after training (Flood and Roberts, 1988).

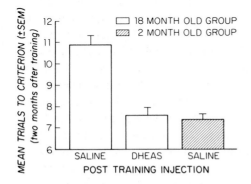

Fig. 2. Effects of subcutaneously injected DHEAS on memory retention in 18-month-old mice. Injections of test solutions were made within 2 min after initial training and testing was performed 2 months after training (Flood and Roberts, 1988).

al., 1984; Ali and Vedeckis, 1987). DHEA and DHEAS also can exert physiological effects when applied directly to neural membranes (Carette and Poulain, 1984) and on EEG activity when injected into animals (Heuser and Eidelberg, 1961; Heuser et al., 1965; Kubli-Garfias et al., 1976, 1982).

It is possible that even the survival of some neurons, endothelial cells, glia, etc. might depend on DHEA, DHEAS, or on one or more of the substances that derive from them. In those cells that have receptors for them, these substances may be required to inhibit the genomic transcription of mRNAs coding for proteins that initiate a self-destruct program (Martin et al., 1988; Truman et al., 1990). When these substances are absent or inadequately available, eventually fatal degenerative processes may begin upon occurrence of functional demands that require coordinated genomic transcriptional responses for recovery from activity to take place. Degenerative processes may not become irreversible as long as the affected cells still possess some receptors for such substances. Restoring adequate levels of the rate-limiting hormones might allow some measure of recovery to take place and could delay cell death.

Prior to searching for molecular mechanisms of their action on retention of learning, it is necessary to determine whether the effects observed are specific to DHEA and DHEAS, themselves, or whether one or more of the several steroids that can be derived from them, or combinations, are the effective substances. To date, the effects of DHEA and DHEAS have been assessed in active and passive avoidance paradigms, which are aversely motivated. In order to ascertain the generality of their effects on learning and memory, it is necessary to extend the study of these substances to tasks that are positively reinforced and on discriminative behavior. Relevant experiments are in progress.

Neither DHEAS (Koo et al., 1983) nor DHEA (E. Roberts and J. Fitten, unpublished observations) appear to be toxic in humans. Although it is not at all certain that what is true for mice is also true for man, it is not unreasonable from the data at hand to suppose that supplementation with DHEA or DHEAS, normal constituents of the blood, might exert salutary effects by helping reestablish effective communication within and among neural subsystems that are inadequately functioning in aging individuals and in those with some major nervous system disorders. With the above in mind, clinical studies with orally administered DHEA are in progress in patients with Alzheimer's disease and multiple sclerosis and in individuals with benign age-related memory loss.

Alzheimer's disease (AD) may be a protein storage disease resulting from genetic or environmentally-induced lysosomal defects: at the core of the problem

Because most often AD occurs coextensively with aging, many pathological features of decybernetization are shared. However, AD cannot be considered in the same category as usual attritional types of aging because, in addition to the general types of aging changes, such as accumulation of lipofuscin (Sohal and Wolfe, 1986), there are some special features. Much effort has been expended on examination of characteristic distributions of the shards found in the brains of those dying of the disease, the neurofibrillary tangles, the neuritic (senile) and amyloid plaques, and the granulovacuolar degenerations. Major molecular insights are coming directly from work with amyloid proteins (see Müller-Hill and Beyreuther, 1989, for review) and studies of interference of axonal transport of the neurofilament complex (Gajdusek, 1985). However, the problems in AD are particularly difficult because they relate not only to molecular and cellular properties of the brain but also to emergent properties of the whole system, such as memory, cognition, and participation in everyday life.

Like a modern metropolis, all cells face waste disposal problems. "The principal organelle responsible for the degradation of cellular waste is the lysosome. It is a common constituent of all cell types of the nervous system and is particularly pro-

minent in neurons . . . . Its function is to fuse with the membrane of waste-containing vacuoles (phagosomes), into which it releases hydrolytic enzymes. The sequestered material is then degraded within the vacuole, and the organelle becomes a secondary lysosome and is usually electron dense and large" (Raine, 1989).

In recent years many genetic disorders have been identified in which specific defects of lysosomal hydrolytic enzymes result in abnormal accumulations of incompletely degraded lipids, glycoproteins, and mucopolysaccharides (Suzuki, 1989), often with major effects on nervous system structure and function. Activities of acid proteases of lysosomes play a major role in protein turnover in cells (Hershko and Ciechanover, 1982; Beynon and Bond, 1986; Mayer and Doherty, 1986; Tanaka, et al., 1986). Intraventricular infusions of protease inhibitors result in accumulation of dense bodies in neurons and glial cells, suggesting that decrease in specific proteases, genetically or environmentally caused, may result in toxic accumulation of undegraded protein material.

In light of the above, it is of great interest that amyloid precursor protein (APP) has been found to be concentrated in secondary lysosomes of pyramidal cortical and hippocampal cells in normal and AD brains and that in the latter "abnormally dense immunostaining in enlarged intracellular domains accompanied a severe atrophy of CA1 neurons. These data suggest that accumulations of APP in lysosomes of particular neurons may, in AD, lead to proteolytic events that form the insoluble 4.2 kDa amyloid peptide" (Benowitz et al., 1989). Also, a peptide derived from the APP may be neurotoxic (Yankner et al., 1989). Although the genes for familial AD and for APP are both on chromosome 21, it is clear that they are at different loci (see Müller-Hill and Beyreuther, 1989, for summary). A mutation of the APP gene is probably not the cause of AD. Rather it seems more productive to begin to look for genetic or environmentally induced defects in the enzymatic machinery involved in degradation of APP.

At the end of its cellular sojourn, APP, possibly a heparan sulfate proteoglycan core protein (Schubert et al., 1988; Shivers et al., 1988), may be secreted as such or may be processed by lysosomal and cytosolic hydrolases to yield amino acids, peptides, and carbohydrates which are secreted, metabolized, or reused. The degradative processing must involve a highly coordinated sequence of desulfation, dephosphorylation, deglycosylation, and proteolytic splitting. If during such processing the formation of an insoluble and indigestible self-aggregating unit should take place, a protein storage disorder could arise (Hook et al., 1984; Kang et al., 1987; Kirschner et al., 1987; Allsop et al., 1988; Dyrks et al., 1988; Salbaum et al., 1988; Selkoe et al., 1988; Müller-Hill and Beyreuther, 1989).

APP, or a fragment thereof, may have proteolytic activity

I suggest that APP, itself, or a subunit of it might be a proteolytic enzyme and might participate in its own processing (Roberts, 1986d). I surmise this from the following. Within the amyloid subunit (residues 597−648 of APP-695) there is embedded the tripeptide Asp-Ser-Gly at residues 603−605 in a region outside of the putative transmembrane portion (residues 624−648) (Kang et al., 1987). This triplet is the same as that which contains the active site serine residue in virtually all serine proteases (Woodbury et al., 1978; Greer, 1981; Reid and Porter, 1981) and which is bound covalently by nexins (Baker et al., 1980). The catalytic site of the serine proteases is characterized by a Ser, His, Asp triad (Kraut, 1977; Carter and Wells, 1988), an oxanion binding site, the three participating residues converging from different parts of the protein chain. In subtilisin from *Bacillus amyloliquefaciens* Ser 221, His 64 and Asp 32 congregate at the catalytic site, although the His and Asp are 157 and 189 residues, respectively, distant from active site Ser 221 in the protein chain. If Ser 604 of APP-695 were an active site Ser of a protease, there would be His 458 and Asp 429, 146 and 175 residues, respectively,

removed from it that might possibly join with Ser to form the active catalytic site. In addition to being degraded by ambient proteases, APP-695 might undergo autoproteolytic splitting as part of its normal metabolic handling (see Power et al., 1986). Interference with coordination of such processes at some stage, e.g., as by interaction with α_1-antichymotrypsin (Abraham et al., 1988), could yield subunits that might self-aggregate or heteroaggregate via exposed β-stranded domains to form the amyloid fibril proteins found in neuritic or cerebrovascular plaques. If an incompletely processed subunit in APP-695 should possess proteolytic activity that could accelerate formation of more of such subunits from APP, the whole process could become self-sustaining and might even be propagated by the spread of such an entity. Normal APP-695 might be incompletely processed to give subunits which can form insoluble aggregates or, either in monomeric or aggregated form, can proteolytically degrade APP-695 to form more units like themselves. If only the native monomeric form of APP-695 ordinarily inhibits its own formation at translational or transcriptional levels in feedback fashion, the inhibition would be lost upon its accelerated degradation or removal by aggregation into insoluble complexes, and an uncontrolled continuous synthesis of the native protein and enhanced expression of the gene coding for it could occur. Thus, a nucleic acid-free protein (a subunit with protease activity) might act in a pseudo-infectious manner on passage from cell to cell or even from one organism to another.

It will be of great interest to determine whether or not a peptide arises during APP processing that possesses proteolytic activity and/or the ability to "infect" neural tissue in vivo or in vitro in such a manner as to cause more of the same material to be produced.

A "constipated" cell is a sick one: the disease may become fatal

Severe disruptions in cellular functions may occur when normal proteins are caused to aggregate in the presence of foreign materials. Vincristine, a plant alkaloid, arrests mitosis by destroying mitotic spindles because at low concentrations it combines with tubulin dimer, inducing self-association of the tubulin into indefinite polymers (Prakash and Timasheff, 1985). Major difficulties may arise when variants of proteins are present whose ability to maintain their native functional state in the full range of operational circumstances is restricted. For example, sickle cell hemoglobin (HbS) is a hemoglobin variant in which there is a single amino acid substitution of valine for glutamate. The solubility of the oxygenated form of HbS is identical with that of the normal form, but deoxy HbS is much less soluble because it aggregates to form filaments or tubules of indeterminately high molecular weight. At low oxygen tension, such as occurs upon exercise, the filaments may aggregate to form fibers and bundles of fibers and distort the shape of the erythrocytes of affected individuals from biconcave disks to sickles of crescent shape. An anemia results because the sickled cells are more fragile and tend to lyse readily. Their altered shape impedes movement through microcapillaries, allowing greater removal of oxygen from them and increasing their tendency to sickling (Perutz, 1978).

Familial amyloidotic polyneuropathies (autosomal dominant) are characterized by extracellular accumulations of amyloid fibrils and progressive disorders of peripheral nerves (Saraiva et al., 1984). In some cases of this disease, the abnormality is attributable to the substitution of methionine for a valine residue in prealbumin (Tawara et al., 1983; Dwulet and Benson, 1984), normally a tetrameric molecule present in serum that separately plays an important role both in transport of vitamin A by forming a protein-protein complex with retinol-binding protein and in transport of thyroid hormones, which bind to it. The above genetic defect in plasma prealbumin leads to the aggregation of the tetramers into amyloid fibrils, the deposition of which in tissues leads to the pathologies found in this group of disorders. It is particularly interesting that the amino acid triplet found in amyloid from AD and Down's syndrome, Asp-Ser-Gly, also is found in both normal and mutant prealbumin (Kanda et al., 1974), although there are no other shared sequences. Amyloid fibrils consisting of protein related to β_2-microglobulin, and entirely different from those above, were deposited in the tissues of a chronic hemodialysis patient with carpal tunnel syndrome (Gejyo et al., 1985).

A variety of data support the proposition that impairment of synchronous slow axonal transport of neurofilament proteins may underlie the pathological manifestations of a number of neurodegenerative disorders, among which are AD, amyotrophic lateral sclerosis, and parkinsonian dementia (Cork et al., 1979; Clark et al., 1980; Gadjusek, 1985). The presence of aluminosilicates and abnormal intracellular amyloid-like polymeric aggregates, alone or together, could lead to incoordinations in the cellular machinery which would result in failure of neurofilament protein transport without block in synthesis, leading to excessive accumulations of neurofilament aggregates in the cell body and initial axon segments and to the physical binding of neurofilament proteins to the amyloid or covalent linkage to it by action of transglutaminase (Selkoe et al., 1982).

It is not beyond reason to imagine the development of suitably genetically engineered, specifically targeted cell "laxatives" that would rescue "constipated" cells from their dilemma. However, much greater knowledge of intracellular protein breakdown will be required than now exists.

Alzheimer's disease may begin in the nose and may be caused by aluminosilicates: a hypothesis revisited (Roberts, 1986d)

The essence of my argument in this matter is that genetic factors may interact with aging changes in the nasal mucociliary apparatus to increase the probability that ubiquitously occurring aluminosilicates may enter sensory neurons of the olfactory epithelium, which appears to be injured in AD (Talamo et al., 1989), and spread transneuronally to several olfactory-related areas of the brain, thereby initiating changes that eventually result in neuronal damage typical of Alzheimer's disease. Aluminosilicates, which are insoluble and highly reactive chemically, were chosen as potential environmental culprits because analyses have shown them to be present in the cores of plaques isolated from brains of AD patients (Masters et al., 1985; Candy et al., 1986).

Many factors which change with age in nasal mucosa could increase the probability that a particular entity, such as aluminosilicate fibers, might enter sensory neurons of the olfactory epithelium directly from the mucosa or from the surrounding CSF, there being direct communication between the external secretions and the CSF in pathological conditions (Bullard et al., 1981; Grundfast et al., 1986) and even to some extent in the normal state (Hasegawa, 1983). In particular, there could be decreases in the rates at which such fibers could be coated with particular acidic glycoproteins found in nasal secretions and moved away from sites of vulnerability by mucociliary action.

Can aluminosilicates enter via the nasal mucosa and lodge in those regions of the brain in which the pathological changes are found in AD? If such movement were shown to take place, it could be determined whether or not pathological changes eventually arise that resemble those seen in the human disorder. However, to date progress has been hampered by lack of suitable isotopes for tracing either Al or Si. Technology now may become available to us by which young and old animals of several species may be exposed in a nose-only manner for prolonged periods to suitably labeled and metered aluminosilicate dusts of known composition and particle size (Snipes, 1983). Hopefully, definitive experiments will be performed in the near future. If aluminosilicates should be shown not to be transported transneuronally, it will be possible to determine whether or not they damage the sensory neurons sufficiently to cause anterograde damage because of an interruption of flow of trophic substances.

Magic bullets or cellular sociology: normal transactions and spinal cord injury

Unquestionably there exists an inherent capacity of injured adult mammalian CNS tissue to undergo repair and regrowth after injury. However, this is rarely, if ever, achieved. Formation of astrocytic and connective tissue scars and progressive necrosis usually have been insuperable impediments to effective regeneration and reinstitution of function. Efforts to develop pharmacological treatments to stimulate tissues repair and regeneration largely have been unsuccessful because of failure to correct the complex and incoordinated pathological responses of the mammalian spinal cord to injury. Much effort is being devoted to identifying specific growth and attachment factors which, when administered, might enable nerve tissue repair to take place. I call this the "magic bullet" approach because choosing to test a particular factor at hand is to engage in a low-probability gamble, there being many factors, known and unknown. Is a more analytical approach possible?

When in the course of their normal activities neurons are depolarized, influx of Na^+ and Ca^{2+} ions occurs. There follow releases of transmitters, neuromodulators, trophic substances, and K^+ ions. These substances are released in amounts related to extent and length of time of neuronal depolarization and serve as quantitative signals to non-neural cells in the vicinity, which become depolarized by the released K^+ ions as well as being variously affected by the other substances. Depolarization in the non-neural cells would result in release from them and transmittal to each other and to neighboring neurons of a variety of trophic substances in amounts that reflect their degree of depolarization and, therefore, the effects on them of the preceding neural activity. The various trophic substances release recovery cascades in the neurons as well as among members of the non-neural community that have receptors for them in such a manner as to allow housekeeping matters to be taken care of and structural and functional adjustments to take place that might be required as a result of the preceding activity.

One of the most important housekeeping matters is the maintenance of cytoplasmic pH (pH_i) within the normal range of $7.0 - 7.3$, since protons are liberated which could acidify the cytoplasm as a consequence of the release of energy-yielding cascades necessary to support the reactions that reestablish transmembrane potential to prestimulus levels. An alkaline shift in pH_i favors increases in cell volume and initiation of growth and proliferation, processes necessary for post-activity reorganization. The shuttling of H^+ ions among ever shifting sources and sinks in all cellular domains makes possible facile traverses of adaptive functional ranges. By affecting protein conformational states and, therefore, activities of structural components, enzymes, transporters, etc., evanescent local accumulations and depletions of protons affect virtually all cell processes.

A key player in pH_i regulation is a TP-independent, electroneutral system of ubiquitous occurrence that exchanges internal protons (H_i) for external Na^+ (Na_o) on a 1:1 basis (Grinstein and Rothstein, 1986; Moolenaar, 1986). The Na_o/H_i^+ exchanger is minimally active at pH $7.0 - 7.3$ and is turned off at higher pH_i; but it becomes increasingly active as pH_i falls below a certain threshold value. A second H^+ binding site, existing only on its cytoplasmic side, allosterically activates the exchanger. When this site is not protonated, the exchanger is inactive. The set point or threshold for protonation of this site and, therefore, for activation of the exchanger coincides with normal physiological pH. Many trophic substances and mitogens, among their other effects, only while they are present activate the Na^+/H^+ exchanger allosterically in such a manner that the set point is raised and a rapid rise in pH_i of $0.1 - 0.3$ pH units occurs. An important property of the exchanger is that it is inhibited by elevation of extracellular H^+ ion concentrations, external H^+ ions (H_o) competing with Na_o for the transport site.

"Trauma to the spinal cord triggers a progressive series of autodestructive events that lead to varying degrees of tissue necrosis and paralysis, depending on the severity of the injury. Pathological changes that occur in traumatized spinal cord tissue include petechial hemorrhage progressing to hemorrhagic necrosis, lipid peroxidation, lipid hydrolyses with subsequent prostaglandin and leukotriene (eicosanoid) formation, loss of Ca^{2+} from the extracellular space and loss of K^+ from the intracellular space; ischemia with consequent decline in tissue O_2 tension and energy metabolites and development of lactic acidosis; edema; and inflammation and neuronophagia by polymorphonuclear leukocytes (PMN)" (Anderson et al., 1985.)

A number of the events in the above litany of spinal cord damage must begin early on, perhaps within 1 min after trauma occurs. I conjecture that among the earliest and most critical among them would be anoxia-consequent decreases in pH in both neurons and non-neural cells, increases in extracellular K^+, and decreases in extracellular Ca^{2+} because of influx of Ca^{2+} into cytoplasmic compartments. The released K^+ ions would cause prolonged depolarization of all cells in the affected region because the restorative $Na^+ - K^+$ ATPase could not be energized. The resultant initial increase in cellular activities would promote further accumulation of H_i and lactate. Accumulation of H_i and H_o would exhaust the supply of the natural bicarbonate buffer and competition of H_o with Na_o would shut down operation of the Na_o/H_i exchanger, making it impossible to return pH_i to the physiological range, let alone to increase it to the higher levels conducive for synthetic recovery reactions to take place. Lactic acid formation would continue, particularly in glial cells (Kraig et al., 1985, 1986a, b), decreasing pH_i and increasing lactate in them eventually to lethal levels. Hydrolytic lysosomal enzymes would become activated at low pH_i. Increases in intracellular Ca^{2+} would release a host of degradative processes, including proteolysis and lipolysis accompanied by free radical generation, which could not be limited by the normal energy-requiring routes for Ca^{2+} extrusion and intracellular sequestration. Attack on membranes by free radicals formed by lipid peroxidation would further decrease their capacity to generate an adequate TP. Finally, accumulations of denatured and degraded cellular debris would attract inflammation-causing neutrophils and phagic response on the part of PMNs. Continuation of these processes would lead to anterograde degeneration and cell death in neurons.

Guth and I (Guth et al., 1985; Roberts, 1987) chose to investigate whether or not prevention of H^+ accumulation would attenuate the pathological changes following spinal cord injury. A brief compression was used to initiate spinal cord injury in rats (mild-crush model) and the injury site was superfused with a solution containing triethanolamine (pK , 7.9; pH, 7.3; 10 mM) 4 times daily for 2 weeks through indwelling polyethylene tubes positioned over the lesion site. The results were compared with those in animals similarly treated with unbuffered physiological saline adjusted to pH 7.3 (Fig. 3). In the animals treated with triethanolamine buffer, there was remarkably greater invasion of the lesion by nerve fibers than in the saline-treated controls, the nerve fibers growing into the lesion site in such profusion that they were no longer oriented longitudinally, but grew rather haphazardly in all directions. Fibers were frequently undulating and varicose and often were arranged in small bundles containing 3 – 6 axons. In the treated animals the onset of necrosis was markedly delayed by comparison with the controls. Macrophages that accumulated in the controls were engorged with cellular debris, while those in the buffer-treated animals did not contain evidence of tissue breakdown. However, when treatment was stopped in the buffer-treated animals, degenerative changes proceeded to take place as in the controls (unpublished). It is unlikely that anoxia due to ischemia was causative in the recapitulation of the degenerative sequence seen from the outset in the controls because extensive revascularization had taken place during the period of buffer treatment. It seems more likely that the buffer treatment enabled the regenerating tissue to be sufficiently normal metabolically so that chemical signals to the waiting macrophages were interpreted by them as coming from essentially normal tissue. Once treatment ceased, signals from the incompletely reconstituted tissue, perhaps protons or lactate, aroused the macrophages to a feeding frenzy, and they ran amok to produce the typical cystic degeneration and cavitation.

Efforts are now under way to develop treatment modalities by which monocytes and macrophages can be primed in such a manner as to elicit from them secretion of growth factors while preventing

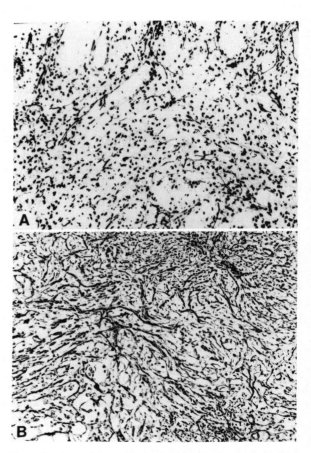

Fig. 3. Sections of tissue of spinal cord taken from rats 2 weeks after compression injury. *A*. Treatment with saline. *B*. Treatment with triethanolamine buffer, pH 7.3. (Guth et al., 1985.)

liberation of cytotoxic agents. Current evidence suggests that it may be possible to switch the differentiation of macrophages from a hostile to a friendly mode, for example, by treatment with *E. coli* bacterial lipopolysaccharide.

Controlling the pH externally, as above, washing out the injured area with saline so as to remove or dilute products of initial injury (Sabel and Stein, 1982; Sabel et al., 1985), administering Ca^{2+} channel blocking agents to prevent catastrophic increases in intracellular Ca^{2+} (Gelbfish et al., 1986), perfusing with growth factors (Williams et al., 1986) or free radical-trapping agents (Demopoulos et al., 1982) or decreasing neural activity (Wilhjelm and Arnfred, 1965; Rothman, 1983) may individually or synergistically attenuate autodestructive processes in injured spinal cord — the danger from within. However, the key to eventually successful regeneration may be in adjusting the relationships between the injured tissue and the overzealous macrophagic defenders — the danger from without.

Comment

In all complex systems dynamic tension exists between influences that maintain the relative freedom of interactions and those that tend to synchronize activities of the constituent units or to isolate them from each other functionally. The health of cells, individuals, and nations often is precarious because the respective systems are walking tightropes between states of freedom without license, tyrannical authority and anarchy. Sometimes it may take but little additional input to tip the balance in catastrophic fashion from one to another of these modes. It is interesting in this light to contemplate some of the easily observable neurotic behavioral and psychic consequences of the irremediable tensions in individual human beings between the demands of instinct and the restrictions of civilization, the ready transitions between political tyranny and revolution that have occurred throughout history and are widely evident today, and the fluctuations in affect that oc-

cur in manic-depressive disorder. The "cure" of a diseased system is similar in principle to the restoration of a fallen acrobat to his tightrope.

There is an urgency to finding solutions to problems related to catastrophes that befall the nervous system. The large numbers of individuals with AD have overwhelmed our capacity to deal with them, with numbers increasing inexorably as the population ages. Memory impairment of all varieties in aging individuals results in untold anguish and great economic losses. What would we do with thousands of individuals who might suffer spinal cord injuries as the result of a major earthquake, as is predicted to take place in California in the not too distant future?[1]

I have proposed that: (1) a key organizing principle of adaptive function is the coupling of variability generation to functional demand; and (2) while cycling freely through all their operational modes, healthy living systems, from cell to society, use their functional capabilities to extents which are sufficient to ensure high probabilities of achieving solutions to the problems with which they are faced. One of the purposes of the present paper was to generate additional variability in outlooks and approaches among those whose activities might contribute to solutions of problems of aging, AD, and spinal cord injury.

Some potential therapeutic approaches have been suggested that might help restore and/or maintain effective communications within and between subsystems which are cybernetically subnormally effective or are completely ineffective in aging and injured neural tissue. With appropriate treatment, restoration of function might be achieved to the extent that there are sufficient numbers of potentially operational units remaining in rate-limiting neural, glial and endothelial systems. Further deterioration of critical aspects of the system

---

[1]Since the completion of this manuscript, a major earthquake shook Northern California on October 17, 1989. The number of spinal cord injuries that resulted is not known. An even more severe earthquake is expected to take place somewhere along the many faults that exist in that state.

might be halted if grossly pathological relationships could be corrected, e.g., by rebalancing the adjustment between the nature and extent of cellular injury and the restorative and destructive potentials residing in the immunological defense systems and in the genome of the injured cell itself. Although it would be expected that at the time of injury some irreversible damage already might have occurred, all damage would not be irreversible. Techniques of early evaluation and treatment should be sought so that therapies could be instituted when reversibility might be greatest. Available treatment modalities give us sufficient tools to begin to make meaningful progress without invoking complex neurosurgical and transplantation technologies that could not possibly be made available to victims of an earthquake or a major train wreck or to large numbers of AD patients. Current results give encouragement to the idea that appropriate manipulation of a relatively small number of key factors may lead to important progress in attempts to achieve recovery from CNS injury.

There are unavoidable weak links in all hypotheses and experimental paths proposed, metaphorically similar to those in plans for voyages to unknown places when choices of destinations and routes depend on maps of doubtful reliability and on anecdotal reports of travellers. Lack of knowledge or faulty information may lead to failure. The routes chosen may lead elsewhere than to the desired goals. But in the process we are learning what questions to ask and at what levels of organization to ask them.

Acknowledgements

Supported in part by grants from the G. Harold and Leila Y. Mathers Foundation, the Ziskin Family Trust and the National Metal Steel Foundation.

References

Abraham, C.R., Selkoe, D.J. and Potter, H. (1988) Immunochemical identification of the serine protease inhibitory α_1-antichymotrypsin in the brain amyloid deposits of Alzheimer's disease. *Cell,* 52: 487 – 501.

Ali, M. and Vedeckis, W.V. (1987) The glucocorticoid receptor protein binds to transfer RNA. *Science,* 235: 467 – 470.

Allsop, D., Wong, C.W., Ikeda, S.-I., Landon, M., Kidd, M. and Glenner, G.G. (1988) Immunohistochemical evidence for the derivation of a peptide ligand from the amyloid β-protein precursor of Alzheimer disease. *Proc. Natl. Acad. Sci. U.S.A.,* 85: 2790 – 2794.

Ames, A., Walseth, T.F., Heyman, R.A., Barad, M., Graeff, R.M. and Goldberg, N.D. (1986) Light-induced increases in cGMP metabolic flux correspond with electrical responses of photoreceptors. *J. Biol. Chem.,* 261: 13034 – 13042.

Anderson, D.K., Demediuk, P., Saunders, R.D., Dugan, L.L., Means, E.D. and Horrocks, L.A. (1985) Spinal cord injury and protection. *Ann. Emerg. Med.,* 83: 816 – 821.

Ashton, D. (1988) *Picasso on Art* (unabridged republication of edition published in New York in 1972), Da Capo Press, New York, 187 pp.

Baker, J.B., Low, D.A., Simmer, R.L. and Cunningham, D.D. (1980) Protease-nexin: a cellular component that links thrombin and plasminogen activator and mediates their binding to cells. *Cell,* 21: 37 – 45.

Benowitz, L.I., Rodriguez, W., Paskevich, P., Mufson, E.J., Schenk, D. and Neve, R.L. (1989) The amyloid precursor protein is concentrated in neuronal lysosomes in normal and Alzheimer disease subjects. *Exp. Neurol.,* 106: 237 – 250.

Beynon, R.J. and Bond, J.S. (1986) Catabolism of intracellular protein: molecular aspects. *Am. J. Physiol.,* 251: C141 – C152.

Bologa, L., Sharma, J. and Roberts, E. (1987) Dehydroepiandrosterone and its sulfated derivative reduce neuronal death and enhance astrocytic differentiation in brain cell cultures. *J. Neurosci. Res.,* 17: 225 – 234.

Bullard, D.E., Crockard, H.A. and McDonald, W.I. (1981) Spontaneous cerebrospinal fluid rhinorrhea associated with dysplastic optic discs and a basal encephalocele. *J. Neurosurg.,* 54: 807 – 810.

Candy, J.M., Klinowski, J., Perry, R., Perry, E.K., Fairbairn, A., Oakley, A.E., Carpenter, T.A., Atack, J.R., Blessed, G. and Edwardson, J.A. (1986) Aluminosilicates and senile plaque formation in Alzheimer's disease. *Lancet,* i: 354 – 357.

Carette, B. and Poulain, D. (1984) Excitatory effect of dehydroepiandrosterone, its sulphate ester and pregnenolone sulphate, applied by iontophoresis and pressure, on single neurones in the septo-preoptic area of the guinea pig. *Neurosci. Lett.,* 45: 205 – 210.

Carter, P. and Wells, J.A. (1988) Dissecting the catalytic triad of a serine protease. *Nature,* 332: 564 – 568.

Chrousos, G.P., Loriaux, D.L. and Lipsett, M.B. (1986) Steroid hormone resistance. Mechanisms and clinical aspects. *Adv. Exp. Med. Biol.,* 196: 1 – 437.

Clark, A.W., Griffin, J.W. and Price, D.L. (1980) The axonal pathology in chronic IDPN intoxication. *J. Neuropathol. Exp. Neurol.,* 39: 42 – 55.

Cordingley, M.G., Riegel, A.T. and Hager, G.L. (1987) Steroid-dependent interaction of transcription factors with the inducible promoter of mouse mammary tumor in vivo. *Cell,* 48: 261 – 270.

Cork, L.C., Griffin, J.W., Munnell, J.F., Lorenz, M.D., Adams, R.J. and Price, D.L. (1979) Hereditary canine spinal muscular atrophy. *J. Neuropathol. Exp. Neurol.,* 38: 209 – 221.

Demopoulos, H.B., Flamm, E.S., Seligman, M.L., Pietronigro, D.D., Tomasula, J. and De Crescito, V. (1982) Further studies on free-radical pathology in the major central nervous system disorders: effect of very high doses of methylprednisolone on the functional outcome, morphology and chemistry of experimental spinal cord impact injury. *Can. J. Physiol. Pharmacol.,* 60: 1415 – 1424.

Dwulet, F.E. and Benson, M.D. (1984) Primary structure of an amyloid prealbumin and its plasma precursor in a heredofamilial polyneuropathy of Swedish origin. *Proc. Natl. Acad. Sci. U.S.A.,* 81: 694 – 698.

Dyrks, T., Weidemann, A., Multhaup, G., Salbaum, J.M., Lemaire, H.-G., Kang, J., Müller-Hill, B., Masters, C.L. and Beyreuther, K. (1988) Identification, transmembrane orientation and biogenesis of the amyloid A4 precursor of Alzheimer's disease. *EMBO J.,* 7: 949 – 957.

Ennis, D.M. (1988) Toward a universal law of generalization. *Science,* 242: 944.

Evans, R.M. (1988) The steroid and thyroid hormone receptor superfamily. *Science,* 240: 889 – 895.

Flood, J.F. and Roberts, E. (1988) Dehydroepiandrosterone sulfate improves memory in aging mice. *Brain Res.,* 448: 178 – 181.

Flood, J.F., Smith, G.E. and Roberts, E. (1988) Dehydroepiandrosterone and its sulfate enhance memory retention in mice. *Brain Res.,* 447: 269 – 278.

Gajdusek, D.C. (1985) Hypothesis: interference with axonal transport of neurofilament as a common pathogenetic mechanism in certain diseases of the central nervous system. *N. Engl. J. Med.,* 312: 714 – 719.

Gejyo, F., Yamada, T., Odani, S., Nakagawa, Y., Arakawa, M., Kunitomo, T., Kataoka, H., Suzuki, M., Hirasawa, Y., Shirahama, T., Cohen, A.S. and Schmid, K. (1985) A new form of amyloid protein associated with chronic hemodialysis was identified as β_2-microglobulin. *Biochem. Biophys. Res. Commun.,* 129: 701 – 706.

Gelbfish, J.S., Phillips, T., Rose, D.M., Wait, R. and Cunningham, J.N., Jr. (1986) Acute spinal cord ischemia: prevention of paraplegia with verapamil. *Circulation,* 74(suppl. I): I5 – I10.

Goldberg, N.D. and Walseth, T.F. (1985) A second role for second messengers: uncovering the utility of cyclic nucleotide hydrolysis. *Biotechnology,* 3: 235 – 238.

Goldberg, N.D., Ames, A., III, Gander, J.E. and Walseth, T.F. (1983) Magnitude of increase in retinal cGMP metabolic flux determined by ^{18}O incorporation into nucleotide α-phosphoryls corresponds with intensity of photic stimulation. *J. Biol. Chem.,* 258: 9213 – 9219.

Greer, J. (1981) Comparative model-building of the mammalian serine proteases. *J. Mol. Biol.,* 153: 1027 – 1042.

Grinstein, S. and Rothstein, A. (1986) Mechanisms of regulation of the Na^+/H^+ exchanger. *J. Membr. Biol.,* 90: 1 – 12.

Grundfast, K.M., Mihail, R. and Majd, M. (1986) Intraoperative detection of cerebrospinal fluid leak in surgical removal of congenital nasal masses. *Laryngoscope,* 96: 211.

Gupta, C., Katsumata, M., Goldman, A.S., Herold, R. and Piddington, R. (1984) Glucocorticoid-induced phospholipase A_2-inhibitory proteins mediate glucocorticoid teratogenicity in vitro. *Proc. Natl. Acad. Sci. U.S.A.,* 81: 1140 – 1143.

Guth, L., Barrett, C.P., Donati, E.J., Smith, M.V., Lifson, M. and Roberts, E. (1985) Enhancement of axonal growth into a spinal lesion by topical application of triethanolamine and cytosine arabinoside. *Exp. Neurol.,* 88: 44 – 55.

Hasegawa, M., Watanabe, I., Hiratsuka, H., Okumura, T. and Inanba, Y. (1983) Transfer of radioisotope from CSF to nasal secretion. *Acta Otolaryngol. (Stockh.),* 95: 359 – 364.

Hershko, A. and Ciechanover, A. (1982) Mechanisms of intracellular protein breakdown. *Annu. Rev. Biochem.,* 51: 335 – 364.

Heuser, G. and Eidelberg, E. (1961) Steroid-induced convulsions in experimental animals. *Endocrinology,* 69: 915 – 924.

Heuser, G., Ling, G.M. and Buchwald, N.A. (1965) Sedation or seizures as dose-dependent effects of steroids. *Arch. Neurol.,* 13: 195 – 203.

Hikosaka, O. and Wurtz, R.H. (1983) Visual and oculomotor functions of monkey substantia nigra pars reticulata. IV. Relation of substantia nigra to superior colliculus. *J. Neurophysiol.,* 49: 1285 – 1301.

Hook, M. (1984) Cell-surface glycosaminoglycans. *Annu. Rev. Biochem.,* 53: 847 – 869.

Kanda, Y., Goodman, D.S., Canfield, R.E. and Morgan, F.J. (1974) The amino acid sequence of human plasma prealbumin. *J. Biol. Chem.,* 249: 6796 – 6805.

Kang, J., Lemaire, H.-G., Unterbeck, A., Salbaum, J.M., Masters, C.L., Grzeschik, K.-H., Multhaup, G., Beyreuther, K. and Müller-Hill, B. (1987) The precursor of Alzheimer's disease amyloid A4 protein resembles a cell-surface receptor. *Nature,* 325: 733 – 736.

Kirkwood, T.B.L. (1989) DNA mutations and aging. *Mutat. Res.,* 219: 1 – 7.

Kirschner, D.A., Inouye, H., Duffy, L.K., Sinclair, A., Lind, M. and Selkoe, D.J. (1987) Synthetic peptide homologous to β protein from Alzheimer disease forms amyloid-like fibrils in vitro. *Proc. Natl. Acad. Sci. U.S.A.,* 84: 6953 – 6957.

Koo, E., Feher, K.G., Feher, T. and Fust, G. (1983) Effect of dehydroepiandrosterone on hereditary angioedema. *Klin. Wochenschr.,* 61: 715 – 717.

Kraig, R.P., Pulsinelli, W.A. and Plum, F. (1985)

Heterogeneous distribution of hydrogen and bicarbonate ions during complete brain ischemia. *Progr. Brain Res.,* 63: 155 – 166.

Kraig, R.P., Petito, C., Plum, F. and Pulsinelli, W. (1986a) Hydrogen ions and ischemic brain damage. *Ann. N.Y. Acad. Sci.,* 481: 372 – 374.

Kraig, R.P., Pulsinelli, W.A. and Plum, F. (1986b) Carbonic acid buffer changes during complete brain ischemia. *Am. J. Physiol.,* 250: R348 – R357.

Kraut, J. (1977) Serine proteases: structure and mechanism of catalysis. *Annu. Rev. Biochem.,* 46: 331 – 358.

Kubli-Garfias, C., Cervantes, M. and Beyer, C. (1976) Changes in multiunit activity and EEG induced by the administration of natural progestins to flaxedil immobilized cats. *Brain Res.,* 114: 71 – 81.

Kubli-Garfias, C., Canchola, E., Arauz-Contreras, J. and Feria-Velasco, A. (1982) Depressant effect of androgens on the cat brain electrical activity and its antagonism by ruthenium red. *Neuroscience,* 7: 2777 – 2782.

Litwack, G., Schmidt, T.J., Miller-Diener, A., Webb, M., Bodine, P., Barnett, C.A., Platt, D. and Baldridge, R.C. (1986) Steroid receptor activation: the glucocorticoid receptor as a model system. *Adv. Exp. Med. Biol.,* 196: 11 – 22.

Lorenz, E.N. (1963) Deterministic non-periodic flow. *J. Atmos. Sci.,* 20: 130 – 141.

Mandell, A.J. (1983) From intermittency to transitivity in neuropsychobiological flows. *Am. J. Physiol.,* 245: R484 – R494.

Martin, D.P., Schmidt, R.E., DiStefano, P.S., Lowry, O.H., Carter, J.G. and Johnson, E.M., Jr. (1988) Inhibitors of protein synthesis and RNA synthesis prevent neuronal death caused by nerve growth factor deprivation. *J. Cell Biol.,* 106: 829 – 844.

Masters, C.L., Simms, G., Weinman, N.A., Multhaup, G., McDonalds, B.L. and Beyreuther, K. (1985) Amyloid plaque core protein in Alzheimer disease and Down syndrome. *Proc. Natl. Acad. Sci. U.S.A.,* 82: 4245 – 4249.

Mayer, R.J. and Doherty, F. (1986) Intracellular protein catabolism: state of the art. *FEBS Lett.,* 198: 181 – 193.

Moolenaar, W.H. (1986) Effects of growth factors on intracellular pH regulation. *Ann. Rev. Physiol.,* 48: 363 – 376.

Morgan, J.I., Cohen, D.R., Hempstead, J.L. and Curran, T. (1987) Mapping patterns of *c-fos* expression in the central nervous system after seizure. *Science,* 237: 192 – 197.

Müller-Hill, B. and Beyreuther, K. (1989) Molecular biology of Alzheimer's disease. *Annu. Rev. Biochem.,* 58: 287 – 307.

Orentreich, N., Brind, J.L., Rizer, R.L. and Vogelman, J.H. (1984) Age changes and sex differences in serum dehydroepiandrosterone sulfate concentrations throughout adulthood. *J. Clin. Endocrinol. Metab.,* 59: 551 – 555.

Parker, L.N. (1989) *Adrenal Androgens in Clinical Medicine,* Academic Press, New York, 615 pp.

Parker, L.N. and Odell, W.D. (1980) Control of adrenal androgen secretion. *Endocr. Rev.,* 1: 392 – 410.

Parker, L.N., Levin, E.R. and Lifrak, E.T. (1985) Evidence for adrenocortical adaptation to severe illness. *J. Clin. Endocrinol. Metab.,* 60: 947 – 953.

Perutz, M.F. (1978) Hemoglobin structure and respiratory transport. *Sci. Am.,* 239: 92 – 125.

Power, S.D., Adams, R.M. and Wells, J.A. (1986) Secretion and autoproteolytic maturation of subtilisin. *Proc. Natl. Acad. Sci. U.S.A.,* 83: 3096 – 3100.

Prakash, V. and Timasheff, S.N. (1985) Vincristine-induced self-association of calf brain tubulin. *Biochemistry,* 24: 5004 – 5010.

Raine, C.S. (1989) Neurocellular anatomy. In: G. Siegel, B. Agranoff, R.W. Albers and P. Molinoff (Eds.), *Basic Neurochemistry,* Raven Press, New York, pp. 3 – 33.

Ratner, S. (1979) The dynamic state of body proteins. In: P.R. Srinivasan, J.S. Fruton and J.T. Edsall (Eds.), *The Origins of Modern Biochemistry. Ann. N.Y. Acad. Sci.,* 325: 189 – 209.

Reid, K.B.M. and Porter, R.R. (1981) The proteolytic activation systems of complement. *Annu. Rev. Biochem.,* 50: 433 – 464.

Roberts, E. (1976) Disinhibition as an organizing principle in the nervous system – the role of the GABA system. Application to neurologic and psychiatric disorders. In: E. Roberts, T.N. Chase and D.B. Tower (Eds.), *GABA in Nervous System Function,* Raven Press, New York, pp. 515 – 539.

Roberts, E. (1986a) What do GABA neurons really do? They make possible variability generation in relation to demand. *Exp. Neurol.,* 93: 279 – 290.

Roberts, E. (1986b) GABA: the road to neurotransmitter status. In: R.W. Olsen and J.C. Venter (Eds.), *Benzodiazepine/GABA Receptors and Chloride Channels: Structural and Functional Properties,* Alan R. Liss, New York, pp. 1 – 39.

Roberts, E. (1986c) Failure of GABAergic inhibition: a key to local and global seizures. *Adv. Neurol.,* 44: 319 – 341.

Roberts, E. (1986d) Alzheimer's disease may begin in the nose and may be caused by aluminosilicates. *Neurobiol. Aging,* 7: 561 – 567. Author's response to commentaries. *Neurobiol. Aging,* 7: 587 – 590.

Roberts, E. (1986e) Guides through the labyrinth of AD: dehydroepiandrosterone, potassium channels, and the C4 component of complement. In: T. Crook, R.T. Bartus, S. Ferris and S. Gershon (Eds.), *Treatment Development Strategies for Alzheimer's Disease,* Mark Powley, Madison, CT, pp. 173 – 219.

Roberts, E. (1987) A systems approach to nerve regeneration. *Progr. Brain Res.,* 71: 209 – 227.

Roberts, E. and Matthysse, S. (1970) Neurobiochemistry at the crossroads of neurobiology. *Annu. Rev. Biochem.,* 39: 777 – 820.

Roberts, E. and Simonsen, D.G. (1962) Free amino acids in animal tissue. In: J.T. Holden (Ed.), *Amino Acid Pools,* Elsevier, Amsterdam, pp. 284 – 349.

Roberts, E., Bologa, L., Flood, J.F. and Smith, G.E. (1987) Effects of dehydroepiandrosterone and its sulfate on brain tissue in culture and on memory in mice. *Brain Res.*, 406: 357 – 362.

Rössler, O.E. (1976) Chaotic behavior in simple reaction systems. *Z. Naturforsch. (A)*, 31: 259 – 264.

Rothman, S.M. (1983) Synaptic activity mediates death of hypoxic neurons. *Science*, 220: 536 – 537.

Sabel, B.A. and Stein, D.G. (1982) Intracerebral injections of isotonic saline prevent behavioral deficits from brain damage. *Physiol. Behav.*, 28: 1017 – 1023.

Sabel, B.A., Labbe, R. and Stein, D.G. (1985) The saline effect: minimizing the severity of brain damage by reduction of secondary degeneration. *Exp. Neurol.*, 88: 95 – 107.

Saffen, D.W., Cole, A.J., Worley, P.F., Christy, B.A., Ryder, K. and Baraban, J.M. (1988) Convulsant-induced increase in transcription factor messenger RNAs in rat brain. *Proc. Natl. Acad. Sci. U.S.A.*, 85: 7795 – 7799.

Salbaum, J.M., Weidemann, A., Lemaire, H.-G., Masters, C.L. and Beyreuther, K. (1988) The promoter of Alzheimer's disease amyloid A4 precursor gene. *EMBO J.*, 7: 2807 – 2813.

Sapolsky, R.M. (1990) Glucocorticoids, hippocampal damage and the glutamatergic synapse. (This volume.)

Saraiva, M.J.M., Birken, S., Costa, P.P. and Goodman, D.S. (1984) Amyloid fibril protein in familial amyloidotic polyneuropathy, Portuguese type. *J. Clin. Invest.*, 74: 104 – 119.

Schoenheimer, R. (1942) *The Dynamic State of Body Constituents*, Harvard University Press, Cambridge, MA, 78 pp.

Schubert, D., Schroeder, R., LaCorbiere, M., Saitoh, T. and Cole, G. (1988) Amyloid β protein precursor is possibly a heparan sulfate proteoglycan core protein. *Science*, 241: 223 – 226.

Selkoe, D.J., Abraham, C. and Ihara, Y. (1982) Brain transglutaminase: in vitro crosslinking of human neurofilament proteins into insoluble polymers. *Proc. Natl. Acad. Sci. U.S.A.*, 79: 6070 – 6074.

Selkoe, D.J., Poslisny, M.B., Joachim, C.L., Vickers, E.A., Lee, G., Fritz, L.C. and Oltersdorf, T. (1988) β-Amyloid precursor protein of Alzheimer disease occurs as 110 – 135-kilodalton membrane-associated proteins in neural and nonneural tissues. *Proc. Natl. Acad. Sci. U.S.A.*, 84: 7341 – 7345.

Shepard, R.N. (1987) Toward a universal law of generalization for psychological science. *Science*, 237: 1317 – 1323.

Shivers, B., Hilbich, C., Multhaup, G., Salbaum, M., Beyreuther, K. and Seeburg, P.H. (1988) Alzheimer's disease amyloidogenic glycoprotein: expression pattern in rat brain suggests a role in cell contact. *EMBO J.*, 7: 1365 – 1370.

Slater, E.P., Anderson, T., Cattini, P., Isaacs, R., Birnbaum, M.J., Gardner, D.G., Eberhardt, N.L. and Baxter, J.D. (1986) Mechanisms of glucocorticoid hormone action. *Adv. Exp. Med. Biol.*, 196: 67 – 80.

Snipes, M.B., Boecker, B.B. and McClellan, R.O. (1983) Retention of monodisperse or polydisperse aluminosilicate particles inhaled by dogs, rats, and mice. *Toxicol. Appl. Pharmacol.*, 69: 345 – 362.

Sohal, R.S. and Wolfe, L.S. (1986) Lipofucsin: characteristics and significance. *Progr. Brain Res.*, 70: 171 – 183.

Sonka, J. (1976) Dehydroepiandrosterone. Metabolic effects. *Acta Univ. Carol. (Med. Monogr.) (Praha)*, 71: 1 – 171.

Suzuki, K. (1989) Genetic disorders of lipid, glycoprotein, and mucopolysaccharide metabolism. In: G. Siegel, B. Agranoff, R.W. Albers and P. Molinoff (Eds.), *Basic Neurochemistry*, Raven Press, New York, pp. 715 – 732.

Talamo, B.R., Rudel, R.A., Kosik, K.S., Lee, V.M.-Y., Neff, S., Adelman, L. and Kauer, J.S. (1989) Pathological changes in olfactory neurons in patients with Alzheimer's disease. *Science*, 337: 736 – 739.

Tam, S.-P., Hache, R.J.G. and Deeley, R.G. (1986) Estrogen memory effect in human hepatocytes during repeated cell division without hormone. *Science*, 234: 1234 – 1237.

Tanaka, R.D., Li, A.C., Fogelman, A.M. and Edwards, P.A. (1986) Inhibition of lysosomal protein degradation inhibits the basal degradation of 3-hydroxy-3-methylglutaryl coenzyme A reductase. *J. Lipid Res.*, 27: 261 – 273.

Tawara, S., Nakazato, M., Kangawa, K., Matsuo, H. and Araki, S. (1983) Identification of amyloid prealbumin variant in familial amyloidotic polyneuropathy (Japanese type). *Biochem. Biophys. Res. Commun.*, 116: 880 – 888.

Thom, R. (1975) *Structural Stability and Morphogenesis* (translated from the French language), Benjamin, Reading, MA, 348 pp.

Truman, J.W., Fahrbach, S. and Kimura, K.-I. (1989) Hormones and programmed cell death: insights from invertebrate studies. (This volume.)

Wheatley, D.N. and Inglis, M.S. (1986) Protein turnover during cell growth: a re-examination of the problem of linear incorporation kinetics of radioactively-labeled amino acids into protein and its relationship to growth characteristics. *Cytobios*, 47: 187 – 210.

Wilhjelm, B.J. and Arnfred, I. (1965) Protective action of some anaesthetics against anoxia. *Acta Pharmacol. Toxicol.*, 22: 93 – 98.

Williams, L.R., Varon, S., Peterson, G.M., Wictorin, K., Fischer, W., Björklund, A. and Gage, F.H. (1986) Continuous infusion of nerve growth factor prevents basal forebrain neuronal death after fimbria fornix transection. *Proc. Natl. Acad. Sci. U.S.A.*, 83: 9231 – 9235.

Woodbury, R.G., Katunuma, N., Kobayashi, K., Titani, K. and Neurath, H. (1978) Covalent structure of a group-specific protease from small rat intestine. *Biochemistry*, 17: 811 – 819.

Yankner, B.A., Dawes, L.R., Fisher, S., Villa-Komaroff, L., Oster-Granite, M.L. and Neve, R.L. (1989) Neurotoxicity of a fragment of the amyloid precursor associated with Alzheimer's disease. *Science*, 245: 417 – 420.

Subject Index

ace Library 3/14